Understanding Pharmacology for Health Professionals

Third Edition

Susan M. Turley

MA (Educ), BSN, RN, RHIT, CMT

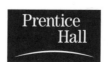

Prentice Hall

Upper Saddle River, New Jersey 07458

Library of Congress Cataloging-in-Publication Data

Turley, Susan M.
  Understanding pharmacology for health professionals / Susan M.
Turley.—3rd ed.
    p. ; cm.
  Includes index.
  ISBN 0-13-041742-4
  1. Pharmacology.   2. Allied health personnel.
    [DNLM: 1. Pharmaceutical Preparations.   2. Drug Therapy—
methods.   3. Pharmacology—methods.   QV 55 T941ua 2003]
  I. Title.
RM300.T85 2003
615'.1—dc21

                                                        2002005780

Notice: The author and the publisher of this volume have taken care to make certain that the doses of drugs and schedules of treatment are correct and compatible with the standards generally accepted at the time of publication. Nevertheless, as new information becomes available, changes in treatment and in the use of drugs become necessary. The reader is advised to carefully consult the instruction and information material included in the package insert of each drug or therapeutic agent before administration. This advice is especially important when using, administering, or recommending new or infrequently used drugs. The author and publisher disclaim all responsibility for any liability, loss, injury, or damage incurred as a consequence, directly or indirectly, of the use and application of any of the contents of this volume.

Publisher: Julie Levin Alexander
Publisher's Assistant: Regina Bruno
Senior Acquisitions Editor: Mark Cohen
Assistant Editor: Melissa Kerian
Editoral Assistant: Mary Ellen Ruitenberg
Senior Marketing Manager: Nicole Benson
Product Information Manager: Rachele Strober
Marketing Assistant: Janet Ryerson
Director of Production and Manufacturing:
  Bruce Johnson
Managing Editor for Production: Patrick Walsh

Production Editor: Karen Berry
Copyeditor: Laura Burgess
Manufacturing Manager: Ilene Sanford
Manufacturing Buyer: Pat Brown
Creative Director: Cheryl Asherman
Cover Design Coordinator: Maria Guglielmo Walsh
New Media Production Manager: Amy Peltier
New Media Project Manager: Stephen Hartner
Formatting: Pine Tree Composition
Printer/Binder: Courier Westford
Cover Printer: Phoenix Color

Pearson Education Ltd., *London*
Pearson Education Australia Pty. Limited, *Sydney*
Pearson Education Singapore, Pte. Ltd.
Pearson Education North Asia Ltd., *Hong Kong*
Pearson Education Canada, Ltd., *Toronto*
Pearson Educación de Mexico, S.A. de C.V.
Pearson Education—Japan, *Tokyo*
Pearson Education Malaysia, Pte. Ltd.
Pearson Education, *Upper Saddle River, New Jersey*

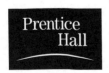

10 9 8 7 6 5 4 3 2 1
ISBN 0-13-041742-4

Presenting the Third Edition of *Understanding Pharmacology for Health Professionals*

TEXTBOOK OVERVIEW

The purpose of this book is to serve as your guide as you study pharmacology. The road of pharmacology is paved with extensive and often unrecognized research on the part of thousands of doctors and scientists around the world; it is built layer by layer on previous discoveries and consists of equal parts hard work, astute observation, and, not infrequently, sudden insights and divinely appointed coincidences. This road is constantly being built anew with each drug discovery.

It is not the purpose of this book to instruct in the prescribing or administration of medication. Rather, its purpose is to provide a framework of knowledge to help you (whether you are a student or a healthcare professional) recognize drug names and drug classes; understand drug actions and the rationale for treatment; discern between sound-alike drugs; understand why side effects, allergic effects, and other effects of drugs occur; and address various current healthcare issues relating to pharmacology and drugs. By providing this foundation of knowledge, you will be prepared to deal with current drugs and also with the myriad of new drugs that are approved each year. With the help of this textbook, the road of pharmacology that stretches ahead of you will become both familiar and nonthreatening, to be traveled frequently in the future.

TEXTBOOK ORGANIZATION AND FEATURES

The arrangement of the chapters by medical specialty or drug category has proven very effective in the past two editions, and this organization was retained in the third edition. Coverage of generic and trade name drugs, drug categories, and drug actions continues to be comprehensive and includes prescription as well as over-the-counter drugs. Each chapter has been newly updated and revised to include the most current drugs and drug information.

The preliminary chapters on the history of drugs, drug legislation, drug design, drug actions, and drug terminology have been revised, updated, and expanded to include additional material and illustrations.

The special features "Did You Know?," "Historical Notes," and "In Depth," popular with students, teachers, and practitioners, have been retained and expanded. Touches of humor throughout this textbook, one of its best-known features, have been retained and expanded.

NEW FEATURES IN THE THIRD EDITION

Focus on Healthcare Issues

This new special feature helps students and teachers explore some of the complex issues in the world of health care and pharmacology that are in the news each day. The Instructor's Manual provides additional material on the pros and cons of controversial issues so that the instructor can guide students in classroom discussion and discovery.

Clinical Scenarios

Excerpts from real medical case histories are accompanied by critical-thinking questions.

Handwritten Prescriptions

These exercises let students test their ability to read and interpret written prescriptions.

Discontinued Drugs

Drugs recently removed from the market are listed in the Glossary and Index and are in a different format to clearly identify them as being discontinued.

Drug Forms and Dosages

The Glossary and Index has been updated and now includes drug forms and dosages for all the listed drugs, except investigational and orphan drugs.

Pronunciation Guide

The Glossary and Index now includes drug pronunciation guides in a "see and say" format.

Web Site

The textbook now has its own Web site that is updated periodically. This site includes new drugs, drugs taken off the market since the publication of the textbook, and discussions of current healthcare issues that pertain to pharmacology. The site also contains quizzes whose results are returned immediately for instant feedback.

A GUIDED TOUR OF CHAPTER FEATURES AND FORMAT

Chapter Contents

A quick look at the organization of the chapter and its component sections.

Learning Objectives

An overall guide to help verify that you have mastered key concepts and terms in the chapter.

Drug Categories

Drugs are grouped into categories according to their therapeutic action or according to the disease process that they treat.

Drug Terminology

Within the narrative text, special drug terms are highlighted in boldface type.

Generic and Trade Name Drugs

Generic and trade name drugs currently on the market are listed for each drug category, and trade name drugs are capitalized while generic drugs are appropriately lowercased.

Did You Know?

This special feature highlights interesting anecdotes or unusual information pertinent to the drugs being discussed.

Historical Notes

This special feature highlights interesting information about the historical basis of pharmacology.

In Depth

This special feature explains technically complex issues pertaining to drug use or action.

Focus on Healthcare Issues

This special feature explores both sides of complex issues in health care today that pertain to pharmacology.

Illustrations

Photographs and line drawings add interest and visual detail to clarify concepts discussed in the text. Cartoons from two nationally known cartoonists enliven the study of pharmacology!

Review Questions

Detailed and thought-provoking questions are provided at the end of each chapter. The answers are included in the Instructor's Manual.

Clinical Scenarios

Excerpts from real medical case histories are presented and accompanied by exercises or questions. The answers are included in the Instructor's Manual.

The Prescription/Physician's Order Record

Handwritten prescriptions and Physician's Order Records are presented for students to read and interpret. The answers are included in the Instructor's Manual.

Spelling Tips

These tips help students watch out for unusual spelling of drug names and the use of internal capitalization in drug names.

A NOTE TO STUDENTS

The Beginnings of Understanding Pharmacology for Health Professionals

Over 15 years ago, I began teaching a course in pharmacology (lecture and clinical lab) in a community college setting. By the third semester of teaching, I had selected, used, and subsequently discarded three different pharmacology textbooks from three different publishers. Some of my objections to these textbooks were that they were:

- Dry and uninteresting
- Out of date
- Inconsistent in the depth of content presented
- Unclear in their explanation of drug actions
- Visually uninviting
- Lacking in humor and anecdotal information

By the fourth semester of teaching pharmacology, I made the decision to write student handouts for each drug chapter to supplement my weekly lecture. I tried to make the explanations of drug action and other advanced topics as clear and straightforward as possible. This often necessitated prolonged research until I was certain I could convey a complicated concept in a concise and understandable way.

After many revisions, additions, and much research, this material became the basis for the first edition of this textbook.

Prior to finishing the first edition, I received a Master of Arts degree in adult education. Having thoroughly studied the techniques of the best educators, I was more convinced than ever that these techniques could be applied to the teaching of pharmacology and that pharmacology could be presented in an interesting, stimulating, challenging, and even humorous way to enhance the total learning experience. I searched for interesting anecdotal material as well as humorous material/cartoons/quotes to enliven the textbook.

Abundant positive feedback from healthcare instructors, students, and professionals from across the country overwhelmingly validated this combination of clear explanations and attention-holding techniques as a successful educational and professional tool.

How to Study This Textbook

As you begin each chapter, do these things first before reading the text:

- Review the Chapter Contents list. This will alert you to all of the topics that will be presented in the chapter.
- Review the Learning Objectives. This will give you key concepts from the chapter and a general idea of what types of information you will be expected to know when you finish the chapter.
- Browse through the pages of the chapter. This will give you an idea of the length of the chapter and more specific information about its contents.
- Look at some of the illustrations and cartoons in the chapter and boxed areas entitled "Did You Know?" and "Historical Notes." These will entice you to begin reading the chapter material!

After you have finished reading the chapter, answer the Review Questions at the end of the chapter. This will help you assess your level of learning and understanding of the chapter material.

I hope this textbook will make your study of pharmacology relevant and interesting! Good luck with your studies!

Practical Applications of Knowledge

It is important that you relate the information you are learning to your own life experiences, either on a personal or professional level. Everyone has at least some familiarity with drugs. In addition, most people have a family member or friend who is taking medication. As you begin to study a particular chapter in this textbook, your instructor may ask you to interview family members or friends about medications they are taking, the symptoms that prompted the prescription of those drugs, and whether or not their symptoms improved (while keeping the person's identity confidential, of course!). You may also want to describe medications you are taking and why, but this is optional (to preserve your privacy). In this way, you become an active participant in the information-gathering process and begin to see yourself as a researcher. The facts you gather will form a mental framework upon which you can place the information you learn about similar drugs as you study. You will remember that your sister takes Flovent for her asthma, that your oldest child uses tetracycline to treat his acne vulgaris, that you use Zyrtec for your seasonal allergies, or that your elderly aunt takes Celebrex for her arthritis and hydrochlorothiazide for her blood pressure. This will be familiar to you as you study the chapters about those drugs and other similar drugs.

Besides a knowledge of drug uses and actions, it is important for you to know how to communicate your knowledge through speaking and writing. This means mastering the pronunciation and spelling of drug names and recognizing common generic drugs and their trade name equivalents.

When I was teaching a pharmacology course at a community college, a student in the Emergency Medical Technician (EMT) Program approached me and asked for assistance in learning to pronounce drug names. The EMTs did not take the pharmacology course I taught, and this student stated that he was being ridiculed when he tried to call the hospital from the ambulance and couldn't correctly pronounce drug names. I made a tape of the pronunciation of the most common generic and trade name drugs for him. He studied it and later reported that he was successfully pronouncing the drug names and that the healthcare professionals he dealt with had noticed his improvement in this area.

The pronunciation of drug names should be practiced during the study of each chapter. Many drug names, particularly the generic names, have multiple syllables, and correct pronunciation requires some practice. Hearing your instructor pronounce the drug name is just the first step. You need to practice pronouncing drug names for yourself. A pronunciation guide for many of the generic and trade name drugs in the textbook can be found in the Glossary and Index.

While studying pharmacology, it is easy to become buried by the sheer volume of drug names, drug facts, and other details. It is important to recognize common generic and trade name drugs for each category of drugs. However, long after you have forgotten some of the specific drug facts, it is critical that you retain the ability to research and find information about new drugs as they come on the market. You need to know how to locate drugs in drug reference books, interpret printed drug information, formulate questions to obtain additional information, contact appropriate individuals (pharmacists, doctors, etc.) or departments to obtain information, and evaluate the strengths and weaknesses of particular drug references or sources of information.

On a personal note, I would encourage you to constantly increase your knowledge of pharmacology during your study of this textbook and also in the future. Be sure to look for new information about drugs and pharmacology in newspapers and magazines and on TV. You can also research particular drug topics on the Internet.

TO

My husband Al for his support and love

My children Daniel, Minh, and Lien

Contents

List of Figures   xiii

Foreword   xv

Preface   xvii

Acknowledgments   xix

About the Author   xxi

Chapter   1. Introduction to Pharmacology   1

Chapter   2. The History of Drugs: An Overview   5

Chapter   3. Drug Legislation   12

Chapter   4. Drug Design, Testing, Manufacturing, and Marketing   21

Chapter   5. Drug Forms and Routes of Administration   33

Chapter   6. Steps in the Drug Cycle   45

Chapter   7. Drug Effects   50

Chapter   8. Drug Terminology   60

Chapter   9. Systems of Measurement   68

Chapter 10. The Prescription   74

Chapter 11. Dermatologic Drugs   82

Chapter 12. Urinary Tract Drugs   102

Chapter 13. Gastrointestinal Drugs   115

Chapter 14. Musculoskeletal Drugs   137

Chapter 15. Cardiovascular Drugs   150

Chapter 16. Emergency Drugs   178

Chapter 17. Anticoagulant and Thrombolytic Drugs   185

Chapter 18. Pulmonary Drugs   192

Chapter 19. Ear, Nose, and Throat (ENT) Drugs   205

Chapter 20. Ophthalmic Drugs   217

Chapter 21. Endocrine Drugs   228

Chapter 22. Antidiabetic Drugs   236

Chapter 23. Obstetric/Gynecologic Drugs   243

Chapter 24. Neurological Drugs   262

Chapter 25. Psychiatric Drugs   279

Chapter 26. Analgesic Drugs   296

Chapter 27. Anti-Infective Drugs   311

Chapter 28. AIDS Drugs and Antiviral Drugs   323

Chapter 29. Antifungal Drugs   334

Chapter 30. Chemotherapy Drugs   337

Chapter 31. Anesthetics   365

Chapter 32. Intravenous Fluids and Blood Products   373

Glossary and Index   387

Figures

Figure 1–1   (photo) Pills

Figure 1–2   (photo) Child receiving immunization

Figure 3–1   Ad for *Cocaine Toothache Drops*

Figure 3–2   Symbol for a Schedule IV drug

Figure 4–1   Chemical structure for hydrochlorothiazide (Esidrix, HydroDIURIL, Oretic), a diuretic

Figure 4–2   Chemical structures of chlordiazepoxide (Librium) and diazepam (Valium)

Figure 4–3   Cartoon by David W. Harbaugh

Figure 4–4   Typical newspaper ad for volunteers for clinical drug trials

Figure 5–1   Scored tablets

Figure 5–2   Cartoon by David W. Harbaugh

Figure 5–3   Cartoon by David W. Harbaugh

Figure 5–4   The prescription drug nystatin (Mycostatin)

Figure 5–5   Cross-section of transdermal patch of Transderm-Nitro

Figure 5–6   (photo) Some patients have difficulty swallowing solid medication

Figure 5–7   (photo) Inhaler

Figure 5–8   The prescription antibiotic gatifloxacin (Tequin)

Figure 7–1   Cartoon by Sidney Harris

Figure 7–2   How agonist and antagonist drugs work

Figure 7–3   Cartoon by David W. Harbaugh

Figure 8–1   Ampule

Figure 8–2   (photo) A butterfly needle

Figure 8–3   (photo) A tuberculin or TB syringe

Figure 8–4   Vial

Figure 9–1   Symbols used in handwritten prescriptions

Figure 10–1   Typical prescription form

Figure 10–2   Cartoon by David W. Harbaugh

Figure 10–3   A prescription

Figure 10–4   A prescription

Figure 12–1   The prescription drug finasteride (Proscar)

Figure 12–2   A prescription

Figure 13–1   (photo) The prescription drug esomeprazole (Nexium)

Figure 13–2   Cartoon by David W. Harbaugh

Figure 14–1   Illustration from the works of Andreas Vesalius

Figure 15–1   (photo) *Digitalis lanata,* or foxglove plant, the original source of the cardiac drug digitalis

Figure 15–2   (photo) Digitalis toxicity

Figure 15–3   Cartoon by David W. Harbaugh

Figure 15–4   (photo) The prescription drug atorvastatin (Lipitor)

Figure 15–5   Physician's Order Record

Figure 17–1   Physician's Order Record

Figure 18–1   (photo) Proventil inhaler

Figure 18–2   (photo) Serevent Diskus

Figure 18–3   (photo) Flovent Diskus

Figure 18–4   A prescription

Figure 19–1   (photo) The prescription drug fexofenadine (Allegra)

Figure 19–2   (photo) The prescription drug budesonide (Rhinocort Aqua)

Figure 20–1   A prescription

Figure 21–1   The prescription drug liotrix (Thyrolar)

Figure 22–1   (photo) Insulin syringe

Figure 23–1   Cartoon by David W. Harbaugh

Figure 24–1   Cartoon by David W. Harbaugh

Figure 25–1   Chemical structures of chlordiazepoxide (Librium) and diazepam (Valium)

Figure 25–2   Chemical structures of the tricyclic antidepressants imipramine (Tofranil) and amitriptyline (Elavil)

Figure 25–3   A prescription

Figure 26–1   Cartoon by David W. Harbaugh

Figure 27–1   Chemical structures of penicillin G and ampicillin

Figure 27–2   (photo) Culture of *Penicillium* mold

Figure 30–1   Chemical structures of folic acid and methotrexate

Figure 30–2   Cartoon by David W. Harbaugh

Figure 30–3   (photo) Vinca (periwinkle), the original source of the chemotherapy drugs vinblastine (Velban) and vincristine (Oncovin)

Figure 32–1   TPN order form

Figure 32–2   (photo) Blood

Figure 32–3   Physician's Order Record

Foreword

The classical Greek word *pharmakon*, on which the term *pharmacology* is based, had three related meanings: "charm," "poison," and "remedy." These variant senses of the word spotlight important aspects of the history of pharmacology.

In the prescientific age, issues of cause-and-effect were frequently assumed without experimental proof. What we now call superstition and magic took the place of more rational modes of thought and action. Primitive healers used natural substances of animal, vegetable, and mineral origin with boundless confidence in their power to cure, even though objective evidence of their efficacy was lacking. And we can be sure that many cures took place through the power of suggestion, a potent force still recognized today as the "placebo effect."

But if some patients recovered after dosing with crude, prehistoric remedies, others were killed outright. It cannot have escaped the early medicine men—or their patients—that some "medicines" were more useful for getting rid of enemies (or inconvenient friends) than for treating the sick. Hence the second meaning of *pharmakon*. Even today the toxicity of drugs is a major problem, for some of our most effective drugs also have the narrowest margins of safety.

Only after centuries of observation and experimentation has medical science achieved an understanding of the ways drugs work and a sound basis for their safe and effective use. The third sense of *pharmakon*, a sense hedged about with a great deal of wishful thinking in primitive times, has thus largely been realized today. And yet in many ways, we have only scratched the surface.

Many medicines achieve their effects not by neatly eliminating or neutralizing the source of symptoms but by inducing abnormalities in body chemistry or function that tend to offset the abnormalities caused by the disease. Except for a few naturally occurring enzymes, hormones, vitamins, and minerals, most substances administered as medicines are foreign to the body and therefore capable of causing annoying side effects and allergic reactions. Clearly this state of affairs leaves much to be desired and presents a continuing challenge to pharmacologic chemists and clinical researchers.

The fact that we don't have a single perfect drug, much less a panacea or cure-all, accounts for the staggering multitude and diversity of imperfect drugs in current use. The great number and variety of drugs are apt to prove daunting at first sight to the student or healthcare professional who undertakes the study of medical therapeutics.

I am sometimes asked, "How can you possibly remember all those drugs?" The answer is simple. I can't, and neither can anyone else. The typical practicing physician has a working knowledge of just one or two drugs in each pharmacologic class—perhaps more in classes pertaining to his or her specialty, perhaps none in classes he or she never has occasion to prescribe. Once a physician is fully familiar with the characteristics, indications, side effects, and dosage of one drug in a pharmacologic class, similar information about all the others in the same class would be excess baggage.

Just as the range of useful information for the practicing physician doesn't include the whole field of pharmacology, students in health care don't need to memorize huge masses of information or endless lists of drugs. What they need is a general understanding of how various kinds of drugs work, their potentials and limitations, some of the reasons for their number and diversity, and the rationale behind their bewildering and often tongue-twisting names.

That is exactly the kind of mental database that *Understanding Pharmacology for Health Professionals* will give you. The author, drawing from her diversified background in nursing, medical transcription, health information management, and education, has produced a clear, well-organized, stimulating textbook that takes the student step-by-step through the whole subject of pharmacology without going into needless complexities or irrelevant details. The facts are accurate and up-to-date, and their logical connections are presented with clarity and simplicity. Historical sidelights and pertinent illustrations keep the interest level high. A concise glossary at the end of the book gives capsule information about hundreds of current drugs.

Understanding Pharmacology for Health Professionals is not only a superb introductory textbook but is also a reference work that you will consult often and with profit.

John H. Dirckx, M.D.

Preface

Pharmacology is a fascinating and multifaceted discipline that impacts both our professional careers and personal lives. From our role as members of the healthcare team to that of consumers, pharmacology plays a part in our lives.

The study of pharmacology covers a broad spectrum of diverse yet interrelated topics, such as botany, molecular chemistry, research, clinical observation, toxicology, legislation, and patient education.

There is an excitement inherent in the study of pharmacology that stretches from understanding the historical use of herbs and plant extracts, to seeing painstaking research produce both unusable products as well as life-saving discoveries, to finally viewing the future with its nearly limitless potential for medical discovery.

Acknowledgments

I wish to acknowledge Mark Cohen, Senior Editor, Health Professions, Prentice Hall, for his support and enthusiasm for the second and third editions of this textbook.

I wish to thank the many teachers who have used this textbook and the students who have studied this textbook, as well as the healthcare professionals who use this textbook as a day-to-day drug reference on the job. Their insightful comments have helped to continuously improve this textbook from edition to edition.

I wish to acknowledge Sally C. Pitman, Linda Campbell, and the staff of Health Professions Institute for their encouragement and faith in the first edition of this textbook. I also wish to thank John H. Dirckx, M.D., for his insightful comments as an expert reviewer for the first edition and author of the Foreword.

About the Author

Susan M. Turley is an experienced educator and practitioner in many areas of health care. She has worked in acute care, managed care, long-term care, and the physician's office and has held positions in nursing, quality management, infection control, medical assisting, medical transcription, and health information management.

As an educator, she has taught college and community college courses in pharmacology and pathophysiology. She has presented numerous staff inservices in acute care, managed care, and long-term care settings and co-presented numerous all-day seminars for teachers throughout the country. She codeveloped the curriculum and training materials for a nationally distributed medical transcription training program and currently works as a consultant in curriculum development and instructor for a distance learning school with health information management and medical transcription programs.

She is the author of numerous medical and educational articles for national journals, and co-author of two funded national healthcare grants.

She has a Master of Arts degree in adult education, a Bachelor of Science degree in nursing, and national certification in the fields of health information management and medical transcription.

Her writing is well-known for its clarity in presenting technically difficult material and for a special blend of in-depth coverage that also includes humor and interesting anecdotes to keep interest high.

1

Introduction
to Pharmacology

CHAPTER CONTENTS

Definition and linguistic origin of terms
Medical uses for drugs
Overview of the structure of this textbook
Review questions

LEARNING OBJECTIVES

After studying this chapter, you should be able to do the following:

1. Describe the linguistic origin of the terms *pharmacology*, *drug*, and *medicine*.
2. Define the term *pharmacology* and other terms related to specialty fields within the field of pharmacology.
3. List and describe the three general areas of medical uses for drugs.

DEFINITION AND LINGUISTIC ORIGIN OF TERMS

Pharmacology

Pharmacology is the study of drugs and their interactions with living organisms. The term *pharmacology* comes from the Greek words *pharmakon* meaning *medicine* and the suffix *-ology* meaning *the study of*. Pharmacology is concerned with the nature of drugs and medications, their actions in the body, drug dosages, side effects, and so forth.

Pharmacology is a general term. Other more specific terms related to specialty fields within the field of pharmacology include:

pharmacodynamics   (how drugs produce their effects)

pharmacokinetics   (mathematical descriptions of drug response based on time and dose)

molecular pharmacology   (the chemical structure of drugs at the molecular level)

toxicology   (the study of the toxic or poisonous effects of drugs)

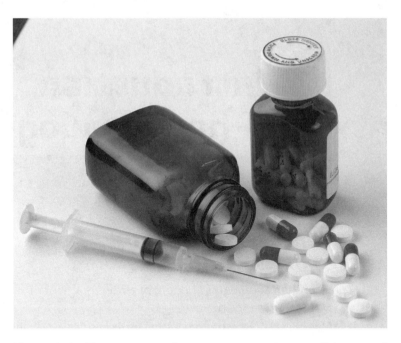

Figure 1–1   Drugs are used to treat symptoms, conditions, and diseases. *Photo reprinted courtesy of Dorling Kindersley.*

Drugs and Medicines

The term *drug* is derived from the Dutch word *droog,* which means *dry,* and refers to the use of dried herbs and plants as the first medicines. The Latin word for *drug* is *medicina,* from which we derive the term *medicine.* A drug or a medicine can be thought of as any nonfood chemical substance that affects the mind or the body. The term *medicine* refers to a drug that is deliberately administered for its medicinal value as a therapeutic, preventative, or diagnostic agent. The term *drug* can be used interchangeably with *medicine,* but can also refer specifically to chemical substances that are not used for their therapeutic, preventative, or diagnostic qualities (e.g., illicit drugs).

MEDICAL USES FOR DRUGS

Drugs have three medical uses.

1. *Therapeutic use.* Drugs are used to control, improve, or cure symptoms, conditions, or diseases of a physiological or psychological nature. Examples of the therapeutic use of drugs include the following:
   - Antibiotics to kill the bacteria that cause an infection
   - Analgesics to control the pain and inflammation of arthritis
   - Hormone replacement therapy for the symptoms of menopause
2. *Preventative use.* Drugs are used to prevent the occurrence of symptoms, conditions, or diseases. Examples of the preventative use of drugs include the following:

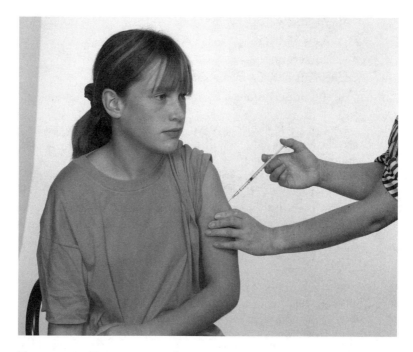

Figure 1–2 Drugs are used to prevent symptoms, conditions, and diseases. The American Academy of Pediatrics issues an annual immunization schedule. All children must receive certain immunizations before they are permitted to enroll in school. *Photo reprinted courtesy of Dorling Kindersley.*

- Vaccination for immunization against childhood diseases
- Drugs taken to prevent motion sickness prior to flying on an airplane

3. *Diagnostic use.* Drugs are used by themselves or in conjunction with radiological procedures and other types of medical tests to provide evidence of a disease process. Examples of the diagnostic use of drugs include the following:
   - Radiopaque dyes used during x-ray procedures
   - Drugs given to simulate cardiac exercise in patients who cannot undergo regular exercise stress testing

OVERVIEW OF THE STRUCTURE OF THIS TEXTBOOK

In Chapters 2 through 10 of this textbook, we discuss the following topics:

Overview of the history of drugs
Drug legislation
Drug design, testing, manufacturing, and marketing
Drug forms and routes of administration

Steps in the drug cycle
Effects of drugs
Drug terminology
Systems of drug measurement
Drug prescriptions

All of these subjects serve as introductory material to build a strong foundation of basic knowledge, which will facilitate the learning of specific drugs introduced in later chapters.

The later chapters follow a common format. Those chapters and the drugs in them are related to a specific body system to facilitate the learning process. The material presented in each of those chapters includes brief historical notes, categories of drugs, pharmaceutical actions, and notes on current therapeutic applications and healthcare issues.

REVIEW QUESTIONS

1. Describe the linguistic origin of the following words:
   pharmacology
   medicine
   drug
2. A knowledge of drug forms, routes of administration, drug effects, and drug measurement is an essential foundation for understanding the action and use of specific drugs. True or False?
3. Describe the three medical uses for drugs and give examples.
4. How are the definitions of *drug* and *medicine* the same? How are they different?

GET CONNECTED

Multimedia Extension Activities

 www.prenhall.com/turley

Use the above address to access the free, interactive Companion Website created for this textbook. Included in the features of this site are drug updates and additional chapter-specific exercises for further practice.

2

The History of Drugs: An Overview

CHAPTER CONTENTS

Ancient drugs
Modern drugs derived from plants, animals, and minerals
Drugs in the 1800s and 1900s
Pharmaceutical milestones
Review questions

LEARNING OBJECTIVES

After studying this chapter, you should be able to do the following:

1. Describe the origin and meaning of the symbol *Rx*.
2. Name at least five drugs historically derived from plant, animal, or mineral sources that are still in use today.
3. Describe the process of the preparation of drugs in the 1800s to early 1900s.
4. Name 10 major pharmaceutical milestones that have occurred since the 1800s.

ANCIENT DRUGS

Pharmacology is one of the oldest branches of medicine. Ancient peoples such as the Sumerians and Egyptians recorded the use of drugs on clay tablets and papyrus as early as 2000 B.C. At that time, diseases were treated with frogs' bile, sour milk, lizards' blood, pigs' teeth, spiders' webs, hippopotamus' oil, and toads' eyelids. The ancient Egyptians applied moldy bread to abrasions, a practice that actually has some therapeutic basis as, many centuries later, penicillin was extracted from a mold. In the early 1800s, an Egyptian medicinal scroll (the Ebers Papyrus) was discovered. It dated back to 1500 B.C. and contained the names of 800 different herbal formulations and prescriptions. The Egyptians also extracted the oil from various plants known for their healing properties. In 1922, when King Tut's tomb was opened, archeologists discovered 350 alabaster jars of plant oils near it. The Aztec Indians of Mexico grew many herbs with medicinal properties. King Montezuma maintained royal gardens of medicinal plants.

Ancient drugs were prepared according to standard recipes that involved drying, crushing, and combining a variety of plants or organic substances. The symbol *Rx*, which comes from the Latin word *recipe* meaning *take*, indicates a **prescription**, the combining of ingredients to form a drug.

The use of some ingredients was based on medical lore and superstition. Some ingredients had therapeutic value and others were worthless. Indeed, some ingredients were actually harmful.

Because little was known about even the most fundamental physical and chemical processes of the body, the therapeutic use of drugs was a matter of much guessing. Medieval physicians prescribed a broad range of medicinals, from herbs to metals (e.g., powdered gold) to addictive substances (e.g., opium). In the 1600s, patients were advised to eat soap to cure blood in the urine and drink mercury in beer to cure intestinal worms.

MODERN DRUGS DERIVED FROM NATURAL SOURCES

There are a number of drugs, based on old prescriptions, that are still in use today.

Drugs Derived from Plants

The medicinal use of the foxglove plant (*Digitalis lanata*) has been noted in 13th-century writings. A derivative, digoxin (Lanoxin), is still used to treat congestive heart failure.

The belladonna plant was the original source of two drugs that are still in use today—atropine and scopolamine. Belladonna means *beautiful lady* in Italian. "Sixteenth century Italian women . . . squeezed the berries of these plants into their eyes to widen and brighten them" (Michael C. Gerald, *Pharmacology: An Introduction to Drugs*, 2nd ed. [Englewood Cliffs, NJ: Prentice Hall, 1981], p. 149, out of print).

Atropine is still used to dilate the pupil in patients with inflammatory conditions of the iris. Scopolamine is used for motion sickness, but has a side effect of blurred vision from paralysis of the muscles of accommodation around the pupil.

Colchicine, a drug still used to treat gout, was used for that same purpose in the sixth century. It was originally derived from the autumn crocus known as *Colchicum autumnale.*

Ephedrine is present in the leaves of a bushy shrub (species name, *Ephedra*), which, when burned, were used by the ancient Chinese to treat respiratory ailments. Today, ephedrine is present in over-the-counter (OTC) bronchodilators.

Many estrogen hormone replacement therapy drugs are derived from yams.

DID YOU KNOW?   Herbs have been a part of all cultures for centuries and have been mentioned frequently in literature. Henbane, a very toxic herb, was supposed to have been the poison that Claudius used to kill his brother, Hamlet's father. "Henbane should not be confused with wolfsbane. Students of literature know wolfsbane to be useful as a vampire repellant (Dracula, 1897); however, we should point out that double-blind studies demonstrating the effectiveness of this plant have not as yet been conducted."

Michael C. Gerald, *Pharmacology: An Introduction to Drugs*, 2nd ed. (Englewood Cliffs, NJ: Prentice Hall, 1981), p. 149, out of print.

The drug galantamine (Reminyl), which is used to treat Alzheimer's disease, is derived from daffodil bulbs.

In addition, many of the gums, oils, and bases in which drugs are dissolved come from plant sources. The drug Accutane, which is used to treat severe cystic acne, contains soybean oil in its capsule. Other drug capsules contain sesame seed oil or olive oil.

Drugs Derived from Animals

Thyroid supplement tablets are composed of dried (desiccated) thyroid gland tissue taken from animals. Thyroid supplements are used to treat patients with hypothyroidism.

The drug Premarin (conjugated estrogens) is derived from **pregnant mare**s' **urine**, and the trade name is formed from letters in that phrase. Premarin is used to relieve the symptoms of menopause.

In the recent past, insulin was derived from the ground-up pancreas of cows or pigs.

FOCUS ON HEALTHCARE ISSUES: Beef and beef/pork insulins have been withdrawn from the market in the United States because bovine spongiform encephalopathy (a fatal disease in cattle) has been linked to outbreaks of an incurable neurological condition in humans known as Creutzfeldt–Jakob disease. Some diabetics who have tried to switch to other types of insulin have found that they have poorly controlled blood sugar levels. Some diabetics have tried to obtain beef/pork insulin from other countries and have petitioned the U.S. government to allow them to continue to use beef/pork insulin.

Lanolin, a common ingredient of topical skin drugs, is obtained from the purified fat of processed sheeps' wool.

Drugs Derived from Minerals

Minerals like calcium and iron are available as individual dietary supplements, and trace minerals like copper, magnesium, selenium, and zinc are included in many multivitamin supplements.

Potassium, in the form of potassium chloride, is given in conjunction with diuretic drugs. (Diuretics cause excretion of excess water from the body; potassium is excreted along with the water.)

The cardiac drug quinapril (Accupril) contains red iron oxide as an inert ingredient in its brown tablets.

Table 2–1 lists the original sources of some common modern drugs.

DRUGS IN THE 1800s AND 1900s

It was not until the 1800s that chemists developed techniques to extract and isolate pure substances from crude drug preparations. The isolation of morphine in 1806 by a German pharmacist marked the beginning of modern drug treatment using chemically pure ingredients.

Table 2–1   **Original Sources of Common Modern Drugs**

Plant, Animal, Mineral Source	Modern Drug
cocoa butter	binder or filler ingredient
foxglove (*Digitalis lanata*)	digoxin
rose hips	vitamin C
belladonna	atropine, scopolamine
willow bark	aspirin
cinchona bark	quinine
opium poppy	morphine
vinca (periwinkle)	vincristine
sharks' liver oil	binder or filler ingredient
snakeroot	reserpine
soy bean oil	binder or filler ingredient
mold	penicillin
minerals	iron, calcium, potassium
yams	estrogen hormone replacement therapy

In the early 1900s, extraction and preparation of drugs was still a time-consuming process that utilized test tubes, filters, and Bunsen burners. Pharmacists at that time had daily duties of preparing drugs from prescriptions. They actually made milk of magnesia, paregoric, and syrup bases for liquid medicines. In addition, they hand-rolled cocoa butter suppositories. They measured drugs in minims, drams, ounces, grains, and scruples.

DID YOU KNOW?   What was the working relationship between the physician and the pharmacist? One hundred years ago, the *Journal of the American Medical Association* published this account:

A physician may be ever so well versed in therapeutics, but if his prescriptions are filled with inert drugs, or drugs varying in strength, his efforts are useless or even dangerous. The pharmacist has greatly aided our efforts in improving the preparation of the various remedies. But the time will come when he should be held responsible not only for the chemic and botanic purity of his preparation, but also for the physiologic activity of those important medicinal agents which cannot be standardized by chemic methods. Probably to the physician the most important duty of the pharmacist is his examination of the crude drugs before they are made up into fluid extracts, tinctures, pills, etc. The ideal preparation is one that possesses activity and elegance to the highest degree.

E. M. Houghton, "How Can We Increase the Therapeutic Relativity of Medicinal Agents (*JAMA* 100 Years Ago)," *JAMA*, 277(13), p. 1088.

Many original drugs are now completely synthetic rather than derived from natural sources. Other natural drugs have undergone chemical modification and molecular restructuring to create new drugs that possess superior pharmaceutical action. In addition, the pharmacist no longer prepares medications but dispenses them and provides patient information and education.

PHARMACEUTICAL MILESTONES

The following list briefly notes some major pharmaceutical milestones dating from the 1800s to the present.

1806	Morphine isolated from crude opium
1899	Aspirin introduced
1908	Sulfanilamide introduced (first anti-infective drug)
1912	Phenobarbital introduced for epilepsy
1913	Vitamins A and B discovered
1922	Insulin isolated
1938	Dilantin introduced for epilepsy
1941	Penicillin introduced (first antibiotic)
1945	Benadryl introduced (first antihistamine)
1948	Cortisone introduced (first corticosteroid)
1952	Thorazine introduced for psychosis
1952	Hydrocortisone introduced (first topical corticosteroid)
1957	Librium introduced for neurosis
1958	Haldol introduced for psychosis
1966	Clotting factors introduced for hemophilia
1967	Inderal introduced for hypertension (first beta-blocker)
1970	Levodopa introduced for Parkinson's disease
1977	Tagamet introduced for peptic ulcers (first H_2 blocker)
1978	First portable insulin pump introduced
1981	Verapamil introduced for arrhythmias (first calcium channel blocker)
1982	First drug made using recombinant DNA technology (human insulin [Humulin])
1983	Topical hydrocortisone approved for over-the-counter sales
1985	ACE inhibitors introduced for hypertension
1985	Seldane introduced for relief of allergy symptoms (first nonsedating antihistamine)
1986	Orthoclone OKT3 introduced (first monoclonal antibody)
1987	Alteplase (Activase) introduced for dissolving blood clots (first tissue plasminogen activator)
1987	AZT (zidovudine, Retrovir) introduced (first AIDS drug)

1992	Proscar introduced for the nonsurgical treatment of benign prostatic hypertrophy (BPH)
1993	Tacrine introduced for Alzheimer's disease
1994	Combination drug therapy introduced for peptic ulcers caused by *Helicobacter pylori*
1995	Cozaar introduced for hypertension (first angiotensin II receptor blocker)
1996	Invirase introduced for AIDS (first protease inhibitor)
1996	Fosamax introduced for osteoporosis (first nonhormonal treatment)
1996	Nicoderm introduced (first prescription-strength drug for stopping smoking available over the counter)
1999	Celebrex introduced for arthritis (first COX–2 inhibitor)
2000	Deciphering of the human genome opens the field of gene therapy in pharmacology
2000	Many decongestants and appetite suppressants withdrawn from the market or reformulated when main ingredient phenylpropanolamine found to cause deaths
2001	Anthrax attack on the United States creates high demand for the antibiotics ciprofloxacin and doxycycline

REVIEW QUESTIONS

1. Give the meaning of and describe the linguistic origin of the symbol *Rx*.
2. Give the name of a medication in current usage that originated from the natural sources listed below:

Natural Source	*Medication*
foxglove plant	
sheeps' wool	
rose hips	
mold	
periwinkle	

3. In what decade were each of the following drugs or drug technologies first introduced? Circle the correct answer.

insulin	1890s	1900s	1910s	1920s	1930s	1940s
penicillin	1890s	1900s	1910s	1920s	1930s	1940s
aspirin	1890s	1900s	1910s	1920s	1930s	1940s
cortisone	1890s	1900s	1910s	1920s	1930s	1940s
vitamin A	1890s	1900s	1910s	1920s	1930s	1940s
Tagamet	1950s	1960s	1970s	1980s	1990s	2000s
Librium	1950s	1960s	1970s	1980s	1990s	2000s
recombinant DNA	1950s	1960s	1970s	1980s	1990s	2000s
Inderal	1950s	1960s	1970s	1980s	1990s	2000s
H_2 blockers	1950s	1960s	1970s	1980s	1990s	2000s
Celebrex	1950s	1960s	1970s	1980s	1990s	2000s

4. Name some ancient "medicines" that seem silly or outrageous to us today.

5. Is it possible that some of the "medicines" you named for Question 4 could be found to have some therapeutic value in the future? State the reason for your answer. Discuss other unusual natural substances that you have heard of that seem to have some therapeutic value.

GET CONNECTED

Multimedia Extension Activities

 www.prenhall.com/turley

Use the above address to access the free, interactive Companion Website created for this textbook. Included in the features of this site are drug updates and additional chapter-specific exercises for further practice.

3

Drug Legislation

CHAPTER CONTENTS

Patent medicines
Origin of drug legislation
Food and Drug Administration (FDA)
Schedule drugs
Orphan drugs
Prescription and over-the-counter (OTC) drugs
Review questions

LEARNING OBJECTIVES

After studying this chapter, you should be able to do the following:

1. Describe the use of patent medicines and the problem they presented in the past for consumer safety.
2. Describe the origin and content of the various drug laws.
3. Describe the function of the Food and Drug Administration (FDA) with respect to approving or removing drugs from the market.
4. Define *schedule drugs* and describe the five categories of controlled substances.
5. Define *orphan drugs*.
6. Differentiate between prescription and over-the-counter (OTC) drugs.

PATENT MEDICINES

From the early history of pharmacology, most physicians attempted to treat patients accurately based on what little scientific knowledge was available to them. As early as 2100 B.C., the Code of Hammurabi gave severe penalties for malpractice.

However, throughout medical history many ineffective and even dangerous medicines have been prescribed. During the 1700s and 1800s, **patent medicines** with such names as *Warner's Safe Cure for Diabetes*, *Dr. Shreve's Anti-Gallstone Remedy*, and *Anti-Morbific Great Liver and Kidney Medicine* were commonly sold without regulation and accompanied by extravagant claims of cures. These medicines often contained one or the other of the addicting drugs opium and morphine without their presence being listed on the label. *Mrs. Winslow's Syrup* for infants' teething pain contained morphine. *Ayer's Cherry Pectoral* for respiratory ailments contained cherry flavoring and heroin.

It is estimated that in the early 1900s one of every 200 Americans was addicted, most of them middle-class women who used these patent medicines for themselves and their children.

HISTORICAL NOTES: Thomas Beecham (1820–1907), an English manufacturer of patent drugs, had this advertisement printed in hymnbooks:

> Hark the herald angels sing
> Beecham's pills are just the thing.
> Peace on earth and mercy mild
> Two for man and one for child.

Marian Ringo, *Nobody Said It Better: 2700 Wise and Witty Quotations about Famous People* (Rand McNally, 1980).

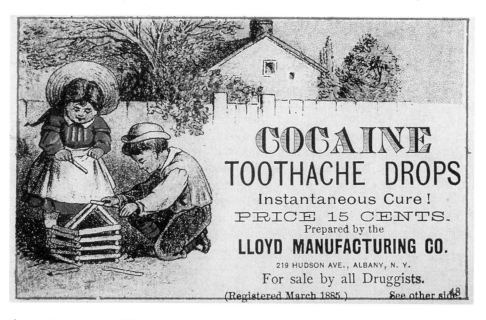

Figure 3–1   An 1885 advertisement for the patent medicine *Cocaine Toothache Drops*. It was not known at that time that cocaine was a highly addictive drug.
Photo reprinted courtesy of the National Library of Medicine, History of Medicine Division.

Warnings against the misuse of drugs, addiction, or drug side effects did not exist. One drug prescribed for respiratory ailments, hydrocyanic acid, caused many deaths. (This poison, which as a gas contains cyanide, is used for legal executions.) "Let the buyer beware" was the prevailing dictum.

THE ORIGIN OF DRUG LEGISLATION

Laws were passed in the 1900s to protect the public from unscrupulous drug sellers as well as from worthless or harmful medicines that were then on the market. The manufacturers of patent medicines strongly opposed drug laws, but public outrage resulted in the passage of **The Food and Drugs Act of 1906**, the first federal drug law. This law required the accurate labeling of drugs to prevent substitution or mislabeling of ingredients. It also stated that only drugs listed in the *United States Pharmacopeia* or *National Formulary* could be prescribed. Nevertheless, many worthless patent medicines remained on the market because the burden of proof lay with the government to show fraud on the part of the seller.

> **DID YOU KNOW?**   The *United States Pharmacopeia (USP)* was compiled by 11 physicians in 1820 and was the first comprehensive drug reference in the United States. A *pharmacopeia* is a collection or compendium of information about all of the drugs in use in a particular country. The *National Formulary (NF)* was first published in 1888 by the American Pharmaceutical Association. Since 1979, these two references have been combined into one volume, called the *USP/NF*. The *USP/NF* contains standards for manufacturing drugs (strength, purity, uniformity, labeling, storage, etc.), as well as information about drugs, dietary supplements, and various types of medical products.

It took a national tragedy to force a much-needed update in The Food and Drugs Act of 1906. Sulfonamide, an early antibacterial drug, was widely used in the United States in 1937. After an extensive advertising campaign aimed at physicians, a Tennessee company marketed this drug in a raspberry-flavored base and called it "Elixir of Sulfonamide." This base had been tested by the manufacturer for flavor and fragrance but not for safety. Elixirs are made from a sweetened alcohol base, but this drug base was an industrial-strength liquid solvent. A number of children died after taking less than 1 ounce of this drug, and over 350 people were poisoned. At that time, a drug manufacturer did not need FDA approval before marketing a drug. In 1938, Congress passed **The Food, Drug, and Cosmetic Act of 1938** that previously had lacked the support it needed to pass. As a result, the government no longer needed proof of fraud to stop the sale of drugs. It could seize products suspected of being toxic. Secondly, the burden of proof was shifted to the drug manufacturers, who were required to provide data based on scientific experiments to show that their product was safe before they were allowed to market it. It became the job of the **Food and Drug Administration (FDA)** to review these data and evaluate the safety of drugs.

In 1951, the **Durham–Humphrey Amendment** to The Food, Drug, and Cosmetic Act defined prescription drugs as those that could be given only to patients under the care of a physician.

In the late 1950s, the drug thalidomide was developed in West Germany and used extensively to treat morning sickness in women early in pregnancy. The FDA refused to approve its use in the United States without further studies. Before these additional studies could be completed by the manufacturer, evidence against the safety of the drug began to accumulate. Over 8,000 babies in Europe were born with deformed limbs ("seal limbs" or phocomelia). This tragedy resulted in the passage of the 1962 **Kefauver–Harris Amendment** to The Food, Drug, and Cosmetic Act, which tightened control on existing prescription drugs and new drugs. It required that drugs be shown to be both safe and effective before being marketed. It also required manufacturers to report adverse side effects from new drugs. Since that time, many drugs have been kept from the market or have been removed from the market because of a lack of safety.

DID YOU KNOW?   Thalidomide was in the news again in 1997 because it was discovered to be useful in treating cancer, AIDS, and leprosy. The potential side effects of this drug are so great that it is only considered as a viable treatment option for life-threatening diseases. The FDA regulates the use of thalidomide in two ways: (1) by limiting the number of physicians who can prescribe it and (2) by requiring women taking the drug not to have sex or to use two forms of birth control if they have sex.

For each new drug, the FDA must weigh the inherent risks of the drug against its potential benefits. To do this thoroughly, the FDA must take the time to complete its review process and issue a final approval (or rejection) of a new drug.

In the early 1990s, FDA approval of a new drug took an average of 34 months. However, for certain critical drugs the process could be much shorter. The first drug (AZT, zidovudine, Retrovir) effective against AIDS was approved by the FDA in 1987 in just 107 days. Despite the rapid handling of many critical drugs, critics still pointed to a time lag in the approval of other new drugs. They argued that some drugs were available in other countries for quite a while before they received approval by the FDA for use in the United States. Inderal, a widely used drug for hypertension and arrhythmias, was available in Europe for nearly 10 years before it was finally approved for use in the United States in 1967.

In response to this criticism, the FDA made a concerted effort to streamline the approval process, particularly with respect to drugs used to treat life-threatening diseases. In 1996, indinavir (Crixivan), a protease inhibitor used to treat AIDS, was approved by the FDA in record time, just 42 days after the new drug application was submitted. In 1997, then-President Clinton signed the **Food and Drug Administration (FDA) Modernization Act**. It gave the FDA the authority to accelerate the approval process for certain types of drugs. In 2000, the average review time for new drugs was less than 15 months. Critically needed drugs (as well as those for whom the manufacturer pays a special fee) can be approved in as little as 6 months.

In addition, the FDA allows physicians to prescribe some investigational drugs even before they are officially approved for marketing. These are drugs for life-threatening diseases for which no other alternative therapy exists. To prescribe these drugs, the FDA requires Emergency and Treatment Investigational New Drug (IND) applications to be filed. These are also known as **Compassionate Use IND** applications. In the 1970s, long before the cardiac drug amiodarone (Cordarone) was on the market (final approval, 1985), cardiologists prescribed it as an investigational new drug to treat patients with life-threatening cardiac arrhythmias that did not respond to other antiarrhythmic drugs. Similarly, the first AIDS drug (AZT, zidovudine, Retrovir) was prescribed for patients before its approval in 1987. This was done under a Compassionate Use IND application.

SCHEDULE DRUGS

Drugs with the potential for abuse and dependence were first regulated by **The Harrison Narcotics Act of 1914.** This Act established the legal framework for controlling these drugs and introduced the drug term *narcotic*. It was replaced in 1970 by **The Comprehensive Drug Abuse Prevention and Control Act**. Title II of this Act, **The Controlled Substances Act,** established the **Drug Enforcement Administration (DEA)** to regulate the manufacturing and dispensing of these drugs. The Act also divided potentially addictive drugs into five categories or schedules based on their potential for physical or psychological dependence. These drugs are known as *schedule drugs* or *controlled substances*.

Schedule I

High potential for abuse

No currently accepted medical use

Examples: PCP, heroin, LSD, marijuana, gamma hydroxybutyrate (GHB), methaqualone, peyote, psilocybin

Schedule II

High potential for abuse

Current medical uses

Severe physical and psychological dependence may result

Examples: Percodan, Demerol, morphine, codeine, cocaine, Dilaudid, Ritalin, methadone

Schedule III

Less potential for abuse than Schedule II drugs

Current medical uses

Moderate physical and psychological dependence may result

Examples: Tylenol with Codeine, paregoric, Vicodin, OxyContin

Schedule IV

Less potential for abuse than Schedule III drugs

Current medical uses

Limited-to-moderate physical and psychological dependence may result

Examples: Darvon, Librium, Valium, phenobarbital, Ambien, Ativan

Schedule V

Limited potential for abuse

Current medical uses

Examples: Lomotil, cough syrups with codeine, Phenergan

FOCUS ON HEALTHCARE ISSUES: There has been a longstanding debate over whether marijuana (a Schedule I drug) should be legally available to treat patients with certain medical conditions. In 1996, voters in California passed Proposition 215 to allow seriously ill patients to use marijuana if approved by their primary care physician. Eight other states passed similar laws. However, the federal law that prohibits the manufacture and distribution of marijuana takes precedence over any state laws.

In November 2000, the U.S. Supreme Court agreed to hear a case that sought an exemption from the federal law for cases of medical necessity. The American Medical Association (AMA) advised that marijuana does provide medical benefit to patients with certain conditions, and many other groups supported the legalization of marijuana to varying extents. In May 2001, however, the Supreme Court issued a decision that federal drug laws that ban the manufacture and distribution of marijuana allow for no exceptions, even for medical necessity.

FOCUS ON HEALTHCARE ISSUES: OxyContin is used to treat moderate-to-severe pain. It was first marketed in 1997. According to law enforcement officials, it has become the fastest growing drug of abuse in history. Abuse of OxyContin has reached epidemic proportions. One official likened it to the crack epidemic in the 1980s.

OxyContin is manufactured as a slow-release tablet to control pain over a long period of time, but abusers chew the tablet to release the full dose of the drug all at once. If the drug is crushed, the powder can be snorted like cocaine or injected like heroin.

Physicians, dentists, chiropractors, podiatrists, nurse practitioners, and other healthcare providers whose state licenses allow may prescribe controlled substances. First, however, they must register with the federal DEA and be issued a DEA certificate and number to prescribe or dispense any schedule (controlled) drug. The provider's DEA number must be clearly written on any prescription for a schedule drug. In addition, some states require the healthcare provider to register with the state agency that controls schedule drugs and be issued a state certificate and number to prescribe or dispense schedule drugs in that state.

The label and packaging for a controlled substance and all of its advertisements must clearly show the drug's assigned schedule. This is written to the right of the drug name as shown in Figure 3–2.

For security purposes, schedule drugs are stored separately from other drugs and kept in a double-locked box or cabinet in the physician's office or on the unit in the hospi-

Figure 3–2   The large *C* stands for *controlled substance*. The number written inside (always a Roman numeral) indicates the assigned schedule number. It is important to remember that a *C* with the Roman numeral IV inside it does not denote that the drug is to be given by the intravenous (I.V.) route, but that the drug is a Schedule IV controlled substance.

tal. Access to the box or cabinet is restricted to those healthcare providers who are licensed to handle controlled substances. A log is kept for each schedule drug. Each dose of a schedule drug that is administered to a patient is noted in the log, along with the date, time, patient's name, amount of the dose, and so forth. Any drug that is wasted or not actually administered to the patient must be accounted for and noted on the log. At the end of the day (or at the end of each shift in the hospital), the log is verified as accurate by two healthcare providers who are licensed to handle controlled substances. Each person independently counts the supply of each controlled substance and then verifies that the count matches the log and matches the count of the other person. Discrepancies in the count are investigated immediately. Theft of a controlled substance must be reported right away to the local police, the state agency for controlled substances, and the federal DEA.

ORPHAN DRUGS

In 1983, **The Orphan Drug Act** was passed. Its purpose was to facilitate the development of new drugs to treat rare diseases. Normally, pharmaceutical companies are reluctant to spend large amounts of time and money to research and test a drug if it will have a limited market. The Orphan Drug Act provides incentives to a drug manufacturer by offering a tax credit (allowing the manufacturer to deduct up to 75% of the cost of clinical trials for the new drug), by simplifying the process of obtaining FDA approval, and by giving the manufacturer exclusive marketing rights for 7 years.

PRESCRIPTION AND OVER-THE-COUNTER (OTC) DRUGS

Prescription drugs are defined as those drugs that are not safe to use except under professional medical supervision and that can only be prescribed by a physician, dentist, nurse practitioner, or other healthcare provider whose license permits this. Prescription drugs are identified on the package label with the inscription "Caution: Federal law prohibits dispensing without a prescription" or "Rx only."

In addition to prescription drugs, the FDA also regulates **over-the-counter (OTC) drugs**. In 1992, the **OTC Drugs Advisory Committee** was created to assist the FDA in reviewing OTC drugs. This Committee consists of physicians and pharmacists as well as one nonvoting member from the drug/cosmetics industry.

An OTC drug is defined as one that can be purchased without a prescription and is generally considered safe for consumers to use if the label's directions and warnings are properly followed. OTC drugs comprise more than half of all the medications used in the United States.

For many years, there was a clear distinction between prescription drugs and OTC drugs. Then in 1983, the topical prescription drug hydrocortisone was approved for OTC sales and many other drugs followed. The OTC Drugs Advisory Committee helps the FDA determine which prescription drugs are appropriate and safe for OTC use. Often the OTC drug is the same as the original prescription drug, but the recommended dosage is just a fraction (often half) of the dosage of the prescription drug.

The FDA approves a prescription drug being reclassified as an OTC drug if (1) the indication for the drug's OTC use is similar to its use as a prescription drug, (2) the patient can easily diagnose and monitor his or her own condition, (3) the drug has a low rate of side effects/toxicity and a low potential for abuse, and (4) use of the drug does not require any special monitoring or ongoing tests.

FOCUS ON HEALTHCARE ISSUES: Supporters of the reclassification of some prescription drugs to an OTC status claim that this will lower drug prices and allow better access to treatment and fewer visits to the doctor. Opponents claim that consumers may actually pay more because health insurance plans will not reimburse the purchase of OTC drugs. They also worry that excessive use of OTC drugs may increase the number of adverse drug–drug interactions and that consumers may try to self-medicate serious illnesses instead of visiting their physicians. In 2001, the manufacturer of lovastatin (Mevacor) asked the FDA to allow this drug to switch from a prescription drug to an OTC drug, but the FDA did not approve this change.

Table 3–1   **Some Prescription Drugs That Are Also OTC Drugs**

Generic Name	Rx Trade Name	OTC Trade Name	Therapeutic Use
butoconazole	Gynazole-1	Femstat 3	vaginal fungal infection
cimetidine	Tagamet	Tagamet HB	heartburn/ulcer
clotrimazole	Mycelex	Gyne-Lotrimin 7	vaginal fungal infection
clotrimazole	Lotrimin	Lotrimin AF	skin fungal infection
cromolyn	Intal	NasalCrom	nasal allergies
famotidine	Pepcid	Pepcid AC	heartburn/ulcer
hydrocortisone	Hycort	Cortizone–5	skin inflammation
ibuprofen	Motrin	Motrin IB	pain
ketoprofen	Orudis	Orudis KT	pain
naproxen	Naprosyn	Aleve	analgesic
nizatidine	Axid	Axid AR	heartburn/ulcer
nicotine	Habitrol	Nicoderm CQ	quit smoking
ranitidine	Zantac	Zantac 75	heartburn/ulcer

REVIEW QUESTIONS

1. In the 1700s and 1800s, patent medicines frequently contained addictive ingredients not listed on the label. Name two such ingredients.

2. Describe the social and consumer safety circumstances that led to the introduction of this drug legislation: The Food and Drugs Act of 1906; The Food, Drug, and Cosmetic Act of 1938; the Kefauver–Harris Amendment of 1962; the FDA Modernization Act of 1987.

3. No drug is entirely safe and without potential side effects and risks. True or False?

4. What federal agency is empowered to review data on a drug's safety and clinical effectiveness and approve drugs for marketing?

5. You are writing an article criticizing the time lag in the United States of the approval of new drugs already in clinical use in other countries. What example might you give to support your position?

6. You are writing an article in rebuttal to the article mentioned in Question 5, defending the time lag as based on appropriate medical caution. What example might you give to support your position?

7. What is a Compassionate Use IND application?

8. Describe (1) how The Controlled Substances Act of 1970 categorized drugs of potential abuse and (2) how healthcare providers are affected by this legislation.

9. Describe how schedule drugs are counted and kept secure in a physician's office or hospital unit.

10. What is the purpose of the 1983 Orphan Drug Act? What three incentives does it offer drug manufacturers to develop orphan drugs?

11. What part of the wording of a drug label tells you that it is a prescription drug?

12. Why was the drug thalidomide, which caused severe birth defects in thousands of babies, allowed on the market again?

13. Discuss these two healthcare issues: (1) OxyContin as a drug of abuse and (2) the legalization of marijuana in cases of medical necessity. Search the Internet and newspapers for recent updates and articles on these two healthcare issues.

GET CONNECTED

Multimedia Extension Activities

 www.prenhall.com/turley

Use the above address to access the free, interactive Companion Website created for this textbook. Included in the features of this site are drug updates and additional chapter-specific exercises for further practice.

4

Drug Design, Testing, Manufacturing, and Marketing

CHAPTER CONTENTS

Drug names (chemical, generic, trade)
Spelling of drug names
Origins of new drugs
Testing of new drugs
Drug patents
Drug manufacturing and quality
Generic drug substitution
Drug recalls
Marketing and drug costs
Review questions

LEARNING OBJECTIVES

After studying this chapter, you should be able to do the following:

1. Describe the chemical, generic, and trade/brand names of a drug.
2. List at least five things that the names of drugs might tell you about those drugs.
3. Name the two ways in which drugs are discovered.
4. Describe how the computer can facilitate drug design.
5. Describe the phases of the testing of new drugs.
6. Explain what is meant by *generic drug substitution*.
7. Define the terms *recombinant DNA technology, drug patent, inert ingredients, therapeutic index, clinical trials, in vivo testing, control group,* and *bioavailability*.
8. Describe the current situation in health care with respect to prescription drug costs.

DRUG NAMES

From the moment of its discovery or design, every drug has a **chemical name** that accurately describes its molecular structure and distinguishes it from all other drugs. The chemical name is used by drug companies and chemists, but is too lengthy and complicated for everyday use by healthcare professionals. The drug company, together with an organization known as the **United States Adopted Names Council**, determines a second name for the drug—its **generic name**. When the FDA gives final approval for marketing, the drug company releases a third name known as the **trade name** or **brand name**. This name is registered with the U.S. Patent Office as a registered trademark. Only the original drug manufacturer has the right to advertise and market the drug under that trade name.

SPELLING OF DRUG NAMES

The accurate spelling of drug names is critical. At the end of each chapter throughout this textbook, there are tips to assist in accurate spelling of drug names. Here is a summary list of tips on drug spellings.

Tip #1: The spelling of some generic drugs reflects their similar chemical structure. All of the following drugs are members of the benzodiazepine class of tranquilizers and are used to treat anxiety and neurosis.

diazepam (Valium)
lorazepam (Ativan)
oxazepam (Serax)

Tip #2: The drug manufacturer selected the drug name to indicate the disease process that the drug will be used to treat.

Azmacort, a drug used to treat asthma
Rythmol, a drug used to treat cardiac arrhythmias
Pepcid, a drug used to treat peptic ulcers

Tip #3: The drug manufacturer selected the drug name to indicate the part of the body that the drug will be used to treat.

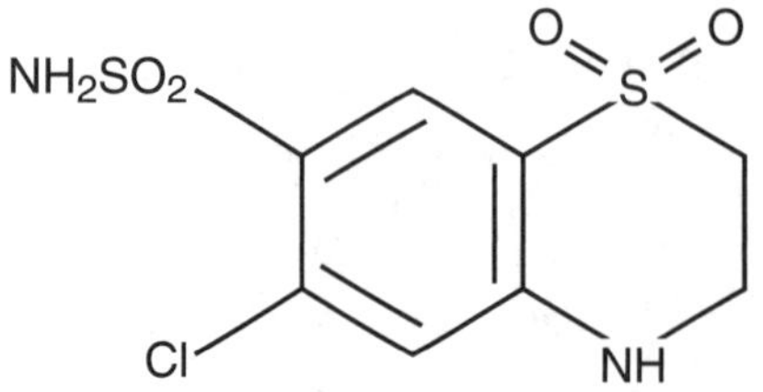

Figure 4–1   Chemical name: 6-chloro-3, 4-dihydro-2H-1, 2, 4-benzothiadiazine-7-sulfonamide 1, 1-dioxide
Generic name: Hydrochlorothiazide
Trade names: Esidrix, HydroDIURIL, Oretic

NasalCrom, a drug used to treat nasal allergies

Bronkaid, a drug used to dilate the bronchial tubes

Tip #4: The drug manufacturer selected the drug name to simplify the generic name while retaining its phonetic sound.

Sudafed (generic drug pseudoephedrine)

Haldol (generic drug haloperidol)

Cipro (generic drug ciprofloxacin

Tip #5: The drug manufacturer selected the drug name to indicate the source of the drug.

Kay Ciel, a drug composed of potassium chloride (**KCl**)

Premarin, a drug obtained from **pre**gnant **mar**e's ur**in**e

basiliximab, a **m**onoclonal **a**nti**b**ody (**MAB**)

Tip #6: The drug manufacturer selected the drug name to indicate the action of the drug.

Elavil, a drug used to elevate depressed mood

Elimite, a drug used to treat scabies (mites)

Flexeril, a skeletal muscle relaxant

Tip #7: The drug manufacturer selected the drug name to indicate that this drug contains several drugs in combination.

Ser-Ap-Es (combines the trade name drugs Serpasil, Apresoline, and Esidrix)

Tip #8: The drug manufacturer selected the drug name to indicate how often the drug is to be taken.

Nitro-Bid, a drug used to treat angina pectoris (twice a day; *b.i.d.* is an abbreviation for the Latin words *bis in die*)

Tip #9: The drug manufacturer selected the drug name to indicate the duration of the drug's action.

Pronestyl-SR, a sustained-release tablet for cardiac arrhythmias

Slow-K, slow-release potassium supplement

Tip #10: The drug manufacturer selected the drug name to indicate the strength of the drug.

Bactrim DS, a **d**ouble-**s**trength dose of the antibiotic

Cortizone-5, a 0.5% hydrocortisone anti-inflammatory topical ointment

Tip #11: The drug manufacturer selected the drug name to indicate the amount of active ingredients.

Tylenol with Codeine No. 2 (contains 15 mg of codeine)

Tylenol with Codeine No. 3 (contains 30 mg of codeine)

Tip #12: The drug manufacturer selected the drug name to reflect the manufacturer's identity.

Wycillin, Wygesic, and Wytensin (Wyeth-Ayerst pharmaceutical company manufacturers these drugs)

Some trade name drugs are particularly difficult to spell because drug manufacturers are not held to any linguistic standards. As noted earlier, Rythmol is used to treat cardiac arrhythmias, and yet the letter *h* found in the word *rhythm* has been deleted from the drug name.

ORIGINS OF NEW DRUGS

The development, testing, manufacturing, and eventual marketing of any drug is a time-consuming and expensive process. In the early 1900s, Paul Ehrlich, a German chemist, tested 605 separate arsenic compounds before finding the first drug known to cure syphilis. This drug was nicknamed "the magic bullet." Today, a pharmaceutical company may evaluate thousands of different chemicals before finding one that moves successfully through all phases of testing and is finally approved by the FDA for release and marketing. In this chapter, we trace the steps from a newly discovered or designed chemical to final FDA approval and clinical use of a drug.

New drugs are discovered in one of two ways.

1. A totally new chemical substance may be discovered in the environment (e.g., in soil samples, plants, marine animals, etc.). Thousands of soil samples have been evaluated for evidence of antibiotic activity. Many new antibiotics have been discovered in this way. The fungus from which the cephalosporin antibiotics are derived was first isolated near a sewer outlet in Sardinia. Streptomycin was first isolated from the stomach of a chicken. As stated in Chapter 2, many drugs still in use today were originally derived from plant, animal, and mineral sources.

2. A totally new chemical may be derived from molecular manipulation of a drug that is already in use. This new chemical may be semisynthetic or totally synthetic. With only very slight molecular changes, the original drug may be significantly changed in a variety of ways that influence absorption, metabolism, half-life, and side effects. For example, penicillin G is derived from the mold *Penicillium chrysogenum*. One of the drug's major drawbacks is that it is destroyed by stomach acid and cannot be administered orally. When the penicillin structure was changed by adding certain chemicals to the vats

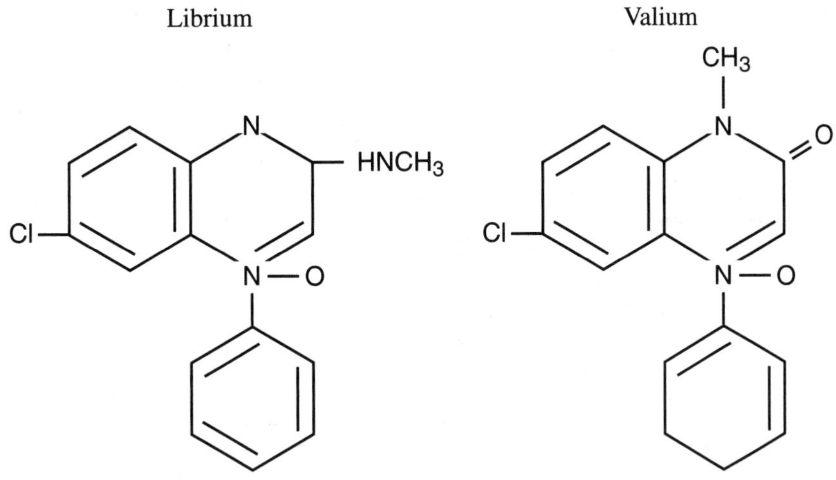

Librium   Valium

Figure 4–2   The similar chemical structures of chlordiazepoxide (Librium) and diazepam (Valium), the first two benzodiazepine tranquilizers. They are still used today to treat anxiety and neurosis.

where the penicillin was fermenting, a semisynthetic penicillin was obtained that was not destroyed by stomach acid. This new penicillin derivative was named *ampicillin.*

In 1957, the first benzodiazepine antianxiety drug was synthesized: chlordiazepoxide (Librium). Working with its basic molecular structure, the same researcher then produced diazepam (Valium). In 1991, when reports of severe cardiac side effects were linked to the then-popular antihistamine terfenadine (Seldane), researchers were able to modify its chemical structure and produce the new drug fexofenadine (Allegra), which has none of those side effects.

In the not-so-distant past, designing a new drug by changing the molecular structure of an existing drug was a slow process of trial and error, using intuition and molecular models made from wood and wire. Now, chemists use computers to aid them in designing new drugs. A computer can process hundreds of variables in chemical structure in a fraction of the time it previously took a chemist to do this manually. The computer can identify those chemicals that would probably not be successful in treating a particular disease before time and money are invested in extensive testing. With computers, chemists can study any molecule, rotating it in three dimensions on the computer screen.

DID YOU KNOW?   A computer can display the molecular structure of any drug from a listing of thousands contained in its database. By looking at and analyzing one of these molecules, scientists can tell if a drug's particular arrangement of atoms is the molecular "key" that will open the "lock," the receptor on the cell membrane. When a scientist wants to know why different-looking drugs act on the same receptor, he can ask the computer to superimpose them all on the screen so he can see how their atoms match up.

"The heart on the computer screen is pounding erratically—severe arrhythmia. But with a few keystrokes, researcher Raimond Winslow adjusts the ion channels and within moments the heart—a three-dimensional model that exists only within the computer—is again beating normally. Winslow, an associate professor of biomedical engineering at The Johns Hopkins University, is developing a detailed computer model that mimics the way the heart works—down to the subcellular level—in order to study serious cardiac arrhythmias and mathematically test the drugs that might cure them. 'There's just an explosion of cellular and molecular data on the properties of heart tissue,' Winslow says. . . . By using computer models of the heart, Winslow says pharmaceutical companies will be able to dramatically narrow their searches for life-saving medicines as well as save millions of dollars now spent on conventional trial-and-error methods. 'If you can tell a company to search for a drug that has a specific effect on a particular channel,' he says, 'that's important, because once these companies know what kind of drug to look for, they have the technology to screen more than 10,000 compounds a day in an effort to find such a drug."

Laurie Palmer, "Plugged In: Computer Modeling Improves Cardiac Care," *Journal of the American Health Information Management Association*, October 1997(68), p. 13.

Recombinant DNA technology (also known as **gene splicing** or **genetic engineering**) represents an ongoing advance in drug development. Aided by computer design, researchers are able, with the use of enzymes, to remove DNA chemically from one organism and transplant it into another organism. The recipient organism, usually a common bacterium that multiplies rapidly, is then directed by the new DNA to produce a particular substance. In huge vats, these bacteria can produce unlimited quantities of drugs. In 1982, human insulin (Humulin) became the first recombinant DNA drug to be approved by the FDA. The **Recombinant DNA Advisory Committee** is a group of physicians and pharmacists who review the clinical trials of genetically engineered new drugs and make recommendations to the FDA.

DID YOU KNOW?   A single bacterium can become two, then four, then eight, then a billion in less than a day. All that's needed is enough food—a standard microbiological medium—for the whole multiplying clan to eat. . . . [They then] mass-produce perfect copies of themselves, . . . continually pumping out the desired product without error."

Doug Stewart, "These Germs Work Wonders," *Reader's Digest*, January 1991, pp. 83–86.

With the deciphering of all 3.2 billion parts of the human genome in June 2000, the field of pharmacology and recombinant DNA technology has now expanded to include the possibility of gene therapy that replaces defective genes in the body at the molecular level!

TESTING OF NEW DRUGS

No matter how a drug was originally discovered or designed, it must be thoroughly tested by the pharmaceutical manufacturer according to certain guidelines specified by the FDA to determine its effectiveness and safety.

Chemical analysis of a drug done in a laboratory in test tubes is known as *in vitro* **testing** (*in vitro* is Latin for *in glass*). Testing carried out in animals or humans is termed *in vivo* **testing** (*in vivo* is Latin for *in living*).

The animal phase of drug testing precedes that of human testing. During animal testing, any toxic effects, side effects, addictions, cancerous tumors, or fetal deformities are noted and evaluated. Also during this phase, the therapeutic index of the drug is calculated. The **therapeutic index (TI)** reflects the relative margin of safety between the dosage that produces a **therapeutic effect** and the dosage that produces a **toxic effect**. Animal studies, however, are not always a reliable indicator as to how well a drug will perform in humans. For example, penicillin causes few side effects in humans, even in fairly high doses, but is toxic to some animals, even in small doses.

When animal studies are completed, the pharmaceutical company applies to the FDA for permission to test the drug in humans in what are known as **clinical trials**. The pharmaceutical company submits an **Investigational New Drug (IND)** application to the FDA to receive permission to begin clinical trials.

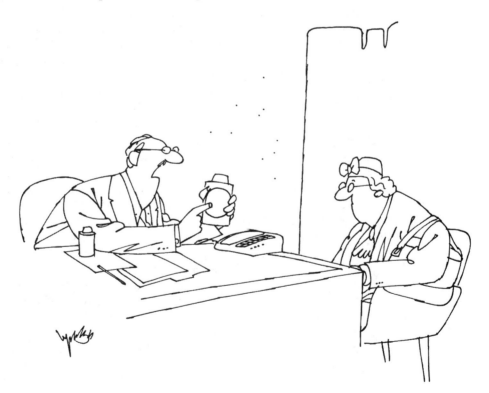

Figure 4–3 *This tonic was tested on 2,000 white mice and they had a ball.* —David W. Harbaugh. *Reprinted with permission.*

EARN $400

Healthy male/female volunteers age 18 to 35 needed now to participate in upcoming inpatient studies. Stay in our pleasant dormitory at Utopia University, with recreational facilities available.

CENTER FOR
VACCINE
DEVELOPMENT
Utopia University

Figure 4–4   A typical newspaper ad seeking volunteers to participate in clinical trials to test a new drug.

There are three phases of human testing. During phase I, about 10 to 100 healthy volunteers are used to study a safe dose range, evaluate side effects, and establish a correct dosage. Absorption, metabolism, and excretion of the drug are also studied. It is not uncommon to see "want-ads" in the classified section of newspapers of large cities for volunteers for these drug studies. Informed consent is mandatory, and during the testing, volunteers are monitored and given medical examinations. Phase I testing of a new drug generally takes 1½ years.

In phase II, the drug is given on an experimental basis to about 50 to 500 patients who actually have the disease that the drug is to treat. This is done to determine the extent of its therapeutic effect. Phase II testing of a new drug usually takes 2 years.

During phase III, the drug is administered to several hundred or several thousand ill patients in exactly the way in which it will be used (dosage, route of administration) once it is on the market. The performance of the drug is compared with that of other drugs currently being used to treat the same disease to evaluate its relative effectiveness. In addition, double-blind studies with the drug and a **placebo** are performed in which neither the patients nor the physician-investigators know which patients are receiving the drug and which **(the control group)** are receiving the placebo. Phase III testing of a new drug usually last 3½ years.

In 1993, the FDA issued guidelines that clinical trials should address the issue of how a drug acts in both men and women. In 1998, Congress extended the standard 17-year patent on new drugs by 6 months for manufacturers who agreed to test their new drugs on children so that pediatric dosages could be better standardized.

Once phase III is completed, the pharmaceutical company submits all of its documentation on the drug to the FDA to await a final decision for approval or denial.

DID YOU KNOW?   The data collected for just one patient in one clinical drug trial can exceed 100 pages of documentation. It takes approximately 12 years for an experimental drug to be approved and the cost of development can exceed $350 million. Only 5 of every 5,000 chemicals tested ever make it to human clinical trials and, of these, only one is actually approved to be marketed.

The complete documentation submitted by pharmaceutical manufacturers to the FDA for approval of a drug can be quite extensive. The ulcer drug cimetidine (Tagamet) is a case in point. After four years of testing, the SmithKline company had accumulated a stack of documents 17 feet high that had to be taken to the FDA in a truck.

Denise Grady, "Bottleneck at the FDA," *Discover*, November 1981, p. 56.

It is the responsibility of the FDA to evaluate a new drug based on the manufacturer's documentation and an examination of the relative risks and benefits of the drug. Only about 20% of the IND applications that are filed with the FDA ever receive final FDA approval for marketing.

Once a drug has received its final approval from the FDA, its ingredients, manufacturing process, labeling, packaging, and dosage cannot be changed. With further clinical trials, however, a drug's indicated uses may be expanded. For example, propranolol (Inderal) was approved by the FDA in 1967 for arrhythmias. In 1973, it was approved for treating hypertension. In 1979, it was approved to treat patients with migraine headaches. Another example of expanded uses: The drug indomethacin (Indocin), a little-used drug for arthritis and gout, was approved in 1985 for use in premature infants to close a patent ductus arteriosus (a heart defect). Although this new clinical indication seems far removed from the drug's original use, it is actually based on the same pharmacologic action—inhibiting the production of prostaglandins.

DRUG PATENTS

A pharmaceutical company is protected by a 17-year patent on any new drug that they develop that is approved by the FDA. This means that, during those 17 years, no other company can manufacture or market an identical drug. However, part of the 17-year patent period is lost during the testing process before the drug is even approved. In 1984, a law was passed that allows the manufacturer to get back up to 5 years of patent protection that were used during the approval process.

When the patent expires at the end of the 17 years, any other pharmaceutical company can manufacture that drug under its original generic name or under a new trade name. The original manufacturer hopes that its new drug will be so successful that its trade name will be firmly entrenched in the minds of prescribing physicians before other drug manufacturers can market other trade name drugs from that same generic drug.

The drug's original trade name can only be used by the original manufacturer. If a generic drug is manufactured by several different pharmaceutical companies, it may be listed under different names: one generic name and several different trade names.

Generic name:	amoxicillin (an antibiotic)
Trade name:	Amoxil (manufactured by GlaxoSmithKline)
	Trimox (manufactured by Bristol-Myers Squibb Company)

Wymox (manufactured by Wyeth–Ayerst)

Generic name: mesalamine (used to treat inflammatory bowel disease)
Asacol (manufactured by Procter & Gamble)
Pentasa (manufactured by Aventis Pharmaceuticals)

Some pharmaceutical companies begin to seek FDA approval for their own version of another manufacturer's popular trade name drug even before the 17-year patent expires. As early as 2001, three different drug companies had produced their version of the popular antidepressant Prozac, even though the original manufacturer's patent does not expire until 2003.

DRUG MANUFACTURING AND QUALITY

The FDA carefully monitors the quality of both the generic and trade name drugs manufactured by all pharmaceutical companies. A generic drug of a certain strength and drug form and the trade name drugs from different manufacturers must all contain exactly the same active drug ingredients and must be able to be administered in exactly the same way. However, the **inert ingredients** (binders, fillers) in each drug can vary, as well as the preservatives, antioxidants, and buffers. In most cases, these variations only minimally affect the disintegration and absorption of the drug. However, in some cases, the inert ingredients do seem to affect the therapeutic action of the drug.

The **bioavailability** of the active drug ingredient can be particularly crucial in drugs with a low therapeutic index (a low margin of safety between the therapeutic and the toxic dose). The inert ingredients can affect the bioavailability of certain drugs. A 1971 study in the *New England Journal of Medicine* compared four preparations of digoxin. All met FDA standards, but the bioavailability of the active drug was much higher for one preparation than for the others. This resulted in blood levels of the drug that ranged from subtherapeutic to toxic.

GENERIC DRUG SUBSTITUTION

In most states under state law, pharmacists are permitted to or must substitute the generic drug for a prescribed trade name drug. If the prescribing physician specifically wants the trade name drug, he or she must indicate that on the prescription, by either checking a box or writing "no substitution" or "dispense as written." The use of generic rather than trade name drugs can result in considerable savings to consumers, but for certain critical drugs—such as digoxin (Lanoxin) for congestive heart failure, phenytoin (Dilantin) for seizures, and anticoagulant drugs—many physicians prefer to rely on the proven therapeutic action a trade name drug. Prescriptions for generic drugs accounted for 13.5% of all new prescriptions in the United States in 1995.

DRUG RECALLS

Each year, the FDA removes certain lots of drugs from the market because of various types of manufacturing defects. A recall can be done for several different reasons.

1. The drug does not remain stable for the whole time preceding its expiration date.
2. The drug is contaminated with particulate matter from the manufacturing process.
3. The drug does not contain the correct amount of active ingredient.

In 1999, the manufacturer of Norplant (an implantable 5-year contraceptive) found that certain lots did not release enough of the drug to prevent pregnancy. The manufacturer notified physicians who were asked to tell their patients with Norplant to use other methods of birth control. In 2000, the manufacturer recalled certain lots of etodolac (Lodine), a drug used to treat arthritis, because the capsules were contaminated with acebutolol, a cardiac drug. It is the responsibility of the drug manufacturer to notify physicians, hospitals, and pharmacies of a drug recall. Once notified, it is the responsibility of the physician, hospital, or pharmacy to dispose of the recalled lots of drugs.

MARKETING AND DRUG COSTS

The marketing of drugs has taken on a new dimension recently. In the past, drug commercials advertised OTC drugs that were widely available in drug stores and supermarkets. Now, approximately half of the television ads for drugs are for prescription drugs. Insurance companies complain that the $1.3 billion spent on drug advertising is prompting consumers to demand new drugs in place of older, less expensive, but equally effective drugs. The insurance companies feel that consumers are watching prescription drug ads and then following the directions to "ask your doctor if [this drug] is right for you." Prescription drugs advertised directly to consumers have more than a 40% growth in annual sales, while other prescription drugs not advertised in this way have a sales growth rate of only 13%. Prescription drugs that have had extensive consumer advertising campaigns include Claritin (an antihistamine), Propecia (for hair loss), Zyrtec (an antihistamine), Pravachol (for high cholesterol levels), Allegra (an antihistamine), Zyban (to stop smoking), Prilosec (for peptic ulcers), Zocor (for high cholesterol levels), Evista (for prevention of osteoporosis), Prozac (for depression), Celebrex and Vioxx (both for arthritis), and Nexium (for gastroesophageal reflux disease).

FOCUS ON HEALTHCARE ISSUES: The Health Care Financing Administration (HCFA) has noted that the cost of prescription drugs, which increased 79% from 1993 to 1999, has been a major factor in rising healthcare costs. During 2000, many of the largest health insurance companies increased their insurance premiums by 10 to 20%, and they attributed these increases primarily to high prescription drug prices. According to *Fortune* magazine, pharmaceutical companies as a whole enjoyed an 18.6% profit margin in 1999, which was greater than that of banks, insurance companies, and telecommunications companies. The pharmaceutical industry claims that this figure is inaccurate because it does not take into account the high expense involved in the research and development of drugs. The American Association for Retired Persons (AARP) disagrees. Both seniors and baby boomers taking care of their senior relatives are complaining to their congressional representatives about the high cost of prescription drugs.

A 2001 study by the National Institute for Health Care Management showed that just two drugs (both heavily advertised and expensive)—Vioxx and Prilosec—accounted for half of the $20.8 billion rise in prescription drug costs from 1999 to 2000.

The president of the National Association of Chain Drug Stores (which represents 94,000 pharmacists and 32,000 drug stores) reported that pharmacists "see first-hand the struggle of seniors having to choose between food and medicine because they lack prescription drug coverage for what have become increasingly complex and effective, but expensive medications." Many seniors rely on the kindness of their primary care physicians to supply them with enough drug samples to last until their next visit, or they decrease the frequency of doses or simply do without the medication.

REVIEW QUESTIONS

1. What are the three names that can be assigned to a drug?
2. The spelling of generic drugs may be similar if they belong to the same drug classification. True or False?
3. List six ways in which pharmaceutical companies select a trade name for a drug.
4. In what two fundamental ways may a new drug be discovered?
5. In general, describe recombinant DNA technology and how it helps pharmaceutical manufacturers produce certain drugs.
6. What is meant by tests that are performed *in vitro*? *in vivo*?
7. What types of drug characteristics/effects are studied during each of the three phases of human testing of a drug prior to FDA approval?
8. Explain the reasoning behind some physicians' decision not to prescribe certain generic drugs for their patients, even though generics are less costly than trade name drugs.
9. How does the computer assist in the designing of new drugs?
10. How can inert ingredients affect the bioavailability of a drug?
11. Name three reasons why a drug can be recalled.
12. Discuss the effects of marketing and the rising costs of prescription drugs in health care.

GET CONNECTED

Multimedia Extension Activities

 www.prenhall.com/turley

Use the above address to access the free, interactive Companion Website created for this textbook. Included in the features of this site are drug updates and additional chapter-specific exercises for further practice.

5

Drug Forms and Routes of Administration

CHAPTER CONTENTS

Drug forms
Routes of drug administration
Review questions
Spelling tips

LEARNING OBJECTIVES

After studying this chapter, you should be able to do the following:

1. Name nine forms in which drugs are manufactured.
2. Name eight routes of drug administration.
3. Describe the advantages and disadvantages of oral administration of a drug.
4. List the sites suitable for subcutaneous and intramuscular injections.
5. Define the special medical terms associated with intravenous administration of a drug.

DRUG FORMS

Before a drug can receive final approval by the FDA, the drug company must clearly state in what form or forms the drug will be manufactured and what routes of administration have been found to be safe and effective. Different forms of a drug are appropriate for different routes of administration. Some drugs are ineffective when administered in a certain form or by a certain route; other drugs may seriously injure the patient if administered in a certain form or by a certain route.

   1. Tablet. This drug form contains dried powdered active drug as well as inert ingredients (binders and fillers) to provide bulk and ensure proper tablet size. A **scored tablet** has an indented line running across it so that it can be easily broken into pieces with a knife to produce an accurate but reduced dose.

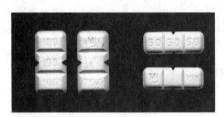

Figure 5–1   A scored tablet can be easily and accurately divided. The prescription drug trazodone (Desyrel Dividose) is used to treat depression. The tablet can be divided into smaller doses according to the patient's need. *Photo reprinted courtesy of Bristol–Myers Squibb Company.*

An **enteric tablet** is covered with a special coating that resists stomach acid but dissolves in the alkaline environment of the small intestine to avoid irritating the stomach (e.g., Ecotrin for pain). A **slow-release tablet** is manufactured to provide a continuous, sustained release of the drug. The drug name often includes the abbreviation **SR (slow release)** or **LA (long acting)** (e.g., Calan SR for migraine headaches, Entex LA for colds). **Caplets** are coated tablets in the form of capsules. Tablets can also be designed to be dis-

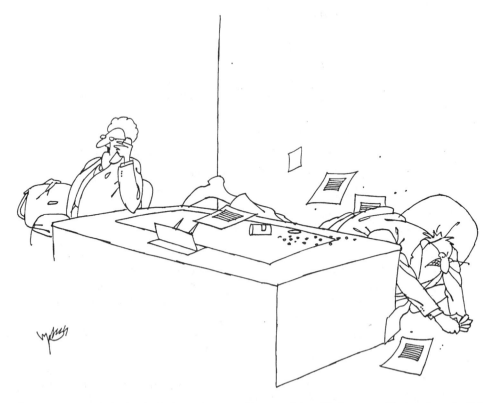

Figure 5–2   *While the doctor's trying to split one of the pills he prescribed, I thought I'd give you a call.*—David W. Harbaugh. *Reprinted with permission.*

solved in water before being taken orally (e.g., Alka-Seltzer effervescent tablets for head colds). Some over-the-counter drugs come in the form of **lozenges**. These round, flat tablets are formed from a hardened base of sugar and water containing the drug and other flavorings. Lozenges are never swallowed, but are allowed to dissolve slowly in the mouth to release the drug topically in the mouth and throat (e.g., Cepacol lozenges for sore throats). A **troche** is an oblong tablet that has a base of sugar and dissolves in the mouth (e.g., nystatin [Mycostatin Pastilles] for yeast infections in the mouth). A *pastille* is another term for a *troche*.

In written prescriptions, *tablet* is sometimes abbreviated as *tab* or *tabs*.

2. Capsule. This drug form comes in two varieties. The first is a soft gelatin shell manufactured in one piece in which the drug is in a liquid form inside the shell (e.g., docusate [Colace, Surfak], a stool softener; fat-soluble vitamins such as A and E). The second type of capsule is a hard shell manufactured in two pieces that fit together and hold the drug, which is in a powdered or granular form. Many nonprescription cold remedies and pain medications were manufactured in this form until some Tylenol capsules were reported to be contaminated with cyanide in the early 1980s. Now, most drug companies manufacture their nonprescription pain medications in a tablet or caplet form. Many prescription drugs, however, are still manufactured as hard-shell capsules. In written prescriptions, *capsule* is sometimes abbreviated as *cap* or *caps*.

3. Cream. A cream is a semisolid emulsion of drug, oil (e.g., lanolin or petroleum), and water, the main ingredient being water. Emulsifying agents are added to keep the oil and water mixed together. Many topical drugs are manufactured in a cream base (e.g., hydrocortisone cream for skin inflammation).

4. Ointment. An ointment is a semisolid emulsion of drug, oil (e.g., lanolin or petroleum), and water, the main ingredient being oil. Many topical drugs are manufactured in an ointment base (e.g., Kenalog ointment for skin inflammation). Specially formulated ophthalmic ointments can be applied topically to the eye without causing irritation.

5. Lotion. A lotion is a semisolid suspension of drug dissolved in a thickened water base (e.g., Keri lotion and calamine lotion for skin dryness and irritation).

6. Gel. A gel is a semisolid suspension in which the drug particles are suspended in a thickened water base (e.g., MetroGel for acne rosacea).

7. Powder. A powder is the finely ground form of an active drug. Powdered drugs can be in capsules but also can be manufactured in glass vials where they must be reconstituted with sterile water before being injected (e.g., intravenous ampicillin, an antibiotic). Powders can also come in packets; the packet is opened and the powder is reconstituted with water for oral use (e.g., Metamucil, a laxative). Powders can also be sprinkled on topically or sprayed on (e.g., Tinactin, an antifungal drug for the skin). Powders can also be inhaled into the lungs with the help of a special inhalation device (e.g., Serevent Diskus, a bronchodilator).

8. Liquid. Liquids come in the form of either solutions or suspensions.

Solutions contain the drug dissolved in a water base. Solutions never need to be mixed as the drug-to-water concentration is always the same in every part of the solution, even after prolonged standing. Solutions come in many forms: elixirs, syrups, tinctures, liquid sprays, and foams.

Elixirs are solutions that contain an alcohol and water base with added sugar and flavoring (e.g., Tylenol elixir for fever and pain). Elixirs are commonly used for pediatric or elderly patients who cannot swallow the tablet or capsule form of a drug.

Syrups are solutions that contain no alcohol and are a concentrated solution of sugar, water, and flavorings. Syrups are sweeter and more viscous (thicker) than elixirs. Most OTC cough medications have a syrup base that not only carries the drug but acts to soothe inflamed mucous membranes in the throat (e.g., guaifenesin [Robitussin] for coughs).

DID YOU KNOW?   Liquid oral medications come in a variety of flavors to please everyone and "help the medicine go down": grape, cherry, bubble gum, pineapple, maple, wine, raspberry, mocha, butterscotch, strawberry, mint, orange, honey lemon, root beer, watermelon, coconut, licorice, banana, and so forth.

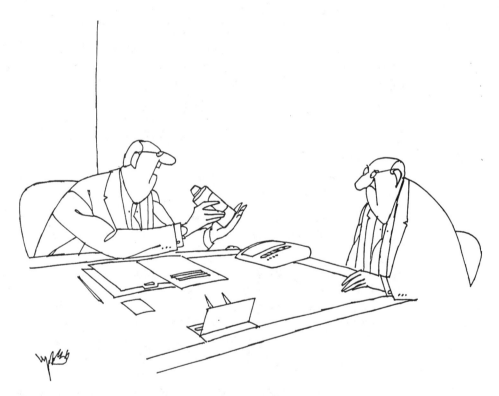

Figure 5–3   *I think you'll like this new medication, . . . it's a little spritzy, sweet and spicy with some bite but not abrupt . . . and it has a rich toasted almond–peach aftertaste with lots of character*—David W. Harbaugh. *Reprinted with permission.*

Liquid sprays contain a solution of drug combined with water or alcohol; they are sprayed by a pump or aerosol propellant. Spray liquid drugs are commonly used for topical application (e.g., Afrin nasal spray, a decongestant).

Foams contain a solution of drug that is expanded by tiny aerosol bubbles (e.g., OTC contraceptive foam).

Suspensions contain fine, undissolved particles of drug suspended in a water base. With prolonged standing, these fine particles gradually settle to the bottom of the container. It is always important to shake suspensions well before using them, a fact that is noted on the label of these drugs (e.g., Maalox antacid). See Figure 5–4. An **emulsion** is a suspension in which the drug is mixed with fat particles and water (e.g., Intralipid intravenous fat solution).

Two general terms used to describe a liquid are *aqueous* (from the Latin word *aqua*, for *water*), meaning *of a watery consistency*, and *viscous*, which designates a nonwatery or thick liquid.

9. Suppository. A suppository is composed of a solid base of glycerin or cocoa butter that contains the drug. It is manufactured in appropriate sizes for rectal or vaginal insertion and in adult and pediatric sizes. Vaginal suppositories are most often used to treat vaginal infections, but can also be inserted into the mouth to treat oral yeast infections.

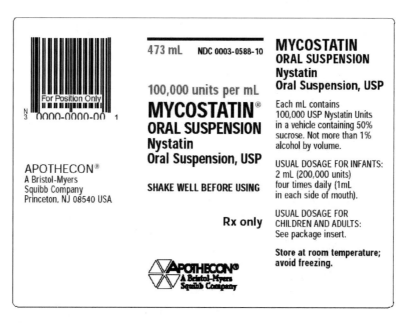

Figure 5–4   The prescription drug nystatin (Mycostatin) is used to treat yeast infections in the mouth. This drug comes in the form of a suspension. Notice the instruction on the label: "Shake well before using." The large drug particles in a suspension tend to settle to the bottom of the container. Shaking redistributes the particles and assures an accurate dosage. *Photo reprinted courtesy of Bristol–Myers Squibb Company.*

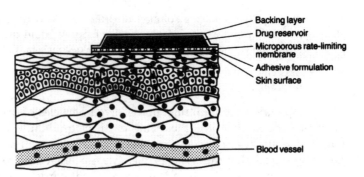

Figure 5–5 Cross-section of a transdermal patch of the drug Transderm-Nitro, which is used to prevent angina. *Illustration reprinted courtesy of Novartis Pharmaceuticals Corp.*

Rectal suppositories can be used to administer drugs to patients who are vomiting and cannot take oral medication.

10. Transdermal. The transdermal form of a drug consists of a multilayered disk consisting of a drug reservoir, a porous membrane, and an adhesive layer to hold it to the skin. The porous membrane regulates the amount of drug released into the skin. These drugs are also known as *transdermal patches.*

11. Pellet/Bead. A drug can be implanted in the body in the form of a pellet or bead that slowly releases the drug to the surrounding tissues (e.g., Norplant for birth control is implanted under the skin; gentamicin beads [Septopal] on a surgical wire are inserted into the bone to treat chronic osteomyelitis).

ROUTES OF DRUG ADMINISTRATION

There are various routes of drug administration. Some drugs are approved for use via more than one route and are manufactured in different forms appropriate for those different routes. Each route of administration has distinct advantages and disadvantages as discussed next. A drug given by one route will be therapeutic; given by another route, it may be ineffective, harmful, or even fatal.

1. Oral. The oral route is the most convenient route of administration and the one most commonly used. Tablets, capsules, and liquids are all given orally. Even patients who have difficulty swallowing a tablet or capsule can usually take the liquid form of a drug without problems. Infants are given drugs in a liquid form that is mixed with a small amount of formula and administered through a nipple. The oral route is routinely abbreviated as **PO** or **p.o.** (Latin for *per os,* meaning *through the mouth*).

Disadvantages of the oral route include the following: Some drugs (e.g., penicillins) are inactivated by stomach acid and cannot be given orally. After oral administration, some drugs (e.g., lidocaine [Xylocaine] for cardiac arrhythmias) are metabolized so quickly by the liver that a therapeutic blood level cannot be achieved. Some drugs (e.g., tetracycline) cannot be taken with certain foods and drinks because they combine chemically to form an insoluble complex. Other drugs (e.g., MAO inhibitors for depression) cannot be taken with certain foods or drinks because they produce adverse side effects.

2. Sublingual. Sublingual administration involves placing the drug (usually in a tablet form) under the tongue and allowing it to slowly dissolve. The tablet is not swallowed (because this would become oral administration). The drug is absorbed quickly through oral mucous membranes and into the large blood vessels under the tongue. The sublingual route provides a faster therapeutic effect than the oral route (e.g., nitroglycerin tablets for treating angina).

3. Nasogastric. This route is used to administer drugs to patients who cannot take oral medications. Nasogastric administration is accomplished with a nasogastric tube that

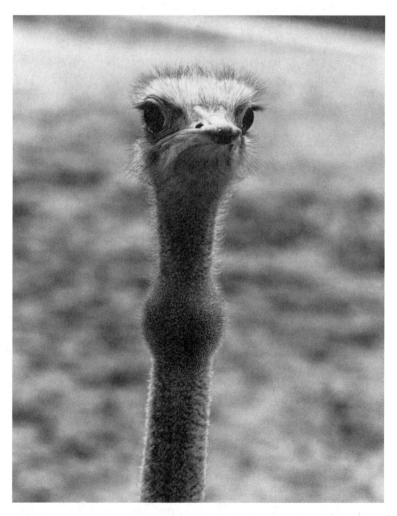

Figure 5–6   Some patients have difficulty swallowing solid medication. *Photo reprinted courtesy of Abbott Laboratories.*

passes from the nose through the esophagus and into the stomach. Only liquid drugs can be given by this route.

4. Gastrostomy or **jejunostomy.** These routes are used to administer drugs to patients who cannot take oral medications. These routes use a surgically implanted feeding tube to deliver liquid drugs directly into the stomach (gastrostomy) or jejunum (jejunostomy).

5. Rectal. This route is reserved for certain clinical situations, such as when the patient is vomiting and/or the medication cannot be given by injection (e.g., Tylenol suppositories). Absorption of a drug via the rectal route of administration is slow and often unpredictable, so this route is not used often. However, the rectal route is the preferred route when drugs are administered locally to relieve constipation (e.g., Fleet enema) or treat hemorrhoids (e.g., Anusol) or ulcerative colitis (Proctofoam-HC).

6. Vaginal. The vaginal route is used to treat vaginal infections and vaginitis by means of creams and suppositories (e.g., Monistat 7 suppositories, Premarin vaginal cream). Contraceptive foams are inserted vaginally as well.

7. Topical. When a drug is applied directly to the skin or to the mucous membranes of the eyes, ears, nose, or mouth, it is administered via the topical route. The effects of the drug are generally local (e.g., bacitracin antibiotic ointment for skin abrasions, Sudafed nasal decongestant spray, Timoptic eye drops for glaucoma).

Some sites of topical administration are abbreviated as follows:

Abbreviation	Latin Meaning	Medical Meaning
A.D./AD	*auris dextra*	right ear
A.S./AS	*auris sinistra*	left ear
A.U./AU	*auris uterque*	both ears
O.D./OD	*oculus dexter*	right eye
O.S./OS	*oculus sinister*	left eye
O.U./OU	*oculus uterque*	both eyes

8. Transdermal. This route of administration differs from the topical route in that the drug is applied to the skin via physical delivery through a porous membrane, and the therapeutic effects are felt systemically, not just at the site of administration. Drugs delivered by the transdermal route are manufactured in the form of a patch. A transdermal patch is worn on the skin and releases the drug slowly over a 24-hour period, providing sustained therapeutic blood levels (e.g., Transderm-Nitro for prevention of angina pectoris).

9. Inhalation. This route of administration involves the inhaling of a drug that is in a gas, liquid, or powder form. The drug is absorbed through the alveoli of the lungs (e.g., nitrous oxide, a general anesthetic; albuterol [Proventil], a bronchodilator).

10. Parenteral. *Parenteral* is a general term taken from two Greek words, *para* and *enteron*, which literally mean *apart from the intestine*. Technically, parenteral administration includes all routes of administration other than oral, but in clinical usage, parenteral administration commonly includes the following routes of administration: subcutaneous, intramuscular, and intravenous, and other less frequently used routes: endotracheal,

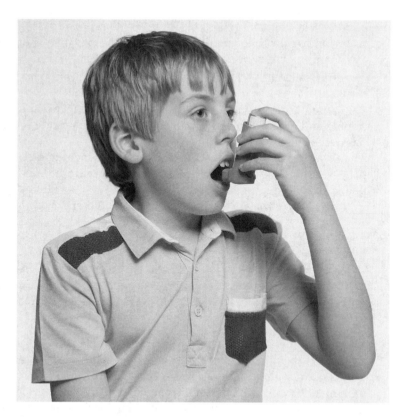

Figure 5–7   A variety of bronchodilators are administered via inhalation using a metered-dose inhaler. *Photo reprinted courtesy of Dorling Kindersley.*

intra-arterial, intra-articular, intracardiac, intradermal, intrathecal, and injection into the umbilical artery or vein.

Subcutaneous administration involves the injection of liquid into the subcutaneous tissue (the fatty layer of tissue just under the dermis of the skin but above the muscle layer) (e.g., insulin for diabetes mellitus, allergy shots). There are few blood vessels in this layer, so drugs are absorbed more slowly by this route than when given by intramuscular injection. Diabetics who inject insulin use approximately 10 to 12 different areas on the upper arms, thighs, and abdomen and rotate the site of each subcutaneous insulin injection. The term *subcutaneous* is abbreviated in various ways as *subQ*, *SQ*, and *subcu*. There is no one official abbreviation.

Intramuscular administration involves the injection of a liquid into the belly (area of greatest mass) of a large muscle. The large muscles of the body are well supplied with blood vessels, and drugs are absorbed more quickly by this route than when given by subcutaneous injection. There are five I.M. injection sites that can be used; injection at other sites can cause damage to adjacent nerves and blood vessels.

- Deltoid, located on the upper arm, lateral aspect.
- Vastus lateralis, located on the midthigh, lateral aspect.

- Rectus femoris, located on the midthigh, anterior aspect.
- Ventrogluteal, located on the side of the hip over the gluteus muscle between the anterior and superior spines of the iliac crest.
- Dorsogluteal, located in the upper outer quadrant of each buttock.

Some drugs cannot be given by intramuscular injection because they are not water soluble and would form precipitate particles in the tissue (e.g., Valium and Librium, antianxiety drugs).

Examples of drugs given intramuscularly include meperidine (Demerol) for severe pain, vitamin B_{12} for pernicious anemia, and aurothioglucose (Solganal), a gold compound used to treat rheumatoid arthritis.

The term *intramuscular* is abbreviated as either *IM* or *I.M.*

DID YOU KNOW?   Fans of the television series *Star Trek* are familiar with the drug delivery system of the future: the hypospray. No needles and no pain!

Intravenous administration of a drug involves the injection of a liquid directly into a vein. The therapeutic effect of drugs given intravenously can often be seen immediately. This is because the drug does not need to be absorbed from tissue or muscle before it can exert an effect. I.V. administration can be done in one of three ways. The injection of a single dose of a drug **(bolus)** can be given through a **port** (rubber stopper) into an existing I.V. line. This is often referred to as *I.V. push* because the drug is manually pushed into the I.V. line in a very short period of time. A drug can also be mixed with the fluid in an I.V. bag or bottle and administered continuously over several hours. This is known as *I.V. drip.* A drug can also be mixed in a very small I.V. bag or bottle and administered over an hour or less by I.V. drip. This small secondary I.V. bag or bottle is connected through tubing to a port in the existing primary I.V. line. This method is known as *I.V. piggyback administration.*

Examples of drugs given intravenously include thiopental (Pentothal) for induction of general anesthesia, diazepam (Valium) to control continuous epileptic seizures, and most chemotherapy drugs.

The term *intravenous* is abbreviated as either *IV* or *I.V.*

Endotracheal. This route is used to give certain drugs (e.g., epinephrine [Adrenalin]) during emergency resuscitation after the patient has been intubated with an endotracheal tube. This route is also used routinely to treat respiratory distress syndrome in newborn infants (e.g., beractant [Survanta], a lung surfactant). The drugs are absorbed through the tissues of the lungs.

Intra-arterial. This route is used for direct injection of a chemotherapy drug into the area of a tumor. Generally, arterial lines are used for continuous monitoring of arterial blood pressure and are not used to administer drugs.

Intra-articular. This route is used to inject certain drugs (e.g., corticosteroids to decrease pain and inflammation) into a joint. The Latin root word *articulo-* means *joint.*

Intracardiac. This route is used only during emergency resuscitation (e.g., epinephrine [Adrenalin] is given through the chest wall into the heart to stimulate the heart muscle during cardiac arrest).

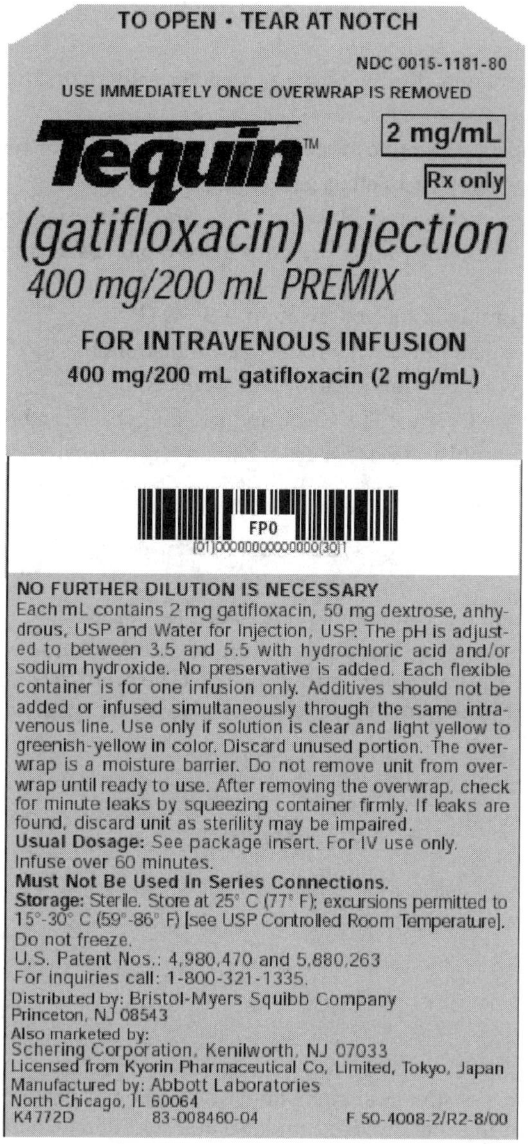

TO OPEN · TEAR AT NOTCH

NDC 0015-1181-80

USE IMMEDIATELY ONCE OVERWRAP IS REMOVED

Tequin™

2 mg/mL

Rx only

(gatifloxacin) Injection
400 mg/200 mL PREMIX

FOR INTRAVENOUS INFUSION

400 mg/200 mL gatifloxacin (2 mg/mL)

FPO
[01]000000000000000(30)1

NO FURTHER DILUTION IS NECESSARY
Each mL contains 2 mg gatifloxacin, 50 mg dextrose, anhydrous, USP and Water for Injection, USP. The pH is adjusted to between 3.5 and 5.5 with hydrochloric acid and/or sodium hydroxide. No preservative is added. Each flexible container is for one infusion only. Additives should not be added or infused simultaneously through the same intravenous line. Use only if solution is clear and light yellow to greenish-yellow in color. Discard unused portion. The overwrap is a moisture barrier. Do not remove unit from overwrap until ready to use. After removing the overwrap, check for minute leaks by squeezing container firmly. If leaks are found, discard unit as sterility may be impaired.
Usual Dosage: See package insert. For IV use only. Infuse over 60 minutes.
Must Not Be Used In Series Connections.
Storage: Sterile. Store at 25° C (77° F); excursions permitted to 15°-30° C (59°-86° F) [see USP Controlled Room Temperature]. Do not freeze.
U.S. Patent Nos.: 4,980,470 and 5,880,263
For inquiries call: 1-800-321-1335.
Distributed by: Bristol-Myers Squibb Company
Princeton, NJ 08543
Also marketed by:
Schering Corporation, Kenilworth, NJ 07033
Licensed from Kyorin Pharmaceutical Co, Limited, Tokyo, Japan
Manufactured by: Abbott Laboratories
North Chicago, IL 60064
K4772D   83-008460-04   F 50-4008-2/R2-8/00

Figure 5–8 The prescription antibiotic gatifloxacin (Tequin), showing the indication for the intravenous route of administration. *Photo reprinted courtesy of Bristol–Myers Squibb Company.*

Intradermal. This route involves the injection of a liquid into the dermis, the layer of skin just below the epidermis. The epidermis itself is less than 1/20 of an inch thick; therefore, when an intradermal injection is correctly positioned, the tip of the needle is still plainly visible through the skin (e.g., Mantoux test for tuberculosis).

Intrathecal. This route involves the injection of a liquid within the sheath or meninges of the spinal cord into the cerebrospinal fluid (e.g., spinal anesthesia). The Greek root word *theka* means *sheath*.

Umbilical artery or vein. This route is accessible only in newborn infants before the umbilical cord has dried. It is used to administer fluids and draw blood. It is generally not used to give drugs. Instead, an I.V. line is inserted peripherally in the hand, foot, or scalp for drug administration.

REVIEW QUESTIONS

1. What is the reason for manufacturing a drug as an enterically coated tablet?
2. What are caplets?
3. Besides tablets and capsules, list five other forms in which drugs are manufactured.
4. Describe the difference between an elixir and a syrup.
5. List two disadvantages encountered when administering some drugs by the oral route.
6. The sublingual route of administration provides more rapid absorption of a drug than the oral route. True or False?
7. What is the English meaning of the abbreviation A.S.? O.U.?
8. A diabetic would inject insulin via what route of administration?
9. Describe three of the five acceptable sites for an I.M. injection.
10. Differentiate between the I.V. push, I.V. drip, and I.V. piggyback methods of administration.
11. List several routes of administration that are considered *parenteral*.

SPELLING TIPS

lozenge   no final *r*, although it is commonly pronounced as "lozenger."

intravenous   not *inter*venous. Note the same with intra-arterial, intracardiac, intradermal, intramuscular, and intrathecal. The prefix *intra-* means *within*. (The prefix *inter-* means *between*. This prefix would give the wrong meaning in these medical words.)

parenteral   not *parental*.

GET CONNECTED

Multimedia Extension Activities

    www.prenhall.com/turley

Use the above address to access the free, interactive Companion Website created for this textbook. Included in the features of this site are drug updates and additional chapter-specific exercises for further practice.

6

Steps in the Drug Cycle

CHAPTER CONTENTS

Steps in the drug cycle
Absorption of drugs
Distribution of drugs
Metabolism of drugs
Excretion of drugs
Review questions

LEARNING OBJECTIVES

After studying this chapter, you should be able to do the following:

1. Describe how drugs administered via the following routes are absorbed: topical, oral, inhalation, rectal/vaginal, and parenteral.
2. Define the role of plasma proteins and the blood–brain barrier in distribution of a drug.
3. Describe how the liver metabolizes drugs.
4. Describe how the kidneys excrete drugs.
5. Describe how drug dosages are adjusted for patients with liver or kidney disease, elderly patients, or premature infants.

STEPS IN THE DRUG CYCLE

Following administration, most drugs go through several steps in a well-defined sequence before being excreted from the body. These steps include:

Absorption from the site of administration
Distribution via the circulatory system
Metabolism
Excretion from the body

ABSORPTION OF DRUGS

Absorption involves the movement of the drug from the site of administration, through tissues, and into the bloodstream. Topical drugs, however, are not absorbed to any great extent, and their therapeutic action is exerted locally at the site of administration. For other drugs, absorption involves several steps.

Tablets, capsules, suppositories, and so on, first disintegrate; this step is omitted with drugs that are in a liquid form.

Drugs given orally dissolve in body fluids (saliva, gastric juice) and are absorbed through the tissue into the blood vessels. The presence or absence of food in the stomach can influence the rate of absorption.

Some drugs are not absorbed at all following oral administration (e.g., neomycin, an antibiotic). This drawback can be overcome by administering the drug via a different route. However, nonabsorption of a drug via the oral route can be a therapeutic advantage. Examples: Neomycin can be given orally to exert its antibiotic effect solely in the intestinal tract to kill intestinal bacteria prior to abdominal surgery. Carafate is given orally to bind directly to stomach ulcers. This drug is not absorbed into the bloodstream but exerts its therapeutic effect locally on the stomach mucosa. Metamucil is not absorbed but binds with water in the intestinal tract to increase stool bulk and relieve constipation.

Following administration of a drug by inhalation, the vaporized liquid is absorbed through the mucous membranes lining the alveoli and into adjacent capillaries. Some drugs given by inhalation exert a topical effect but may also produce systemic side effects. Inhaled general anesthetic gases exert only a systemic effect.

Following rectal or vaginal administration, a suppository melts and releases the drug topically to the mucous membranes. The rate of absorption with rectal administration is rather slow and variable; therefore, it is often reserved for topical drug applications (e.g., Anusol to treat hemorrhoids) in which the rate of absorption is not critical.

Injections (intradermal, subcutaneous, intramuscular) of liquid drugs are absorbed from body tissues into adjacent blood vessels.

Only intravenous injections entirely bypass the step of absorption because the drug is administered directly into the bloodstream.

DISTRIBUTION OF DRUGS

Once a drug has been adsorbed into the bloodstream, it is distributed throughout the body via the circulatory system. As a drug dose enters the bloodstream, some of the drug binds to circulating **plasma proteins,** such as **albumin.** Plasma proteins have indentations in their molecular surface that permit drug molecules to bind to them. The drug molecules that are bound to plasma proteins are essentially pharmacologically inactive as they are carried through the bloodstream.

As the portion of the drug that did not bind to plasma proteins moves from the blood into body tissues to exert a therapeutic effect, some of the bound drug is released from the plasma proteins to maintain an equilibrium of unbound drug in the bloodstream.

Unbound drug that moves into body tissues comes in contact with cell membranes where it exerts an effect by interacting with a **receptor.** This process will be discussed in the next chapter.

One area of the body where drugs may not be distributed following absorption is in the central nervous system. Theoretically, the brain tissues are protected by the so-called **blood–brain barrier** that is thought to exist between the blood vessels in the brain and the surrounding brain tissue. However, some drugs, like antihistamines and morphine-type drugs, are able to pass through the blood–brain barrier and cause effects such as drowsiness and euphoria, respectively. General anesthetics also cross the blood–brain barrier to produce unconsciousness. Sometimes the blood–brain barrier actually excludes the very drugs needed to correct disease conditions in the brain. Parkinson's disease is due to a deficiency of the **neurotransmitter** dopamine in the brain. Although dopamine can be administered orally, it cannot cross the blood–brain barrier to be therapeutically effective in the brain. Fortunately another drug, levodopa, which is structurally different, can cross the blood–brain barrier, where it is then converted to dopamine to correct the deficiency.

At one time, it was thought that the placenta formed a barrier to protect the developing fetus from harmful drugs. It is now known that the placenta allows nearly all drugs to pass from the maternal circulation to the fetus. Each year, many infants are born addicted or with birth defects due to the action of drugs taken by their mothers.

METABOLISM OF DRUGS

The process of metabolism is also known as **biotransformation** because the drug is transformed or metabolized from its original active form to a less active, or even inactive, form. This process is accomplished by the action of enzymes.

The liver is the principal organ of metabolism, although other organs metabolize certain drugs to a limited degree. Drugs absorbed through the mucous membrane of the stomach or intestines enter the bloodstream via the portal vein. Before this vein empties into the general circulation, it passes through the liver. Therefore, drugs given by the oral route, absorbed from the GI tract, and carried in the bloodstream to the liver are immediately subjected to metabolism by liver enzymes. This initial metabolism by the liver is referred to as the **first-pass effect**—the drug must first pass through the liver before it can reach the general circulation. For some drugs, the first-pass effect is so extensive that most of the drug dose is immediately metabolized.

> **DID YOU KNOW?**   Lidocaine (Xylocaine), a drug used to treat cardiac arrhythmias, cannot be given orally because the first-pass effect removes all of the active drug and no therapeutic effect can be achieved systemically.

Some drugs (e.g., chloral hydrate, a sedative) are administered in an inactive form and remain inactive until they are metabolized. It is the **metabolite** of these drugs that actually exerts a therapeutic effect.

Because the liver is the principal organ for drug metabolism, any decrease in liver function affects the rate of drug metabolism. Standard drug dosages need to be adjusted downward to compensate for the prolonged pharmacologic action of unmetabolized drug in the bloodstreams of these types of patients: patients with liver diseases, elderly patients with degenerative liver changes associated with aging, and premature infants with immature livers.

> **DID YOU KNOW?**   Chronotherapy (the word root *chrono-* is Latin for *time*) attempts to coordinate the administration and metabolism of a drug to the body's own biological rhythms. Certain diseases like hypertension or asthma tend to be worse at certain times of the day. If an antihypertensive drug is taken at bedtime, it is metabolized and reaches its highest therapeutic levels in the early morning, just when the blood pressure rises dramatically and there is an increased incidence of heart attacks and strokes.

EXCRETION OF DRUGS

The excretion of drugs is a necessary step in ridding the body of waste products (inactive drug **metabolites**) or in removing active drugs that are not metabolized by the liver. The principal organ involved in the excretion of drugs is the kidney, although other organs are involved to a limited degree. The lungs excrete certain general anesthetics as the patient exhales. Also, trace amounts of drugs are excreted in saliva, tears, and sweat.

> **DID YOU KNOW?**   Trace amounts of drugs are also excreted in breast milk. While the amount of drug in breast milk may be insignificant when compared with the total amount of drug excreted by the kidneys, it can be enough of a dose to significantly affect a nursing baby.

A drug is not automatically excreted by the kidney just because it reaches the kidney. A drug that remains bound to albumin, which is a large molecule, cannot pass through the glomerular membrane in the nephron of the kidney. That drug remains bound to albumin in the blood and is returned to the general circulation. However, unbound drug exists as a molecule that is small enough to pass through the glomerular membrane. Once through the glomerular membrane, a further distinction is made between **water-soluble drugs** and **fat-soluble drugs.** An unbound water-soluble drug is excreted in the urine because of its affinity for the water content of urine. An unbound fat-soluble drug is more attracted to the lipid (fat) structure of the renal tubule wall than to the urine. Most of the unbound fat-soluble drug is reabsorbed into the renal tubules and returned to the bloodstream. Eventually, the fat-soluble drug is metabolized by the liver into a more water-soluble form that can be excreted in the urine. Without the action of the liver, it is difficult for a fat-soluble drug to be excreted by the kidneys. Indeed, it has been estimated that some fat-soluble barbiturates could remain in the bloodstream for years if the liver did not metabolize them to a water-soluble form.

Poor renal function can significantly prolong the effects of some drugs. Patients with renal disease and elderly patients with physiologically decreased levels of kidney function are prescribed lower dosages of drugs to prevent toxic symptoms due to decreased rates of drug excretion.

REVIEW QUESTIONS

1. Describe the steps of absorption, distribution, metabolism, and excretion of a drug that is administered orally.
2. What is meant by the term *first-pass effect?*
3. How do plasma proteins such as albumin regulate the amount of drug circulating in the bloodstream?
4. What is the theoretical function of the blood–brain barrier?
5. Give two reasons why standard drug dosages may need to be decreased for elderly patients.
6. Give two reasons why drugs reaching the kidney may not be excreted in the urine.
7. What is chronotherapy and how is it useful in determining when to administer drugs?
8. Define these terms: *biotransformation, albumin,* and *metabolite.*

GET CONNECTED

Multimedia Extension Activities

 www.prenhall.com/turley

Use the above address to access the free, interactive Companion Website created for this textbook. Included in the features of this site are drug updates and additional chapter-specific exercises for further practice.

7

Drug Effects

CHAPTER CONTENTS

Local versus systemic effects of drugs
Therapeutic effects of drugs
Side effects of drugs
Adverse effects of drugs
Toxic effects of drugs
Allergic reactions to drugs
Idiosyncratic reactions to drugs
Basis of drug effects
Drug–drug and drug–food interations
Review questions

LEARNING OBJECTIVES

After studying this chapter, you should be able to do the following:

1. Differentiate between a local and systemic drug effect.
2. Define these terms: *therapeutic effect, side effect, adverse effect*, and *target organ*.
3. Describe two actions the physician might take to reverse drug toxicity.
4. Describe the physiologic response that occurs during an allergic drug reaction.
5. Define the terms *receptor, agonist, antagonist, synergism*, and *antagonism*.

LOCAL VERSUS SYSTEMIC EFFECTS OF DRUGS

Basically, drugs act in one of two ways, either locally or systemically. A local effect is limited to the site of administration and those tissues immediately surrounding it. Most drugs applied topically exert a local effect (e.g., nasal sprays and topical creams and ointments). A few drugs applied topically exert a systemic effect (e.g., Transderm-Nitro transdermal patch).

A systemic effect is not limited to the site of administration but can be felt throughout the body to varying degrees. Drugs given intravenously or intramuscularly always exert a systemic effect. Drugs given subcutaneously exert either a local effect or systemic effect, depending on the type of drug. Drugs taken orally usually exert a systemic effect. (In the previous chapter, we discussed how some oral drugs are not absorbed into the bloodstream but only exert a local effect in the gastrointestinal tract.) Inhaled drugs exert either a local effect or a systemic effect, depending on the type of drug. Drugs given vaginally exert a local effect. Drugs given rectally exert either a local or a systemic effect, depending on the type of drug.

The same drug given via different routes can exert either a local or a systemic effect. For example, lidocaine (Xylocaine) is gargled for topical anesthesia, injected subcutaneously for local anesthesia, or given intravenously to act systemically in treating cardiac arrhythmias. The antihistamine diphenhydramine (Benadryl) can be purchased over the counter as a spray or cream for topical application to relieve itching; it can also be purchased as a capsule and taken orally to act systemically to relieve allergy symptoms.

THERAPEUTIC EFFECTS OF DRUGS

The **therapeutic effect** is the drug's main action for which it was prescribed by the physician or other healthcare provider. The therapeutic effect of the drug is selected to cure a disease (e.g., an antibiotic), decrease disease symptoms (e.g., insulin), prevent a disease (e.g., a vaccine), or diagnose a disease.

Most medical problems and diseases cannot be treated by a drug that acts only at the site of administration; they must be treated with a drug that acts systemically. The action of that drug is directed toward the specific area of the body with the medical problem or disease—often toward a **target organ** (e.g., the heart, in patients being treated for congestive heart failure).

The therapeutic effect is not always directed toward a target organ. For example, when a physician prescribes antibiotics, the therapeutic effect is intended to destroy or inhibit the growth of disease-causing bacteria within the body.

Sometimes the therapeutic effect is actually one of the side effects of the drug. Many antihistamines, when given orally for allergies, can produce drowsiness. However, this side effect of drowsiness can be utilized as a therapeutic effect when an antihistamine is incorporated into a medication for insomnia.

The perfect drug would have a complete therapeutic effect perfectly suited to its medical purpose and no other effects. Unfortunately, the perfect drug does not exist.

SIDE EFFECTS OF DRUGS

When a drug acts systemically, it exerts an effect not only on the target organ but also on other body tissues. Drug effects other than the therapeutic effect are termed **side effects.** Side effects can be mild and short-lived, moderate and annoying, or severe enough that the drug must be discontinued.

It should be noted that no drug is entirely safe and without potential side effects and risks. Even one of the oldest and most widely used OTC drugs—aspirin—can cause serious side effects such as gastric ulcer.

The drug manufacturer compiles a list of common side effects as a new drug is tested. If the side effects are severe, the FDA may not approve the drug.

Examples of side effects vary widely with the type of drug. Some drugs produce few side effects, but most drugs are associated with at least one or two side effects that are frequently observed after administration of the drug. Common gastrointestinal side effects include anorexia, nausea, vomiting, or diarrhea. A common side effect of codeine is constipation. Common central nervous system side effects include drowsiness, excitement, or depression. Some antidepressant medications cause significant side effects of blurred vision, dry mouth, and fatigue. Common side effects of chemotherapy drugs may include nausea, vomiting, chills, fever, and loss of hair. These side effects are more severe than those of other drugs, but are tolerated because the chemotherapy drug is used to treat cancer—a life-threatening condition. Categories of chemically related drugs often produce a pattern of similar side effects because they activate the same receptors.

Once on the market, the advertisements, informational literature, prescribing information, and package inserts for the drug must list the side effects.

ADVERSE EFFECTS OF DRUGS

Severe side effects are often referred to as **adverse effects.** Adverse effects are not as commonly observed as side effects, so some adverse effects only become apparent after a drug has been on the market for some time and has been prescribed for large numbers of patients.

In 2000, the FDA proposed regulations to make the prescribing information provided with drugs easier for doctors to use. The FDA acknowledged that too few doctors read these lengthy, fine-print information sheets. The new revised drug information begins with a section describing the most important warnings for not prescribing a drug for particular types of patients and ends with a patient-counseling checklist that the doctor can review with the patient. Seven of the 11 drugs taken off the market from 1997 to 2000 were discontinued because doctors kept prescribing them for certain types of patients despite warnings to the contrary in the drug information, and adverse effects occurred.

The FDA can remove a drug from the market even after it has been approved if there are adverse effects. In 1982, Oraflex was hailed as a breakthrough drug in the treatment of arthritis. Within three months, 500,000 prescriptions had been written for it. This nonsteroidal anti-inflammatory drug (NSAID) needed to be taken only once daily (due to its long **half-life** of 25 to 32 hours). However, two months later, the FDA began receiving reports of the deaths of a number of elderly patients who had been taking Oraflex. It was found that, in these patients, the half-life of the drug could increase dramatically to as long as 100 hours (due to slower metabolism and excretion in the elderly), producing toxic symptoms and death. The Oraflex label did not clearly state the need to reduce dosages in elderly patients. This drug was removed from the market by the FDA, and due to adverse publicity, the manufacturer chose not to relabel the drug but instead discontinued it.

In 1997, the FDA removed from the market one of the two drugs in the widely popular "fen-phen" combination drug treatment for weight control. Fenfluramine (Pondimin) was removed from the market; the other drug, phentermine (Fastin), was allowed to remain on the market as an appetite suppressant. At the same time, the chemically related drug dexfenfluramine (Redux) was taken off the market. Both fenfluramine (Pondimin) and dexfenfluramine (Redux) were linked to cases of primary pulmonary arterial hypertension and damage to the heart valves. Before it was taken off the market, Redux had been prescribed for 2 million people.

Often an adverse effect is so unusual and seemingly unrelated to the drug's therapeutic action that it takes some time before a causal relationship is established.

FOCUS ON HEALTHCARE ISSUES: Isotretinoin (Accutane) is a vitamin A-type drug that was first approved by the FDA in 1982 for the treatment of severe cystic acne vulgaris. It was not until 2001 that the FDA required patients to sign a consent form prior to taking Accutane because of a possible link with suicide attempts and suicides. See Chapter 11, "Dermatologic Drugs," for a Focus on Healthcare Issues feature that describes how this affected one family.

Adverse drug reactions account for 2 to 5% of all hospital admissions. It is estimated that up to 2 million Americans are hospitalized annually because of adverse drug effects and as many as 100,000 to 140,000 die as a result.

Physicians can report adverse effects by using a special form provided by the FDA.

TOXIC EFFECTS OF DRUGS

Toxic effects result when serum levels of a drug rise above the therapeutic level to higher levels that are toxic. Before FDA approval, the pharmaceutical manufacturer must show that a drug does not produce toxic effects when administered in therapeutic doses. However, when a drug has a low **therapeutic index** (a narrow margin of safety between the therapeutic dose and the toxic dose)—such as the heart medication digoxin (Lanoxin)—it is not uncommon to see toxic symptoms, particularly in elderly patients.

When toxic symptoms occur, the physician may elect to decrease the dosage of the drug, lengthen the time between doses, or discontinue the drug altogether. Patients on drugs that are known to frequently cause toxic effects are also scheduled for blood tests to monitor drug levels and other laboratory tests to monitor particular organs that might be affected. The antibiotics gentamicin (Garamycin) and kanamycin (Kantrex) are known to exert toxic effects on the ear **(ototoxicity)** and kidneys **(nephrotoxicity).** Patients on these drugs are given audiograms to monitor hearing acuity and blood tests to assess kidney function. Liver function tests are done for patients on cholesterol-lowering drugs (Lipitor, Mevacor, Pravachol, Zocor) because these drugs can have a toxic effect on the liver.

ALLERGIC REACTIONS TO DRUGS

Allergic reactions to drugs are another type of effect but differ from side effects, adverse effects, or toxic effects in that they have a different underlying cause: the systemic release of **histamine** that occurs even when a drug is at therapeutic levels. The term *allergy* was introduced in the early 1900s. An allergy is a reaction that occurs when the body's im-

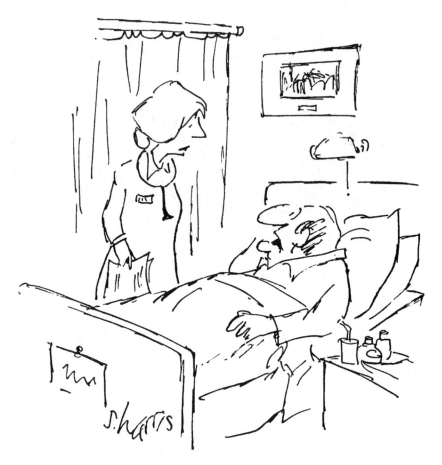

Figure 7–1 *I stopped taking the medicine because I prefer the original disease to the side effects.*—Sidney Harris, 1981, *American Scientist* magazine. *Reprinted with permission.*

mune system identifies a foreign substance (an **antigen**) and initiates an antibody response against it. The antigen (pollen, dust, food, or a drug) does not provoke an allergic reaction in everyone, but only in certain hypersensitive people. The presence of the **antigen** combined with an **antibody** stimulates the release of **histamine.**

Histamine produces mild to severe allergic symptoms, depending on the amount released. Mild allergic reactions are characterized by itching, swelling, redness, sneezing, and wheezing. Severe to life-threatening allergic reactions involve bronchospasm, edema, shock, and death. The severest symptoms of an allergic reaction are collectively termed **anaphylaxis** or **anaphylactic shock.** Anaphylactic shock is not common, but is most often associated with the antibiotic penicillin, although other drugs may also produce it. Interestingly, a patient may take several courses of penicillin before any allergic reaction occurs. Once a patient is sensitized to a particular drug, even a small dose can trigger an allergic reaction. In addition, some drugs show cross-allergies to other drug groups because of similarities in their molecular structures. For example, patients allergic to penicillin should avoid other drugs in the penicillin group, such as ampicillin, and may also exhibit hypersensitivity to cephalosporin antibiotics (Keflex, Velosef, Ceclor) because of their similar chemical structure.

The patient's drug allergies are listed in the medical record. When a patient has no drug allergies, this is also noted as *NKDA (no known drug allergies).*

IDIOSYNCRATIC REACTIONS TO DRUGS

A **drug idiosyncrasy** is a type of reaction that is not a side effect, adverse reaction, or allergic reaction. It is an individual's unique reaction to a drug, and it may have its basis in genetics. Certain genetic factors cause variations in the metabolism and action of a drug. For example, after an identical oral dose of a tricyclic antidepressant drug was given to a group of patients, it was found that there was a 10- to 40-fold variation in blood concentrations of the drug. Another idiosyncratic reaction is that of malignant hyperthermia (a sudden, uncontrolled elevation in body temperature that occurs in 1 out of 20,000 patients given the inhaled general anesthetic halothane).

BASIS OF DRUG EFFECTS

Drug effects are initiated through **receptors.** Receptors are special protein molecules located on the cell membranes of every cell. They are specifically designed to interact with natural body chemicals (hormones, enzymes, neurotransmittors), but they can also interact with drugs. There are many different kinds of receptors located on cells throughout the body.

You can think of a receptor as a type of lock and the drug as a type of key. A certain drug can unlock (or activate) a receptor. In fact, several drugs may be able to unlock one type of receptor. Chemically similar drugs may activate the same receptor to produce similar effects. A drug that is able to unlock or activate a receptor and produce an effect is known as an **agonist.**

Some drugs appear to fit a certain receptor but cannot actually unlock or activate the receptor to produce an effect. These drugs are known as **antagonists** or **blockers.** When an antagonist drug combines with a receptor, it is similar to inserting the wrong key into a lock. The key may fit, but it cannot be turned to unlock the lock. An antagonist drug may fit with a receptor, but it does not activate it. Instead, its therapeutic action is to occupy the receptor site and block body chemicals or other drugs from activating the receptor.

It should also be noted that one drug can act as a master key to unlock or activate several different types of receptors. This accounts for the various therapeutic and side effects that can be produced throughout the body by just one drug.

There are many types of receptors throughout the body, but these three types are commonly involved in drug therapy. Adrenergic receptors are part of the sympathetic nervous system and are activated by the natural neurotransmitters epinephrine, norepinephrine, and dopamine or by drugs. Cholinergic receptors are part of the parasympathetic nervous system and are activated by the natural neurotransmitter acetylcholine. H_1 and H_2 receptors are activated by histamine.

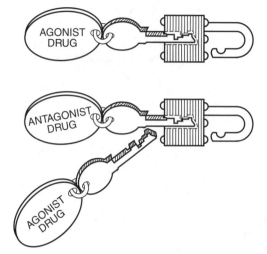

Figure 7–2   How agonist and antagonist drugs work. An agonist drug (key) un-locks or activates a receptor (lock). An antagonist drug (key) occupies or blocks a re-ceptor (lock) but does not ac-tivate it.

DRUG–DRUG AND DRUG–FOOD INTERACTIONS

Many patients take more than one drug on a daily basis. In particular, elderly patients with chronic medical problems may consume a number of medications several times a day. In addition, many patients take both prescription drugs and several OTC drugs of their own choice. This is known as *polypharmacy.* Polypharmacy increases the likelihood of a drug–drug interaction.

DID YOU KNOW?   Although Elvis Presley officially died of a heart attack in 1977, the State Board of Medical Examiners found that his physician had prescribed some 12,000 pills—tranquilizers, stimulants, sedatives, and painkillers—for him in the last 18 months prior to his death.

When administered simultaneously, some drugs interact with each other in a partic-ular way to either accentuate or diminish the action of each. There are two types of drug–drug interactions: synergism and antagonism. **Synergism** involves two drugs com-bining to produce an effect greater than the independent effect of each drug. In many cases, synergism is beneficial. Tylenol is taken with codeine to provide more complete pain relief than either drug alone can provide. A potassium-wasting diuretic is taken with a potassium-sparing diuretic to achieve effective water loss while conserving potassium. However, an undesirable type of synergism can also occur. One well-publicized undesir-able drug combination is that of alcohol and tranquilizers or alcohol and antihistamines. In both cases the drug's side effect of drowsiness is heightened by the sedative effect of al-cohol, often with fatal results. Prozac (an antidepressant) and alcohol taken by the chauf-feur driving Princess Diana contributed to the car accident in which she was tragically killed in 1997.

DID YOU KNOW?   Astemizole (Hismanal) and terfenadine (Seldane) were hailed as superior to older antihistamines because they were nonsedating. After they had been on the market for some time, the FDA required them to carry a warning label that they should not be used by patients taking the antibiotic erythromycin or the antifungal drugs ketoconazole or itraconazole. Taking just a little more than the prescribed dose of either of these antihistamines in combination with the antibiotic or antifungal drug could cause a fatal cardiac arrhythmia. Not long after that, both drugs were removed from the market.

Another type of drug–drug interaction is known as **antagonism:** two drugs combine to produce an effect that is less than the intended effect for either drug. When the antibiotic tetracycline is taken with an antacid, these two drugs combine to form an insoluble complex that prevents either of them from exerting a therapeutic effect.

Antagonistic **drug–food interactions** also occur. Tetracycline also cannot be taken with milk because it forms an insoluble complex. MAO inhibitors, a class of antidepressant drugs, cannot be taken with foods rich in the amino acid tyramine because of a chemical reaction that causes hypertension, headaches, and possible stroke. Tyramine is present in aged cheeses, alcoholic beverages, bananas, liver, avocados, and chocolate, and patients taking MAO inhibitors must avoid these foods.

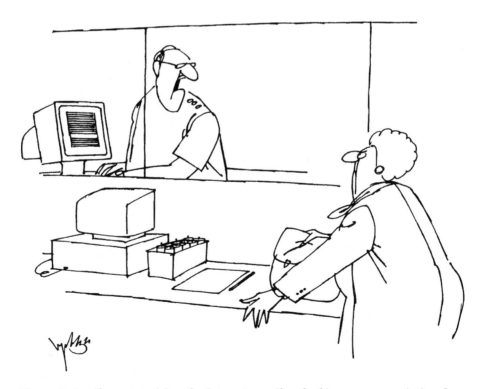

Figure 7–3   *I'm not cruising the Internet . . . I'm checking your prescription drug interactions.*—David W. Harbaugh. *Reprinted with permission.*

REVIEW QUESTIONS

1. Describe the difference between local and systemic drug effects.
2. Give an example of a drug that can act either locally or systemically to produce a therapeutic effect depending on the route of administration.
3. Differentiate between a drug's therapeutic effect and its side effect.
4. List several common side effects involving the GI tract and the central nervous system.
5. How does a toxic effect differ from a side effect?
6. Define the term *therapeutic index*.
7. What is the basis for all of the symptoms associated with an allergic reaction?
8. Describe the lock-and-key concept as it pertains to a drug and a receptor.
9. Give an example of a synergistic drug–drug interaction and of an antagonistic drug–drug interaction.
10. Examine several drug advertisements in magazines or medical journals. What type of information is provided about the drug, its actions, and its side effects or adverse effects? How does the artwork or photography in the ad enhance the drug's appeal to physician prescribers or consumers?
11. What is polypharmacy?
12. Review the excerpt below, which is from a real case history, and use the Glossary/Index at the back of this textbook to identify the category that each of the drugs belongs to. Is this patient at risk for drug–drug interactions?

CLINICAL SCENARIO

This is a 76-year-old white female who is currently taking Accupril 20 mg q.d., Actos 45 mg q.d., aspirin 81 mg q.d., Catapres-TTS-1 one patch weekly, monthly B_{12} injections, Lasix 40 mg q.d. (we will increase to 80 mg q.d. today), Glucotrol XL 10 mg q.d., Humulin N 12 units q.a.m. (we will decrease to 8 units q.a.m. today), K-Dur 10 mEq. q.d., Lanoxin 0.125 mg q.d., lorazepam 0.5 mg b.i.d., Metamucil p.r.n., Prozac 20 mg q.d., Zantac 150 mg b.i.d., Risperdal 0.5 mg q.h.s., Serevent inhaler 2 puffs q.12h., Synthroid 0.2 mg q.d., Vioxx 12.5 mg q.d., Zaroxolyn 10 mg q.d., and Ambien 5 mg q.h.s. p.r.n. She presents today with increasing fatigue, fever, and a productive cough. She is to begin Levaquin 250 mg q.d. for 10 days.

Drug	Drug Category
Accupril	_____
Actos	_____
aspirin	_____
Catapres-TTS-1	_____
B_{12}	_____
Lasix	_____
Glucotrol XL	_____
Humulin N	_____
K-Dur	_____
Lanoxin	_____

Drug	Drug Category
lorazepam	
Metamucil	
Prozac	
Zantac	
Risperdal	
Serevent	
Synthroid	
Vioxx	
Zaroxolyn	
Ambien	
Levaquin	

GET CONNECTED

Multimedia Extension Activities

 www.prenhall.com/turley

Use the above address to access the free, interactive Companion Website created for this textbook. Included in the features of this site are drug updates and additional chapter-specific exercises for further practice.

8

Drug Terminology

CHAPTER CONTENTS

Selected terminology relating to drugs, drug classes, and drug administration

LEARNING OBJECTIVES

After studying this chapter, you should be able to do the following:

1. Define common terms used in pharmacology that apply to drugs, drug classes, and drug administration.
2. Apply this knowledge to your study of the next chapters in this textbook.

Familiarize yourself with these terms so that you will understand their meaning when they are presented later in this textbook.

acetylcholine: The principal neurotransmitter of the parasympathetic nervous system, acetylcholine activates cholinergic receptor sites throughout the body. Its action is blocked by anticholinergic drugs.

addiction: An acquired physical or psychological dependence on a drug characterized by the habitual use of the drug, the tendency to increase the drug dose to experience the same or greater effects, increasing tolerance to the effects, and the appearance of withdrawal symptoms when deprived of the drug. Drugs with addictive potential are legally referred to as *controlled substances* or *schedule drugs*.

adrenergic: A receptor for the sympathetic nervous system that is activated by the neurotransmitter norepinephrine. There are three common types of adrenergic receptors often mentioned in pharmacology: alpha, $beta_1$, and $beta_2$.

ampule: A small, slender, all-glass container with a narrow neck, an ampule contains certain liquid drugs for injection or intravenous use only (see Figure 8–1.) The ampule is broken open by placing an alcohol swab around the neck (narrowest part) and briskly snapping both ends of the ampule. An ampule contains enough drug for one dose. Once an ampule is opened, the drug inside it is not saved or reused because it does not contain any preservative. Ampules often contain drugs used in emergency re-

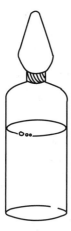

Figure 8–1   An ampule.

suscitation such as epinephrine (Adrenalin) or calcium chloride. The term *ampule* has no proper abbreviation and should always be written in full.

analgesic: A drug that selectively suppresses pain without producing sedation.

analog: A drug obtained by slightly modifying the molecular structure of another drug. Analogs are created for the purpose of changing the original drug's characteristics in order to produce a new, improved drug with fewer side effects or a stronger therapeutic action.

anesthetic, general: A drug that eliminates pain and voluntary muscle control by inducing unconsciousness.

anesthetic, local: A drug that eliminates pain perception in a limited area because of its local action on sensory nerves.

antibiotic: A drug used to treat infection by killing (bactericidal) or inhibiting the growth (bacteriostatic) of disease-causing (pathogenic) bacteria.

anticholinergic: A drug that opposes the action of acetylcholine (a neurotransmitter for the parasympathetic nervous system) at the site of cholinergic receptors. Anticholinergic drugs exert a predictable set of side effects known as *anticholinergic side effects*. The ABCs of anticholinergic side effects: A—anticholinergic; B—blurred vision, bladder retention; C—constipation; D—dry mouth.

antidepressant: A psychotherapeutic drug that produces mood elevation.

antiemetic: A drug that prevents or relieves vomiting. (*Emesis* means *vomiting*.)

antifungal: A drug used to treat fungal infections.

antihistamine: A drug used to decrease the symptoms of inflammation caused by histamine released during an allergic reaction.

antihypertensive: A drug that lowers high blood pressure (hypertension).

anti-inflammatory: A drug used to decrease symptoms of inflammation by inhibiting the release of prostaglandins.

antineoplastic: A drug that is selectively toxic to rapidly dividing cells such as malignant cells and is used to treat cancer. (*Neoplasm* means *tumor*.)

antipruritic: A drug that prevents or relieves itching. (*Pruritus* means *itching*.)

antiseptic: A drug that inhibits the growth of bacteria, but does not destroy them. Antiseptics are used topically, not internally.

antispasmodic: A drug used to stop the spasm of voluntary or involuntary muscles.

antitussive: A drug that suppresses coughing. (*Tussis* is Latin for *cough*.)

antiviral: A drug used to treat viral infections.

bactericidal: An adjective used to describe a drug that kills bacteria. Most antibiotics are bactericidal.

bacteriostatic: An adjective used to describe a drug that inhibits the growth of bacteria but does not kill them. Some antibiotics are bacteriostatic.

bioavailability: That portion of the total drug dose, after absorption, that is actually available to interact with receptors and produce a therapeutic effect. Bioavailability is determined by a number of factors influencing absorption, including drug composition (inert fillers and buffers), particle size, and stomach pH.

bore: See *needle*.

bronchodilator: A drug that relaxes the smooth muscle around the bronchi and dilates them to increase air flow into the lungs.

butterfly needle: See *needle*.

CD: An abbreviation for *controlled dose*. The drug contains beads both for immediate release and extended release.

cholinergic: A receptor for the parasympathetic nervous system that is activated by the neurotransmitter acetylcholine.

corticosteroid: A drug that decreases severe inflammation or itching by suppressing the response of the immune system.

CR: An abbreviation for *controlled release*. A part of the name of sustained release, long-acting drugs (e.g., Norpace CR).

decongestant: A drug that decreases congestion of the mucous membranes in the sinuses and nose.

dextrorotary: A term used to describe the position of a drug molecule when light passed through it is bent to the right. (*Dextro-* is Latin for *right*.) The generic name of some drugs indicates that they are dextrorotary: dextromethorphan, dextroamphetamine. Also see *isomer*.

diluent: An agent such as sterile normal saline or sterile water that is used to reconstitute the powdered form of a drug to prepare it for injection (e.g., bacteriostatic diluent that has a preservative to retard bacterial growth). The word *diluent* is frequently misspelled and mispronounced as *dilutent* because of its association with *dilute*.

disinfectant: An agent (not a drug) that is used to kill microorganisms on surfaces and instruments.

diuretic: A drug used to treat edema and hypertension by causing the kidneys to excrete more sodium and water.

drug of choice: A drug that has been shown to be of particular clinical value in treating a specific disease state. It is preferred above all other similar drugs because of its superior therapeutic effect. The drug of choice can change when a new drug is introduced and is found to be superior to the older drug.

drug tolerance: A decreased susceptibility to the effects of a drug because of continued use. See also *addiction*.

DS: An abbreviation for *double strength*. A part of the name of some drugs that contain a double dosage in one tablet or capsule (e.g., Bactrim DS).

Duracap: A term used to designate a time-release capsule (e.g., Theobid Duracaps).

ER: An abbreviation for *extended release*.

expectorant: A drug that thins mucus in the respiratory tract to make it easier to cough it up.

Extencaps/Extentabs: A term used to designate a time-release capsule or tablet (e.g., Donnatal Extentabs).

gauge: See *needle*.

Gyrocap: A term used to designate a slow-release capsule (e.g., Slo-Phyllin Gyrocaps).

half-life: The time required for drug levels in the serum to decrease from 100% to 50%. The half-life of a drug can be significantly prolonged when liver or kidney disease decreases metabolism and excretion of a drug. The shorter a drug's half-life, the more frequently it must be administered to sustain therapeutic levels. Drugs with a short half-life may be manufactured in a slow-release form to provide sustained drug levels with less frequent doses. Digoxin (Lanoxin) has a half-life of approximately 30 hours. Elderly patients with decreased liver and kidney function often develop toxicity from this drug.

hypodermic: A nonspecific term for any injection administered under the skin, or for the syringe used to give the injection.

Infatab: A term used to designate a chewable tablet that contains a pediatric-size dosage of a drug (e.g., Dilantin Infatab).

insulin syringe: A special syringe designed to measure only insulin. It is calibrated in units, not in milliliters as are all other syringes.

isomer: A drug that has the same chemical formula and the identical types and numbers of atoms in its molecule as another drug, but has those atoms arranged in a different way— either with different chemical bonds or in a different structural relationship to each other. Dextrorotary and levorotary drugs are isomers with identical chemical structures. Their major difference lies in their ability to reflect light in opposite directions because their chemical structures are mirror images of each other. This has significance because, in one case (that of the dextro and levo isomers of amphetamine), the dextro isomer is several times more potent than the levo isomer as a central nervous system stimulant. (M. C. Gerald, *Pharmacology: An Introduction to Drugs*, 2nd ed. [Englewood Cliffs, NJ: Prentice Hall, 1981], p. 302, out of print).

Kapseals: A term used to designate a banded capsule (Dilantin Kapseals).

Liqui-Gels or **Liquigels:** A term used to designate a capsule with a liquid drug inside (e.g., Alka-Seltzer Plus Allergy Liqui-Gels).

LA: An abbreviation for *long acting*. A part of the trade name of sustained-release, long-acting drugs (e.g., Entex LA).

levorotary: A term used to describe the position of a drug molecule when light passed through it is bent to the left. The word *levo* means *left* (*laevus* is Latin for *left*). The generic name of some drugs indicates that they are levorotary: levodopa. *Levorotary* can be abbreviated as *L* as in L-dopa and L-asparaginase. See also *isomer*.

loading dose: If the therapeutic effect of a drug is desired immediately to treat a medical disease, a large dose of the drug may be administered at once. This is known as a *loading dose*. The loading dose is generally twice the maintenance dose. Digoxin (Lanoxin) is often given in a loading dose to patients in acute congestive heart failure. The loading dose is given only once; the maintenance dose is then used for subsequent treatment. See *maintenance dose*.

maintenance dose: The maintenance dose is the standard dose prescribed by the physician for any drug. The maintenance dose is generally one-half the loading dose. See *loading dose*.

mydriatic: A drug that dilates the pupil of the eye.

needle: Needles are classified according to gauge and length. The **gauge** is the inside diameter of the needle. The lower the gauge number, the larger the inside diameter will be. For example, a 15-gauge needle is used for blood donation to allow the blood to flow freely through the needle and to decrease turbulence and damage to the red blood

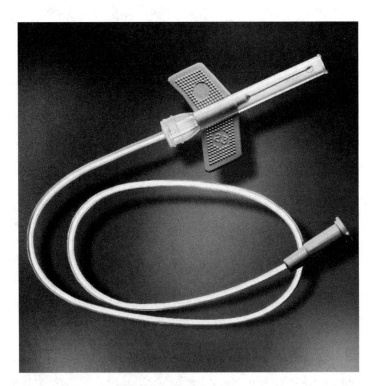

Figure 8–2   A butterfly needle, 23 gauge, with extension tubing. *Photo reprinted courtesy of BD (Becton, Dickinson, and Company).*

cells. An 18- to 22-gauge needle is used for intramuscular injections in adults. A 27-gauge needle is used for an intravenous line in a premature infant. The inside diameter of a needle is also known as the **bore**. The term *bore* is synonymous with *gauge*, but the bore is designated only as either small or large. A **butterfly needle** is a specially designed needle of short length and high gauge with color-coded tabs of plastic on each side of the needle. These tabs facilitate control of the needle during insertion. This needle gets its name because the tabs on either side of the needle make it appear like the wings of a butterfly. Butterfly needles are most often used to start intravenous lines on premature infants or on elderly patients with poor veins.

pathogen: An agent (bacteria, virus, etc.) that causes disease.

peak level: The highest serum level achieved following a single dose of a drug, as determined by a blood test. If the peak level is too high, the patient can develop toxicity. If the peak level is too low, there will not be a therapeutic effect.

placebo: The term *placebo* means *I will please* in Latin. A placebo, of itself, has no pharmacologic action. It exerts no therapeutic effect, and produces no side effects. Placebos are used in **double-blind clinical trials** in which neither the researcher nor the patient knows whether the medication given was the drug being tested or was a placebo. Placebos are commonly sugar pills or injections of sterile normal saline solution. Interestingly, while it is physiologically impossible for a placebo to exert any pharmacologic effect, patients often report a decrease in certain types of symptoms and can even experience "side effects" when given a placebo. These effects are quite real and demonstrate that, in some situations, the power of suggestion can produce changes within the body that closely mimic the pharmacologic action of an actual drug.

prophylaxis: This term is from a Greek word meaning *to keep guard before*. A drug given prophylactically is administered before the onset of a disease or other condition to prevent its occurrence (e.g., birth control pills, flu shots, and vaccines; penicillin G is given prophylactically to patients with a history of rheumatic heart disease prior to undergoing surgery or a tooth extraction).

prototype: The original type or kind of a drug from which all other drugs in that same category were developed. For example, chlorpromazine (Thorazine) is the prototype of all phenothiazine derivatives used to treat psychosis. The prototype drug does not always remain the drug of choice for treatment. It may be replaced by newer drugs.

racemic: This term describes a drug that is composed of equal amounts of dextrorotary and levorotary isomers. (Sample dictation: The patient was treated with racemic epi. Note: "Epi" is a slang term for *epinephrine*.)

Repetabs: A term used to designate a sustained-release tablet (e.g., Trinalin Repetabs).

SA: An abbreviation for *sustained action*. A part of the name of sustained-release, long-acting drugs (e.g., Choledyl SA).

Sequels: A term used to designate a slow-release capsule (e.g., Ferro-Sequels).

SolTab: Trade name for a tablet that disintegrates into a solution in the mouth within 30 seconds (e.g., Remeron SolTab).

Spansules: A term used to designate a slow-release capsule (e.g., Compazine Spansules).

Sprinkle: A term used to designate a long-acting capsule that can be swallowed or opened up; the granules of the drug can be sprinkled on soft food and eaten (e.g., Humibid DM Sprinkle).

SR: An abbreviation for *slow release* or *sustained release*. A part of the trade name of sustained release, long-acting drugs (e.g., Pronestyl-SR).

TB syringe: See *tuberculin syringe*.

Tembids: A term used to designate a sustained-release tablet (e.g., Isordil Tembids).

therapeutic index: The therapeutic index is calculated during animal testing of any new drug. It reflects the relative margin of safety between the dose needed to produce a therapeutic effect and the dose that produces toxic effects. The higher the therapeutic index number is, the more desirable because it indicates that the drug has a wide margin of safety. For example, penicillin has a therapeutic index of greater than 100. The therapeutic index of digoxin (Lanoxin) is less than 2, and it is not uncommon for patients given a therapeutic dose to exhibit symptoms of toxicity.

Titradose: A term used to designate a scored tablet that can be divided into smaller doses, allowing the physician to **titrate** the dose (e.g., Isordil Titradose).

titrate: To determine the smallest dosage that will produce the desired therapeutic effect for a particular individual.

trough level: The lowest serum level of a drug that occurs just before the next dose is to be given, as deteremined by a blood test. If the trough level is too low, this indicates that the drug is at a subtherapeutic level and the dosage needs to be increased.

tuberculin syringe or **TB syringe:**   A small syringe often manufactured with an attached 25-gauge needle. The tuberculin syringe only holds a total of 1 mL. It is used to administer the Mantoux test for tuberculosis, hence its name. It is also used for pediatric injections and for allergy injections.

vasodilator: A drug that relaxes the smooth muscle of blood vessels to improve blood flow.

vasopressor: A drug that constricts the smooth muscle of blood vessels to increase the blood pressure.

vial: A small glass bottle containing a liquid or powder for injection. It has a rubber stopper in the cap that allows diluent to be injected to reconstitute a powdered drug.

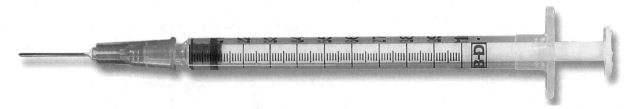

Figure 8–3   A tuberculin or TB syringe is calibrated in hundredths of a milliliter (mL) and holds a total of 1 mL. *Photo reprinted courtesy of BD (Becton, Dickinson, and Company).*

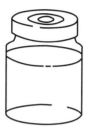

Figure 8–4 A vial.

The rubber stopper also allows repeated doses of the drug to be withdrawn from the same vial.

XR: An abbreviation for *extended release*.

GET CONNECTED

Multimedia Extension Activities

 www.prenhall.com/turley

Use the above address to access the free, interactive Companion Website created for this textbook. Included in the features of this site are drug updates and additional chapter-specific exercises for further practice.

9

Systems of Measurement

CHAPTER CONTENTS

Apothecary system of drug measurement
Metric system of drug measurement
Other drug measurement systems
Number forms and symbols
Dosage schedules
Dosage calculations
Review questions
Spelling tips

LEARNING OBJECTIVES

After studying this chapter, you should be able to do the following:

1. Describe the apothecary system of drug measurement.
2. Describe the metric system of drug measurement.
3. Name at least three common metric abbreviations used in drug dosages.
4. Describe these drug measurement systems: units, inches, drops, milliequivalents, percentages, and ratios.
5. Recognize number symbols for drug dosages and translate them correctly.
6. Define Latin abbreviations indicating frequency of dosing.
7. Describe how dosage calculations are made for adults, children, patients on chemotherapy, and burn patients.

In the early history of pharmacology, the measurement of drug doses was crude and imprecise. The powdered, dried herbs in many prescriptions contained varying amounts of active drug that could not be measured accurately.

APOTHECARY SYSTEM OF DRUG MEASUREMENT

In the 1700s, the apothecary system was brought to the United States from England. The term *apothecary* comes from a Greek word and refers to a person who combines and dispenses drugs. Some apothecary measurements are still in use today. These include the liquid measurements of pint, quart, and gallon. Apothecary measurements for calculating doses of drugs included the minim, grain, scruple, and dram. (The standard of a grain was originally based on the average weight of one grain of wheat.) In past years, the apothecary measurements of minim, scruple, and dram were discontinued, but grain (gr) is still used. Desiccated thyroid is the only drug that is manufactured in equivalent apothecary and metric doses. See Figure 21–1.

METRIC SYSTEM OF DRUG MEASUREMENT

The metric system was invented by the French in 1790. It is based on the length of a meter, which was originally calculated by dividing the earth's circumference by 10 million. The use of the metric system was made legal but not mandatory in the United States in 1866. In 1975, Congress passed the Metric Conversion Act, but with the exception of scientists, doctors, and other professionals in scientific fields, few laypersons use the metric system on a regular basis.

The metric system is officially known as the International System of Units (SI). The abbreviation is derived from the original French name, *Système International d'Unites*. The SI was officially adopted as the exclusive unit of measurement by the American Medical Association on July 1, 1988. The SI metric system is based on the kilogram (for weight measurements), the liter (for volume measurements), and the meter (for length measurements). Metric weight measurements include the kilogram, gram, milligram, and microgram. Each of these differs by a factor of 1000.

1 kilogram (kg)	= 1000 grams (*Kholioi* is Greek for *one thousand*.)
1 gram(g)	= 1000 milligrams (*Mille* is Latin for *one thousand*.)
1 milligram (mg)	= 1000 micrograms (mcg) (*Mikros* is Greek for *small* and stands for *one million*. A microgram is one-millionth of a gram.)

Drug weight measurements are not expressed in terms of kilograms. Kilograms are more appropriately used to describe a person's weight (e.g., a 110-pound woman weighs 50 kilograms). Extremely premature infants may be measured in grams (e.g., a 900-gram premature infant weighs about 2 pounds). Most drugs are measured not in grams but in milligrams (mg) and occasionally in micrograms (mcg).

The metric system also includes the liquid measurements of liter and milliliter. Drugs are not prescribed by the liter; however, the milliliter (mL) is used frequently.

1 liter = 1000 milliliters

For example, a common dose for the antacid Maalox is 30 mL. The Mantoux intradermal test for tuberculosis involves the injection of 0.1 mL of solution.

The basic measurement of length in the metric system is the meter, as noted earlier. The centimeter is equivalent to 1/100 of a meter. When a cube is formed that is 1 cm long on each side, it becomes a measurement of volume known as the *cubic centimeter* (cm³ or cc). This volume measurement is equivalent to the volume contained in a milliliter, and the two volume abbreviations *mL* and *cc* are used interchangeably.

OTHER DRUG MEASUREMENT SYSTEMS

Other types of drug measurement systems include units, inches, drops, milliequivalents, percentages, ratios, and household measurements.

1. Unit. The dosages of certain drugs are measured by a special designation called a *unit*. Some penicillins, some vitamins, and all types of insulin are measured in units. The exact value of a unit varies from drug to drug. A unit of penicillin was standardized in 1944 as 0.6 mcg of penicillin G based on its ability to cause a ring of growth inhibition of a certain size around a bacterial colony. A unit of insulin is defined on the weight basis of pure insulin, with 28 units equaling 1 mg. Insulin is manufactured in solutions with 100 units per milliliter, abbreviated as U-100.

2. Inch. Only one commonly prescribed drug is measured in inches, and that is nitroglycerin ointment (Nitro-Bid, Nitrol), a cardiac drug used to treat angina pectoris. Individual calibrated papers are supplied with each tube of ointment so that the patient can accurately measure each dose. The ointment is squeezed onto the paper along the measuring line which is marked off in ½-inch increments. The prescribed dose may range from ½ inch to 4 inches or more.

3. Drop. The Latin word for *drop* is *gutta*, and the abbreviation for *drop* is *gtt*. Eye and ear liquid medications are prescribed in the number of drops to be given.

4. Milliequivalent (mEq). An equivalent is the molecular weight of an ion divided by the number of hydrogen ions it reacts with. A milliequivalent is 1/1000 of an equivalent. Doses of electrolytes like potassium are measured in milliequivalents, although the doses can also be given in milligrams.

5. Percentage. A percentage is one part in relationship to the whole, based on a total of 100. Thus a 10% solution would be composed of 10 mL of drug in a total of 100 mL of solution. A 2.5% preparation of the steroid ointment triamcinolone (Aristocort, Kenalog) would contain 25 mg of drug in 1,000 mg of white petrolatum base.

6. Ratio. A ratio expresses the relationship between the concentrations of two substances together in solution. A ratio is expressed as two numbers with a colon mark between them. For example, epinephrine for intracardiac injection during resuscitation is supplied in a ratio of 1:10,000 (or one part epinephrine to 10,000 parts of solution). Epinephrine with a local anesthetic for subcutaneous injection is supplied in a ratio of 1:100,000.

7. Household measurement. The household system of measurement is an unofficial system that patients use in their homes for measuring drugs. It includes everyday teaspoons and tablespoons. This is an inaccurate measurement system because there is no standard size for teaspoons and tablespoons. In fact, a teaspoon can hold anywhere from 4 to 7 mL of liquid. Many OTC medicines (e.g., cough syrup) have instructions on the label to measure the dose in teaspoons, but the package includes either a standardized plastic medicine cup or medicine spoon with teaspoon markings.

NUMBER FORMS AND SYMBOLS

Measurements in the metric system are never expressed in fractions. Metric numbers less than 1 are written as decimals and always have a zero added to the left of the decimal point (e.g., 0.5 mg, not .5 mg). The decimal point must be placed carefully, as an error in placement can mean a 10-fold increase or decrease in the drug dose.

Roman numerals were often used with the old apothecary measurements. Today, Roman numerals can be used in handwritten prescriptions, at the discretion of the physician writing the prescription. The Roman numeral is not written in standard form as I, II, III, or IV, but is handwritten as shown in Figure 9–1.

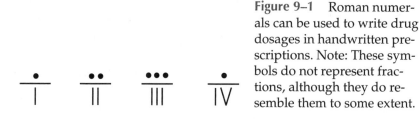

Figure 9–1   Roman numerals can be used to write drug dosages in handwritten prescriptions. Note: These symbols do not represent fractions, although they do resemble them to some extent.

Some numbers written after a drug name are an integral part of the drug's name and do not indicate the amount of the drug to be taken.

> Catapres-TTS-1 (a transdermal patch that releases 0.1 mg/24 hours, used to treat hypertension)
> Tylenol with Codeine No. 3 (a combination drug containing 300 mg of Tylenol and 30 mg of codeine)

DOSAGE SCHEDULES

Drugs are measured not only in terms of the amount of the dosage but also in terms of the frequency of the dosage. There are a number of commonly used abbreviations that indicate the frequency of administration. These abbreviations are based on Latin words (see Table 9–1).

DOSAGE CALCULATIONS

The standard adult dosage for a drug is appropriate for most adults and is calculated to encompass a range that includes the weight of most adult patients. However, patients who are elderly, extremely thin, or extremely obese and fall outside this range may need to have their drug dosage adjusted.

Table 9–1   Latin Abbreviations That Indicate Frequency of Administration

Abbreviation	Latin Translation	Medical Meaning
a.c.	*ante cibum*	before meals
ad lib.	*ad libitum*	as needed
b.i.d.	*bis in die*	twice a day
c̄	*cum*	with
h.s.	*hora somni*	at bedtime (hour of sleep)
n.p.o., NPO	*nil per os*	nothing by mouth
p.c.	*post cibum*	after meals
p.r.n.	*pro re nata*	as needed
q.d.	*quaque die*	every day
q.h.	*quaque hora*	every hour
q.h.s.	*quaque hora somni*	at bedtime (hour of sleep)
q.i.d.	*quater in die*	four times a day
q.o.d.	(informal usage)	every other day
s̄	*sine*	without
t.i.d.	*ter in die*	three times a day

Pediatric dosages, especially those for infants and premature babies, must be calculated with great accuracy. Dosages calculated on the basis of age alone cannot be individually tailored to each child. Therefore, a pediatric drug dose is often calculated based on the total body weight of the patient, not the age. Because the weight of a child increases regularly, the dosage needs to be adjusted periodically when the child is on long-term medication. Pediatric drug dosages are expressed as **mg/kg/day** (milligrams of drug needed per kilograms of body weight per 24-hour period).

Chemotherapy drug dosages are calculated based on the patient's total body surface area. This method customizes the dosage for each patient to maximize the effectiveness of the drug while minimizing its severe side effects. Chemotherapy drug dosages are expressed as **mg/m²** (milligrams per meter squared).

REVIEW QUESTIONS

1. Name the two metric measurements used for drug dosages.
2. A milliliter is equivalent in volume to a cubic centimeter. True or False?
3. Give the definition of these common abbreviations.
   a.c.
   b.i.d.
   g
   h.s.
   mcg
   mg

mL
mEq
p.r.n.
q.i.d.
t.i.d.

4. Name three drugs measured in units.

5. Is there a standard measurement for a unit? Explain your answer.

6. Name one drug measured in inches. Why do you think dermatology drugs that are also available in an ointment form are not measured in inches?

7. Pediatric drug dosages are individually calculated on the basis of what criterion?

8. Chemotherapy drug dosages are individually calculated on the basis of what criterion?

SPELLING TIPS

milliequivalent   often mispronounced as "millequivalent." The abbreviation *mEq* is unusual for its internal capitalization.

GET CONNECTED

Multimedia Extension Activities

 www.prenhall.com/turley

Use the above address to access the free, interactive Companion Website created for this textbook. Included in the features of this site are drug updates and additional chapter-specific exercises for further practice.

10

The Prescription

CHAPTER CONTENTS

Prescriptions and medication orders
Verbal orders, standing orders, and automatic stop orders
Component parts of a prescription and medication order
Review questions
Spelling tips

LEARNING OBJECTIVES

After studying this chapter, you should be able to do the following:

1. Describe the difference between and similarities of the prescription and medication order.
2. List four ways to prevent theft of prescription pads from a medical office.
3. Describe how verbal medication orders are taken in a hospital setting.
4. Name and describe the 12 component parts of a prescription or medication order.

PRESCRIPTIONS AND MEDICATION ORDERS

The term *prescription* comes from the Latin word *praescriptio*, meaning *a written order*. By law, all drugs are classified as either prescription or nonprescription. Prescription drugs can only be ordered by a physician, dentist, or other appropriately licensed healthcare provider. OTC (nonprescription) drugs do not need a prescription and can be purchased by any adult.

A **prescription** is the written record of a physician's order to the pharmacist to dispense medication to a patient. The prescription is written on a single preprinted sheet from a prescription pad, or it may be typed into the office's computer and a printed copy given to the patient.

DID YOU KNOW?   It is not an uncommon occurrence for people to steal prescription pads and write prescriptions for drugs of abuse. To prevent theft of prescription pads, medical office staff should take these precautions.

1. Store extra prescription pads in a locked drawer or closet.
2. Have the physician carry just one prescription pad on his or her person from examining room to examining room.
3. Never leave a prescription pad on the counter or in an unlocked drawer in an examining room.
4. The physician should sign the prescription form only at the time he or she writes the prescription. The physician should never pre-sign blank prescription forms.

All prescriptions written in the medical office should also be recorded in a medications list in the patient's medical record for future reference.

A **medication order** is the written record of a physician's order to the pharmacist to dispense medication to a patient who is in a hospital or other healthcare facility. The medication order is written on a chart-sized preprinted form known as the **physician's order record** or **medication order sheet,** which is located in the patient's medical record.

All prescriptions and medication orders must be written in ink. Whether written on a prescription pad or on a facility's medication order sheet or printed out on a computer-generated sheet, the prescription is considered a legal document.

DID YOU KNOW?   About 2.5 billion prescriptions were filled in the United States in 1998, and there were 3.75 billion drugs ordered and administered to patients in the hospital.

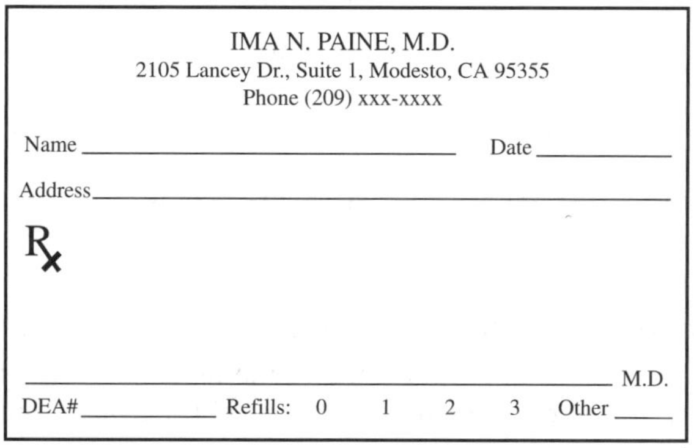

IMA N. PAINE, M.D.
2105 Lancey Dr., Suite 1, Modesto, CA 95355
Phone (209) xxx-xxxx

Name _____   Date _____

Address_____

R℞x

_____ M.D.

DEA#_____   Refills: 0   1   2   3   Other _____

Figure 10–1   An example of a prescription form used in a medical office.

OTHER TYPES OF DRUG ORDERS

Verbal Orders

In cases in which the physician cannot see the patient in the medical office (e.g., on weekends), the physician may verbally give a prescription over the telephone to a pharmacist. When the prescription is for a drug that is not a controlled substance, the pharmacist can fill the prescription without a written prescription and without the physician's signature.

When a patient has been admitted to the hospital, a physician who is already on the medical staff and is responsible for the patient's care may give a verbal medication order over the telephone to a licensed nurse who then writes the order on the medication order sheet and marks it as a **verbal order (V.O.)** The physician must then come to the facility to personally sign the order within a specified amount of time. Verbal orders are also known as **telephone orders**.

Standing Orders

These are a group of specific orders that are usually preprinted on the facility's medication order sheet. They often pertain to a protocol of treatment related to a specific disease or surgical procedure and contain certain common orders that pertain to any patient who has that disease or surgical procedure. For example, all patients admitted for bowel surgery would have standing orders for an enema, a clear liquid diet, an antibiotic to kill bacteria in the bowel, and no food (NPO) after midnight before the surgery.

In addition to the standing orders, the physician would also write individualized medication orders based on the patient's current medical needs and ongoing disease processes (diabetes, hypertension, etc.).

Automatic Stop Orders

This type of medication order originates not with the physician but with the hospital pharmacy. Medication orders for certain types of drugs (e.g., controlled substances) are only valid for a certain number of days. (The exact number of days is determined by the hospital's Pharmacy Committee.) When the medication order expires, the physician must write an entirely new medication order so that the patient can continue to receive that drug.

All medication orders carry an automatic stop order that is activated whenever a patient goes to surgery, is transferred to another unit within the hospital, or is transferred out to another facility or to home.

COMPONENT PARTS OF A PRESCRIPTION AND MEDICATION ORDER

Prescriptions and medication orders are composed of several distinct parts as described next.

1. **Identifying information about the prescriber.**

   Prescription. The physician's name (and the name of the medical group), office address, and phone number are preprinted at the top of the prescription form to positively identify the prescriber.

   Medication Order. This information is not included on the physician's order record.

> **DID YOU KNOW?**   In a hospital or other healthcare facility, the physician's name and office address are not needed on the order sheet because the physician is already a member of the facility's medical staff. Prior to joining the medical staff, each physician must provide his or her name, office address, home address, phone numbers, social security number, medical license and DEA numbers, educational background, board certification, and other identifying information in a written application that is kept on file in the facility's medical staff services office. No physician is permitted to write orders, including medication orders, unless he or she is already an approved member of that facility's medical staff.

2. **Identifying information about the patient.**

    Prescription. The patient's first and last name and his or her address are handwritten on the prescription form by the physician to positively identify the patient.

    Medication Order: This information is located at the top right-hand or left-hand corner of the order sheet. This information is imprinted by using the patient's hospital card (like a credit card) that was created at the time of the patient's admission.

3. **Date.**

    Prescription. The physician writes the full date (month/day/year) on the prescription form.

    Medication Order. The physician writes the full date next to each medication order or with each group of orders.

4. **Rx.** This symbol stands for the Latin word *recipe*, meaning *take*. Prescriptions were, at one time, actually recipes listing several ingredients to be crushed and mixed by the pharmacist before dispensing.

    Prescription. Most prescription pads come with a large preprinted *Rx* just to the left of the area where the prescription itself will be handwritten.

    Medication Order. The *Rx* symbol is not preprinted on the order sheet because the page is large and it is used to order other types of treatments and services (physical therapy, social services, etc.) besides drugs.

5. **Drug name.**

    Prescription. The physician may write either the drug's generic or trade name on the prescription form. The chemical name of a drug is not used in writing a prescription.

    Medication Order. Same.

6. **Drug strength.**

    Prescription. The first number after the drug name indicates the actual amount of drug in each unit (e.g., capsule or tablet). This part of the prescription may be omitted if the drug is available in only one strength. The physician must prescribe a drug strength that corresponds exactly to the strengths in which the drug is manufactured. For example, if the drug is manufactured in 25-mg and 50-mg dosages, the physician cannot write a prescription for an 80-mg dose. However, if the drug is manufactured as a scored tablet, the physician can write a prescription for exactly one-half of the amount in one tablet, knowing that that dosage can easily be obtained by dividing the scored tablet in two. This cannot be done with other types of drug forms, such as unscored tablets or capsules.

    Medication Order. Same.

7. **Quantity to be dispensed.**

   Prescription. The symbol # is read as *number* and indicates to the pharmacist the total number of capsules, tablets, milliliters, or ounces of drug to dispense to the patient. Sometimes the physician will preface the number sign with the abbreviation for the word *dispense* (e.g., Disp. #30). The total amount dispensed equals the length of the prescribed treatment multiplied by the number of doses to be taken each day.

   Medication Order. The physician does not indicate the total number of capsules, tablets, milliliters, or ounces of drug to dispense, as the medication order continues as long as the patient is in the hospital (with the exception of certain drugs like controlled substances). Only the amount of medication needed for one day is dispensed to each unit's medication room or medication cart by the hospital pharmacy.

8. **Directions for use.**

   Prescription. The abbreviation *Sig.* stands for the Latin word *signetur*, meaning *write on the label*. It indicates that the directions for using the drug will follow. These are the directions the pharmacist is to type on the label of the prescription bottle that is given to the patient. The physician writes these directions using Latin abbreviations; however, when the prescription is filled, the directions for use are translated into English so the patient can understand them. These directions describe the **amount of the dose** (e.g., 1 tablet), **route of administration** (e.g., P.O.), and **frequency of the dose** (e.g., b.i.d.). Note: Sometimes the abbreviation *Sig.* is written as just *S* or may not be written at all on the prescription.

   Medication Order. The abbreviation *Sig.* is often not included. The physician writes the directions using Latin abbreviations. These directions describe the amount of the dose, route of administration, and frequency of the dose.

9. **Signature line.**

   Prescription. At the bottom of a prescription form, there is a preprinted line with *M.D.* at the far right-hand side if the provider is an M.D. The physician must sign his or her name on that line for the prescription to be valid.

   Medication Order. The physician signs his or her name and title directly below the last medication order, not at the bottom of the sheet. This prevents anyone from illegally inserting additional medication orders at a later time above the physician's signature.

10. **Refills.**

    Prescription. The physician indicates how many times the patient is permitted to refill the prescription before he or she must be re-evaluated medically. On some prescription forms, there is a preprinted box that says *refills* followed by the numbers 1, 2, and 3. The physician simply circles the appropriate number to indicate how many refills are indicated. The number of refills may also be written out (e.g., Refills x 2). Refills of schedule drugs are limited by law.

    Medication Order. The physician does not indicate the number of refills because the pharmacy continues to send the medication to the unit as long as the patient is in the hospital.

11. **Generic substitution.**

    Prescriptions. Some states mandate that the pharmacist must fill each prescription with a generic drug. If the physician wants the prescription filled with a trade name drug, he or she must specifically indicate this either by writing the trade name and

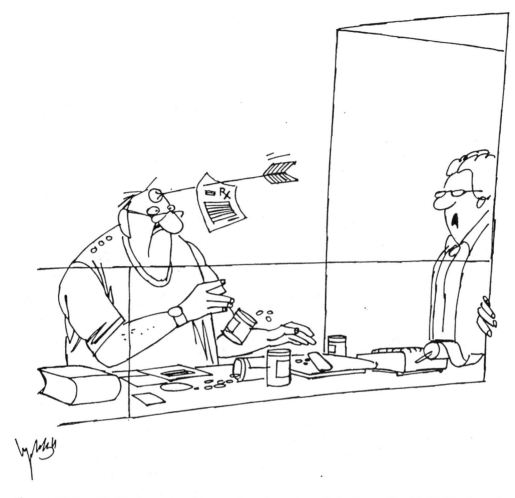

Figure 10–2 *That's from a customer who refuses to wait in line.*—David W. Harbaugh. *Reprinted with permission.*

checking a box stating "Dispense as Written" or by writing the trade name and also writing "No substitutions."

Medication Order. Each hospital has its own formulary that contains all of the drugs that are stocked by the hospital pharmacy. The hospital pharmacist will dispense the generic equivalent of a drug unless the physician specifically requests a particular trade name.

12. **DEA number.** Dispensing of prescription drugs with a potential for abuse or physical/psychological dependence (i.e., schedule drugs or controlled substances) is restricted under The Controlled Substances Act of 1970.

Prescription. For schedule drugs, the physician's assigned DEA number must be included for the prescription to be valid. Many preprinted prescription forms provide a specific line for this information. Prescriptions for drugs that are not controlled substances do not require the physician's DEA number.

Medication Order. The physician does not need to provide his or her DEA number when writing a medication order for a controlled substance. When the physician became a member of the medical staff, his or her DEA certification was verified, and it is re-verified on an ongoing basis.

REVIEW QUESTIONS

1. Define these terms and symbols: *Rx*, *#*, *Sig.*, and *DEA*.
2. How does a prescription differ from a medication order?
3. Describe how verbal orders for medications are handled in a hospital setting.
4. What precautions should be taken to prevent theft of prescription pads from the medical office?
5. What precaution is taken to prevent prescriptions for schedule drugs from being written by an unlicensed individual?
6. What precaution is taken to prevent additional medication orders from being illegally inserted at a later time after the physician signs the medication order sheet?
7. How can a physician indicate that he or she wants the patient to receive a trade name drug?
8. Identify the component parts of the prescriptions in Figures 10–3 and 10–4. Write down any component parts that are missing. Use the Glossary/Index at the end of this textbook to help you verify the spelling of the name of the drug; write down its name and its therapeutic action. Verify that the drug is available in a strength that matches the dosage prescribed. Translate the directions for use into English and write them as they would appear on the prescription bottle given to the patient.

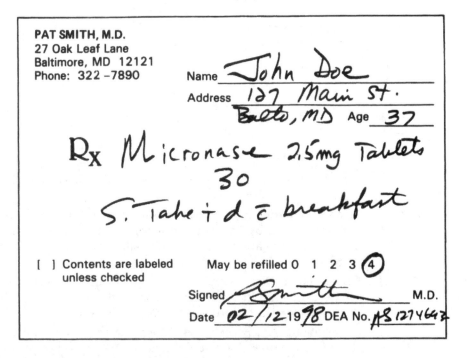

Figure 10–3   A prescription. *Reprinted courtesy of Marvin Stoogenke,* The Pharmacy Technician, *2nd ed. (Upper Saddle River, NJ: Brady/Prentice Hall, 1998), p. 34.*

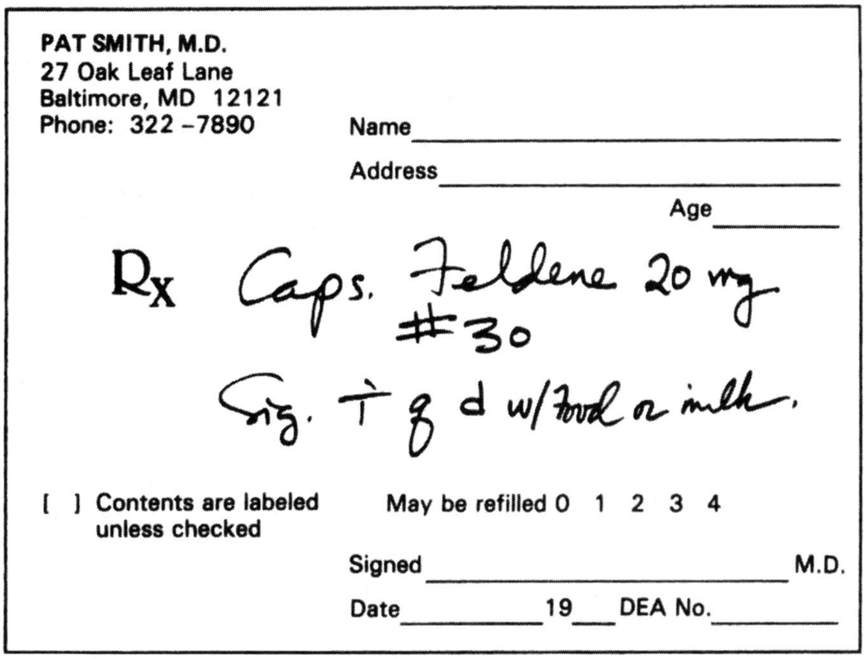

PAT SMITH, M.D.
27 Oak Leaf Lane
Baltimore, MD 12121
Phone: 322 –7890   Name_____

                     Address_____

                                              Age_____

R$_x$ *Caps. Feldene 20 mg*
        #30

        Sig. ī q d w/food or milk.

[ ] Contents are labeled   May be refilled 0   1   2   3   4
    unless checked

                     Signed_____ M.D.

                     Date_____ 19___ DEA No._____

Figure 10–4 A prescription. *Reprinted courtesy of Marvin Stoogenke,* The Pharmacy Technician, *2nd ed. (Upper Saddle River, NJ: Brady/Prentice Hall, 1998), p. 376.*

SPELLING TIPS

prescription   not "perscription," although it is pronounced this way by some people.

GET CONNECTED

Multimedia Extension Activities

www.prenhall.com/turley

Use the above address to access the free, interactive Companion Website created for this textbook. Included in the features of this site are drug updates and additional chapter-specific exercises for further practice.

11

Dermatologic Drugs

CHAPTER CONTENTS

Drugs used to treat acne vulgaris

Drugs used to treat acne rosacea

Drugs used to treat psoriasis

Drugs used to treat bacterial infections of the skin

Drugs used to treat fungal and yeast infections of the skin

Drugs used to treat viral infections of the skin

Drugs used to treat inflammation and itching

Drugs used to treat scabies and pediculosis

Drugs used to treat burns and skin ulcers

Miscellaneous dermatologic drugs

Review questions

Spelling tips

LEARNING OBJECTIVES

After studying this chapter, you should be able to do the following:

1. Name several categories of topical drugs.
2. Describe the therapeutic actions of drugs used to treat acne vulgaris, acne rosacea, psoriasis, itching, scabies, and burns.
3. Describe the therapeutic actions of topical corticosteroids, topical antibiotics, and topical antifungal drugs.
4. Given the generic and trade name of a dermatologic drug, identify what drug category it belongs to or what disease it is used to treat.
5. Given a dermatologic drug category, identify several generic and trade name drugs within that category.
6. Identify the Historical Notes or Did You Know? section in this chapter that you found most interesting.
7. Discuss the controversy surrounding an adverse effect of Accutane.

Because of the superficial nature and location of most dermatologic diseases, they respond well to topical drug therapy. Mild cases of skin diseases such as acne; psoriasis; poison ivy; contact dermatitis; superficial bacterial, fungal, yeast, and viral infections; parasitic infections; diaper rash; and so forth, can be successfully treated with topical drugs. However, drugs that act systemically may be necessary when dermatologic diseases become widespread or particularly severe. For example, a variety of OTC topical drugs are effective in providing relief from mild, localized cases of poison ivy. However, a widespread case of poison ivy with large areas of open, weeping lesions is difficult to treat with topical medication. A drug that acts systemically, such as an oral corticosteroid or antihistamine, may be prescribed to relieve the inflammation and severe itching.

This chapter describes common OTC and prescription drugs used topically and systemically to treat dermatologic diseases. Topical dermatologic drugs are available as creams, lotions, liquids, ointments, gels, and shampoos. Dermatologic drugs that act systemically are available as capsules, tablets, and liquids and are given orally or by injection.

DRUGS USED TO TREAT ACNE VULGARIS

Acne vulgaris is the form of acne that is commonly seen during adolescence. Drugs used to treat acne vulgaris include creams, lotions, liquids, and gels. These drugs are applied topically to cleanse away oil and dead skin (keratolytic action), close the pores (astringent action), inhibit the growth of skin bacteria (antiseptic action), and kill skin bacteria (antibiotic action). Ointments are not usually used to treat acne because their high oil content tends to clog the pores of the skin.

Topical OTC Drugs for Acne Vulgaris

These drugs have either a keratolytic action or an antibiotic action. The number in the trade name refers to the strength of the drug expressed as a percentage.

> benzoyl peroxide (Benzac 5, Benzac 10, Benzac AC 2½, Benzac AC 5, Benzac AC 10, Benzac AC Wash 2½, Benzac AC Wash 5, Benzac AC Wash 10, Benzac W 5, Benzac W 10, Benzac W Wash 5, Benzac W Wash 10, Clearasil Maximum Strength, Desquam-E, Desquam-E 5, Desquam-E 10, Desquam-X 5, Desquam-X 5 Wash, Desquam-X 10, Desquam-X 10 Wash, Fostex 10% BPO, Fostex 10% Wash, Neutrogena Acne Mask, Oxy 10 Maximum Strength Advanced Formula, Oxy 10 Wash, Triaz)
>
> salicylic acid (Clearasil Medicated Deep Cleanser, Pernox Lathering Abradant Scrub, PROPApH Foaming Face Wash, PROPApH Peel-off Acne Mask)
>
> triclosan (Stri-Dex Anti-Bacterial Foaming Wash)

DID YOU KNOW?   Salicylic acid is also used for its keratolytic action to remove corns and calluses on the feet.

Topical Vitamin A-Type Drugs for Acne Vulgaris

Vitamin A-type drugs cause epithelial cells to multiply more rapidly. This rapid turnover prevents pores from becoming clogged.

adapalene (Differin)
tazarotene (Tazorac)
tretinoin (Avita, Retin-A, Retin-A Micro)

DID YOU KNOW?   Tretinoin, under the trade name Renova, is also used topically to decrease fine wrinkle lines on the face, particularly around the eyes, and areas of hyperpigmentation.

Topical Antibiotics for Acne Vulgaris

azelaic (Azelex, Finevin)
chlortetracycline (Aureomycin)
clindamycin (Cleocin T, C/T/S)
erythromycin (A/T/S, Emgel, Eryderm, Erygel, Staticin, T-Stat)
meclocycline (Meclan)
tetracycline (Achromycin)

Topical Combination Drugs for Acne Vulgaris

These drugs combine antibiotics (benzoyl peroxide, clindamycin, erythromycin) or a keratolytic drug (sulfur).

BenzaClin (benzoyl peroxide, clindamycin)
Benzamycin (benzoyl peroxide, erythromycin)
Sulfoxyl Regular, Sulfoxyl Strong (benzoyl peroxide, sulfur)

Oral Antibiotics for Acne Vulgaris

These tetracycline-group oral antibiotics are used for systemic treatment of more severe cases of acne vulgaris to kill bacteria in the deeper layers of the skin.

minocycline (Dynacin, Minocin, Vectrin)
tetracycline (Panmycin, Sumycin, Tetracyn, Tetralan)

Oral Vitamin A-Type Drugs for Severe Cystic Acne Vulgaris

Severe cystic acne unresponsive to antibiotic treatment may be treated topically with a form of vitamin A. These drugs cause epithelial cells to multiply more rapidly. This rapid turnover prevents pores from becoming clogged and infected and decreases cyst formation.

isotretinoin (Accutane)

FOCUS ON HEALTHCARE ISSUES: Isotretinoin (Accutane) is believed to cause the unusual adverse effect of suicide attempts.

On that snowy January day last year, Brandon Troppman seemed to be loving life. He put on a new shirt and combed his hair just so before heading to the mall to hang out with his high school sweetheart. . . . At 6:30 that evening, he talked on the phone with his best friend, laughing and making his friend laugh, as always. An hour later, Brandon hanged himself from a rod in his bedroom closet. . . . [He] hadn't appeared depressed, never abused drugs or alcohol, never talked of suicide. In the months after his death, his parents reached a conclusion that now seems inescapable to them: The popular acne drug Accutane, they believe, led to their son's suicide.

The FDA has received reports of at least 66 suicides, 55 suicide attempts, and more than 1,300 cases of psychiatric problems among . . . the half million people a year [who] use the drug.

[Congressman Bart Stupak from Michigan] publicly blamed the drug for his 17-year-old son's suicide. [During his own investigation], he found an internal 1988 FDA memo that stated: "Given all the pieces of evidence available, it is difficult to avoid the conclusion that Accutane use . . . is associated with severe psychiatric disease in some patients."

Gary Gately, "A Drug's Dark Side," *The Sun*, March 4, 2001. (Baltimore, MD) p. N1.

DID YOU KNOW?   A deficiency of vitamin A can cause abnormal changes in the epithelial cells of the skin. Isotretinoin is structurally similar to a metabolite of vitamin A. Tretinoin is a form of vitamin A. Isotretinoin and tretinoin are used to treat acne vulgaris. Acitretin is a metabolite of a form of vitamin A; acitretin (Soriatane) is used to treat psoriasis.

DID YOU KNOW?   Oral contraceptives (birth control pills) have been found to be effective in treating acne vulgaris. Drug manufacturers are now advertising this desirable effect along with these drugs' main therapeutic effect of birth control.

DRUGS USED TO TREAT ACNE ROSACEA

Acne rosacea is an adult form of acne characterized by pustules with erythema and small, dilated blood vessels of the face. It involves excess secretion of sebum and is exacerbated by heat, stress, and skin irritation. It is treated with a topical drug that has antibacterial and anti-inflammatory properties.

metronidazole (MetroGel, MetroLotion)

DID YOU KNOW?   Metronidazole also has antiprotozoal and antibacterial actions. Metronidazole (Flagyl, Protostat) is taken orally to treat intestinal amebiasis, dysentery, and vaginal *Trichomonas*. Metronidazole (MetroGel-Vaginal) is applied topically to treat vaginal infections with *Hemophilus* and *Gardnerella*. Metronidazole (Helidac) is used to treat peptic ulcers caused by *Helicobacter pylori*.

DRUGS USED TO TREAT PSORIASIS

Psoriasis is a chronic skin condition that is characterized by scaly, raised, silvery-red patches on the skin. It is often resistant to treatment. In psoriasis, the skin is abnormal at the cellular level, exhibiting an accelerated rate of epithelial cell division and abnormal keratinocytes.

Topical Coal Tar Derivatives for Psoriasis

Coal tar lotions, gels, shampoos, and bath liquids help to decrease the rate of epidermal cell production, correct abnormalities of the keratinocytes, cleanse away dead skin (keratolytic action) and decrease itching (antipruritic action).

AquaTar
Balnetar
Denorex, Extra Strength Denorex
Estar
Neutrogena T/Derm, Neutrogena T/Gel
Tegrin for Psoriasis, Tegrin Medicated, Tegrin Medicated for Psoriasis
Zetar

HISTORICAL NOTES: Coal tar, a by-product of the processing of bituminous coal, contains over 10,000 different chemical ingredients. It has been used since the 1800s to treat psoriasis.

Topical Vitamin A-Type Drugs for Psoriasis

tazarotene (Tazorac)

Topical Vitamin D-Type Drugs for Psoriasis

The red, scaly patches of psoriasis are caused by abnormal keratinocytes within the skin. Synthetic vitamin D-type drugs are applied topically; they activate vitamin D receptors in the keratinocytes and slow the abnormal cell growth.

calcipotriene (Dovonex)

Topical Corticosteroids for Psoriasis

Topical corticosteroids decrease the inflammation and itching associated with psoriasis. For a discussion of topical corticosteroids, see the section in this chapter entitled "Drugs Used to Treat Inflammation and Itching."

Other Topical Drugs for Psoriasis

Other topical drugs for psoriasis act to decrease the rate at which epithelial cells divide.

anthralin (Anthra-Derm, Drithocreme, Micanol)

Oral Vitamin A-Type Drugs for Psoriasis

Systemic drugs are used to treat severe psoriasis that cannot be controlled by topical drugs. These drugs are given orally, and their exact mechanism of action in treating psoriasis is not known.

acitretin (Soriatane)

Other Oral Drugs for Psoriasis

These drugs are only used to treat severe, disabling psoriasis that has not responded to other types of drug therapy. These drugs decrease the rate at which epithelial cells divide (methotrexate) or suppress the activity of T lymphocytes in the autoimmune response.

alefacept (Amevive)
cyclosporine (Neoral)
efalizumab (Xanelim)
hydroxyurea (Hydrea, Mylocel)
methotrexate (Rheumatrex, Rheumatrex Dose Pack)
sirolimus (Rapamune)

DID YOU KNOW?   Methotrexate is also a well-known chemotherapy drug that inhibits DNA synthesis. This slows down the reproduction of rapidly dividing cells such as cancer cells. Cyclosporine is a well-known immunosuppressant given to patients after organ transplantation to prevent rejection of the donor organ.

Psoralens for Psoriasis

Severe, disabling psoriasis may also be treated by exposure to ultraviolet light in combination with a drug that sensitizes the skin to the effects of ultraviolet light. These drugs are collectively known as *psoralens*. This combined treatment damages cell DNA and decreases the rate of cell division.

methoxsalen (Oxsoralen-Ultra, 8-MOP)

Treatment that combines methoxsalen and ultraviolet light is known as psoralen/ultraviolet wavelength A (PUVA).

DRUGS USED TO TREAT BACTERIAL INFECTIONS OF THE SKIN

Topical Antibiotic Drugs

These drugs are used topically to treat minor, superficial bacterial skin infections. They act to inhibit the growth of or kill bacteria by blocking their ability to maintain a cell wall. Topical antibiotics are manufactured as gels, lotions, creams, ointments, and sprays.

> bacitracin (Baciguent)
> gentamicin (Garamycin)
> mupirocin (Bactroban, Bactroban Nasal)
> neomycin (Myciguent)

HISTORICAL NOTES: Bacitracin is only administered topically because it can produce toxic effects when given systemically. This drug was developed from a strain of bacteria found growing in a culture of wound drainage taken from a patient named Margaret Tracy. The drug name *bacitracin* was formed from the bacteria's name and the patient's name: ***Bacillus* subtilis + *Tracy* + *in*.**

DID YOU KNOW?   Mupirocin (Bactroban, Bactroban Nasal) has a special use in treating outbreaks of methicillin-resistant *Staphylococcus aureus* (MRSA) in healthcare facilities. The ointment is applied inside the nose of healthcare providers to prevent resistant bacteria from being transferred from the provider's nose and hands to the patient.

Topical Antibiotic Combination Drugs

These drugs combine the antibiotics bacitracin, neomycin, and polymyxin B.

> Mycitracin Triple Antibiotic (bacitracin, neomycin, polymyxin B)
> Neosporin, Maximum Strength Neosporin (bacitracin, neomycin, polymyxin B)
> Polysporin (bacitracin, polymyxin B)

These drugs combine two antibiotics with a corticosteroid (hydrocortisone) to treat inflammation.

> Cortisporin (hydrocortisone, neomycin, polymyxin B)

For serious or widespread bacterial skin infections, various systemic antibiotics can be prescribed. For oral antibiotic drugs, see Chapter 27, "Anti-Infective Drugs."

FOCUS ON HEALTHCARE ISSUES: The Soap and Detergent Association reported that approximately 45% of hand and body wash products contain antibacterial compounds. Another study showed that 75% of liquid soaps and 30% of bar soaps contain antibacterial compounds. Small amounts of antibacterial compounds in a wide variety of products, as well as those antibiotics that are routinely added to animal feed, are believed to have contributed to the rise of antibiotic-resistant bacteria.

DRUGS USED TO TREAT FUNGAL INFECTIONS OF THE SKIN

Topical Antifungal Drugs

Fungal infections such as ringworm (tinea corporis), athlete's foot (tinea pedis), jock itch (tinea cruris), and fungal infections of the nails (onychomycosis) can be effectively treated with topical antifungal drugs. These drugs alter the cell wall of the fungus and disrupt enzyme activity, resulting in cell death. These OTC and prescription drugs are manufactured in cream, ointment, lotion, and shampoo forms.

butenafine (Mentax)
ciclopirox (Loprox, Penlac Nail Lacquer)
clioquinol
clotrimazole (Cruex, Desenex, Lotrimin, Lotrimin AF 1%)
econazole (Spectazole)
haloprogin (Halotex)
ketoconazole (Nizoral, Nizoral A-D)
miconazole (Lotrimin AF 2%, Micatin, Monistat-Derm, Prescription Strength Desenex, Ting)
naftifine (Naftin)
oxiconazole (Oxistat)
sulconazole (Exelderm)
terbinafine (Lamisil AT, Lamisil DermGel)
tolnaftate (Absorbine Athlete's Foot Cream, Absorbine Footcare, Aftate for Athlete's Foot, Aftate for Jock Itch, Tinactin, Tinactin for Jock Itch)
triacetin (Fungoid, Fungoid Creme, Fungoid Tincture)

Note: The ending *-azole* is common to generic antifungal drugs.

Topical Antifungal Combination Drugs

This drug combines an antifungal drug with a corticosteroid to decrease inflammation.

Lotrisone (betamethasone, clotrimazole)

Systemic Antifungal Drugs

When topical fungal skin infections are extensive or become severely embedded in the nails, the following antifungal drugs may be given orally to exert a systemic effect.

> griseofulvin (Fulvicin P/G, Fulvicin U/F, Grisactin, Grisactin Ultra, Griseofulvin Ultramicrosize)
> itraconazole (Sporanox)
> ketoconazole (Nizoral)
> terbinafine (Lamisil)

DRUGS USED TO TREAT YEAST INFECTIONS OF THE SKIN

Yeast infections of the skin are usually caused by *Candida albicans*. You will notice that some of the same drugs used to treat fungal infections are also used to treat yeast infections. This is because yeasts are closely related (biologically) to fungi.

Topical Antiyeast Drugs

The following topical OTC and prescription drugs are used to treat yeast infections of the skin.

> amphotericin B (Fungizone)
> clotrimazole (Lotrimin)
> econazole (Spectazole)
> ketoconazole (Nizoral, Nizoral A-D)
> miconazole (Monistat-Derm)
> nystatin (Mycostatin, Nilstat)

Topical Antiyeast Combination Drugs

These drugs combine the antiyeast drugs clotrimazole or nystatin with a corticosteroid (betamethasone, triamcinolone) to decrease inflammation.

> Lotrisone (betamethasone, clotrimazole)
> Mycolog-II (nystatin, triamcinolone)
> Mytrex (nystatin, triamcinolone)

Serious or widespread yeast infections generally involve more body systems than just the skin. For oral antiyeast drugs used systemically to treat these infections, see Chapter 29, "Antifungal Drugs."

DRUGS USED TO TREAT VIRAL INFECTIONS OF THE SKIN

Herpes simplex virus type 2 infections involving the genital area are considered to be a sexually transmitted disease (STD), while type 1 infections involve just the areas of the face and mouth and are known as *cold sores*. Type 1 and type 2 lesions are treated topically or with oral drugs that act systemically. Both the topical and the oral drugs interfere with DNA synthesis and keep the virus from reproducing.

Topical Drugs for Herpes Simplex Type I Infections

> acyclovir (Zovirax)
> docosanol (Abreva)
> penciclovir (Denavir)

For oral antiviral drugs used systemically to treat herpes simplex type I infections, see Chapter 28, "AIDS Drugs and Antiviral Drugs."

Topical Drugs for Herpes Zoster Infections

Herpes zoster virus infections, also known as *shingles*, are due to a reemergence of the same virus that first caused chickenpox in the patient.

The lesions of herpes zoster are particularly painful. The following topical drugs treat the pain associated with these lesions by exerting a local anesthetic effect.

> capsaicin (Capsin, Zostrix, Zostrix-HP)
> lidocaine (Lidoderm Patch)

DID YOU KNOW?   **Capsaicin** is a derivative of the habanero hot pepper plant! This variety of hot peppers is so caustic that it will burn your hand if you touch it without wearing protective gloves. The amount of capsaicin in a hot pepper is measured in Scoville units, which were devised in 1912 by the pharmacist Thomas Scoville. Habanero hot peppers are rated the highest of all peppers—100,000 to 300,000 Scoville units. This means that you can still feel the heat when you taste a solution that only has 1 part habanero pepper in 100,000 to 300,000 parts of a sugar water and alcohol mix.

For oral antiviral drugs used systemically to treat herpes zoster infections, see Chapter 28, "AIDS Drugs and Antiviral Drugs."

Topical Drugs for Common Warts

The human papilloma virus causes both common warts (verrucae) and genital warts (condyloma acuminatum). For a discussion of the drugs used to treat genital warts, a sexually transmitted disease (STD), see Chapter 23, "Obstetric/Gynecologic Drugs."

The following OTC and prescription drugs are applied topically to common warts.

> monochloroacetic acid (Mono-Chlor)
> salicylic acid (Compound W, Dr Scholl's Clear Away Plantar, Dr Scholl's Wart Remover, DuoFilm, DuoPlant, Wart-Off)
> trichloroacetic acid (Tri-Chlor)

DRUGS USED TO TREAT INFLAMMATION AND ITCHING

Topical Corticosteroids

Topical corticosteroids, both OTC and prescription, are indicated to relieve contact dermatitis, poison ivy, and insect bites and to treat psoriasis, seborrhea, and eczema. These drugs come in several strengths and in several forms (ointment, gel, lotion, cream, and aerosol). Some common OTC and prescription generic and trade name topical corticosteroid drugs include:

alclometasone (Aclovate)

amcinonide (Cyclocort)

betamethasone (Alphatrex, Betatrex, Diprolene, Diprolene AF, Diprosone, Luxiq, Maxivate, Psorion, Teladar)

clobetasol (Cormax, Olux, Temovate)

clocortolone (Cloderm)

desonide (DesOwen, Tridesilon)

desoximetasone (Topicort, Topicort LP)

dexamethasone (Decadron, Decaspray)

diflorasone (Florone, Florone E, Maxiflor, Psorcon E)

fluocinolone (Derma-Smoothe/FS, Flurosyn, Synalar, Synalar-HP)

fluocinonide (Lidex, Lidex-E)

flurandrenolide (Cordran, Cordran SP)

fluticasone (Cutivate)

halcinonide (Halog, Halog-E)

halobetasol (Ultravate)

hydrocortisone (Cortaid Intensive Therapy, Cortaid with Aloe, Cort-Dome, Cortizone-5, Cortizone-10, Dermacort, Dermolate, Hycort, Hytone, Lanacort 5, Lanacort 10, Locoid, Maximum Strength Bactine, Maximum Strength Caldecort, Maximum Strength Cortaid, Maximum Strength KeriCort-10, Pandel, Scalpicin, T/Scalp, Westcort)

mometasone (Elocon)

prednicarbate (Dermatop)

triamcinolone (Aristocort, Aristocort A, Flutex, Kenalog, Kenalog-H)

Intradermal Corticosteroids

Some corticosteroids are injected directly into individual skin lesions.

betamethasone (Celestone Soluspan)

dexamethasone (Dalalone D.P., Dalalone L.A., Decadron-LA)

methylprednisolone (Depo-Medrol, Depopred-40)

prednisolone (Predalone 50)

triamcinolone (Aristocort Intralesional, Aristospan Intralesional, Kenalog-10, Tac-3)

Note: The endings *-sone*, *-olone*, and *-onide* are common to generic corticosteroids.

Systemic Corticosteroids

Severe or widespread dermatitis, inflammation, allergic skin conditions, or itching may be treated with oral corticosteroid drugs that exert a systemic effect.

> dexamethasone (Decadron, Hexadrol)
> methylprednisolone (Medrol)
> triamcinolone (Aristocort, Kenacort)

IN DEPTH: *Steroid* is a general term encompassing a number of hormones produced by the body. *Corticosteroids* include those hormones produced by the cortex of the adrenal gland. Within this large group, there are corticosteroids that specifically act to suppress the immune system's response to tissue damage, decreasing tissue inflammation and itching. Hydrocortisone, introduced in 1952, was the first topical corticosteroid. In 1983, hydrocortisone was also the first corticosteroid approved in a nonprescription strength for OTC sales. As a group, both topical and systemic corticosteroids are known as *anti-inflammatory drugs*.

Topical Antihistamines

These drugs inhibit inflammation, redness, and itching due to the release of histamine (hence the name *antihistamine*) during an allergic skin reaction such as contact dermatitis. As a group, these drugs are also known as *antipruritics* (*pruritus* means *itching*).

> diphenhydramine (Benadryl, Benadryl Itch Relief, Benadryl Itch Relief Children's Formula, Benadryl Itch Stopping Maximum Strength, Benadryl Itch Stopping Children's Formula, Benadryl Itch Stopping Original Strength, Dermamycin, Maximum Strength Benadryl 2%, Maximum Strength Benadryl Itch Relief)
> doxepin (Zonalon)

DID YOU KNOW? Doxepin is also a tricyclic antidepressant marketed under the trade name Sinequan.

Topical Combination Antihistamines

These drugs combine the antihistamine/antipruritic drugs diphenhydramine or pyrilamine with the astringents calamine and zinc oxide to decrease oozing and exudates and the topical anesthetic benzocaine.

Caladryl (calamine, diphenhydramine)

Caladryl Clear (diphenhydramine, zinc oxide)

Calamycin (benzocaine, calamine, pyrilamine, zinc oxide)

Ziradryl (diphenhydramine, zinc oxide)

For oral antihistamine drugs used systemically to treat allergic reactions of the skin, see Chapter 19, "Ear, Nose, and Throat (ENT) Drugs."

DID YOU KNOW?   Chronic itching and hives may be treated with an antihistamine in combination with the H_2 blocker cimetidine (Tagamet) that blocks another type of histamine receptor.

Topical Anesthetic Drugs

Topical anesthetics provide brief periods of anesthesia to a limited depth in the skin. These drugs provide temporary symptomatic relief for various skin disorders including minor burns, sunburns, rashes, insect bites, and so forth.

benzocaine (Americaine Anesthetic, Bicozene, Dermoplast, Lanacane, Solarcaine, Solarcaine Medicated First Aid)

butamben (Butesin)

dibucaine (Nupercainal)

lidocaine (Solarcaine Aloe Extra Burn Relief, Unguentine Plus, Xylocaine, Zilactin-L)

pramoxine (Tronothane)

tetracaine (Pontocaine, Viractin)

Topical Combination Anesthetic Drugs

These drugs contain vrious topical anesthetics and the antiseptic benzalkonium.

Bactine Antiseptic Anesthetic (benzalkonium, lidocaine)

Cetacaine (benzocaine, butamben, tetracaine)

EMLA (lidocaine, prilocaine)

Medi-Quik (benzalkonium, lidocaine)

Note: Also see the previous section, "Topical Drugs for Herpes Zoster Infections," for a discussion of anesthetic drugs specifically used to treat the pain of shingles.

Other Topical Drugs for Inflammation and Itching

A and D (contains vitamins A and D to promote healing)

Aveeno (topical oatmeal and lanolin solution used as a lotion or in bath water)

Aveeno Anti-Itch (contains calamine)

Burow's solution (Domeboro) (applied as a wet dressing, acts as an astringent. Not a trade name, this drug is named for the German surgeon Dr. Burow.)

calamine (common ingredient in other topical combination drugs)

Desitin (used to treat diaper rash, contains zinc oxide to dry the skin, lanolin, and cod liver oil with vitamin A to promote healing)

dexpanthenol (Panthoderm)

pimecrolimus (Elidel)

zinc oxide (astringent to dry areas of oozing and to protect the skin, common ingredient in other topical combination drugs)

> **JUST FOR FUN!** What's Your I.Q. (Itch Quotient)? Visit this Web site and take a short quiz on itching: causes and common misconceptions. Sponsored by the Lanacane Itch Information Center, *www.lanacane.com/whatsyrIQ.html.*

DRUGS USED TO TREAT SCABIES AND PEDICULOSIS

Drugs Used to Treat Scabies

This skin condition is caused by tiny parasites called mites that tunnel under the skin and cause itchy lesions. (The scalp is rarely infected.) These topical OTC and prescription drugs are used to treat scabies.

crotamiton (Eurax)

lindane

permethrin (Acticin, Elimite, Nix)

> **DID YOU KNOW?** Scabies in humans is caused by the same parasite that causes mange in dogs!

Drugs Used to Treat Pediculosis

This skin condition is caused by an infestation of lice and their eggs that can be found on both the scalp and body. Lice are easily transmitted from one person to another by means of combs and hats. These topical OTC and prescription drugs are applied to the body as a cream or lotion; a shampoo is used to treat the scalp.

lindane

malathion (Ovide)

permethrin (Acticin, Elimite, Nix)

R & C

RID
Step 2
Tegrin-LT
Tisit, Tisit Blue

DID YOU KNOW?   Nonprescription drugs used to treat lice contain the active ingredient pyrethrin, which is derived from chrysanthemums. The drug acts on the nervous system of the parasite to paralyze it. Pyrethrin is a common ingredient in flea powder for dogs as well!

The term *nitpicking*, meaning *to point out and criticize tiny details*, comes from the process of picking through the hair looking for lice eggs which are called *nits*.

DRUGS USED TO TREAT BURNS AND SKIN ULCERS

Burns and skin ulcers present unique problems in medical management. They may contain a large amount of necrotic (dead) tissue that must be removed (debrided) before new tissue can form (granulation). In addition, the affected area may produce a large amount of exudate (drainage) that must be removed in order to promote healing and prevent infection.

Topical Drugs for Debridement

Topical enzymes dissolve scar tissue and necrotic tissue and allow new tissue to begin to form at the base of the burn or ulcer.

collagenase (Santyl)
papain (Accuzyme, Panafil)
trypsin (Dermuspray, Granulderm, Granulex, GranuMed)

DID YOU KNOW?   Trypsin is an enzyme in the stomach that digests dietary protein.

Topical Drugs to Absorb Exudate

dextranomer (Debrisan)
DuoDerm
IntraSite
Sorbsan

DID YOU KNOW?   Dextranomer (Debrisan) contains tiny polymer beads of dextran that absorb amounts of wound drainage equal to four times their size. Sorbsan contains absorbent calcium fibers.

Topical Drugs to Stimulate Granulation

These drugs stimulate the formation of healthy, new granulation tissue.

becaplermin (Regranex)

DID YOU KNOW?   Becaplermin (Regranex) was created by taking a gene that produces a certain type of growth factor in cells and, through recombinant DNA technology, inserting it into a yeast cell.

Topical Antibiotics for Burns

These drugs are used specifically to treat extensive burns to keep them from becoming infected.

mafenide (Sulfamylon)
nitrofurazone (Furacin)
silver sulfadiazine (Silvadene)

DID YOU KNOW?   The active ingredient in silver sulfadiazine (Silvadene) is actually the chemical element of silver in an ion form.

Other Topical Drugs for Burns and Wounds

These drugs promote healing and neutralize the odor from wounds.

chlorophyll derivative (Chloresium)

MISCELLANEOUS DERMATOLOGIC DRUGS

ACU-dyne: A topical brown iodine-containing anti-infective drug used as a hand wash and preoperative surgical skin prep.

AgNO₃: See *silver nitrate*.

alitretinoin (Panretin):   This topical vitamin A-type drug is used to treat the skin lesions of Kaposi's sarcoma in AIDS patients. It acts by inhibiting the growth of these cancerous cells.

aminolevulinic acid (Levulan Kerastick):   This topical drug is used to treat actinic keratoses. It is used in conjunction with exposure to a special blue light (BLU-U) of a specific wavelength. The blue light causes a chemical reaction with the drug and this destroys the abnormal skin cells.

Betadine: A topical brown iodine-containing anti-infective drug used as a hand wash and preoperative surgical skin prep. In ointment form, it is placed on the skin around the insertion site of an I.V. line or a catheter. The active drug ingredient is iodine.

bexarotene (Targretin):   Topical and oral drug used to treat the cancerous skin lesions of cutaneous T-cell lymphoma.

chlorhexidine (Betasept, Hibiclens, Hibistat):   Topical anti-infective hand wash and preoperative surgical skin scrub.

chloroxine (Capitrol):   This topical antibacterial drug is used as a shampoo to treat seborrheic dermatitis of the scalp.

ciprofloxacin (Cipro, Cipro I.V.):   Antibiotic used to treat cutaneous anthrax from bioterrorism.

diclofenac (Solaraze):   Topical drug used to treat actinic keratoses.

dihydroxyacetone (Chromelin Complexion Blender):   This drug is applied topically to darken the skin in patients with vitiligo (loss of normal skin pigmentation). It must be reapplied each day to affected areas of the skin.

desipramine (Norpramin):   Antidepressant used to treat urticaria.

doxepin (Sinequan, Sinequan Concentrate):   Antidepressant used to treat urticaria.

doxycycline (Doryx, Vibramycin, Vibramycin I.V., Vibra-Tabs):   Antibiotic used to treat cutaneous anthrax from bioterrorism.

dutasteride: Used to treat male pattern baldness.

eflornithine (Vaniqa):   Topical cream used to slow the growth of unwanted facial hair in women.

finasteride (Propecia):   Used to treat male pattern baldness, this drug is given orally. It blocks an enzyme that converts testosterone (male sex hormone) into another male hormone that causes hair follicles to atrophy.

DID YOU KNOW?   Finasteride, under the trade name Proscar, is also used to treat benign prostatic hypertrophy (BPH). The drug blocks the enzyme that converts testosterone (male sex hormone) into another male hormone that causes the cells of the prostate gland to hypertrophy.

fluorouracil (Efudex): This topical drug is used to treat keratoses and superficial basal cell carcinomas by causing cellular necrosis of the lesion.

gentian violet: This topical antibacterial and antifungal drug is a deep purple liquid dye. It is sometimes applied to the umbilical cord stump and around the navel of newborns to prevent a bacterial or fungal infection from developing as the cord dries.

hexachlorophene (pHisoHex): This topical antibacterial skin cleanser generated controversy years ago when it caused seizures in newborns with areas of open skin due to diaper rash. (The hexachlorophene was readily absorbed through the broken skin and reached toxic levels in the blood.)

hydroquinone (Esoterica, Melanex, Porcelana): This topical drug is used to lighten hyperpigmented areas of the skin like freckles and age spots.

interferon gamma-1b (Actimmune): This drug is used to treat the skin infections of chronic granulomatous disease.

methoxsalen (Oxsoralen): This topical drug, in conjunction with exposure to ultraviolet light, is used to treat hypopigmented skin areas in vitiligo.

minoxidil (Rogaine): This topical drug is used to treat male and female pattern baldness. It acts to dilate arteries in the scalp to increase blood flow and stimulate hair growth. It must be applied twice daily for at least four months before an effect is seen. It is not effective in all patients. If it does produce hair growth, the drug must be continued indefinitely to maintain that growth.

DID YOU KNOW?   Minoxidil, under the trade name Loniten, is also given orally to treat hypertension. It acts by dilating the arteries and decreasing the blood pressure.

HISTORICAL NOTES: For thousands of years, men have smeared smelly stuff on their scalps in a vain attempt to beat back baldness. Cleopatra reportedly anointed Caesar with a concoction of bear grease, burned mice, deer marrow, and horse teeth. Other remedies have included pigeon droppings, horseradish, and buffalo dung. Minoxidil (Rogaine) was the first medicine scientifically shown to stimulate hair growth.

Joe Graedon and Teresa Graedon, "People's Pharmacy," *The Sun*, April 15, 1997. (Baltimore, MD) p. 3F.

nortriptyline (Aventyl, Pamelor): Antidepressant used to treat urticaria.

oxychlorosene (Clorpactin WCS-90): A topical antibacterial, antifungal, and antiviral solution used to irrigate wounds and fistulas.

pHisoDerm: Despite the similarity of its name to pHisoHex, this soapless skin cleanser contains no hexachlorophene.

silver nitrate (chemical formula $AgNO_3$): This topical antiseptic drug also has caustic qualities. It is used to cauterize the skin to remove warts and granulomatous tissue.

sulfacetamide (Sebizon): This topical anti-infective drug is used to treat seborrheic dermatitis.

tacrolimus (Protopic): A topical nonsteroidal ointment used to treat eczema.

trioxsalen (Trisoralen): This oral drug is used in conjunction with exposure to ultraviolet light to cause pigmentation of the skin. It is used to treat vitiligo, a skin condition that is characterized by patchy areas of loss of skin pigmentation.

REVIEW QUESTIONS

1. Explain why some dermatologic diseases (such as poison ivy) may be treated with either topical or systemic drugs.
2. How does the anti-inflammatory and antipruritic action of an antihistamine differ from that of a corticosteroid? Why is it not appropriate to treat all kinds of itching diseases with an antihistamine?
3. Coal tar preparations and psoralens are prescribed for what dermatologic disease?
4. The drug minoxidil is used to treat both baldness and hypertension. True or False?
5. What type of drug treatment is prescribed when the nails have a severe, embedded fungal infection?
6. What is the difference between acne vulgaris and acne rosacea and how do the prescribed treatments differ?
7. Name four categories of drugs used to treat psoriasis and give examples of drugs in each category.
8. Name two categories of drugs used to treat itching and give examples of drugs in each category.
9. What condition is Rogaine used to treat, and what is its therapeutic action?
10. To what category of drugs does each of these drugs belong and what is its therapeutic action?
    clotrimazole (Lotrimin)
    isotretinoin (Accutane)
    metronidazole (MetroGel)
    nystatin (Nilstat)
    triamcinolone (Aristocort)

SPELLING TIPS

alclometasone (the generic name has an *l* after the *a*); Aclovate (the trade name does not).

ACU-dyne, AquaTar, PROPApH   Unusual internal capitalization.

Benzamycin (with an *a*) but benzocaine (with an *o*).

Cortizone-5, Cortizone-10   Spelled with a *z* unlike the sound-alike drug *cortisone*.

Dermacort (with an *a*) but Dermolate (with an *o*).

DesOwen   Unusual internal capitalization.

DuoDerm   Unusual internal capitalization.

gentamicin (generic) but Garamycin (trade).

IntraSite   Unusual internal capitalization.

MetroGel, MetroLotion   Unusual internal capitalization.

pHisoDerm, pHisoHex   Unusual internal capitalization.
Psorcon, Psorion   Silent *p*.

The endings *-sone*, *-olone*, and *-onide* are common to generic corticosteroids.

GET CONNECTED

Multimedia Extension Activities

   www.prenhall.com/turley

Use the above address to access the free, interactive Companion Website created for this textbook. Included in the features of this site are drug updates and additional chapter-specific exercises for further practice.

12

Urinary Tract Drugs

CHAPTER CONTENTS

Diuretics

Potassium supplements

Drugs used to treat urinary tract infections (UTIs)

Urinary tract analgesic drugs

Urinary tract antispasmodic drugs

Drugs used to treat benign prostatic hypertrophy (BPH)

Drugs used to treat erectile dysfunction

Immunosuppressant drugs used for kidney transplantation

Miscellaneous urinary tract drugs

Review questions

Spelling tips

LEARNING OBJECTIVES

After studying this chapter, you should be able to do the following:

1. Name several categories of urinary tract drugs.
2. Describe the therapeutic effect of diuretics and potassium supplements.
3. Describe the therapeutic effect of drugs used to treat urinary tract infections (UTIs), urinary tract pain, urinary tract spasm, benign prostatic hypertrophy (BPH), and erectile dysfunction.
4. Given the generic and trade name of a urinary tract drug, identify what drug category it belongs to or what disease it is used to treat.
5. Given a urinary tract drug category, identify several generic and trade name drugs within that category.
6. Identify the Historical Notes or Did You Know? section in this chapter that you found most interesting.

Urinary tract drugs include diuretics, potassium supplements (taken concurrently with some diuretics), urinary tract antibiotics and other anti-infective drugs, urinary tract analgesics, urinary tract antispasmodics, drugs for benign prostatic hypertrophy (BPH), and drugs for erectile dysfunction.

DIURETICS

The kidneys filter the circulating blood, extracting waste products, water, sodium, potassium, and various other substances. The kidneys then retain or excrete the nonwaste products, depending on the needs of the body. Diuretic drugs act to block sodium from being reabsorbed back into the bloodstream. As the sodium is excreted in the urine, it holds water to it because of osmotic pressure. By causing extra sodium and water to be excreted, diuretics are useful in the treatment of hypertension, congestive heart failure, and renal failure.

Diuretics are divided into several groups—thiazide diuretics, loop diuretics, and potassium-sparing diuretics—on the basis of the site of the drug's action within the kidney.

Thiazide Diuretics

Thiazide diuretics act at the loop of Henle and the distal renal tubule within the nephron. They increase the excretion of sodium (and therefore water) in the urine.

> bendroflumethiazide (Naturetin)
> benzthiazide (Exna)
> chlorothiazide (Diuril)
> hydrochlorothiazide (abbreviation HCTZ) (Esidrix, HydroDIURIL, Microzide, Oretic)
> hydroflumethiazide (Diucardin)
> indapamide (Lozol)
> methyclothiazide (Aquatensen, Enduron)
> polythiazide (Renese)
> quinethazone (Hydromox)
> trichlormethiazide (Diurese, Metahydrin, Naqua)

Note: The ending *-thiazide* is common to generic thiazide diuretics.

DID YOU KNOW?   The trade name Exna gives a clue as to the drug's diuretic action. The prefix *ex-* means *coming out*, and *Na* is the chemical symbol for *sodium*.

Other Diuretic Drugs

Other diuretics closely related in structure and action to the thiazide diuretics include:

> chlorthalidone (Hygroton)
> metolazone (Mykrox, Zaroxolyn)

Loop Diuretics

Loop diuretics act at the site of the proximal and distal tubules as well as the loop of Henle (hence their name). They block the reabsorption of sodium into the bloodstream so that it is excreted along with water into the urine.

> bumetanide (Bumex)
> ethacrynic acid (Edecrin)
> furosemide (Lasix)
> torsemide (Demadex)

Potassium-Sparing Diuretics

Both thiazide and loop diuretics cause sodium and water to be excreted, but they also cause potassium to be excreted as well. The excessive loss of potassium can cause serious side effects, including cardiac arrhythmias. Potassium-sparing diuretics cause sodium but not potassium to be excreted in the urine. Patients who take a thiazide or loop diuretic may be given potassium supplements, or they may take a potassium-sparing diuretic alone or in combination with the other diuretics.

> amiloride (Midamor)
> spironolactone (Aldactone)
> triamterene (Dyrenium)

Combination Diuretic Drugs

> Aldactazide (hydrochlorothiazide, spironolactone)
> Dyazide (hydrochlorothiazide, triamterene)
> Maxzide (hydrochlorothiazide, triamterene)
> Moduretic (hydrochlorothiazide, amiloride)

POTASSIUM SUPPLEMENTS

Potassium supplements are frequently prescribed for patients taking thiazide and loop diuretics to avoid potassium depletion. Although some foods, such as bananas, are rich in potassium, dietary sources alone are usually not sufficient to replenish potassium loss caused by diuretics. Potassium supplements are manufactured as liquids (patients often object to the taste), powders, effervescent tablets (to be dissolved in water), capsules, and tablets. Dosages are measured in milliequivalents (mEq).

> K + 8, K + 10
> K + Care, K + Care ET
> Kaon
> Kaon-Cl 10
> Kaon-Cl 20%
> Kay Ciel

K-Dur 10, K-Dur 20
K-Lor
Klor-Con, Klor-Con 8, Klor-Con 10, Klor-Con/EF, Klor-Con/25
Klorvess
Klotrix
K-Lyte, K-Lyte/Cl, K-Lyte/Cl 50, K-Lyte DS
K-Tab
Micro-K Extencaps, Micro-K LS, Micro-K 10 Extencaps
Slow-K
Ten-K

Note: The presence of *K* in every trade name refers to K^+, the chemical symbol for *potassium.*

DRUGS USED TO TREAT URINARY TRACT INFECTIONS (UTIs)

Urinary tract infections (UTIs) are treated with drugs that are particularly effective against *E. coli,* a gram-negative pathogen from the gastrointestinal (GI) tract and a frequent cause of UTIs.

Antibiotics for UTIs

There are several classes of antibiotics that act systemically to treat UTIs.

Many penicillin-type drugs (like ampicillin) and most cephalosporin drugs (like cefaclor) are indicated for the treatment of UTIs. For a complete list of the antibiotic drugs included in these categories, see Chapter 27, "Anti-Infective Drugs."

Quinolone antibiotics are a class of drugs that is only used to treat UTIs.

cinoxacin (Cinobac)
nalidixic acid (NegGram)

Note: The trade name *NegGram* was selected by the manufacturer because the drug is effective against gram-negative bacteria.

Fluoroquinolone antibiotics are similar in chemical structure to the quinolones. Some drugs in this class are specifically indicated for the treatment of UTIs and related types of infections such as prostatitis.

ciprofloxacin (Cipro)
enoxacin (Penetrex)
gatifloxacin (Tequin)
levofloxacin (Levaquin)
lomefloxacin (Maxaquin)
norfloxacin (Noroxin)
ofloxacin (Floxin)

Other Antibiotic-Type Drugs for UTIs

These drugs act systemically but have a special affinity for the tissues of the urinary tract. Fosfomycin is actually excreted unchanged (and in a still-active form) in the urine.

fosfomycin (Monurol)

nitrofurantoin (Furadantin, Macrobid, Macrodantin)

trimethoprim (Proloprim, TMP)

Sulfonamide Drugs for UTIs

These drugs are not true antibiotics because they only inhibit the growth of bacteria but do not kill them as antibiotics do. These drugs inhibit one step in the formation of folic acid by certain bacteria. Bacteria that do not synthesize folic acid are not susceptible to the action of sulfonamides. These drugs are used to treat UTIs as well as many other types of infections. Sulfonamides are also called *sulfa drugs*.

sulfadiazine

sulfamethoxazole (Gantanol, SMX)

sulfisoxazole (Gantrisin Pediatric)

Combination Drugs for UTIs

These drugs combine the antibiotic trimethoprim with the sulfa drug sulfamethoxazole. The trimethoprim blocks one step in the synthesis of folic acid by bacteria; the sulfamethoxazole blocks the next step in the same process. Used in combination, these two drugs work synergistically. They are indicated for the treatment of UTIs as well as other types of infections.

Bactrim, Bactrim DS, Bactrim IV, Bactrim Pediatric

Septra, Septra DS, Septra IV

Other Drugs for UTIs

This drug acts like an antibiotic in that it kills bacteria, although it is not an antibiotic. In the urine, it is changed to ammonia and formaldehyde, and these chemicals actually kill the bacteria.

methenamine (Hiprex, Urex)

This drug inhibits an enzyme in particular bacteria that are able to split urea and cause UTIs.

acetohydroxamic acid (Lithostat)

This drug helps to acidify the urine to inhibit the growth of bacteria.

ascorbic acid (vitamin C)

URINARY TRACT ANALGESIC DRUGS

UTIs, interstitial cystitis, and other urinary tract diseases produce symptoms of burning with frequent and painful urination. Urinary tract analgesics exert a local pain-relieving effect on the mucosa of the urinary tract, even though these drugs are given orally.

dimethyl sulfoxide (DMSO, Rimso-50)
pentosan (Elmiron)
phenazopyridine (Pyridium, Urogesic)

URINARY TRACT ANTISPASMODIC DRUGS

Irritation in the urinary tract from infection, catheterization, kidney stones, or overactive bladder can result in ureteral spasms, renal colic, spasm of the bladder sphincter, and urinary retention or urinary incontinence. Antispasmodic drugs relax the smooth muscle in the wall of the urethra and bladder and promote normal bladder function.

bethanechol (Myotonachol)
flavoxate (Urispas)
L-hyoscyamine (Anaspaz, Cystospaz, Cystospaz-M)
neostigmine (Prostigmin)
oxybutynin (Ditropan, Ditropan XL)

COMBINATION URINARY TRACT DRUGS

These drugs combine a urinary tract analgesic (phenazopyridine), a urinary tract antispasmodic (L-hyoscyamine), and a urinary tract anti-infective (methenamine) with a sedative or methylene blue.

Dolsed (L-hyoscyamine, methenamine, methylene blue)
Pyridium Plus (L-hyoscyamine, phenazopyridine, sedative)
Trac Tabs 2X (L-hyoscyamine, methenamine, methylene blue)
Urised (L-hyoscyamine, methenamine, methylene blue)
Urogesic Blue (L-hyoscyamine, methenamine, methylene blue)

DID YOU KNOW? Pyridium turns the urine bright orange. Dolsed, Trac Tabs 2X, Urised, and Urogesic Blue turn the urine a blue-green color because of the presence of methylene blue. Methylene blue, a dye, is an anti-infective drug that has an affinity for the tissues of the urinary tract.

DRUGS USED TO TREAT BENIGN PROSTATIC HYPERTROPHY (BPH)

Benign prostatic hypertrophy (BPH) is common in men over age 50, with the incidence increasing with age. Symptoms include difficulty initiating urination, hesitancy, and decreased urinary stream. The prostate enlarges due to the hormonal influence of dihydrotestosterone. Testosterone, acted on by an enzyme in prostatic cells, is converted to dihydrotestosterone. It is dihydrotestosterone that is responsible for causing the prostate gland to hypertrophy.

This drug inhibits dihydrotestosterone and reduces its level and its effect on prostatic cells. The drug needs to be taken for 6 to 12 months to determine its effectiveness in decreasing the size of the prostate; if effective, treatment must continue indefinitely.

finasteride (Proscar)

DID YOU KNOW?   Finasteride (Proscar) was approved in 1992 as the first nonsurgical treatment for BPH. Finasteride, under the trade name Propecia, is also given orally to treat male pattern baldness, but at a lower dose than that of Proscar. The hormone (dihydrotestosterone) that causes BPH is also responsible for causing male pattern baldness.

A group of drugs known as **alpha$_1$-receptor blockers** are also used to treat BPH. These drugs block alpha$_1$ receptors located in the smooth muscle of the urethra and prostate. This causes the smooth muscle to relax and allows urine to flow more easily. Because there are only a few of these receptors in the neck of the bladder, the drug does not relax the muscle of the bladder neck or cause incontinence.

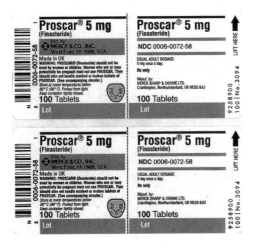

Figure 12–1   The prescription drug finasteride (Proscar) is used to treat benign prostatic hypertrophy (BPH). *Photo reprinted courtesy of Merck & Co, Inc.*

alfuzosin (UroXatral)

doxazosin (Cardura)

prazosin (Minipress)

tamsulosin (Flomax)

terazosin (Hytrin)

DID YOU KNOW?   Doxazosin and terazosin are also given for high blood pressure. The drug action relaxes the smooth muscle of the arteries, lowering the blood pressure.

This drug is the first of a class known as *5-alpha-reductase enzyme inhibitors* used to treat BPH. The drug acts by inhibiting two different enzymes that convert testosterone to dihydrotestosterone.

dutasteride

DID YOU KNOW?   **Saw palmetto**, a small palm tree that is native to the coast of the southeastern United States, is effective in treating BPH. Its fruit was used by the Seminole Indians to treat genitourinary conditions. It is available as an OTC product.

DRUGS USED TO TREAT ERECTILE DYSFUNCTION (ED)

Once a topic that men hesitated to discuss, even with their own physicians, erectile dysfunction (ED) and its treatment have become the subject of numerous newspaper articles and television commercials. There are two types of drugs used to treat this condition.

Through a series of steps, sexual stimulation activates the chemical cGMP, which relaxes the smooth muscles of the arteries in the penis, increases blood flow, and creates an erection. Afterwards, an enzyme metabolizes cGMP and the erection resolves. This drug, given orally, inhibits the enzyme that inactivates cGMP.

sildenafil (Viagra)

This drug acts locally to relax the smooth muscles of the arteries in the penis, increase blood flow, and create an erection. After receiving training from a physician, the patient either injects the drug (Caverject, Edex) into the side of the penis or inserts a pellet (Muse) into the urethra.

alprostadil (Caverject, Edex, Muse)

DID YOU KNOW?   Viagra was approved in 1998. Since that time, physicians in the United States have written 17 million prescriptions for it. Even former presidential candidate Bob Dole appeared in a television commercial, candidly discussing ED and urging viewers to ask their doctor about appropriate treatment.

IMMUNOSUPPRESSANT DRUGS USED FOR KIDNEY TRANSPLANTATION

Kidney transplants are performed on patients who are in acute or chronic renal failure and on dialysis. The closer the match of tissue types between the donor and the recipient, the greater the chance that the transplantation will be successful. All kidney transplant patients (except those who receive a kidney from an identical twin) must take an immunosuppressant drug daily for the rest of their lives. These drugs suppress the immune system's response to the foreign tissue type of the donor organ.

> azathioprine (Imuran)
> basiliximab (Simulect)
> cyclosporine (Gengraf, Neoral, Sandimmune, SangCya)
> daclizumab (Zenapax)
> muromonab-CD3 (Orthoclone OKT3)
> mycophenolate (CellCept)
> sirolimus (Rapamune)
> tacrolimus (Prograf)

DID YOU KNOW?   Cyclosporine is a metabolite of a naturally occurring fungus. Both basiliximab and daclizumab are monoclonal antibodies produced by recombinant DNA technology. Notice the ending *-mab*, common to these two generic drugs, which refers to the standard abbreviation for *monoclonal antibody* (MAB).

DID YOU KNOW?   The first successful human kidney transplant occurred in 1954 in the United States between identical twins. It was not until the FDA approval of the antirejection drug cyclosporine in 1984 that transplantation of kidneys from cadavers or unrelated living donors could be performed successfully.

There are approximately 13,000 kidney transplants performed each year in the United States. However, there are about 47,000 people in the United States who are on the transplant list, waiting for a suitable donor kidney to become available.

MISCELLANEOUS URINARY TRACT DRUGS

betamethasone (Alphatrex, Diprosone, Maxivate): Topical corticosteroid used to treat phimosis and nonretractable foreskin.

Calcibind: Used to prevent the formation of calcium kidney stones, only in patients with absorptive hypercalciuria.

calcifediol (Calderol): Used to treat patients on dialysis who have hypocalcemia.

calcitriol (Calcijex, Rocaltrol): Used to treat patients on dialysis who have hypocalcemia.

captopril (Capoten): An ACE inhibitor used to treat nephropathy in diabetic patients and slow the development of renal failure.

cyclophosphamide (Cytoxan, Cytoxan Lyophilized, Neosar): Used to treat pediatric nephrotic syndrome.

darbepoetin alfa (Aranesp): A protein manufactured by recombinant DNA techniques; this drug stimulates the production of red blood cells. It is structurally similar to the erythropoietin normally produced by the kidney. Used to treat anemia in patients with chronic renal failure.

desmopressin (DDAVP, Stimate): A synthetic replacement of antidiuretic hormone (ADH) from the posterior pituitary, it is administered via a nasal spray as replacement therapy. Studies have shown that many patients who habitually bed-wet have low levels of ADH.

docetaxel (Taxotere): Chemotherapy drug used to treat cancer of the bladder.

duloxetine: Used to treat stress urinary incontinence.

dyclonine (Dyclone): Topical anesthetic solution applied to the urethra prior to a cystoscopic procedure.

enalapril (Vasotec, Vasotec I.V.): An ACE inhibitor used to treat nephropathy in diabetic patients.

epoetin alfa (Epogen, Procrit): A protein manufactured by recombinant DNA techniques; this drug stimulates the production of red blood cells. It is structurally similar to the erythropoietin normally produced by the kidney. Used to treat anemia in patients with chronic renal failure.

epoetin beta (Marogen): A protein manufactured by recombinant DNA techniques; this drug stimulates the production of red blood cells. It is structurally similar to the erythropoietin normally produced by the kidney. Used to treat anemia in patients with chronic renal failure.

imipramine (Tofranil): Tricyclic antidepressant used to treat childhood bed-wetting.

iron sucrose (Venofer): Used to treat iron deficiency anemia in hemodialysis patients.

lidocaine (Anestacon, Xylocaine): Topical anesthetic jelly applied to the urethra prior to a cystoscopic procedure.

K-Phos: Combination potassium and phosphorus drug used to acidify the urine and prevent the formation of calcium kidney stones.

mannitol (Osmitrol):   Diuretic given intravenously to treat acute renal failure by stimulating the production of urine.

mannitol (Resectisol):   Irrigation solution used during urologic surgical procedures.

methylene blue (Urolene Blue):   Used to treat oxalate kidney stones.

Oncophage: Vaccine for renal cell carcinoma.

paclitaxel (Taxol):   Chemotherapy drug used to treat polycystic kidney disease.

paroxetine (Paxil):   Used to treat premature ejaculation.

potassium citrate (Polycitra-K, Urocit-K):   Used to prevent the formation of uric acid kidney stones in patients with gout.

potassium citrate/sodium citrate (Polycitra, Polycitra-LC):   Used to prevent the formation of uric acid kidney stones in patients with gout.

Renacidin: Irrigation solution used to dissolve calcium or magnesium kidney stones in patients who can't have surgery. It is instilled via a nephrostomy tube and/or catheter.

sevelamer (Renagel):   Used to decrease serum phosphatase in hemodialysis patients with end-stage renal disease.

Suby's Solution G: Irrigation solution used to dissolve phosphate stones in the bladder in patients who can't have surgery. It is instilled via a catheter.

succimer (Chemet):   Used to treat cystine kidney stones.

terodiline (Micturin):   Used to treat urinary incontinence. Investigational drug.

Thymoglobulin: Immunoglobulin used to treat rejection of donor kidney after organ transplantation.

tiopronin (Thiola):   Used to prevent the formation of cystine kidney stones in patients with cystinuria.

tolterodine (Detrol, Detrol LA):   Used to treat overactive bladder and symptoms of frequency and incontinence. This drug amplifies the signal that the bladder normally receives from the central nervous system to stop the flow of urine out of the bladder.

vincristine (Vincasar PFS):   Chemotherapy drug used to treat Wilm's tumor.

REVIEW QUESTIONS

1. Describe the therapeutic action of various diuretics and how these drugs are useful for treating hypertension.
2. Why do so many potassium supplements contain the letter *K* in the trade name of the drug?
3. Why do patients on a diuretic often need to take potassium supplements?
4. What is the most common cause of UTIs?
5. How does the action of sulfonamides differ from that of antibiotics?
6. What symptoms are urinary analgesics prescribed to treat?
7. Give examples of two drugs that color the urine.
8. Name the three categories of diuretics and give examples of drugs in each category.
9. What disease is finasteride (Proscar) used to treat?

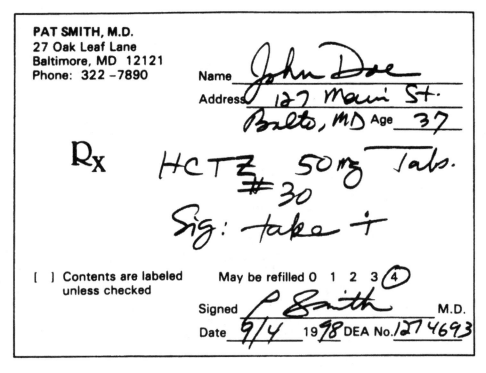

Figure 12–2   A prescription. *Reprinted courtesy of Marvin Stoogenke,* The Pharmacy Technician, *2nd ed. (Upper Saddle River, NJ: Brady/Prentice Hall, 1998), p. 37.*

10. How do alpha$_1$-receptor blockers work to treat BPH?
11. To what category of drugs does each of the following belong?
    cinoxacin (Cinobac)
    Klorvess
    phenazopyridine (Urogesic)
    furosemide (Lasix)
12. How do drugs used to treat ED exert their effect?
13. Identify the component parts of the prescription in Figure 12–2. Write down any component parts that are missing. Use the Glossary/Index at the end of this textbook to help you verify the spelling of the name of this drug. Write down its name, what this abbreviation stands for, and the drug's therapeutic action. Verify that the drug is available in a strength that matches the dosage prescribed. Translate the rest of the prescription into plain English.

SPELLING TIPS

CellCept, SangCya   Unusual internal capitalization.

epoetin alfa   An unusual spelling of the Greek letter *alpha.*

Dyazide   Spelled *Dy,* not *Di* as in *diuretic.*

NegGram   Unusual internal capitalization.

HydroDIURIL   Unusual use of all capital letters in the second part of the drug name.

Kay Ciel   When dictated, it is often not recognized as a trade name drug, but is mistakenly transcribed as *KCl*, an abbreviation of the chemical name *potassium chloride*.

Urispas, Anaspaz, Cystospaz   Sound-alike endings with different spellings.

UroXatral   Unusual internal capitalization.

The ending *-thiazide* is common to generic thiazide diuretics.

GET CONNECTED

Multimedia Extension Activities

 www.prenhall.com/turley

Use the above address to access the free, interactive Companion Website created for this textbook. Included in the features of this site are drug updates and additional chapter-specific exercises for further practice.

13

Gastrointestinal Drugs

CHAPTER CONTENTS

Drugs used to treat peptic ulcer disease
Drugs used to treat *H. pylori* infections
Drugs used to treat gastroesophageal reflux disease (GERD)
Drugs used to treat gastrointestinal (GI) spasm
Drugs used to treat diarrhea
Laxatives
Drugs used to treat ulcerative colitis
Gastric stimulants
Antiemetics
Drugs used to treat gallstones
Drugs used to treat obesity
Liquid nutritional supplements
Miscellaneous gastrointestinal drugs
Review questions
Spelling tips

LEARNING OBJECTIVES

After studying this chapter, you should be able to do the following:

1. Name several categories of gastrointestinal drugs.
2. Describe the therapeutic action of drugs used to treat peptic ulcers, gastroesophageal reflux disease (GERD), diarrhea, ulcerative colitis, obesity, and gallstones.
3. Describe the therapeutic action of antacids, laxatives, antiemetics, and H_2 blockers.
4. Given the generic and trade name of a gastrointestinal drug, identify what drug category it belongs to or what disease it is used to treat.
5. Given a gastrointestinal drug category, identify several generic and trade name drugs within that category.

6. Identify the Historical Notes or Did You Know? section in this chapter that you found most interesting.

Gastrointestinal drugs are used to treat disease conditions of the esophagus, stomach, and intestines, such as ulcers, diarrhea, constipation, ulcerative colitis, and so forth.

DRUGS USED TO TREAT PEPTIC ULCER DISEASE

A peptic ulcer is an ulcer located anywhere in the esophagus, stomach, or duodenum. Peptic ulcers in the stomach are specifically known as *gastric ulcers.* All peptic ulcers are caused by irritation of the mucous membrane lining of the gastrointestinal tract. This irritation is caused by excessive amounts of hydrochloric acid, which strip away the protective mucus of the mucous membrane, and the subsequent action of pepsin, a protein-digesting enzyme, that begins to break down the underlying membrane. Aspirin, nonsteroidal anti-inflammatory drugs (NSAIDs), alcohol, and caffeine also irritate the mucous membranes and can contribute to ulcer formation. Several types of drugs are used to treat peptic ulcers. These include antacids, H$_2$ blockers, antispasmodics, and others.

Antacids for Peptic Ulcer Disease

Antacids were the original, and for many years the only, treatment for peptic ulcers. They are weak bases that exert a therapeutic effect by neutralizing hydrochloric acid. This raises the pH of the stomach contents, which decreases mucous membrane irritation and also inhibits the action of pepsin. Antacids contain aluminum, magnesium, calcium, sodium, or a combination of these as the active ingredients. Antacids are available without a prescription.

Antacids containing aluminum as the active ingredient include:

AlternaGEL
Alu-Cap
Alu-Tab
Amphojel
Basaljel

Antacids containing magnesium as the active ingredient include:

Phillips' Milk of Magnesia, Concentrated Phillips' Milk of Magnesia

Antacids containing calcium as the active ingredient include:

Alka-Mints
Chooz
Maalox Antacid Caplets
Mylanta Lozenges
Titralac, Titralac Extra Strength, Titralac Plus
Tums, Tums Ultra, Extra Strength Tums E-X

DID YOU KNOW?   The use of calcium-containing antacids can provide an additional benefit to women by supplementing calcium intake—so say drug advertisements! In reality, the use of calcium-containing antacids should not take the place of adequate calcium intake in the diet.

Combination Antacids for Peptic Ulcer Disease

These antacids contain aluminum, calcium, magnesium, and/or sodium bicarbonate. In addition, some contain simethicone to relieve flatulence and gas or aspirin or acetaminophen for pain relief. Simethicone acts by changing the surface tension of air bubbles trapped in the GI tract to allow them to be expelled.

Advanced Formula Di-Gel (calcium, magnesium, simethicone)

Bromo Seltzer (acetaminophen, sodium bicarbonate)

Di-Gel (aluminum, magnesium, simethicone)

Double Strength Gaviscon-2 (aluminum, magnesium, sodium bicarbonate)

Extra Strength Maalox, Extra Strength Maalox Plus (aluminum, magnesium, simethicone)

Gaviscon Extra Strength Relief Formula Liquid (aluminum, magnesium, simethicone)

Gaviscon Liquid (aluminum, magnesium)

Gaviscon Tablets, Gaviscon Extra Strength Relief Formula Tablets (aluminum, calcium, magnesium, sodium bicarbonate)

Gelusil (aluminum, magnesium, simethicone)

Maalox, Maalox Therapeutic Concentrate (aluminum, magnesium)

Mylanta Gelcaps, Mylanta Supreme (calcium, magnesium)

Mylanta Liquid (aluminum, simethicone)

Mylanta Tablets, Mylanta Double Strength (aluminum, magnesium, simethicone)

Original Alka-Seltzer, Extra Strength Alka-Seltzer (aspirin, sodium bicarbonate)

Riopan (aluminum, magnesium)

Riopan Plus, Riopan Plus Double Strength (aluminum, magnesium, simethicone)

Rolaids (calcium, magnesium)

Titralac Plus (calcium, simethicone)

DID YOU KNOW?   Baking soda (sodium bicarbonate) in water is an old home remedy for indigestion. Although sodium bicarbonate neutralizes acid, it is not recommended as a long-term treatment for indigestion because of the large amounts of sodium it contains, which are absorbed systemically. Physicians recommend the prudent use of salt (sodium), even for patients without hypertension and other medical conditions. One dose of regular Alka-Seltzer contains 958 mg of sodium. For patients on a low-salt diet, this could equal their recommended allowance of sodium for the entire day.

Simethicone is also available by itself, but it has no antacid action.

Gas-X, Extra-Strength Gas-X
Maalox Anti-Gas
Mylanta Gas, Maximum Strength Mylanta Gas
Mylicon
Phazyme, Phazyme 95, Phazyme 125

H_2 Blockers for Peptic Ulcer Disease

Histamine acts on special histamine receptors (known as H_2 receptors) located in the parietal cells of the stomach to cause the release of hydrochloric acid. Drugs that block these receptors and prevent the release of acid are known as H_2 blockers and are used to treat heartburn, peptic ulcers, and gastroesophageal reflux disease (GERD). H_2 blockers are prescription drugs, but some are also available as OTC drugs.

cimetidine (Tagamet, Tagamet HB 200)
famotidine (Pepcid, Pepcid AC, Pepcid AC Acid Controller, Pepcid RPD)
nizatidine (Axid AR, Axid Pulvules)
ranitidine (Zantac, Zantac 75, Zantac EFFERdose, Zantac GELdose)

Note: The ending *-tidine* is common in generic names of H_2 blockers.

Combination H_2 Blockers for Peptic Ulcer Disease

This drug combines an H_2 blocker and two antacids.

Pepcid Complete (famotidine, calcium, magnesium)

HISTORICAL NOTES: The therapeutic effect of antihistamines has been known since diphenhydramine (Benadryl) was introduced in 1945. It was known that histamine was released during an allergic reaction (causing red, itching eyes, sneezing, and a runny nose) and that antihistamine drugs could prevent these symptoms. It was also known that histamine was released in the stomach, where it stimulated the production of hydrochloric acid. In this case, the release of histamine was not related to an allergic reaction and could not be prevented by antihistamine drugs. Therefore it was postulated that histamine acted upon two different receptors, designated as H_1 and H_2 receptors.

Researchers at Smith, Kline & French pharmaceutical company began to search for a drug that could block the action of histamine on H_2 receptors in the stomach. Such a drug would prevent the release of acid and would be useful in the treatment of ulcers. By rearranging the chemical structure of a molecule of histamine, they developed a drug that combined with H_2 receptors but did not activate them, thus effectively "blocking" both the receptors and the release of acid. A drug that "blocks" a receptor is known as an **antagonist.** The first H_2 blocker was named **cimetidine.** For the trade name, Smith, Kline & French combined syllables from *antagonist* and *cimetidine* to make **Tagamet,** which was released in 1977.

DID YOU KNOW?   Chronic itching and hives may be treated with an antihistamine in combination with the H_2 blocker cimetidine (Tagamet) that blocks the H_2 type of histamine receptor.

Proton Pump Inhibitors for Peptic Ulcer Disease

Unrelated to H_2 blockers, proton pump inhibitors decrease gastric acid by blocking the final step of acid production within the gastric parietal cell. This final step involves an enzyme system known as the *proton pump,* hence the name of this drug category.

lansoprazole (Prevacid)
omeprazole (Prilosec)
rabeprazole (Aciphex)

Note: For a complete list proton pump inhibitors, see the section "Drugs Used to Treat Gastroesophageal Reflux Disease (GERD)" later in this chapter.

DID YOU KNOW?   Horses get gastric ulcers too! Now omeprazole is available in a cinnamon-flavored oral paste under the trade name GastroGard just for horses!

Other Drugs for Peptic Ulcer Disease

Patients on long-term therapy with aspirin or NSAIDs can develop gastric ulcers. This is a common side effect because aspirin and NSAIDs inhibit the formation of prostaglandins. Prostaglandins normally protect the gastric mucosa. When aspirin and NSAIDs suppress the action of prostaglandins, they also remove its protective action on the gastric mucosa. Drugs that are synthetic prostaglandins protect the gastric mucosa when natural prostaglandin is inhibited by aspirin or NSAIDs.

misoprostol (Cytotec)

This drug is unrelated to either antacids or H_2 blockers. It acts topically only on the actual surface of the ulcer. It is attracted to areas of mucous membrane that are draining fluid that is high in protein. The drug binds directly to these areas, forming a protective layer or "bandage" over the ulcer, allowing it to heal.

sucralfate (Carafate)

DRUGS USED TO TREAT H. PYLORI INFECTIONS

Helicobacter pylori are helical (curved) bacteria with flagella. They live in the gastric or duodenal mucosa and are the cause of many peptic ulcers. Successful treatment involves using a combination of antibiotic drugs, bismuth, and either an H_2 blocker or a proton pump inhibitor. Antibiotics and bismuth disrupt the cell wall that surrounds this bacterium, causing cell death.

Antibiotics for H. Pylori Infections

amoxicillin (Amoxil, Trimox, Wymox)

clarithromycin (Biaxin, Biaxin XL)

metronidazole (Flagyl, Flagyl ER, Flagyl 375, Flagyl IV RTU, Protostat)

tetracycline (Panmycin, Sumycin, Tetracyn, Tetralan)

DID YOU KNOW?   Metronidazole is used to treat many different conditions besides *H. pylori* infection. Metronidazole (Flagyl, Protostat) is taken orally to treat intestinal amebiasis, dysentery, and vaginal *Trichomonas*. Metronidazole (MetroGel-Vaginal) is applied topically as a gel to treat vaginal infections due to *Hemophilus* or *Gardnerella*. Metronidazole (MetroGel) is applied topically as a gel to treat acne rosacea.

H₂ Blockers and Proton Pump Inhibitors for H. pylori Infections

See other sections in this chapter that describe the therapeutic action of these classes of drugs. Only the proton pump inhibitors esomeprazole (Nexium), lansoprazole (Prevacid), and omeprazole (Prilosec) are indicated for the treatment of *H. pylori* infections.

Combination Drugs for H. pylori Infection

Helidac (bismuth, metronidazole, tetracycline)

Prevpac (amoxicillin, clarithromycin, lansoprazole)

Tritec (bismuth, ranitidine)

DID YOU KNOW?   Bismuth is an important component of a combined drug approach to treating *H. pylori* infection. Bismuth is an antibacterial drug. The bismuth found in Tritec and the bismuth found in the OTC drug Pepto-Bismol are identical in structure and dose. However, Pepto-Bismol alone is not indicated for the treatment of *H. pylori* infections. Bismuth must be taken as part of a combined drug regimen to be effective in treating *H. pylori* infections.

DRUGS USED TO TREAT GASTROESOPHAGEAL REFLUX DISEASE (GERD)

Gastroesophageal reflux disease (GERD) occurs when stomach acid refluxes or flows back into the esophagus, causing irritation and pain.

Proton Pump Inhibitors for GERD

Proton pump inhibitors decrease the production of hydrochloric acid in the stomach. Proton pump inhibitors are used to treat GERD as well as peptic ulcer disease and *H. pylori* infections (as discussed previously). Another proton pump inhibitor, pantoprazole, is only used to treat GERD.

  esomeprazole (Nexium)
  lansoprazole (Prevacid)
  omeprazole (Prilosec)
  pantoprazole (Protonix, Protonix I.V.)
  rabeprazole (Aciphex)

DID YOU KNOW?   Following FDA approval of esomeprazole (Nexium), the manufacturer launched an extensive advertising campaign on TV and in magazines. Consumers were encouraged to ask their doctor about the "purple pill." This drug even has its own Web site: www.purplepill.com.

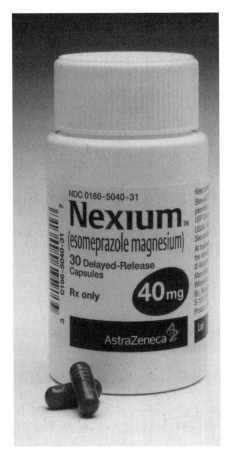

Figure 13–1   The prescription drug esomeprazole (Nexium) is used to treat gastroesophageal reflux disease. This drug is known by consumers as the "purple pill."
Photo reprinted courtesy of AstraZeneca Pharmaceuticals LP.

GI Stimulants for GERD

GI stimulants increase the rate of gastric emptying in order to keep excess acid from accumulating in the stomach.

metoclopramide (Maxolon, Reglan)

DRUGS USED TO TREAT GASTROINTESTINAL (GI) SPASM

Intestinal conditions such as irritable bowel syndrome, spastic colon, diverticulitis, and even peptic ulcers can be accompanied by abdominal pain due to spasms of the smooth muscle of the GI tract. These spasms can be relieved by antispasmodic drugs, which are also known as *anticholinergic drugs.* Anticholinergic drugs exert their therapeutic action in the following way. Muscle contraction and peristalsis in the GI tract are controlled by the parasympathetic nervous system through the release of the neurotransmitter acetylcholine. Acetylcholine acts on cholinergic receptors to stimulate muscular contractions and begin peristalsis to move food through the GI tract. If peristalsis is too strong and causes spasms (as in the disease conditions mentioned earlier), anticholinergic drugs can be given to block the effects of acetylcholine to stop the spasms and slow peristalsis.

clidinium (Quarzan)
dicyclomine (Bentyl, Di-Spaz)
glycopyrrolate (Robinul, Robinul Forte)
L-hyoscyamine (Anaspaz, Gastrosed, Levbid, Levsin, Levsin Drops, Levsin/SL, Levsinex Timecaps)
mepenzolate (Cantil)
methantheline (Banthine)
methscopolamine (Pamine)
propantheline (Pro-Banthine)
tridihexethyl (Pathilon)

Combination Antispasmodic Drugs

These drugs combine an antispasmodic drug with the central nervous system sedative phenobarbital or the antianxiety drug Librium.

Bellergal-S (antispasmodic drug [belladonna], phenobarbital)
Donnatal, Donnatal Extentabs (L-hyoscyamine, scopolamine, phenobarbital)
Librax (clidinium, Librium)

DRUGS USED TO TREAT DIARRHEA

Antidiarrheal drugs produce a therapeutic effect by slowing peristalsis in the intestinal tract or by absorbing extra water from diarrhea stools. Some antidiarrheal drugs exert their effect because they contain opium or related narcotic drugs. Although these drugs have pain-relieving properties, a common side effect is constipation. This side effect then becomes the therapeutic effect in treating diarrhea.

Narcotic Drugs for Diarrhea

Antidiarrheal drugs that contain opium or related narcotic drugs are classified as controlled substances (Schedule III, IV, or V drugs) with an assigned schedule that depends on the actual addictive qualities of that particular drug.

difenoxin (Motofen)
diphenoxylate (Lomotil)
opium (paregoric)

Nonnarcotic Drugs for Diarrhea

loperamide (Imodium A-D, Kaopectate II, Pepto Diarrhea Control)

Antibiotics for Diarrhea

These drugs are used to treat bacterial or protozoal diarrhea or traveler's diarrhea.

ciprofloxacin (Cipro)
doxycycline (Doryx, Vibramycin, Vibra-Tabs)

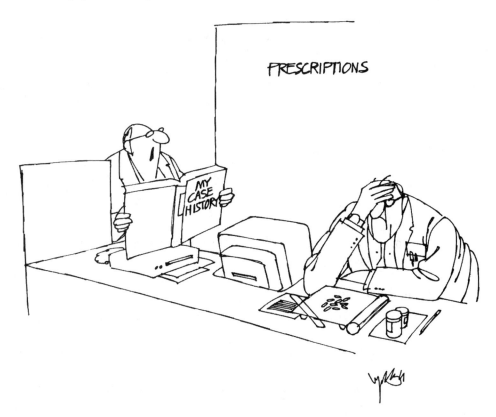

Figure 13–2 —David W. Harbaugh. *Reprinted with permission.*

furazolidone (Furoxone)

trimethoprim/sulfamethoxazole (Bactrim, Septra)

Other Drugs for Diarrhea

These drugs contain kaolin/pectin or a claylike powder (attapulgite) to absorb excess water within the GI tract.

attapulgite (Children's Kaopectate, Donnagel, Kaolin with Pectin, Kaopectate Advanced Formula, Kaopectate Maximum Strength, Parepectolin, Rheaban Maximum Strength)

Kaodene Non-Narcotic (bismuth, kaolin, pectin)

This drug has anti-inflammatory and antimicrobial activity.

bismuth (Pepto-Bismol, Pepto-Bismol Maximum Strength)

Drugs Used to Treat Diarrhea and Wasting Disease in AIDS

These drugs are discussed in Chapter 28, "AIDS Drugs and Antiviral Drugs."

LAXATIVES

Laxatives are used for short-term treatment of constipation, with attention also given to adequate water intake, dietary fiber/bulk, and other measures to promote regularity. OTC laxatives are frequently overused and even abused.

There are several classifications of laxatives. These include magnesium laxatives, irritant/stimulant laxatives, bulk-producing laxatives, stool softeners, mechanical laxatives, and others.

Magnesium Laxatives

Magnesium laxatives contain magnesium as their active ingredient. By the process of osmosis, they attract water from the bloodstream into the intestines to soften the stool.

Epsom salt

milk of magnesia (M.O.M.) (Phillips' Milk of Magnesia, Concentrated Phillips' Milk of Magnesia)

Irritant/Stimulant Laxatives

Irritant/stimulant laxatives act directly on the intestinal mucosa to stimulate peristalsis.

bisacodyl (Correctol, Dulcolax, Feen-a-mint, Fleet Laxative, Modane)

cascara

sennosides (ex-lax, ex-lax chocolated, Fletcher's Castoria, Maximum Strength ex-lax, Senokot, SenokotXTRA)

Bulk-Producing Laxatives

Bulk-producing laxatives contain indigestible dietary fiber and other substances that absorb and hold water in the intestines. The action of this type of laxative is the most natural and safest of all the laxatives.

> methylcellulose (Citrucel)
> polycarbophil (FiberCon, Mitrolan)
> psyllium (Fiberall, Metamucil, Modane Bulk, Perdiem Fiber Therapy)

Stool Softener Laxatives

Stool softeners are emulsifiers that allow fat in the stool to mix with water to make the stool soft.

> docusate (Colace, ex-lax stool softener, Modane Soft, Phillips' Liqui-Gels, Surfak Liquigels)

Mechanical Laxatives

Mechanical laxatives directly stimulate the urge to defecate by their physical presence in the lower colon.

> glycerin (Colace suppository, Fleet Babylax)
> carbon dioxide-releasing suppository (Ceo-Two)

Other Laxatives

> castor oil
> mineral oil
> lactulose (Chronulac)

Combination Laxatives

> Doxidan (stool softener, irritant/stimulant laxative)
> Haley's M-O (magnesium laxative, mineral oil)
> Perdiem Overnight Relief (bulk-producing laxative, irritant/stimulant laxative)
> Peri-Colace (stool softener, irritant/stimulant laxative)
> Senokot-S (stool softener, irritant/stimulant laxative)

Bowel Evacuants/Enemas

These laxatives are given orally to evacuate the colon prior to surgical or endoscopic procedures. Some kits also include a suppository or enema. The use of a bowel evacuant along with an enema is referred to as a *bowel prep.*

> Evac-Q-Kwik
> Fleet Prep Kit 1, Fleet Prep Kit 2, Fleet Prep Kit 3
> polyethylene glycol-electrolyte solution (CoLyte, GoLYTELY, NuLytely, OCL)

polyethylene glycol (PEG) solution (MiraLax)
X-Prep Bowel Evacuant Kit-1, X-Prep Bowel Kit-2, X-Prep Liquid

These drugs are given as enemas to evacuate the lower colon prior to a procedure or to provide relief from constipation.

Fleet, Fleet Bisacodyl, Fleet Mineral Oil

DRUGS USED TO TREAT ULCERATIVE COLITIS

Ulcerative colitis is a chronic disease characterized by abdominal pain, diarrhea, rectal bleeding, and abscesses. The cause is unknown. Besides the antispasmodic drugs described previously, ulcerative colitis is also treated with anti-inflammatory drugs.

Aminosalicyclic Acid (ASA) Drugs for Ulcerative Colitis

The chemical compound aminosalicylic acid (ASA) decreases intestinal inflammation by blocking the production of prostaglandins. These drugs contain 4-ASA or 5-ASA as the active ingredient or contain an ingredient that is metabolized to 5-ASA by bacteria in the colon. These drugs may be taken orally or administered rectally as a suppository or as a solution.

balsalazide (Colazal)
4-aminosalicylic acid (Pamisyl, Rezipas)
mesalamine (5-aminosalicylic acid) (Asacol, Canasa, Pentasa, Rowasa)
olsalazine (Dipentum)
sulfasalazine (Azulfidine, Azulfidine EN-tabs)

Topical Corticosteroids for Ulcerative Colitis

These drugs are corticosteroids that exert a more powerful anti-inflammatory effect than 5-ASA. They are administered as a solution or an aerosol foam that is placed into the rectum.

hydrocortisone (Cortenema, Cortifoam)

GASTRIC STIMULANTS

For certain disease conditions such as diabetic gastroparesis, to facilitate emptying of the intestines prior to x-rays, to facilitate excretion of barium after an x-ray, or to prevent distention and paralytic ileus after major abdominal surgery, patients may be given a gastric stimulant. These drugs enhance the natural action of acetylcholine (described previously), thereby increasing peristalsis in the GI tract.

dexpanthenol (Ilopan)
metoclopramide (Maxolon, Reglan)

ANTIEMETICS

Antiemetic drugs are used to control nausea and vomiting associated with many different diseases. Bacterial or viral illnesses can directly irritate vomiting centers in the GI tract. Some drugs, radiation, or chemotherapy can have a systemic effect that irritates the GI tract or stimulates the chemoreceptor trigger zone and vomiting center in the brain. Surgery, particularly abdominal surgery, can temporarily stop peristalsis. As fluids accumulate in the GI tract, they cause distension and trigger postoperative nausea and vomiting. Patients who are actively vomiting can be given antiemetic drugs in the form of a rectal suppository.

Some drugs used to treat nausea and vomiting block dopamine from activating receptors in the wall of the GI tract and in the chemoreceptor trigger zone and vomiting center in the brain.

> buclizine (Bucladin-S Softabs)
> chlorpromazine (Thorazine)
> cyclizine (Marezine)
> hydroxyzine (Vistaril)
> perphenazine (Trilafon)
> phosphorated carbohydrate solution (Emetrol)
> prochlorperazine (Compazine)
> promethazine (Phenergan)
> thiethylperazine (Torecan)
> trimethobenzamide (Tigan)

DID YOU KNOW?   The antiemetic drugs chlorpromazine (Thorazine) and perphenazine (Trilafon) are also used to treat intractable hiccoughs.

Chemotherapy drugs kill rapidly dividing cancer cells, but they also affect the rapidly dividing cells in the mucous membrane of the GI tract, causing irritation. These drugs also directly stimulate the vomiting center in the brain. In addition, some chemotherapy drugs cause the release of serotonin in the small intestine, which stimulates the vomiting reflex. The nausea and vomiting in response to chemotherapy can be so severe and prolonged that, without antiemetic treatment, the patient may elect to discontinue life-saving chemotherapy. Therefore, antiemetic drugs are often given prophylactically prior to beginning chemotherapy. These drugs, many of which are serotonin blockers, are used specifically to treat the nausea and vomiting associated with chemotherapy, although any of the general antiemetic drugs described previously may also be prescribed.

> chlorpromazine (Thorazine)
> dolasetron (Anzemet)

domperidone (Motilium)

dronabinol (Marinol)

granisetron (Kytril)

metoclopramide (Maxolon, Reglan)

ondansetron (Zofran, Zofran ODT)

DID YOU KNOW?   *ODT* stands for *orally disintegrating tablet.*

DID YOU KNOW?   The antiemetic drug dronabinol (Marinol) is derived from the marijuana plant. The Latin name for the marijuana plant is *Cannabis sativa*, and the active components in marijuana that produce physical and psychological effects are termed *cannabinoids.* The drug dronabinol (Marinol) is a cannabinoid. It is also known by its chemical name **delta-9-tetrahydrocannabinol**, abbreviated **delta-9-THC** or just **THC.** In addition to its use as an antiemetic, dronabinol (Marinol) is also used as an appetite stimulant for patients with AIDS.

See Focus on Healthcare Issues in Chapter 3, "Drug Legislation," for an overview of the debate to legalize marijuana.

Antiemetics for Vertigo or Motion Sickness

Vertigo is a sensation of lightheadedness, dizziness, and whirling caused by irritation or infection in the inner ear that upsets balance and stimulates the vomiting center. Motion sickness occurs when the repetitive motions of a car or airplane overstimulate the inner ear. Drugs used to treat vertigo and motion sickness act either by inhibiting inner ear stimuli from reaching the chemoreceptor trigger zone and the vomiting center in the brain or by reducing the sensitivity of the inner ear to motion.

buclizine (Bucladin-S Softabs)

cyclizine (Marezine)

dimenhydrinate (Children's Dramamine, Dramamine)

diphenhydramine (Benadryl)

meclizine (Antivert, Antivert/25, Antivert/50, Bonine)

promethazine (Phenergan)

scopolamine (Transderm-Scop)

Note: All of these drugs are given orally with the exception of scopolamine (Transderm-Scop); it is manufactured as a small transdermal patch that is worn behind the ear.

DRUGS USED TO TREAT GALLSTONES

Patients who are unable to undergo surgery to remove gallstones may be given drugs to help dissolve the stones. Those drugs (except monoctanoin) are given orally and must be taken for 6 months or longer to achieve a full therapeutic result. Monoctanoin is given via continuous infusion for 2 to 10 days through a catheter or T-tube into the common bile duct. Although these drugs are effective, gallstones do recur in 50% of the patients treated.

chenodiol (Chenix)
monoctanoin (Moctanin)
ursodiol (Actigall)

DRUGS USED TO TREAT OBESITY

Drugs used to treat obesity either keep fat from being utilized by the body or suppress the appetite.

Lipase Inhibitors for Obesity

This drug chemically bonds to the enzyme lipase so that it cannot break down dietary fat in the intestines. The fat is excreted rather than being absorbed by the body.

orlistat (Xenical)

Appetite Suppressants for Obesity

Similar in chemistry to amphetamines but with less addictive properties, these drugs suppress the appetite by affecting dopamine or serotonin levels in the satiety center of the brain. Appetite suppressants are also known as *anorexiants*. The use of these drugs is limited to short-term treatment of exogenous obesity, in conjunction with dietary restrictions. Patients may develop drug dependence and experience withdrawal symptoms if these drugs are discontinued abruptly because they are Schedule III and Schedule IV drugs.

benzphetamine (Didrex)
diethylpropion (Tenuate, Tenuate Dospan)
phendimetrazine (Plegine, Prelu-2)
phentermine (Fastin)
sibutramine (Meridia)

This antidepressant is used to treat obesity, in conjunction with dietary restrictions.

bupropion (Wellbutrin, Wellbutrin SR)

DID YOU KNOW?   The popular appetite suppressants Acutrim and Dexatrim were taken off the market because they contained phenylpropanolamine. This drug caused hundreds of hemorrhagic strokes and some deaths. Americans took 6 billion doses of phenylpropanolamine in 2000. It was also found in many cold and cough preparations.

DID YOU KNOW?   In 1997, the FDA removed from the market the popular weight control drugs fenfluramine (Pondimin) and dexfenfluramine (Redux). The widely popular "fen-phen" combination treatment for weight control (18 million prescriptions in 1996 alone) consisted of fenfluramine (Pondimin) and another appetite suppressant, phentermine (Fastin), which was not taken off the market. Dexfenfluramine (Redux) was introduced in June 1996. Nearly 2 million Americans took it before it was removed from the market. Fenfluramine and dexfenfluramine were linked to cases of primary pulmonary hypertension and valvular heart disease.

LIQUID NUTRITIONAL SUPPLEMENTS

In the past, liquid nutritional supplements were given to patients whose only intake was via a nasogastric or gastrostomy tube or to patients with a chronic disease who needed more calories in a concentrated form. Now, some of these liquid nutritional supplements (Boost, Compleat, Ensure, Resource) are being advertised as part of a normal diet for healthy, active adults who are too busy to eat. This change in marketing emphasis was no doubt prompted by the huge number of baby boomers now entering their older years! Other liquid nutritional supplements are specially formulated to meet the nutritional needs of patients with GI disorders (Peptamen), liver failure (Hepatic-Aid II, Travasorb Hepatic Diet), renal failure (Amin-Aid, Suplena), pulmonary problems (Pulmocare, Respalor), diabetes (Choice dm, Glucerna), AIDS or trauma (Advera, TraumaCal), or the needs of older children with phenylketonuria (PKU) (Phenex-2). Liquid nutritional supplements come as ready-to-drink liquids, concentrated liquids, powders, or puddings and are available in a variety of flavors.

Advera
Amin-Aid
Boost
Choice dm
Citrotein
Compleat Modified Formula
Criticare HN
Ensure, Ensure HN, Ensure High Protein, Ensure Plus, Ensure Plus HN
Forta Drink, Forta Shake

Glucerna
Hepatic-Aid II
Impact
Introlite
Isocal, Isocal HCN, Isocal HN
Isosource, Isosource HN
Isotein HN
Jevity
Kindercal
Lipisorb
Lonalac
Meritene
Nepro
Optimental
Osmolite, Osmolite HN
Peptamen
Phenex-2
Portagen
Pulmocare
Replete
Resource, Resource Plus
Respalor
Suplena
Sustacal, Sustacal Basic, Sustacal Plus
Sustagen
TraumaCal
Travasorb, Travasorb Hepatic Diet, Travasorb HN. Travasorb MCT, Travasorb STD
TwoCal HN
Ultracal
Vivonex T.E.N.

INFANT FORMULAS AND FOODS

The milk protein in infant formulas is processed so that it is nearly as digestible as mother's milk. Infant formulas are usually fortified with iron. Some formulas (Gerber Soy Formula, Isomil, Nursoy, ProSobee, Soyalac) use soy protein for infants who are allergic to cow milk protein. Other formulas are for infants who are lactose intolerant (Enfamil LactoFree, Isomil, Nutramigen, ProSobee), have other digestive/malabsorption disorders (Alimentum, Pregestimil), or have PKU (Lofenalac, Phenex-1).

Alimentum
Bonamil Infant Formula with Iron

Carnation Follow-Up, Carnation Good Start

Enfamil, Enfamil LactoFree, Enfamil Next Step, Enfamil with Iron

Gerber Baby Formula with Iron, Gerber Soy Formula

Isomil, Isomil DF, Isomil SF

Lofenalac

Nursoy

Nutramigen

PediaSure

Phenex-1

Pregestimil

ProSobee

RCF

Similac, Similac Low-Iron, Similac PM 60/40, Similac with Iron

SMA, SMA Iron Fortified, SMA Lo-Iron Infant Formula

Soyalac

MISCELLANEOUS GASTROINTESTINAL DRUGS

activated charcoal: Administered orally or by NG tube, this drug absorbs toxic substances or drugs ingested accidentally or during suicide attempts.

atenolol (Tenormin):   Used to prevent rebleeding from esophageal varices in patients with cirrhosis.

baclofen (Lioresal):   Used to treat intractable hiccoughs.

benzocaine (Americaine Anesthetic):   Topical anesthetic placed on instruments prior to nasogastric intubation, laryngoscopy, esophagoscopy, and sigmoidoscopy.

budesonide (Entocort EC):   Corticosteroid anti-inflammatory drug used to treat Crohn's disease.

celecoxib (Celebrex):   This NSAID and COX-2 inhibitor drug, commonly used to treat osteoarthritis, is also used to decrease the number of colon polyps in patients with familial adenomatous polyposis.

clonidine (Catapres, Catapres-TTS-1, Catapres-TTS-2, Catapres-TTS-3):   Alpha-receptor blocker used to treat ulcerative colitis.

Cotazym, Cotazym-S: Combination drug replacement therapy for the digestive enzymes amylase, lipase, and protease.

cromolyn (Gastrocrom):   Given orally, this mast cell stabilizer prevents the release of histamine and is used to treat patients with food allergies to prevent the occurrence of systemic allergic symptoms.

cyclosporine (Gengraf, Neoral, Sandimmune, SangCya):   Immunosuppressant given to liver transplant patients to prevent rejection of the donor liver.

dehydrocholic acid (Cholan-HMB, Decholin):   Used to thin bile secretions in patients prone to bile duct obstruction.

dexloxiglumide: Used to treat irritable bowel syndrome.

Donnazyme: Combination drug replacement therapy for the digestive enzymes pancreatin, lipase, protease, and amylase.

dyclonine (Dyclone):   Topical anesthetic drug used in the throat prior to esophagoscopy.

ethanolamine (Ethamolin):   A sclerosing drug that is injected locally into esophageal varices to stop bleeding.

glutamic acid: Replacement therapy for low levels of gastric acid in patients with pernicious anemia, allergies, and stomach cancer.

Gustase, Gustase Plus: Combination drug replacement therapy for the digestive enzymes amylase and protease.

hepatitis A vaccine (Havrix, Vaqta)

hepatitis B vaccine (Engerix-B, Recombivax HB)

hydrocortisone (Anusol-HC, Anusol HC-1, Cort-Dome High Potency, Proctocort, ProctoCream-HC):   Topical anti-inflammatory drug for hemorrhoids and perianal itching.

Infalyte: Given orally to children to replace water and electrolytes lost from vomiting and diarrhea.

infliximab (Remicade):   A monoclonal antibody created with recombinant DNA technology that is used to treat the intestinal inflammation of Crohn's disease.

interferon alfa-2a (Roferon-A):   Used to treat hepatitis C.

interferon alfa-2b (Intron A):   Used to treat hepatitis C.

interferon alfacon-1 (Infergen):   Used to treat chronic hepatitis C.

interferon beta-1a (Avonex):   Used to treat non-A, non-B hepatitis.

iodoquinol (Yodoxin):   Used to treat intestinal amebiasis.

ipecac syrup: Used to treat poisonings by inducing vomiting. This drug has been abused by patients with anorexia nervosa and bulimia who use self-induced vomiting to control their weight.

lactulose (Cephulac):   Used to decrease blood ammonia levels in patients with liver disease and encephalopathy.

MCT (medium chain triglycerides):   An easily digested nutritional supplement derived from coconut oil. It is often given to infants or adults who have digestive problems to provide extra calories.

meropenem (Merrem IV):   Carbapenem antibiotic used to treat a ruptured appendix and peritonitis.

morrhuate (Scleromate):   A sclerosing drug that is injected locally into esophageal varices to stop bleeding.

muromonab-CD3 (Orthoclone OKT3):   Monoclonal antibody to human T lymphocytes that acts as an immunosuppressant and is given to transplant patients to prevent rejection of the donor liver.

mycophenolate (CellCept):   Immunosuppressant drug given to transplant patients to prevent rejection of the donor liver.

nadolol (Corgard):   Used to prevent rebleeding from esophageal varices in patients with cirrhosis.

nitazoxanide (NTZ) (Cryptaz):   Used to treat protozoal diarrhea.

> **DID YOU KNOW?**   Massive protozoal (*Cryptosporidium parvum*) contamination of water supplies in Las Vegas and Milwaukee caused 400,000 cases of protozoal diarrhea. It is estimated that 45 million people in the United States are exposed to protozoa-contaminated water each year.

octreotide (Sandostatin, Sandostatin LAR Depot):   Used to treat severe diarrhea caused by irritable bowel syndrome, AIDS-related diarrhea, carcinoid tumors, VIPomas, short-bowel syndrome, dumping syndrome, or chemotherapy.

Pancrease, Pancrease MT 4, Pancrease MT 10, Pancrease MT 16, Pancrease MT 20, Pancrease MT 25:   Combination drug replacement therapy for the digestive enzymes amylase, lipase, and protease.

paromomycin (Humatin):   Aminoglycoside antibiotic used to treat intestinal amebiasis and hepatic coma.

Pedialyte Solution, Pedialyte Freezer Pops: Given orally to children to replace water and electrolytes lost from vomiting and diarrhea.

peginterferon alfa-2b (PEG-Intron):   Used to treat chronic hepatitis C.

pirenzepine (Gastrozepine):   Used to treat peptic ulcers. Investigational drug.

pramoxine (Anusol, ProctoFoam NS, Tronolane):   Topical anesthetic used to treat hemorrhoids.

Preparation H, Preparation H Cooling Gel: Topical drug used to treat hemorrhoids.

Proctofoam-HC: Combination drug with hydrocortisone and a local anesthetic to treat hemorrhoids.

propranolol (Inderal, Inderal LA):   Used to prevent rebleeding from esophageal varices in patients with cirrhosis; used to prevent gastric bleeding in patients with portal hypertension.

Rebetron: Combination of interferon and an antiviral drug used to treat hepatitis C.

Rectagene, Rectagene Medicated Rectal Balm, Rectagene II: Topical drug used to treat hemorrhoids.

> **DID YOU KNOW?**   Both Preparation H and Rectagene contain sharks' liver oil.

roxatidine (Roxin):   Used to treat peptic ulcers. Investigational drug.

scopolamine (Scopace):   Given orally to treat excessive peristalsis of the GI tract in irritable bowel syndrome.

sodium tetradecyl (Sotradecol):   A sclerosing drug that is injected locally into esophageal varices to stop bleeding.

tacrolimus (Prograf):   Immunosuppressant given to transplant patients to prevent rejection of the donor liver.

tegaserod (Zelmac):   A 5-HT$_4$ (serotonin) blocker used to treat irritable bowel syndrome in women. Serotonin is involved in pain perception and GI motility.

terlipressin (Glypressin):   A sclerosing drug that is injected locally into esophageal varices to stop bleeding.

thalidomide (Thalomid):   Used to treat Crohn's disease.

thymalfasin (Zadaxin):   Used to treat hepatitis B.

Twinrix: Combination hepatitis A and hepatitis B vaccine.

Ultrase MT 12, Ultrase MT 18, Ultrase MT 20:   Combination drug replacement therapy for the digestive enzymes amylase, lipase, and protease.

Viokase: Combination drug replacement therapy for the digestive enzymes amylase, lipase, and protease.

Wyanoids Relief Factor: Topical drug used to treat hemorrhoids.

zinc oxide (Nupercainal, Tronolane suppositories):   Topical astringent drug used to treat hemorrhoids.

Zymase: Combination drug replacement therapy for the digestive enzymes amylase, lipase, and protease.

REVIEW QUESTIONS

1. Describe the therapeutic action of H$_2$ blockers.
2. How was the trade name Tagamet selected by the manufacturer?
3. How does the therapeutic action of Carafate differ from that of H$_2$ blockers?
4. Some drugs used to control diarrhea contain opium. True or False?
5. What is unusual about the antiemetic drug Marinol?
6. How do antiemetics exert their therapeutic effect?
7. Describe how 5-aminosalicylic acid is used to treat ulcerative colitis.
8. Name the four categories of laxatives and give examples of drugs from each category.
9. Name three categories of drugs used to treat *H. pylori* infection and give examples of drugs from each category.
10. To what category of drugs does each of these drugs belong?
    Lomotil
    Donnatal
    mesalamine (Asacol, Canasa, Pentasa, Rowasa)
    Mylanta
    nizatidine (Axid AR, Axid Pulvules)
    omeprazole (Prilosec)
    prochlorperazine (Compazine)
    ursodiol (Actigall)

SPELLING TIPS

antacids   Although antacids have an anti-acid effect, the *i* is omitted from *anti* in the correct combined spelling.

Alterna**GEL** but Ampho**jel** and Basal**jel**.

AlternaGEL, CoLyte, GoLYTELY, NuLytely   Unusual internal capitalization.

Compleat   Different spelling than its description as a **complete** nutritional supplement.

Zantac EFFERdose, Zantac GELdose   Unusual internal capitalization.

The ending *-tidine* is common to generic H$_2$ blockers.

GET CONNECTED

Multimedia Extension Activities

 www.prenhall.com/turley

Use the above address to access the free, interactive Companion Website created for this textbook. Included in the features of this site are drug updates and additional chapter-specific exercises for further practice.

14

Musculoskeletal Drugs

CHAPTER CONTENTS

Drugs used to treat osteoarthritis
Drugs used to treat rheumatoid arthritis
Drugs used to treat osteoporosis
Skeletal muscle relaxants
Drugs used to treat tremors
Drugs used to treat gout
Drugs used to treat phantom limb pain
Miscellaneous musculoskeletal drugs
Review questions
Spelling tips

LEARNING OBJECTIVES

After studying this chapter, you should be able to do the following:

1. Name several categories of musculoskeletal drugs.
2. Describe the therapeutic effect of drugs used to treat arthritis, osteoporosis, and gout.
3. Describe the therapeutic effect of skeletal muscle relaxants.
4. Given the generic and trade name of a musculoskeletal drug, identify what drug category it belongs to or what disease it is used to treat.
5. Given a musculoskeletal drug category, identify several generic and trade name drugs within that category.
6. Identify the Historical Notes or Did You Know? section in this chapter that you found most interesting.

Drugs prescribed to treat musculoskeletal conditions such as osteoarthritis, rheumatoid arthritis, osteoporosis, muscle spasms, gout, bursitis, and tendinitis include aspirin, other salicylates, nonsteroidal anti-inflammatory drugs (NSAIDs), gold salts, skeletal muscle relaxants, and so forth. Aspirin and other analgesics used to relieve the pain of minor musculoskeletal conditions (contusions, strains, sprains) are discussed in Chapter 26, "Analgesic Drugs."

DRUGS USED TO TREAT OSTEOARTHRITIS

Osteoarthritis (also known as *degenerative joint disease*) causes pain when cumulative damage ("wear and tear") causes degeneration of the cartilage and the bone ends inside the joint. The weightbearing joints (hips and knees) as well as those joints that are used constantly (fingers) are the first to exhibit signs of osteoarthritis. Inflammation can occur when the synovial membrane of the joint becomes involved or when the damaged bone ends form bony spicules that irritate adjacent tissues.

Drugs used to treat osteoarthritis reduce pain (by inhibiting the production of prostaglandins) and reduce inflammation. These drugs include salicylates (such as aspirin), nonsteroidal anti-inflammatory drugs (NSAIDs), and COX-2 inhibitors. In addition, corticosteroids may be used. None of these drugs, however, can reverse the cartilage and bone damage that has already occurred in the joint.

Salicylates for Osteoarthritis

This class of drugs includes aspirin, the oldest drug used to treat osteoarthritis. Aspirin is also known as *acetylsalicylic acid (ASA)*. The analgesic and anti-inflammatory therapeutic actions of the salicylates are useful in treating the symptoms of osteoarthritis.

> aspirin (Arthritis Foundation Pain Reliever, Ecotrin, Ecotrin Maximum Strength, Empirin, Extended Release Bayer 8-Hour Caplets, Extra Strength Bayer Enteric 500 Aspirin, Genuine Bayer Aspirin, Maximum Bayer Aspirin, Norwich Extra-Strength)
> choline salicylate (Arthropan)
> choline salicylate/magnesium salicylate (Trilisate)
> diflunisal (Dolobid)
> salsalate (Disalcid)

Because salicylate drugs such as aspirin are irritating to the stomach, and long-term therapy with such drugs has been shown to cause peptic ulcers, some manufacturers have taken precautions to reduce this irritation. Ecotrin is manufactured as an enteric-coated tablet that does not dissolve in stomach acid; it dissolves only when it comes in contact with the higher pH environment of the duodenum. Aspirin is often combined with an antacid, as described next.

Combination Salicylates for Osteoarthritis

Aspirin is combined with an antacid to raise the pH of the stomach, inhibit the action of pepsin, and neutralize stomach acid, all of which prevent the formation of peptic ulcers during aspirin therapy.

> Arthritis Pain Formula
> Ascriptin, Ascriptin A/D, Ascriptin Extra Strength

Bayer Buffered Aspirin, Bayer Plus Extra Strength

Bufferin, Tri-Buffered Bufferin

Cama Arthritis Pain Reliever

Acetaminophen for Osteoarthritis

Although acetaminophen is an analgesic like aspirin, it lacks the ability to inhibit the production of prostaglandins and has no anti-inflammatory action. However, the American College of Rheumatology recommends using acetaminophen to treat osteoarthritis because it is the drug of choice for treating musculoskeletal pain in older patients and has fewer side effects compared to NSAIDs, even though it cannot treat the inflammation associated with osteoarthritis.

acetaminophen (Aspirin Free Anacin Maximum Strength, Panadol, Tylenol, Tylenol Arthritis, Tylenol Arthritis Extended Relief, Tylenol Extra Strength, Tylenol Regular Strength)

Nonsteroidal Anti-Inflammatory Drugs (NSAIDs) for Osteoarthritis

NSAIDs inhibit the production of prostaglandins for an analgesic effect, and they also have an anti-inflammatory effect. NSAIDs have less of a tendency than aspirin to cause stomach irritation or peptic ulcers. NSAIDs are structurally similar enough to aspirin that some patients who are allergic to aspirin should not take NSAIDs. The following NSAIDs are used to treat osteoarthritis.

diclofenac (Cataflam, Voltaren, Voltaren-XR)

etodolac (Lodine, Lodine XL)

fenoprofen (Nalfon Pulvules)

flurbiprofen (Ansaid)

ibuprofen (Advil, Advil Liqui-Gels, Haltran, Motrin, Motrin IB)

indomethacin (Indocin, Indocin SR)

ketoprofen (Orudis, Orudis KT, Oruvail)

meclofenamate

meloxicam (Mobic)

nabumetone (Relafen)

naproxen (Aleve, Anaprox, Anaprox DS, EC-Naprosyn, Naprosyn)

oxaprozin (Daypro)

piroxicam (Feldene)

sulindac (Clinoril)

tolmetin (Tolectin 200, Tolectin 600, Tolectin DS)

DID YOU KNOW?   Indomethacin (Indocin) is given intravenously to premature infants who have persistent fetal circulation with a patent ductus arteriosus. The process by which Indocin helps to close the patent ductus arteriosus and establish normal circulation is not known.

Note: The ending *-profen* is common to some generic nonsteroidal anti-inflammatory drugs.

Combination Nonsteroidal Anti-Inflammatory Drugs for Osteoarthritis

This drug combines a nonsteroidal anti-inflammatory with a synthetic prostaglandin drug that protects the gastric mucosa and prevents the formation of peptic ulcers.

Arthrotec (diclofenac, misoprostol)

COX-2 Inhibitors for Osteoarthritis

These drugs, which also belong to the larger category of NSAIDs, selectively inhibit the cyclooxygenase-2 (COX-2) enzyme to decrease the production of prostaglandins and relieve pain.

celecoxib (Celebrex)
rofecoxib (Vioxx)
valdecoxib (Bextra)

IN DEPTH: Prostaglandins, which are present throughout the body and exert various effects, were so named because they were originally isolated from semen from the prostate gland.

Prostaglandins play a role in causing pain in osteoarthritis and rheumatoid arthritis. When body tissue is damaged, cells are destroyed. The contents of the cells spill into the interstitial fluid. There, the cyclooxygenase (COX) enzyme converts one of the intracellular chemicals into prostaglandins. The prostaglandins then stimulate pain receptors in that area. The greater the amount of tissue damage, the more prostaglandins are produced and the greater the sensation of pain. The joints have a large number of pain receptors and damage in the joints can cause chronic, severe pain.

By inhibiting the cyclooxygenase (COX) enzyme, fewer prostaglandins are produced to activate pain receptors.

There are two types of cyclooxygenase (COX) enzyme: COX-1 and COX-2. The COX-1 enzyme plays a role in platelet aggregation and in regulating blood flow and gastric acid levels in the stomach. Aspirin and NSAIDs inhibit COX-1, which blocks the production of prostaglandins that cause pain, but also disrupts the protective action of COX-1 on the stomach. This is why aspirin and NSAIDs can cause stomach upset and peptic ulcers. COX-2 is produced only in response to pain and inflammation. It then produces prostaglandins and this causes pain. Celecoxib, rofecoxib, and valdecoxib selectively inhibit just COX-2 and are known as *COX-2 inhibitors*. Because COX-2 inhibitors do not inhibit the COX-1 enzyme, they do not cause stomach upset and peptic ulcers.

Corticosteroids for Osteoarthritis

Natural corticosteroids, produced in the adrenal cortex, have a powerful anti-inflammatory action. Corticosteroid drugs also have a powerful anti-inflammatory effect and are given orally to treat acute episodes of osteoarthritis associated with inflammation of the synovial membrane. Because of the side effects associated with prolonged oral use, corticosteroid drugs are only used to treat acute exacerbations. For a complete list of oral corticosteroid drugs, see Chapter 21, "Endocrine Drugs."

Corticosteroids can also be injected directly into the joint (intra-articular administration) to relieve pain and inflammation. They can also be injected in the soft tissue near the joint to relieve bursitis and tendinitis. Betamethasone can also be injected into the joint to relieve gouty arthritis.

> betamethasone (Celestone Soluspan)
>
> dexamethasone (Dalalone, Dalalone D.P., Dalalone L.A., Decadron, Decadron-LA, Hexadrol)
>
> hydrocortisone (Hydrocortone)
>
> methylprednisolone (Depo-Medrol, Depopred-40, Depopred-80)
>
> prednisolone (Hydeltrasol, Key-Pred 25, Key-Pred 50, Key-Pred-SP, Predalone 50, Prednisol TBA)
>
> triamcinolone (Aristocort Forte, Aristospan Intra-articular, Kenalog-40)

Other Drugs For Osteoarthritis

Hyaluronic acid is secreted by the synovial membrane of a joint and helps to maintain the lubricating quality of the synovial fluid. These drugs, derivatives of hyaluronic acid, are injected into the joints of patients with osteoarthritis.

> hyaluronic acid derivative (Hyalgan, Synvisc)
>
> sodium hyaluronate (Supartz)

DID YOU KNOW?   Hyaluronic acid derivatives are manufactured from the combs of chickens.

DRUGS USED TO TREAT RHEUMATOID ARTHRITIS

Rheumatoid arthritis produces symptoms of inflammation, swelling, pain, joint deformity, and loss of joint function. It is caused by an autoimmune reaction that targets the joints and cartilage as well as other tissues and organs; the body's own macrophages attack and destroy cartilage and connective tissues. Rheumatoid arthritis is thought to be triggered by a virus.

Salicylates, NSAIDs, and COX-2 Inhibitors for Rheumatoid Arthritis

Rheumatoid arthritis can be treated with many of the same drugs used to treat osteoarthritis. All of the salicylates, NSAIDs, and COX-2 inhibitors described previously (with the exception of meloxicam and rofecoxib) are used to treat rheumatoid arthritis.

None of these drugs is more effective than the other in treating rheumatoid arthritis; the therapeutic effect of the drugs varies from patient to patient. Acetaminophen is used to treat osteoarthritis but not rheumatoid arthritis, because rheumatoid arthritis is associated with a large amount of inflammation against which acetaminophen is not effective.

Salicylates, NSAIDs, and COX-2 inhibitors are the first line of treatment for rheumatoid arthritis. If these drugs fail to control the symptoms, gold compounds may be added to the treatment regimen.

Gold Compounds for Rheumatoid Arthritis

Gold compounds contain actual gold (from 29 to 50% of the total drug) in capsules or in solution for injection. Gold compounds are used to treat active rheumatoid arthritis. These drugs inhibit macrophages that attack the joints and other organs, but cannot reverse damage that has already occurred.

>   auranofin (Ridaura)
>   aurothioglucose (Solganal)
>   gold sodium thiomalate (Aurolate)

Other Drugs for Rheumatoid Arthritis

This drug was originally used (and still is used) to treat malaria but, because it inhibits the immune system, it has been effective in treating rheumatoid arthritis.

>   hydroxychloroquine (Plaquenil)

This drug is human interleukin-1 that is produced through recombinant DNA technology.

>   anakinra (Kineret)

The mechanism of the therapeutic action of these drugs in treating rheumatoid arthritis is not known, but they are effective in reducing joint and tissue inflammation, pain, and swelling.

>   etanercept (Enbrel)
>   infliximab (Remicade)
>   leflunomide (Arava)
>   methotrexate (Rheumatrex, Rheumatrex Dose Pack)
>   sulfasalazine (Azulfidine, Azulfidine EN-tabs)

DID YOU KNOW?   Leflunomide (Arava) has a very long half-life. Traces of the drug can still be found in the body 6 months after the last dose. It is not recommended for use in patients who have decreased liver function because this would prolong the half-life even more.

DID YOU KNOW?   Phenylbutazone (Butazolidin) is commonly used in race horses to reduce inflammation. Its slang name is *bute*. It is illegal to race a horse who is being treated with phenylbutazone, and post-race urine tests are done to look for this drug. In the past, this drug was used to treat arthritis in humans, but was replaced by NSAIDs and finally taken off the market in 1996.

DRUGS USED TO TREAT OSTEOPOROSIS

Osteoporosis (in Latin, *osteo* means *bone;* in Greek, *poros* means *pore*) is a thinning of the bone due to demineralization. Osteoporosis is much more common in women than men, and most common in postmenopausal women. Before menopause, bone is continually being formed and broken down. As estrogen levels decrease in menopause, the rate of bone formation decreases but the rate of bone breakdown remains constant. This causes the bones to slowly and progressively thin. Additional risk factors for osteoporosis include Caucasian or Asian race, slender build, smoking, and alcohol abuse. Osteoporosis is prevented or treated by giving estrogen (to decrease bone breakdown), supplementing calcium, and increasing exercise (to stimulate bone growth).

DID YOU KNOW?   An estimated 1.3 million fractures due to osteoporosis occur annually in the United States: 25% of postmenopausal women have spinal compression fractures from osteoporosis and 15% have hip fractures. Healthcare costs for hip fractures alone exceeded $7 billion in 1995.

Osteoporosis affects about 25 million women and men in the United States. Supermodel Lauren Hutton has been featured in drug advertisements for hormone replacement therapy (estrogen). She states that she disregarded her physician's advice to begin hormone replacement therapy when she experienced hot flashes at the beginning of menopause. The following year, when she found her height had decreased by 1 inch (due to bone loss), she started hormone replacement therapy.

I. Skaer, "Prevention and Treatment of Osteoporosis," *Pharmacy and Therapeutics*, 1995 (20) p. 88.

For hormone replacement therapy and estrogen drugs, see Chapter 23, "Obstetric/Gynecologic Drugs."

Drugs That Inhibit Bone Resorption for Osteoporosis

The hormone calcitonin is normally produced by the thyroid gland and regulates calcium and the rate of bone resorption (breakdown). This drug has the same action as calcitonin. It is derived from salmon calcitonin, which is more potent than human calcitonin.

calcitonin-salmon (Miacalcin)

These drugs decrease the rate of bone resorption by inhibiting osteoclasts (cells that break down bone).

alendronate (Fosamax)
etidronate (Didronel)
pamidronate (Aredia)
risedronate (Actonel)

> **DID YOU KNOW?**   These drugs are also used to treat Paget's disease (a chronic, progressive disease characterized by bone breakdown with excessive rebuilding and deformed bones).

This drug belongs to the class of drugs known as *selective estrogen receptor modulators* (SERMs). It activates estrogen receptors to decrease the rate of bone resorption.

raloxifene (Evista)

Calcium Supplements for Osteoporosis

OTC calcium supplements are numerous. In addition, milk with added calcium is available in the dairy section of the supermarket. Also, the antacid Tums, which uses calcium to neutralize stomach acid, has advertised that it has a secondary therapeutic effect of calcium supplementation for women.

SKELETAL MUSCLE RELAXANTS

Acute musculoskeletal conditions such as strains, sprains, and "pulled muscles" are treated with analgesics and anti-inflammatory drugs; however, the physician may also elect to prescribe a skeletal muscle relaxant in addition to rest and physical therapy. Skeletal muscle relaxants specifically relieve muscle spasm and stiffness.

carisoprodol (Soma)
chlorphenesin (Maolate)
chlorzoxazone (Paraflex, Parafon Forte DSC)
cyclobenzaprine
diazepam (Valium)
metaxalone (Skelaxin)
methocarbamol (Robaxin, Robaxin-750)
orphenadrine (Norflex)

These skeletal muscle relaxants are used to treat severe muscle spasticity in patients with multiple sclerosis, cerebral palsy, stroke, or spinal cord injury.

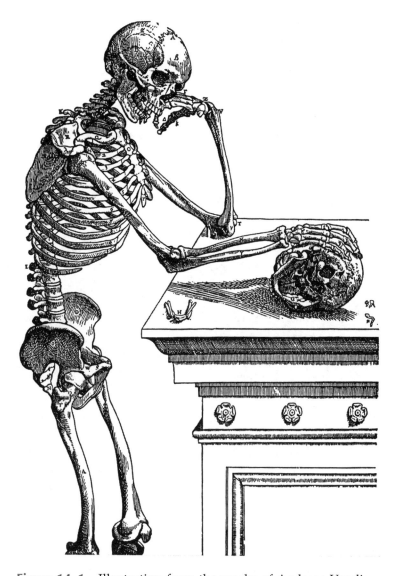

Figure 14–1 Illustration from the works of Andreas Vesalius. *J.B. Saunders and C. O'Malley,* The Illustrations from the Works of Andreas Vesalius of Brussels *(New York, NY: Dover Publications, 1950), p. 87.*

baclofen (Lioresal)
dantrolene (Dantrium)
diazepam (Valium)
L-baclofen (Neuralgon)
tizanidine (Zanaflex)

Combination Skeletal Muscle Relaxants

These drugs contain a skeletal muscle relaxant with the analgesic aspirin and/or the narcotic analgesic codeine.

>   Norgesic (orphenadrine, aspirin)
>   Robaxisal (methocarbamol, aspirin)
>   Soma Compound (carisoprodol, aspirin)
>   Soma Compound with Codeine (carisprodol, aspirin, codeine)

DRUGS USED TO TREAT TREMORS

Beta-blockers block the action of epinephrine at beta receptors and have been found to be helpful in the treatment of essential familial tremor (small involuntary, rhythmic movements of the head and neck), a condition that seems to be hereditary.

>   metoprolol (Lopressor, Toprol-XL)
>   nadolol (Corgard)
>   propranolol (Inderal, Inderal LA)
>   timolol (Blocadren)

DRUGS USED TO TREAT GOUT

Gout is caused by a metabolic defect that allows uric acid to accumulate in the blood. The kidneys are unable to excrete the excess uric acid, and it crystallizes within the joints, causing pain and inflammation. Drugs used to treat gout act either by increasing the excretion of uric acid in the urine or by inhibiting enzymes that produce uric acid in the blood.

>   allopurinol (Zyloprim)
>   colchicine
>   probenecid
>   sodium thiosalicylate (Rexolate)
>   sulfinpyrazone (Anturane)

These drugs help prevent the formation of uric acid stones in the kidneys.

>   potassium citrate (Polycitra-K, Urocit-K)
>   potassium citrate/sodium citrate (Polycitra, Polycitra-LC)

In addition, several nonsteroidal anti-inflammatory drugs (NSAIDs) have been found to be of particular benefit in treating gout and gouty arthritis.

>   indomethacin (Indocin, Indocin SR)
>   naproxen (Aleve, Anaprox, Anaprox DS, EC-Naprosyn, Naprosyn)
>   sulindac (Clinoril)

DRUGS USED TO TREAT PHANTOM LIMB PAIN

After an amputation, most patients experience pain that seems to come from the amputated limb. Nerve impulses coming from just above the area of amputation are interpreted by the brain as being from the missing limb. This pain diminishes over time, but is treated with tricyclic antidepressants that have been found to be effective in treating different types of pain.

> amitriptyline (Elavil)
> amoxapine
> desipramine (Norpramin)
> doxepin (Sinequan, Sinequan Concentrate)
> imipramine (Tofranil, Tofranil-PM)
> nortriptyline (Aventyl, Aventyl Pulvules, Pamelor)
> protriptyline (Vivactil)

MISCELLANEOUS MUSCULOSKELETAL DRUGS

Absorbine Power Gel: Topical irritant drug used to mask the pain of arthritis and muscular aches.

Acthar Gel (ACTH hormone):   Hormonal drug used to treat rheumatoid arthritis.

amiprilose (Therafectin):   Investigational drug used to treat rheumatoid arthritis.

Ben-Gay Original Ointment, Ben-Gay Regular Strength, Ben-Gay SPA, Ben-Gay Ultra Strength, Arthritis Formula Ben-Gay, Vanishing Scent Ben-Gay: Topical irritant drug used to mask the pain of arthritis and muscular aches.

botulinum toxin type A (Botox, Dysport):   Used to treat cervical dystonia (torticollis), muscle contractions that cause neck pain and abnormal head position; used to treat muscle contractures in patients with cerebral palsy.

botulinum toxin type B (Myobloc):   Used to treat cervical dystonia (torticollis), muscle contractions that cause neck pain and abnormal head position.

bupivacaine (Marcaine):   Local anesthetic injected into the joint cavity following arthroscopic surgery to relieve postoperative pain.

calcitonin-human (Cibacalcin):   Calcium-regulating hormone used to treat Paget's disease.

capsaicin (Capsin, Zostrix, Zostrix-HP):   Topical irritant drug used to mask the pain of arthritis.

captopril (Capoten):   Used to treat rheumatoid arthritis.

carprofen (Rimadyl):   NSAID; investigational drug for osteoarthritis and rheumatoid arthritis. Already used by veterinarians for dogs and cats.

clonidine (Catapres, Catapres-TTS-1, Catapres-TTS-2, Catapres-TTS-3):   Alpha-receptor blocker used to treat restless legs syndrome.

dapsone: Used to treat rheumatoid arthritis.

Decadron with Xylocaine: Combination corticosteroid anti-inflammatory and anesthetic drug injected to treat bursitis and tenosynovitis.

Eucalyptamint, Eucalyptamint Maximum Strength: Topical irritant drug used to mask the pain of arthritis and muscular aches.

Flexall Ultra Plus, Maximum Strength Flexall 454:   Topical irritant drug used to mask the pain of arthritis and muscular aches.

gentamicin (Septopal):   Used to treat osteomyelitis; antibiotic beads on a wire that is surgically implanted.

HuMax-CD4:   Investigational drug used to treat rheumatoid arthritis.

hydroxychloroquine (Plaquenil):   In addition to rheumatoid arthritis, this drug is also used to treat systemic lupus erythematosis (a chronic, progressive disease characterized by joint and muscle pain and degeneration of connective tissue).

Icy Hot, Icy Hot Arthritis Therapy, Icy Hot Balm: Topical irritant drug used to mask the pain of arthritis and muscle aches.

interferon beta-1a (Avonex, Rebif):   Interferon is produced in the body in response to a viral infection. This drug is used to treat juvenile rheumatoid arthritis (which may be triggered by a virus, although the exact cause is unknown).

interleukin-1 (Antril):   Used to treat juvenile rheumatoid arthritis.

isoxicam (Maxicam):   NSAID used to treat osteoarthritis or rheumatoid arthritis. Investigational drug.

mazindol (Sanorex):   Used to treat Duchenne's muscular dystrophy.

misoprostol (Cytotec):   Given to patients on long-term aspirin or NSAIDs to prevent the common side effect of peptic ulcers. Aspirin and NSAIDs inhibit the formation of prostaglandins; prostaglandins normally act to protect the gastric mucosa. Misoprostol is a synthetic prostaglandin that protects the gastric mucosa when natural prostaglandin is inhibited by arthritis drugs.

Musterole Deep Strength Rub: Topical irritant drug used to mask the pain of arthritis and muscle aches.

pamidronate (Aredia):   Inhibits the breakdown of bone; in addition to osteoporosis, this drug is used to treat hypercalcemia of malignancy, metastatic bone lesions from breast cancer and multiple myeloma, and Paget's disease.

paroxetine (Paxil):   Used to treat fibromyalgia.

Sportscreme Ice Gel: Topical irritant drug used to mask the pain of arthritis and muscular aches.

tenidap (Enable):   Anti-inflammatory cytokine inhibitor used to treat rheumatoid arthritis. Investigational drug.

Therapeutic Mineral Ice, Therapeutic Mineral Ice Exercise Formula: Topical irritant drug used to mask the pain of arthritis and muscular aches.

tiludronate (Skelid):   Inhibits the breakdown of bone; used to treat Paget's disease.

zoledronic acid (Zometa):   Used to treat Paget's disease. Investigational drug.

REVIEW QUESTIONS

1. Give the meaning of these abbreviations: ASA, COX, NSAID.
2. Contrast the therapeutic action of aspirin with that of acetaminophen.
3. How does enteric-coated aspirin help prevent gastric ulcers in arthritis patients?
4. Name several trade names for the generic drug ibuprofen.
5. Indocin is a NSAID used to treat both arthritis in the elderly and patent ductus arteriosus in premature infants. True or False?
6. Why are gold salts useful in treating rheumatoid arthritis but not osteoarthritis?
7. List the medical conditions for which a skeletal muscle relaxant drug might be prescribed.
8. Describe the action of the various types of drugs used to treat gout.
9. Name the categories of drugs used to treat arthritis and give examples of drugs from each category.
10. Name the categories of drugs used to treat osteoporosis, describe their actions, and give examples of drugs in each category.
11. To what category of drugs does each of these drugs belong?
    alendronate (Fosamax)
    allopurinol (Zyloprim)
    auranofin (Ridaura)
    carisoprodol (Soma)
    celecoxib (Celebrex)
    triamcinolone (Aristocort Forte, Aristospan Intra-articular)

SPELLING TIPS

Several gold salt drug names contain *au*, the chemical symbol for gold: **au**ranofin, Rid**aura**, **au**ro-thioglucose.

Vioxx Double *x*.

GET CONNECTED

Multimedia Extension Activities

 www.prenhall.com/turley

Use the above address to access the free, interactive Companion Website created for this textbook. Included in the features of this site are drug updates and additional chapter-specific exercises for further practice.

15

Cardiovascular Drugs

CHAPTER CONTENTS

Drugs used to treat congestive heart failure (CHF)
Drugs used to treat angina pectoris
Drugs used to treat myocardial infarction (MI)
Drugs used to treat arrhythmias
Antihypertensive drugs
Drugs used to treat hypertensive crisis
Drugs used to treat peripheral vascular disease
Drugs used to treat hyperlipidemia
Miscellaneous cardiovascular drugs
Review questions
Spelling tips

LEARNING OBJECTIVES

After studying this chapter, you should be able to do the following:

1. Name several categories of cardiovascular drugs.
2. Describe the therapeutic action of drugs used to treat congestive heart failure, angina, arrhythmias, and hyperlipidemia.
3. Describe the therapeutic action of antihypertensive drugs and peripheral vasodilators.
4. Given the generic and trade name of a cardiovascular drug, identify what drug category it belongs to or what disease it is used to treat.
5. Given a cardiovascular drug category, identify several generic and trade name drugs within that category.
6. Identify the Historical Notes or Did You Know? section in this chapter that you found most interesting.

Cardiovascular drugs are used to treat a variety of conditions, including congestive heart failure (CHF), angina pectoris, arrhythmias, hypertension, hypertensive crisis, and hyperlipidemia.

DRUGS USED TO TREAT CONGESTIVE HEART FAILURE (CHF)

Congestive heart failure (CHF) occurs when the heart muscle is weakened and unable to adequately pump blood. Right-sided heart failure results in a backup of blood from the right ventricle into the venous circulation, producing liver enlargement and edema in the extremities. Left-sided heart failure results in a backup of blood from the left ventricle into the pulmonary circulation, producing pulmonary edema.

Cardiac Glycosides for Congestive Heart Failure (CHF)

The cardiac glycosides have a molecular structure that consists of chains of glucose sugars known as *glycosides*, hence the name *cardiac glycosides*.

DID YOU KNOW?   Cardiac glycosides are extracted from dried foxglove plants (*Digitalis lanata*) (see Figure 15–1). The term *digitalis* refers collectively to cardiac glycosides as a class of drugs and digoxin as a specific drug. Physicians often use a slang term—*dig* (pronounced "dij")—for digoxin.

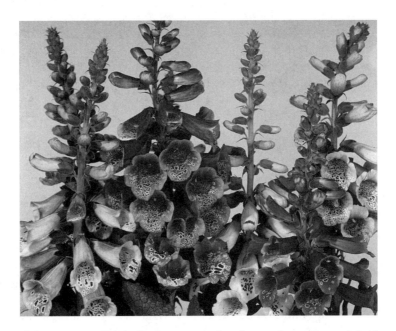

Figure 15–1   *Digitalis lanata*, or foxglove plant, the original source of the cardiac drug digitalis. *Photo reprinted courtesy of W. Atlee Burpee Company, Warminster, PA.*

HISTORICAL NOTES: In the 1500s, foxglove was given the botanical name *Digitalis,* which referred to its fingerlike flowers (like the digits of the hand). In the 1780s, an English physician published a book on foxglove and its medical uses. He stated, "My opinion was asked concerning a family recipe for the cure of dropsy [an old term for the symptoms of congestive heart failure]. I was told that it had long been kept a secret by an old woman in Shropshire who had sometimes made cures after the more regular practitioners had failed. I was informed also that the effects produced were violent vomiting. . . . This medicine was composed of 20 or more different herbs; but it was not very difficult for one conversant in these subjects to perceive that the active herb could be no other than foxglove."

Michael C. Gerald, *Pharmacology: An Introduction to Drugs,* 2nd ed. (Englewood Cliffs, NJ: Prentice Hall, 1981), p. 402, out of print.

IN DEPTH: Cardiac glycosides are used to treat CHF; this application is based on the two separate medical effects of cardiac glycosides: They make the heart pump more slowly but more efficiently.

Negative chronotropic effect. This refers to the ability of cardiac glycosides to slow the heart rate. Cardiac glycosides cause the release of acetylcholine, which depresses the SA node and slows electrical conduction. Note: *Chrono-* refers to *time.*

Positive inotropic effect. This refers to the ability of cardiac glycosides to increase the strength of cardiac contractions. Cardiac glycosides inhibit the flow of positive sodium ions into the cell, which allows positive calcium ions to enter instead. The increased level of intracellular calcium results in a stronger contraction of the cells of the myocardium. Note: *Ino-* refers to *(cardiac muscle) fibers.*

In combination, the negative chronotropic effect and the positive inotropic effect allow the heart to pump more efficiently and fill completely before the next contraction—an important therapeutic action for patients with CHF.

The cardiac glycosides used to treat CHF include:

digoxin (Lanoxicaps, Lanoxin)

Digitalis toxicity from cardiac glycosides is a serious and frequent adverse effect. Nearly one-third of patients taking a cardiac glycoside develop symptoms of digitalis toxicity. This is because these drugs have a low **therapeutic index** (i.e., there is a narrow margin between the therapeutic dose and the toxic dose) and a long **half-life,** which is even more prolonged in elderly patients with decreased kidney function. Symptoms of toxicity may include a pulse rate below 60 beats per minute, confusion, restlessness, nausea/vomiting, diarrhea, yellow-green halos around lights (see Figure 15–2), or hallucinations.

To prevent toxic effects, physicians periodically order blood tests to monitor the drug level to make sure it is therapeutic. These tests are often referred to as "dig levels"

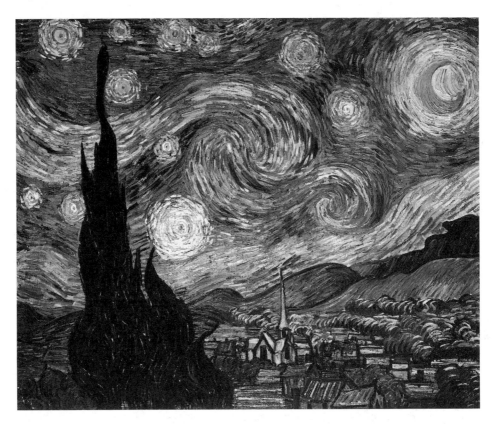

Figure 15–2 Digitalis toxicity. Vincent van Gogh's "The Starry Night" (1889) is felt by some physicians to show evidence of digitalis toxicity in the way the Dutch painter depicted yellow-green halos around the stars. Van Gogh (1853–1890) suffered from mania and epilepsy and may have been given digitalis for lack of a more specific drug therapy available at that time. *GOGH, Vincent van. The Starry Night. (1889) Oil on canvas, 29 × 36 1/4" (73.7 × 92.1 cm). The Museum of Modern Art, New York. Acquired through the Lillie P. Bliss Bequest. Photograph © 2002 The Museum of Modern Art, New York.*

(pronounced *"dij"*). Symptoms of toxicity may be treated in one of three ways: (1) decrease the dosage of the cardiac glycoside; (2) change the dosage of the cardiac glycoside to a less frequent schedule; or in severe cases, (3) administer a drug, such as those listed next, that binds with and inactivates the cardiac glycoside in the gastrointestinal tract or in the bloodstream.

cholestyramine (LoCHOLEST, LoCHOLEST Light, Prevalite, Questran, Questran Light)
colestipol (Colestid)
digoxin immune Fab (Digibind)

DID YOU KNOW?   Digibind is obtained from sheep that have been treated to produce antibodies against the basic molecule of digoxin. The trade name drug Digidote originates from *digi* for *digitalis* and *dote* for *antidote*. The term *Fab* in the generic drug name stands for *fragment, antibody binding*.

Diuretics for Congestive Heart Failure (CHF)

Diuretics are often combined with cardiac glycosides to treat patients with CHF. Diuretics act to increase the excretion of sodium and water to reduce edema, a common symptom of CHF. For a complete discussion of diuretics, see Chapter 12, "Urinary Tract Drugs."

ACE Inhibitors for Congestive Heart Failure (CHF)

Angiotensin-converting enzyme (ACE) inhibitors block the enzyme that converts angiotensin I to angiotensin II, a vasoconstrictor. By blocking this enzyme, ACE inhibitors cause vasodilation, decrease the blood pressure, and decrease pulmonary vascular and peripheral resistance against which the heart must pump. ACE inhibitors may be used in conjunction with diuretics and digitalis to treat CHF.

> captopril (Capoten)
> enalapril (Vasotec, Vasotec I.V.)
> fosinopril (Monopril)
> lisinopril (Prinivil, Zestril)
> quinapril (Accupril)
> ramipril (Altace)

Calcium Channel Blockers for Congestive Heart Failure (CHF)

Calcium channel blockers block the movement of calcium ions into myocardial cells and the smooth muscle cells in blood vessel walls. These drugs decrease the heart rate and blood pressure.

> felodipine (Plendil)
> nicardipine (Cardene, Cardene I.V., Cardene SR)
> nifedipine (Adalat, Adalat CC, Procardia, Procardia XL)
> verapamil (Calan, Calan SR, Covera-HS, Isoptin, Isoptin SR, Verelan, Verelan PM)

Other Drugs for Congestive Heart Failure (CHF)

These drugs increase the strength of contraction of the heart muscle but do not belong to the cardiac glycoside class. These drugs are prescribed for patients who have not responded to treatment with cardiac glycosides and diuretics.

> inamrinone
> milrinone (Primacor)

This drug blocks beta$_1$ and beta$_2$ receptors in the heart to decrease the heart rate and blood pressure. A more detailed description of beta-blocker therapeutic action and beta receptors is provided later in this chapter.

propranolol (Inderal, Inderal LA)

This drug blocks both alpha and beta receptors to decrease the heart rate and cardiac output.

carvedilol (Coreg)

This drug blocks just alpha$_1$ receptors to dilate the blood vessels and decrease the blood pressure.

prazosin (Minipress)

This angiotensin II receptor blocker dilates the blood vessels and decreases the blood pressure.

valsartan (Diovan)

See the section on antihypertensive drugs later in this chapter for a description of the therapeutic action of alpha- and beta-blockers and angiotensin II receptor blockers.

This drug belongs to a new class of drugs known as *human B-type natriuretic peptides (hBNP)*. It binds to receptors on the smooth muscle of blood vessels and causes them to dilate, decreasing the blood pressure. This drug is used to treat severely decompensated CHF.

nesiritide (Natrecor)

> **DID YOU KNOW?** Nesiritide (Natrecor) is manufactured from *E. coli* bacteria using recombinant DNA technology.

DRUGS USED TO TREAT ANGINA PECTORIS

The pain of angina pectoris occurs when cells of the myocardium receive insufficient oxygenated blood to meet their needs. This can be caused by an increased need for oxygen during exercise or stress. It can also be due to an increased **afterload** (the pressure of the arterial system against which the heart must pump) or an increased **preload** (the pressure of the pulmonary circulatory system and the pressure in the left ventricle during diastole). Angina can also occur because of plaques in the coronary arteries, spasm of the coronary arteries, or vasoconstriction from smoking, which decreases the supply of oxygen to the heart. The pain of angina pectoris denotes cellular ischemia but not cellular death. If untreated, however, this ischemia can progress to cellular death (i.e., a myocardial infarction [MI]).

Drugs used to treat angina include nitrates, beta-blockers, and calcium channel blockers, as discussed next.

Nitrates for Angina Pectoris

As a group, nitrates act as vasodilators throughout the circulatory system. By dilating veins, they reduce preload and thereby decrease the need of the myocardium for oxygen. By dilating arteries, they decrease systemic vascular resistance and arterial blood pressure. They also increase the flow of oxygenated blood through the coronary arteries.

The most frequently prescribed nitrate is nitroglycerin. Nitrates can be administered in several different ways. However, not every nitrate can be administered by every route listed below.

Administration Routes

sublingually as a spray
sublingually as a tablet
translingually as a spray
transmucosally between the cheek and gum (buccal) as a tablet
inhaled through the nose
orally as a chewable tablet
orally as a sustained-release capsule or tablet
transdermally as a patch
topically as an ointment (measured in inches)
intravenously

Drugs

amyl nitrite (Amyl Nitrite Aspirols)
isosorbide dinitrate (Isordil, Isordil Titradose, Isordil Tembids, Sorbitrate)
isosorbide mononitrate (Imdur)
nitroglycerin (Deponit, Minitran, Nitro-Bid, Nitro-Bid IV, Nitrodisc, Nitro-Dur, Nitrogard, Nitrol, Nitrolingual, Nitrong, Nitrostat, Transderm-Nitro, Tridil)

DID YOU KNOW? Physicians often dictate "nitro paste" when the correct drug form is actually nitroglycerin ointment. Topical nitroglycerin (Nitro-Bid, Nitrol) is applied to the skin using an applicator paper that has a measuring line on it. The ointment dosage is measured in inches!

Beta-Blockers for Angina Pectoris

Although nitrates, particularly nitroglycerin, are the standard for antianginal therapy, beta-blockers may also be prescribed. Beta-blockers act to decrease the heart rate, which in turn decreases the need of the myocardium for oxygen; this decreases anginal pain. A more detailed description of beta-blocker action and beta receptors is provided later in this chapter.

atenolol (Tenormin)

bisoprolol (Zebeta)

carteolol (Cartrol)

esmolol (Brevibloc)

metoprolol (Lopressor, Toprol-XL)

nadolol (Corgard)

propranolol (Inderal, Inderal LA)

Note: The ending *-olol* is common to generic beta-blockers.

Note: Not all beta-blockers are indicated for treating angina; beta-blockers are also used to treat hypertension and arrhythmias. These applications are discussed later in this chapter.

This drug blocks both beta and alpha$_1$ receptors to lower the blood pressure.

carvedilol (Coreg)

Calcium Channel Blockers for Angina Pectoris

Calcium channel blockers may be used in conjunction with nitrates or beta-blockers to treat angina. Calcium channel blockers relax the smooth muscle of the blood vessels to decrease arterial pressure (the pressure against which the heart must pump). This decreases the heart's need for oxygen. Calcium channel blockers also dilate the coronary arteries and prevent coronary artery spasm that can trigger angina.

amlodipine (Norvasc)

bepridil (Vascor)

diltiazem (Cardizem, Cardizem CD, Cardizem SR, Dilacor XR, Tiamate)

nicardipine (Cardene, Cardene I.V., Cardene SR)

nifedipine (Adalat, Adalat CC, Procardia, Procardia XL)

verapamil (Calan, Calan SR, Covera-HS, Isoptin, Isoptin SR, Verelan, Verelan PM)

Note: The ending *-ipine* is common to generic calcium channel blockers.

IN DEPTH: On a cellular level, calcium channel blockers act in the following way. The pumping contraction of the heart muscle as well as the contraction of smooth muscles in the blood vessels depends on the flow of calcium ions from outside to inside each cell. These calcium ions move into the cell in a specific way, through what are known as *calcium channels*. Calcium channel blockers prevent the movement of calcium from outside the cell through these channels to inside the cell. With less calcium inside the cell, it contracts less strongly and less often. This effect is felt throughout the body as smooth muscles in the blood vessels relax, the blood pressure decreases, and the heart muscle contracts less forcefully and less frequently.

DRUGS USED TO TREAT MYOCARDIAL INFARCTION (MI)

When the cellular ischemia associated with angina pectoris is not treated, it may progress to cellular death (i.e., an MI).

For thrombolytic drugs given at the time of a heart attack, see Chapter 17, "Anticoagulant and Thrombolytic Drugs."

Certain ACE inhibitors can increase survival rate when given within 24 hours of an MI.

captopril (Capoten)

lisinopril (Prinivil, Zestril)

quinapril (Accupril)

Long-term studies have shown that some drugs can prevent the occurrence of a second heart attack.

aspirin (Bayer Low Adult Strength, Ecotrin, Ecotrin Adult Low Strength, Empirin, Genuine Bayer Aspirin, Halfprin 81, Heartline, St. Joseph Adult Chewable Aspirin)

atenolol (Tenormin)

metoprolol (Lopressor, Toprol-XL)

propranolol (Inderal, Inderal LA)

timolol (Blocadren)

For patients who have already had an MI, the beta-blockers atenolol, metoprolol, propranolol, and timolol can be prescribed to reduce the risk of a second heart attack.

DID YOU KNOW?   Certain antidepressants have been found to reduce the risk of a second heart attack. These drugs, known as *selective serotonin reuptake inhibitors (SSRIs)*, include the commonly prescribed drugs Prozac, Paxil, Luvox, and Zoloft. Depression is a known risk factor for heart disease, but these drugs have another recently discovered therapeutic effect: preventing platelets from forming blood clots, the most common cause of heart attacks.

DRUGS USED TO TREAT ARRHYTHMIAS

Cardiac arrhythmias are caused by abnormalities in the conduction of electrical impulses from the SA node through the AV node, bundle of His, and Purkinje system in the heart. Disruptions in this conduction pattern and changes in the normal period of time between beats (the refractory period) result in various arrhythmias involving the atria or ventricles. Arrhythmias can manifest as bradycardia (abnormally slow heart rate), tachycardia (abnormally fast heart rate), atrial flutter (very rapid contraction of the atria not coordinated with the ventricles), ventricular fibrillation (ineffective, extremely rapid contractions of the ventricles), or irregularly spaced beats (bigeminy, premature contractions, heart block).

This drug is used to treat bradycardia by inhibiting acetylcholine and increasing conduction through the SA node.

atropine

Antiarrhythmic drugs that treat flutter or fibrillation exert a therapeutic effect by acting at different times during the electrical cycle of the heart. (This cycle can be visualized graphically on an electrocardiogram. Depolarization of the atria and ventricles corresponds to the P and QRS waves, respectively; repolarization of the ventricles corresponds to the T wave.) Some antiarrhythmic drugs exert their effect during depolarization; other antiarrhythmic drugs exert their effect during repolarization, when the cell returns to its original resting state. The action of each drug is based on slowing the rapid flow of positive sodium ions from outside the cell, through the cell membrane, to inside the cell.

These antiarrhythmic drugs are only used to treat atrial arrhythmias.

clonidine (Catapres, Catapres-TTS-1, Catapres-TTS-2, Catapres-TTS-3)
dofetilide (Tikosyn)
ibutilide (Corvert)

DID YOU KNOW?   The antiarrhythmic drug Corvert takes its name from the terms *cor* (Latin for *heart*) and *vert* for *convert* (the arrhythmia).

These antiarrhythmic drugs are only used to treat ventricular arrhythmias.

adenosine (Adenocard)
amiodarone (Cordarone)
bretylium
disopyramide (Norpace, Norpace CR)
lidocaine (Xylocaine HCl IV for Cardiac Arrhythmias)
mexiletine (Mexitil)
moricizine (Ethmozine)
procainamide (Procanbid, Pronestyl, Pronestyl-SR)
propafenone (Rythmol)
tocainide (Tonocard)

Lidocaine (LidoPen Auto-Injector) is self-injected by cardiac patients to treat their own life-threatening cardiac arrhythmias.

These antiarrhythmic drugs are used to treat both atrial and ventricular arrhythmias.

flecainide (Tambocor)
quinidine (Quinaglute Dura-Tabs, Quinidex Extentabs)

DID YOU KNOW?   The antiarrhythmic drug lidocaine (Xylocaine) is also a topical anesthetic. Its action topically is similar to its antiarrhythmic action in that it inhibits the flow of sodium into the cell. In the heart, this slows the electrical impulse that normally causes the heart to contract.

As an anesthetic, lidocaine actually stops electrical impulses along sensory nerves. With no impulses traveling along sensory nerves, there is no transmission/perception of pain.

Beta-Blockers for Arrhythmias

In addition to the standard antiarrhythmic drugs described earlier, beta-blockers are also prescribed for ventricular arrhythmias. They act by blocking beta receptors in the heart from responding to epinephrine. Epinephrine is normally released by the sympathetic nervous system and acts to increase the heart rate. By blocking the effects of epinephrine at beta receptors in the heart, beta-blockers are effective in slowing the heart rate and controlling arrhythmias. Beta-blockers are only indicated for ventricular arrhythmias.

> acebutolol (Sectral)
>
> atenolol (Tenormin)
>
> bisoprolol (Zebeta)
>
> esmolol (Brevibloc)
>
> metoprolol (Lopressor, Toprol-XL)
>
> nadolol (Corgard)
>
> pindolol (Visken)
>
> propranolol (Inderal, Inderal LA)
>
> sotalol (Betapace, Betapace AF)
>
> timolol (Blocadren)

Calcium Channel Blockers for Arrhythmias

By blocking the movement of calcium in and out of the SA node, these drugs cause the heart to beat more slowly and inhibit arrhythmias.

> diltiazem (Cardizem, Cardizem CD, Cardizem SR, Dilacor XR, Tiamate)
>
> verapamil (Calan, Calan SR, Covera-HS, Isoptin, Isoptin SR, Verelan, Verelan PM)

Other Drugs for Arrhythmias

Cardiac glycoside drugs have an antiarrhythmic effect. They cause the release of acetylcholine, which depresses the SA node and slows electrical conduction. This therapeutic effect is used to treat atrial flutter/fibrillation.

> digoxin (Lanoxicaps, Lanoxin)

This drug is used to treat ventricular arrhythmias caused by digitalis toxicity.

edetate (Endrate)

ANTIHYPERTENSIVE DRUGS

Hypertension (HTN) is a condition that manifests itself as an increase in systolic and/or diastolic blood pressure. HTN is caused by arteriosclerosis, kidney disease, or other diseases, or it may have no identified cause; this last type is known as *essential hypertension*. HTN is defined as a systolic blood pressure of greater than or equal to 140 mmHg and a diastolic blood pressure of greater than or equal to 90 mmHg.

The treatment of HTN follows what is known as a stepped-care approach. Life-style changes are suggested first: patients are asked to restrict the use of salt in cooking and at the table, or the physician may prescribe a low-salt diet to place a limit on total dietary sodium intake. In addition, the patient may be asked to lose weight, exercise, and stop smoking. If these measures cannot control the blood pressure, drugs may be added to the treatment regimen. An antihypertensive drug, often a diuretic, is prescribed first. If a satisfactory reduction in blood pressure is not achieved, a second antihypertensive drug, such as a beta-blocker, is added. Beta-blockers may also be selected as the first step of treatment. Other drugs, such as calcium channel blockers, ACE inhibitors, angiotensin II receptor blockers, alpha-receptor blockers, or vasodilators may be added.

Diuretics for Hypertension (HTN)

By promoting the excretion of sodium and water, diuretics decrease the total blood volume, which lowers the blood pressure. For a complete discussion of the therapeutic action of this class of drugs, see Chapter 12, "Urinary Tract Drugs."

Beta-Blockers for Hypertension (HTN)

Beta-blockers cause the heart to beat less frequently and dilate the blood vessels; these actions contribute to lowering the blood pressure.

IN DEPTH: Beta receptors are special protein molecules located on the cell membrane of the heart cells and in the smooth muscle surrounding the blood vessels and bronchi. Beta receptors in the heart are designated $beta_1$ or β_1 receptors. Those in the smooth muscle of blood vessels or bronchi are designated $beta_2$ or β_2 receptors. Beta receptors are stimulated by epinephrine released by the sympathetic nervous system (in response to stress or danger). When $beta_1$ receptors in the heart are stimulated, they cause the heart rate to increase. When $beta_2$ receptors in smooth muscle are stimulated, they cause the blood vessels to constrict. These two responses result in a rise in blood pressure. In addition, when $beta_2$ receptors in the smooth muscle of the bronchi are stimulated, they cause the bronchi to relax, increasing air flow to the lungs. All of these responses prepare the body to respond to stress or danger by "fight or flight."

In response to stress or danger, these effects are desirable. However, in patients with HTN or angina pectoris, these effects are undesirable. Therefore these patients are given drugs to block the action of epinephrine on beta receptors. These drugs are known as *beta-blockers*. Beta-blockers produce the opposite effect of the action of epinephrine.

Drugs that block both beta$_1$ and beta$_2$ receptors are termed *nonselective beta-blockers*. Some beta-blockers are more selective in their action and block only beta$_1$ receptors in the heart; these drugs are termed *cardioselective beta-blockers*.

Hypertensive patients with asthma are not treated with a nonselective beta-blocker because the beta$_2$ blocking action would cause bronchial constriction. Cardioselective beta-blockers that have no effect on the bronchi would be prescribed for hypertensive asthmatic patients.

Nonselective Beta-Blockers for Hypertension (HTN)

carteolol (Cartrol)

nadolol (Corgard)

penbutolol (Levatol)

pindolol (Visken)

propranolol (Inderal, Inderal LA)

timolol (Blocadren)

Cardioselective Beta-Blockers for Hypertension (HTN)

acebutolol (Sectral)

atenolol (Tenormin)

betaxolol (Kerlone)

bisoprolol (Zebeta)

esmolol (Brevibloc)

metoprolol (Lopressor)

Note: The ending *-olol* is common to many generic beta-blockers.

DID YOU KNOW?   Several beta-blockers (atenolol, metoprolol, nadolol, propranolol, and timolol) are prescribed to prevent migraine headaches. These drugs act on beta receptors in blood vessels in the brain to limit the tendency of the vessels to overdilate during a migraine.

Several beta-blockers are prescribed to treat performance anxiety (stage fright). Professional musicians, actors, and even professional golfers use beta-blockers to block the symptoms of excess epinephrine (dry mouth, tremor, cold extremities, GI upset, inability to concentrate) that impair their ability to perform.

Calcium Channel Blockers for Hypertension (HTN)

Calcium channel blockers exert a therapeutic effect by relaxing the smooth muscle of blood vessels and causing them to dilate, thereby decreasing blood pressure.

amlodipine (Norvasc)
diltiazem (Cardizem, Cardizem CD, Cardizem SR, Dilacor XR, Tiamate)
felodipine (Plendil)
isradipine (DynaCirc, DynaCirc CR)
nicardipine (Cardene, Cardene I.V., Cardene SR)
nifedipine (Adalat, Adalat CC, Procardia, Procardia XL)
nisoldipine (Sular)
verapamil (Calan, Calan SR, Covera-HS, Isoptin, Isoptin SR, Verelan, Verelan PM)

ACE Inhibitors for Hypertension (HTN)

Angiotensin-converting enzyme (ACE) inhibitors have an antihypertensive action that is distinctly different from that of the other drugs described previously. They act by dilating arterial blood vessels and also decreasing blood volume in the following ways.

IN DEPTH: The body has its own natural blood pressure-regulating system. In response to low blood pressure, the kidneys secrete renin, which then helps to synthesize angiotensin I. Angiotensin I is a relatively inactive substance until, when acted upon by angiotensin-converting enzyme, it becomes angiotensin II, a strong vasoconstrictor. Angiotensin II not only constricts blood vessels to raise the blood pressure, it also stimulates the adrenal glands to produce aldosterone. Aldosterone, by inhibiting the excretion of sodium and water from the kidneys, increases the blood volume and raises the blood pressure.

ACE inhibitors, when used to treat hypertension, prevent angiotensin-converting enzyme from changing angiotensin I into angiotensin II. Without angiotensin II, the blood vessels dilate and the blood pressure lowers. Without angiotensin II, the adrenal glands do not produce extra aldosterone, the blood volume decreases, and this also lowers the blood pressure.

ACE inhibitors used to treat HTN include:

benazepril (Lotensin)
captopril (Capoten)
enalapril (Vasotec, Vasotec I.V.)
fosinopril (Monopril)
lisinopril (Prinivil, Zestril)
moexipril (Univasc)
perindopril (Aceon)

quinapril (Accupril)

ramipril (Altace)

trandolapril (Mavik)

Note: The ending *-pril* is common to generic ACE inhibitors.

Angiotensin II Receptor Blockers for Hypertension (HTN)

This class of drugs binds to the same receptor as angiotensin II does and thus blocks angiotensin II from activating the receptor. (This is in contrast to ACE inhibitors that block the enzyme that produces angiotensin II.) When angiotensin II is blocked, the blood vessels dilate and the blood pressure decreases.

candesartan (Atacand)

eprosartan (Teveten)

irbesartan (Avapro)

losartan (Cozaar)

telmisartan (Micardis)

valsartan (Diovan)

Note: The ending *-sartan* is common to generic angiotensin II receptor blockers.

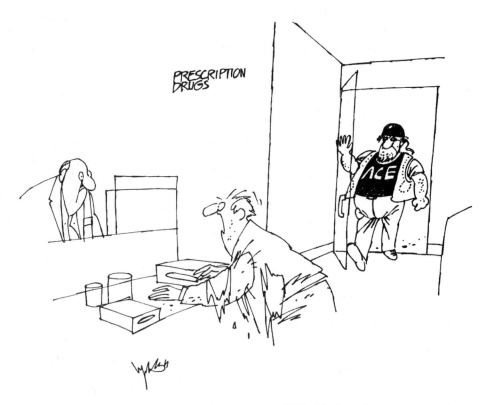

Figure 15–3 *Quick . . . ACE inhibitors.*—David W. Harbaugh. *Reprinted with permission.*

Vasopeptidase Inhibitors (VPIs) for Hypertension (HTN)

This class of drugs inhibits neutral endopeptidase (NEP), an enzyme that regulates blood pressure.

omapatrilat (Vanlev)

Other Drugs for Hypertension (HTN)

Receptors in the sympathetic nervous system consist of both **alpha** (alpha$_1$, alpha$_2$) and **beta** (beta$_1$ and beta$_2$) **receptors.** When activated by norepinephrine, alpha receptors contract the smooth muscle in blood vessels and raise the blood pressure. The role of beta receptors in constricting blood vessels and raising blood pressure has been previously described.

These drugs block alpha$_1$ and all beta receptors. This relaxes the smooth muscle in blood vessels and lowers the blood pressure.

carvedilol (Coreg)
labetalol (Normodyne, Trandate)

Other antihypertensive drugs block just alpha$_1$ receptors. All of the alpha$_1$ receptors are located in the peripheral blood vessels in both arteries and veins. Blocking these receptors causes both the arteries and veins to dilate, and this lowers the blood pressure.

doxazosin (Cardura)
prazosin (Minipress)
terazosin (Hytrin)

Note: The ending *-azosin* is common to generic alpha$_1$-receptor blockers.

Other antihypertensive drugs block just alpha$_2$ receptors. Alpha$_2$ receptors are located in the brain. Blocking these receptors decreases the number of nerve impulses traveling from the sympathetic nervous system to the heart and blood vessels. This causes the heart rate to decrease and the blood vessels to dilate, which lowers the blood pressure.

guanabenz (Wytensin)
guanfacine (Tenex)

Other antihypertensive drugs block all alpha$_1$ and alpha$_2$ receptors.

clonidine (Catapres, Catapres-TTS-1, Catapres-TTS-2, Catapres-TTS-3)
methyldopa (Aldomet)

DID YOU KNOW?   Clonidine has also been used to relieve the symptoms of nicotine withdrawal in patients who want to stop smoking.

These drugs deplete the store of norepinephrine in the adrenal medulla or block its release so that it cannot stimulate alpha receptors in the heart and blood vessels.

> guanadrel (Hylorel)
> guanethidine (Ismelin)
> reserpine

These drugs alter the movement of calcium in the smooth muscle cells of the blood vessels. By relaxing smooth muscle, the blood vessels dilate and the blood pressure decreases. Note: Although calcium channel blockers act in a similar way these two categories of antihypertensive drugs are not related to each other.

> hydralazine (Apresoline)
> minoxidil (Loniten)

DID YOU KNOW?   Minoxidil is also marketed under the trade name Rogaine and is used to treat male pattern baldness. Applied topically, its vasodilator action reestablishes blood flow to hair follicles, resulting in new hair growth in some patients.

This drug belongs to a new class of antihypertensive drugs known as *renin inhibitor drugs*. Normally, renin produced by the kidneys changes angiotensinogen to angiotensin I, which is then converted to angiotensin II, a powerful vasoconstrictor. By blocking renin, angiotensin II is never created, and the blood pressure falls.

> aliskiren

Because of its side effects, this drug is only used to treat severe HTN.

> mecamylamine (Inversine)

Combination Drugs for Hypertension (HTN)

The following drugs combine two different antihypertensives.

> Lexxel Extended-Release Tablet (enalapril, felodipine)
> Lotrel (amlodipine, benazepril)
> Teczem Extended-Release Tablet (enalapril, diltiazem)

The following drugs combine an antihypertensive with a diuretic.

> Accuretic (quinapril, hydrochlorothiazide)
> Aldoclor-150, Aldoclor-250 (methyldopa, chlorothiazide)

Aldoril-15, Aldoril-25, Aldoril D30, Aldoril D50 (methyldopa, hydrochlorothiazide)

Apresazide 25/25, Apresazide 50/50, Apresazide 100/50 (hydralazine, hydrochlorothiazide)

Atacand HCT (candesartan, hydrochlorothiazide)

Avalide (irbesartan, hydrochlorothiazide)

Capozide 25/15, Capozide 25/25, Capozide 50/15, Capozide 50/25 (captopril, hydrochlorothiazide)

Combipres 0.1, Combipres 0.2, Combipres 0.3 (clonidine, chlorthalidone)

Corzide 40/5, Corzide 80/5 (nadolol, bendroflumethiazide)

Diovan HCT (valsartan, hydrochlorothiazide)

Enduronyl, Enduronyl Forte (deserpidine, methyclothiazide)

Esimil (guanethidine, hydrochlorothiazide)

Hyzaar (losartan, hydrochlorothiazide)

Inderide 40/25, Inderide 80/20, Inderide LA 80/50, Inderide LA 120/50, Inderide LA 160/50 (propranolol, hydrochlorothiazide)

Lopressor HCT 50/25, Lopressor HCT 100/25, Lopressor HCT 100/50 (metoprolol, hydrochlorothiazide)

Lotensin 5/6.25, Lotensin HCT 10/12.5, Lotensin HCT 20/12.5, Lotensin HCT 20/25 (benazepril, hydrochlorothiazide)

Metatensin #4 (reserpine, trichlormethiazide)

Micardis HCT (telmisartan, hydrochlorothiazide)

Minizide 1, Minizide 2, Minizide 5 (prazosin, polythiazide)

Prinzide, Prinzide 12.5, Prinzide 25 (lisinopril, hydrochlorothiazide)

Rauzide (rauwolfia, bendroflumethiazide)

Renese-R (reserpine, polythiazide)

Salutensin, Salutensin-Demi (reserpine, hydroflumethiazide)

Ser-Ap-Es (hydralazine, reserpine, hydrochlorothiazide)

Tenoretic 50, Tenoretic 100 (atenolol, chlorthalidone)

Timolide 10-25 (timolol, hydrochlorothiazide)

Vaseretic 5-12.5, Vaseretic 10-25 (enalapril, hydrochlorothiazide)

Zestoretic (lisinopril, hydrochlorothiazide)

Ziac (bisoprolol, hydrochlorothiazide)

DRUGS USED TO TREAT HYPERTENSIVE CRISIS

A patient in hypertensive crisis exhibits an extremely high blood pressure; this is a life-threatening emergency. Beta-blockers, calcium channel blockers, peripheral vasodilators, and other drugs with different therapeutic actions are all potent vasodilators that can quickly lower the blood pressure when given intravenously.

diazoxide (Hyperstat IV)
enalapril (Vasotec I.V.)

fenoldopam (Corlopam)

hydralazine

labetalol (Normodyne, Trandate)

nicardipine (Cardene I.V.)

nitroglycerin (Nitro-Bid IV, Tridil)

nitroprusside (Nitropress)

phentolamine (Regitine)

trimethaphan (Arfonad)

DID YOU KNOW?   In the past, nifedipine (Adalat, Procardia) was used to treat severe HTN/hypertensive crisis by puncturing the capsule with a pin and squirting the drug under the tongue. This is no longer recommended by the manufacturer.

DRUGS USED TO TREAT PERIPHERAL VASCULAR DISEASE

Peripheral vasodilators are used to increase peripheral blood flow to treat diseases such as arteriosclerosis obliterans, Buerger's disease, Raynaud's disease, and diabetic peripheral vascular insufficiency. These drugs selectively dilate deep blood vessels in skeletal muscles rather than those in the skin.

ethaverine

isoxsuprine (Vasodilan)

papaverine

Patients with peripheral vascular disease often experience intermittent claudication (calf pain caused by ischemia) when they exercise. This drug improves blood flow by decreasing the thickness of the blood and increasing RBC flexibility.

pentoxifylline (Trental)

DRUGS USED TO TREAT HYPERLIPIDEMIA

Hyperlipidemia is a general term encompassing both hypercholesterolemia (increased levels of serum cholesterol) and hypertriglyceridemia (increased levels of serum triglycerides). Hyperlipidemia is one of several well-defined risk factors for atherosclerosis.

Normally, cholesterol is produced by the liver; a certain amount of cholesterol is needed by the body for the production of hormones and bile and as a component of skin and nerve fibers. However, excess dietary intake of cholesterol can cause elevated serum cholesterol levels. Dietary sources of cholesterol include foods of animal origin, such as meats, egg yolks, bacon, shrimp, cream, lard, and so forth. Some patients develop extremely high serum cholesterol levels, not because of excess dietary intake, but because they have a genetic disorder. They have too few receptors on the cell membranes for cholesterol to bind to, and so cholesterol levels in the blood remain high.

Triglycerides are produced by the liver and are used to make subcutaneous fat to cushion and protect the body. Excess dietary intake of nonanimal fats can result in excessive storage of fat in the body and high triglyceride levels in the blood. Dietary sources of triglycerides include oils, margarine, and sugar. Also of interest is that excess dietary intake of sugar is converted into triglycerides.

DID YOU KNOW?   Alcoholics often have extremely elevated serum triglyceride levels. Alcoholic beverages contain no nutrients except sugar. The large amount of calories consumed in drinking alcoholic beverages is converted to triglycerides.

Just as water and oil do not mix, so fats or lipids (cholesterol and triglycerides) do not mix with the serum portion of the blood. To be transported through the blood, cholesterol and triglycerides must bind to certain proteins that can carry them in the serum. These carrier molecules, a combination of lipids and proteins, are known as **lipoproteins.** There are three types of lipoproteins found in the body, and their functions are quite different.

High-density lipoproteins (HDLs). This lipoprotein carries serum cholesterol to the liver where it is excreted in the bile; therefore, high levels of HDL are desirable.

Low-density lipoproteins (LDLs). This lipoprotein carries serum cholesterol to the cells where it is metabolized for energy. However, it can also deposit serum cholesterol on artery walls to form arteriosclerotic plaques; thus, high levels of LDL are undesirable.

Very low-density lipoproteins (VLDLs). This lipoprotein carries triglycerides; high levels of VLDL are undesirable.

Dietary therapy rather than drug therapy is the first choice of treatment for hyperlipidemia. In addition, these lifestyle changes may be recommended: exercise, weight loss, decreased alcohol consumption, or cessation of smoking.

Bile Acid Sequestrants for Hypercholesterolemia

Normally, some of the cholesterol in bile is reabsorbed back into the bloodstream from the small intestine. Bile acid sequestrant drugs cause the bile to become an insoluble complex. The cholesterol within the bile is then excreted in the feces rather than being reabsorbed back into the bloodstream.

cholestyramine (LoCHOLEST, LoCHOLEST Light, Prevalite, Questran, Questran Light)

colesevelam (Welchol)

colestipol (Colestid)

HMG-CoA Reductase Inhibitors for Hypercholesterolemia

HMG-CoA reductase is an enzyme that acts during one of the steps in the production of cholesterol in the body. HMG-CoA reductase inhibitor drugs block this step. They also increase the amount of HDL. Because the phrase *HMG-CoA reductase inhibitors* is rather awkward, this class of drugs is also known as **statins** because all the generic drug names in this class end in *-statin*. Patients on these drugs are periodically monitored for liver function abnormalities.

atorvastatin (Lipitor)

fluvastatin (Lescol, Lescol XL)

lovastatin (Mevacor)

pravastatin (Pravachol)

simvastatin (Zocor)

DID YOU KNOW?   In 2001, the manufacturer of lovastatin (Mevacor) asked the FDA to allow this drug to switch from a prescription drug to an OTC drug, but the FDA would not approve this change.

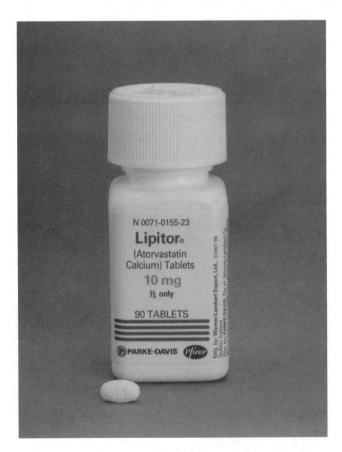

Figure 15–4   The prescription drug atorvastatin (Lipitor), an HMG-CoA reductase inhibitor used to treat hypercholesterolemia. *Photo reprinted courtesy of Pfizer Inc., New York.*

Other Drugs for Hyperlipidemia

Drugs that reduce serum triglyceride levels act by decreasing the production of triglycerides in the liver and by inhibiting the synthesis of and/or accelerating the breakdown of VLDL. This results in lower serum levels of triglycerides and less VLDL to act as a carrier for triglycerides. Fenofibrate (Tricor) also decreases serum cholesterol and LDL levels.

clofibrate (Atromid-S)
fenofibrate (Tricor)
gemfibrozil (Lopid)

Niacin is a B vitamin that is used to treat hypercholesterolemia. Omega-3 fatty acids are a nutritional supplement used to treat hypertriglyceridemia.

niacin (Niaspan)
omega-3 fatty acids (Promega Pearls Softgels, Promega Softgels)
Cholestin

Combination Drugs for Hyperlipidemia

Advicor (lovastatin, niacin)

DID YOU KNOW? Omega-3 fatty acids are found in the oil of cold water fish. While the American Heart Association recommends eating fish, it does not endorse the use of fish oil supplement. Cholestin is a food supplement that can be purchased without a prescription. It contains red yeast that has been fermented either on rice or honeybee pollen. Its active ingredient is a naturally occurring form of the cholesterol-lowering prescription drug lovastatin. Cholestin (under the name Hong Qu) has been used in China for over 2000 years for cardiovascular health.

EMERGENCY CARDIAC DRUGS

Emergency drugs used in cardiovascular resuscitation are discussed in Chapter 16, "Emergency Drugs."

ANTICOAGULANT AND THROMBOLYTIC DRUGS

Anticoagulant and thrombolytic drugs are discussed in Chapter 17, "Anticoagulant and Thrombolytic Drugs."

MISCELLANEOUS CARDIOVASCULAR DRUGS

abciximab (ReoPro):   Platelet aggregation inhibitor used to prevent blood clots in patients with unstable angina or MIs, or in patients who are undergoing angioplasty or atherectomy.

acetazolamide (Diamox, Diamox Sequels):   Used to treat the edema of CHF.

alprostadil (prostaglandin E1, Prostin VR Pediatric):   A prostaglandin drug used to treat newborn infants with congenital heart defects. The drug keeps the ductus arteriosus open to provide oxygenated blood to the body until surgical correction can be accomplished.

> **DID YOU KNOW?**   Alprostadil (prostaglandin E1, Caverject, Muse) is used to treat erectile impotence. This drug relaxes smooth muscle in the penis and lets blood flow in to create an erection.

alteplase (Activase):   Tissue plasminogen activator used to dissolve blood clots from an MI.

amoxicillin: Used prophylactically to prevent bacterial endocarditis in patients with congenital heart disease or rheumatic heart disease undergoing dental procedures and other surgery.

anistreplase (Eminase):   Thrombolytic enzyme used to dissolve blood clots that cause an MI.

aprotinin (Trasylol):   Hemostatic drug that decreases perioperative blood loss in patients undergoing coronary artery bypass grafting.

cardioplegic solution (Plegisol):   Electrolyte solution injected into the aorta to induce cardiac arrest at the beginning of open heart surgery.

celiprolol (Selecor):   Selective beta$_2$-blocker for hypertension and angina pectoris. Investigational drug.

Chromagen: Combination oral vitamin B$_{12}$, intrinsic factor, and iron drug used to treat iron deficiency anemia and pernicious anemia.

cifenline (Cipralan):   Used to treat arrhythmias. Investigational drug.

cilazapril (Inhibace):   ACE inhibitor used to treat HTN and CHF. Investigational drug.

cilostazol (Pletal):   Vasodilator used to treat intermittent claudication in patients with peripheral vascular disease.

clopidogrel (Plavix):   Platelet aggregation inhibitor used to reduce the risk of MI in patients with atherosclerosis and a history of MIs.

cyanocobalamin (Nascobal):   Vitamin B$_{12}$ used to treat treat pernicious anemia. Vitamin B$_{12}$ is necessary for RBC formation. Absorption of dietary vitamin B$_{12}$ depends on the presence of intrinsic factor in the stomach. When levels of intrinsic factor are decreased, as in pernicious anemia, B$_{12}$ is given nasally or by I.M. injection.

cyclosporine (Gengraf, Neoral, Sandimmune, SangCya): Immunosuppressant drug given to transplant patients to prevent rejection of the donor heart.

dexrazoxane (Zinecard): Used to prevent cardiomyopathy in patients receiving doxorubicin chemotherapy.

dilevalol (Unicard): Beta-blocker used to treat HTN. Investigational drug.

dipyridamole (Persantine): A coronary artery vasodilator for patients with coronary artery disease who cannot tolerate an exercise stress test. Normally, exercise on a treadmill is used to induce angina. Because these patients cannot exercise, dipyridamole is given to dilate the arteries, causing the heart rate to increase. This will provoke angina in these patients and result in a positive test. Also, this drug is a platelet aggregation inhibitor used to prevent blood clots after cardiac valve replacement surgery.

dobutamine (Dobutrex): Vasopressor used to treat decompensated CHF.

dopamine (Intropin): Vasopressor used to treat decompensated CHF.

eptifibatide (Integrilin): Platelet aggregation inhibitor used to prevent blood clots in patients with unstable angina or MIs, or in patients who are undergoing angioplasty or atherectomy.

ethaverine: Peripheral vasodilator used to treat blood vessel spasm in peripheral vascular disease.

Ferotrinsic: Combination oral vitamin B_{12}, intrinsic factor, and iron drug used to treat iron deficiency anemia and pernicious anemia.

Ferrlecit: Used to treat iron deficiency anemia in hemodialysis patients.

hydroxocobalamin: Vitamin B_{12} given by I.M. injection to treat pernicious anemia.

indecainide (Decabid): Antiarrhythmic drug. Investigational drug.

indomethacin (Indocin I.V.): NSAID used to close a patent ductus arteriosus in premature infants with persistent fetal circulation. The mechanism by which it exerts its action is not known.

isoproterenol (Isuprel): Used to treat heart block.

isoxsuprine (Vasodilan): Peripheral vasodilator used to treat peripheral vascular disease and Raynaud's disease.

Kayexalate: Used to treat hyperkalemia.

lacidipine (Lacipil): Calcium channel blocker used to treat HTN. Investigational drug.

midodrine (ProAmatine): Alpha$_1$-receptor stimulator used to treat orthostatic hypotension.

morphine (Astramorph PF, Duramorph, Infumorph, Kadian, MS Contin, MSIR, OMS Concentrate, Oramorph SR, RMS, Roxanol, Roxanol 100, Roxanol Rescudose, Roxanol T): Narcotic analgesic used to treat dyspnea in patients with severe CHF.

morrhuate (Scleromate): Sclerosing drug injected into varicose veins of the lower extremities to obliterate the veins.

muromonab-CD3 (Orthoclone OKT3): Monoclonal antibody to human T lymphocytes that acts as an immunosuppressant and is given to transplant patients to prevent rejection of the donor heart.

mycophenolate (CellCept):   Immunosuppressant drug given to transplant patients to prevent rejection of the donor heart.

nitrendipine (Baypress):   Calcium channel blocker used to treat HTN. Investigational drug.

papaverine: Peripheral vasodilator used to treat blood vessel spasm of the coronary arteries and peripheral vascular disease.

pinacidil (Pindac):   Vasodilator used to treat HTN. Investigational drug.

Pronemia Hematinic Capsule: Combination oral vitamin B_{12}, intrinsic factor, and iron drug used to treat iron deficiency anemia and pernicious anemia.

reteplase (Retavase):   Tissue plasminogen activator used to dissolve blood clots from an MI.

sodium tetradecyl (Sotradecol):   Sclerosing drug injected into varicose veins of the lower extremities to obliterate the veins.

streptokinase (Streptase):   Thrombolytic enzyme used to dissolve blood clots from an MI or deep venous thrombosis.

tacrolimus (Prograf):   Immunosuppressant drug given to transplant patients to prevent rejection of the donor heart.

tenecteplase (TNKase):   Tissue plasminogen activator used to dissolve blood clots from an MI.

tirofiban (Aggrastat):   Platelet aggregation inhibitor used to prevent blood clots in patients with unstable angina or MIs, or in patients who are undergoing angioplasty or atherectomy.

tolazoline (Priscoline):   Used to decrease persistent pulmonary hypertension in newborns with persistent fetal circulation who cannot maintain adequate levels of oxygenation.

TriHemic 600:   Combination oral vitamin B_{12}, intrinsic factor, and iron drug used to treat iron deficiency anemia and pernicious anemia.

Trinam: Vascular endothelial growth factor gene contained within a biodegradable device. It is used to prevent intimal hyperplasia within blood vessels that have been surgically anastomosed.

Trinsicon: Combination oral vitamin B_{12}, intrinsic factor, and iron drug used to treat iron deficiency anemia and pernicious anemia.

vesnarinone (Arkin-Z):   Used to treat CHF. Investigational drug.

REVIEW QUESTIONS

1. What two basic therapeutic effects do cardiac glycosides exert on the heart?

2. As a student of both pharmacology and art history, what insightful comment might you make concerning Vincent van Gogh's painting, "The Starry Night"?

3. The ending *-olol* is common to generic calcium channel blockers. True or False?

4. Beta-blockers can be used to treat angina, HTN, and arrhythmias. True or False?

5. Name five routes by which nitroglycerin can be administered.

6. Sheep's antibodies: Digibind = foxglove: _____.
   A. Digitalis plant
   B. Lanoxin
   C. DynaCirc
   D. Inderal

7. What drug used to treat ventricular arrhythmias is also commonly used as a local anesthetic?

8. Describe the difference in the therapeutic action of nonselective beta-blockers and cardioselective beta-blockers.

9. How do bile acid sequestrants exert a therapeutic effect in patients with hyperlipidemia?

10. If a patient exhibits symptoms of digitalis toxicity, what three interventions may the physician choose from?

11. Name the categories of drugs used to treat angina and give an example of a drug from each category.

12. Name the categories of drugs used to treat HTN and give an example of a drug from each category.

13. To what category does each of these drugs belong?
    atenolol (Tenormin)
    atropine
    carvedilol (Coreg)
    diltiazem (Cardizem)
    losartan (Cozaar)
    quinapril (Accupril)
    timolol (Blocadren)
    Zestoretic

14. Define these abbreviations: ACE, CHF, "dig," Fab, HTN.

CLINICAL SCENARIO

Uncontrolled arrhythmias can cause syncope (dizziness). Review this patient's admission Physician's Order Record (see Figure 15–5) and answer the following questions. Use the Glossary/Index at the end of this textbook to verify the spelling of drug names.

What drug allergies does the patient have?

What two medications are prescribed for this patient?

What are the full names of these drugs?

Write the instructions for the drug route and administration in plain English.

SPELLING TIPS

arrhythmia   Often misspelled with just one *r*.
Catapres   Only one *s*.
LoCHOLEST   Unususal internal capitalization.
Cholestin but Colestid   (sound-alikes).

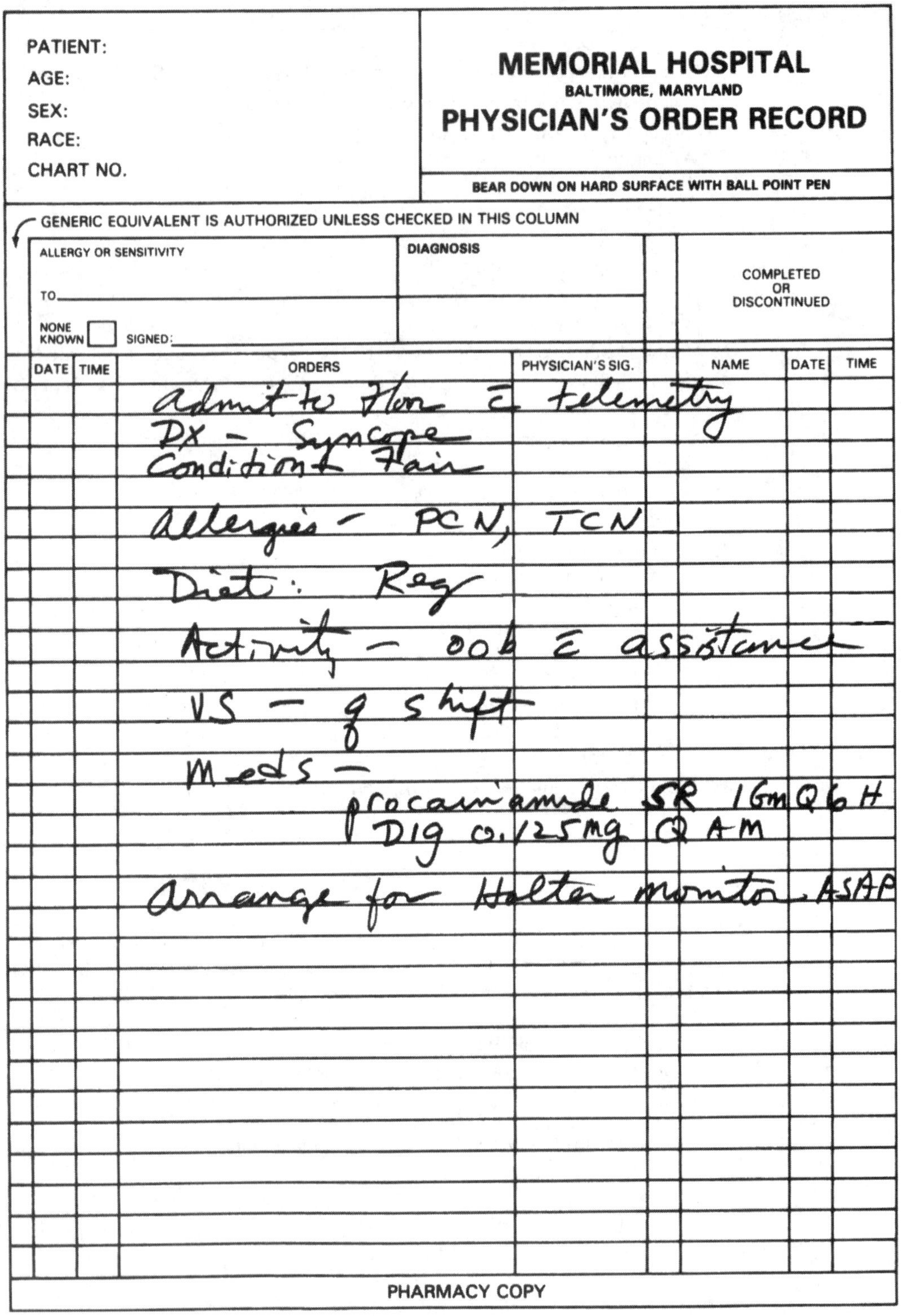

PATIENT:
AGE:
SEX:
RACE:
CHART NO.

MEMORIAL HOSPITAL
BALTIMORE, MARYLAND
PHYSICIAN'S ORDER RECORD

BEAR DOWN ON HARD SURFACE WITH BALL POINT PEN

GENERIC EQUIVALENT IS AUTHORIZED UNLESS CHECKED IN THIS COLUMN

ALLERGY OR SENSITIVITY
TO
NONE KNOWN ☐ SIGNED:

DIAGNOSIS

COMPLETED OR DISCONTINUED

DATE	TIME	ORDERS	PHYSICIAN'S SIG.		NAME	DATE	TIME
		admit to Flor c̄ telemetry					
		DX – Syncope					
		Condition: Fair					
		Allergies – PCN, TCN					
		Diet: Reg					
		Activity – OOB c̄ assistance					
		VS – q shift					
		Meds –					
		procainamide SR 1Gm Q6H					
		DIG 0.125mg Q AM					
		arrange for Holter monitor ASAP					

PHARMACY COPY

Figure 15–5 Physician's Order Record. *Reprinted courtesy of Marvin Stoogenke,* The Pharmacy Technician, *2nd ed. (Upper Saddle River, NJ: Brady/Prentice Hall, 1998), p. 32.*

Combipres   Only one *s*.

DynaCirc   Unusual internal capitalization.

Lopressor   Double *s*.

Minipress   Double *s*.

Nitro-Bid   Unusual internal capitalization.

Nitropress   Double *s*.

Rythmol   Does not have an *h* like *rhythm*.

Vaseretic but Vasotec.   *Vase*- but *Vaso*-.

The ending *-olol* is common to generic beta-blockers.

The ending *-opine* is common to generic calcium channel blockers.

The ending *-pril* is common to generic ACE inhibitors.

GET CONNECTED

Multimedia Extension Activities

 www.prenhall.com/turley

Use the above address to access the free, interactive Companion Website created for this textbook. Included in the features of this site are drug updates and additional chapter-specific exercises for further practice.

16

Emergency Drugs

CHAPTER CONTENTS

Routes of administration for emergency drugs
Drugs for emergency resuscitation
Drugs used after successful resuscitation
Drugs used to treat overdose or suicide attempts
Drugs used to treat anaphylactic shock
Miscellaneous emergency drugs
Review questions
Spelling tips

LEARNING OBJECTIVES

After studying this chapter, you should be able to do the following:

1. Describe several routes for administering emergency drugs.
2. Describe the therapeutic action of several drugs used during and after emergency resuscitation.
3. Describe the therapeutic action of drugs used to treat overdose, suicide attempts, and anaphylactic shock.
4. Identify the Did You Know? section in this chapter that you found most interesting.

There are several types of life-threatening emergencies that require prompt intervention with drugs: cardiac or respiratory arrest, shock from infection or trauma, anaphylaxis, or drug overdose. Unless these problems can be corrected within a matter of minutes, oxygen levels in the blood decrease, carbon dioxide and lactic acid levels in the blood increase, the blood pH becomes more acidic, cell metabolism in the vital organs slowly comes to a halt, and the patient dies.

Basic life support measures as performed in **cardiopulmonary resuscitation (CPR)** involve mechanically circulating the blood and inflating the lungs. **Advanced cardiac life support (ACLS)** includes the use of drug therapy. A **crash cart** containing all necessary emergency drugs and resuscitative equipment is available in every patient area in the hospital and in physicians' offices and clinics.

ROUTES OF ADMINISTRATION FOR EMERGENCY DRUGS

The routes used to administer emergency drugs are different than the routes normally used to administer drugs. This is because of the need to have the drugs take immediate effect at a systemic level. In an emergency, most routes of administration result in too slow an absorption rate for the drug to produce therapeutic results before the patient dies.

Intravenous

Drugs are injected into an I.V. line and given by **I.V. push** or **bolus** to produce a maximum drug effect in the shortest period of time. Following successful resuscitation, continuous I.V. drip infusion is used. The I.V. route is by far the most common route for administering emergency drugs.

Endotracheal

Drugs are administered by placing the solution into an endotracheal tube. As the lungs are mechanically ventilated, the drug solution is pushed into the lungs, where it is rapidly absorbed by the lung tissue and carried through the pulmonary capillaries to the bloodstream. Therapeutic systemic drug levels can be attained, but only certain drugs can be administered by this route.

> **DID YOU KNOW?**   Nurses use the acronym NAVEL, as outlined in the *ACLS Guidelines,* to help them remember which drugs are appropriate to give via an endotracheal tube.
>
> | | |
> |---|---|
> | N | naloxone (Narcan) |
> | A | atropine |
> | V | Valium (diazepam) |
> | E | epinephrine (Adrenalin) |
> | L | lidocaine (Xylocaine HCl for Cardiac Arrhythmias) |

Intracardiac

Intracardiac injection is not used frequently, but can be valuable when other routes have failed to produce a therapeutic result. This route carries with it the risk of pneumothorax, cardiac tamponade, or coronary artery laceration if the injection is not properly placed into the left ventricular chamber.

atropine
calcium chloride
epinephrine (Adrenalin)
isoproterenol (Isuprel)

DRUGS FOR EMERGENCY RESUSCITATION

Drugs for Severe Arrhythmias

Lidocaine is indicated for the management of life-threatening ventricular fibrillation and is the drug of choice in resuscitative efforts for patients with this problem. It inhibits the flow of sodium into the cell; this slows the electrical impulse that causes the heart to fibrillate. This drug has no therapeutic effect if the heart is in asystole.

lidocaine (Lidocaine HCl for Cardiac Arrhythmias)

Atropine blocks the action of acetylcholine released from the vagus nerve. The vagus nerve is part of the parasympathetic nervous system with branches that innervate the myocardium at the SA and AV nodes. When acetylcholine is released, the heart rate slows. Atropine is used specifically to treat severe bradycardia and bradyarrhythmia.

atropine

Drugs for Asystole

Epinephrine is released by the sympathetic nervous system in response to pain, danger, or stress. Epinephrine prepares the body to respond with either "flight or fight" by causing the following changes.

- Constriction of peripheral blood vessels due to stimulation of alpha receptors. This raises the blood pressure.
- Increased heart rate and cardiac output due to stimulation of beta$_1$ receptors in the heart muscle.
- Relaxation of bronchial smooth muscle due to stimulation of beta$_2$ receptors. This causes bronchodilation and increased air flow to the lungs.

During a cardiac arrest, if the heart is in ventricular fibrillation, epinephrine (Adrenalin) makes the myocardium more responsive to the use of a defibrillator to restore normal rhythm. If the heart has completely stopped beating (asystole), epinephrine can actually stimulate contractions of the myocardium. Epinephrine also constricts the blood vessels. Thus, while epinephrine stimulates the heart to beat, it also helps to maintain blood pressure and perfusion to the heart and brain to improve the chances of a successful resuscitative effort.

epinephrine (Adrenalin)

> **DID YOU KNOW?**   The slang term for *epinephrine* is "epi."

Drugs for Metabolic Acidosis

During cardiac and respiratory arrest, the blood pH decreases rapidly as carbon dioxide and waste products accumulate in the blood. In this environment of severe acidosis, emergency drugs lose their effectiveness. These drugs correct the acidosis by buffering excess hydrogen ions and returning the blood pH to within a normal range. There is controversy as to the true effectiveness of sodium bicarbonate. It may actually increase acidosis through a chemical reaction that releases more CO_2 into the blood. The American Heart Association guidelines recommend using it only after other measures have failed.

    sodium bicarbonate
    tromethamine (Tham)

> **DID YOU KNOW?**   Sodium bicarbonate (Alka-Seltzer, Bromo Seltzer) is also given orally as an antacid to neutralize excess acid in the stomach.

Calcium Chloride

Calcium chloride is used to stimulate the myocardium to contract more forcefully and may even stimulate a contraction when the heart is in asystole and has failed to respond to epinephrine.

DRUGS USED AFTER SUCCESSFUL RESUSCITATION

Vasopressors

This class of drugs is used to increase the blood pressure after the patient has been resuscitated. All of these drugs stimulate beta$_1$ receptors to increase the heart rate; they also stimulate alpha receptors in the blood vessels to produce vasoconstriction and raise the blood pressure.

    dobutamine (Dobutrex)
    dopamine (Intropin)
    epinephrine (Adrenalin)
    isoproterenol (Isuprel)
    norepinephrine (Levophed)

Vasopressors also have the desirable effect of maintaining blood flow to the kidneys so that kidney ischemia from hypotension does not later result in renal failure, which would complicate an otherwise successful resuscitative effort.

DRUGS USED TO TREAT OVERDOSE OR SUICIDE ATTEMPTS

Any drug or substance, when ingested in large amounts, can be toxic and fatal. Treatment consists of removing the drug from the stomach, or binding the ingested drug to another substance to make it inert, and/or inactivating the drug in the bloodstream.

Emetics

Drugs that induce vomiting are useful only if the patient is conscious and will not aspirate vomited stomach contents. Emetics are not helpful if the overdose drug has already been absorbed from the stomach into the bloodstream.

> ipecac syrup

Absorbents

Drugs that absorb toxic substances and bind them so that they cannot be absorbed into the bloodstream are administered orally or via a nasogastric tube to patients who are unconscious. This treatment is not helpful if the overdose drug has already been absorbed from the stomach into the bloodstream.

> activated charcoal

Narcotic Antagonists

An overdose of a narcotic drug can be reversed by giving a narcotic antagonist or blocker intravenously. Narcotic antagonists compete for the same receptor sites as the narcotic, block the receptors, and decrease the narcotic drug's effects, particularly that of respiratory depression. (See Chapter 26, "Analgesic Drugs," for a list of generic and trade name narcotic drugs.)

> nalmefene (Revex)
> naloxone (Narcan)
> naltrexone (ReVia, Trexan)

Tranquilizer Antagonists

An overdose of a benzodiazepine-type antianxiety drug can be reversed by giving this antagonist or blocker intravenously. The antagonist competes for the same receptor sites as the tranquilizer, blocks the receptors, and decreases the tranquilizer's effects. (See Chapter 25, "Psychiatric Drugs," for a list of generic and trade name benzodiazepine drugs.)

> flumazenil (Romazicon)

Antidepressant Antagonists

An overdose of a tricyclic-type antidepressant can be reversed by giving this antagonist or blocker intravenously. The antagonist competes for the same receptor sites as the antidepressant, blocks the receptors, and decreases the antidepressant's effects. (See Chapter 25, "Psychiatric Drugs," for a list of generic and trade name tricyclic antidepressants.)

physostigmine (Antilirium)

Other Drugs for Overdose

Drugs used to reverse digoxin toxicity or overdose are discussed in Chapter 15, "Cardio-vascular Drugs."

Acetaminophen (Tylenol) overdose is treated with this drug. It protects the liver, the main site of symptoms from acetaminophen overdose. The exact mechanism of its action is not known.

acetylcysteine (Mucomyst)

Ethylene glycol (antifreeze) used recreationally or swallowed accidentally can result in central nervous system damage, blindness, or death. Methanol (wood alcohol) is found in commercial solvents and paints. Sometimes, an alcoholic will drink methanol instead of ethanol (liquor). In the body, methanol is metabolized into formaldehyde, the same chemical used by pathologists to preserve biopsied tissue specimens. An overdose of either ethylene glycol or methanol can be treated with this drug.

fomepizole (Antizol)

This drug is used to treat pesticide poisoning or an overdose of anticholinesterase drugs used to treat myasthenia gravis.

pralidoxime (Protopam)

DRUGS USED TO TREAT ANAPHYLACTIC SHOCK

Any allergic reaction involves the release of histamine. In anaphylaxis, massive amounts of histamine are released, resulting in extensive generalized vasodilation. If untreated, this causes a severe enough drop in blood pressure to produce shock. Histamine is also a powerful bronchoconstrictor. The massive amounts of histamine released during anaphylaxis can actually decrease air movement in and out of the lungs so completely that the patient suffocates unless treatment occurs within minutes. Treatment involves constricting the blood vessels to maintain a normal blood pressure and relaxing bronchial smooth muscle to allow adequate air flow. Both actions are achieved by these drugs:

epinephrine (Adrenalin)
EpiPen Auto-Injector
EpiPen Jr. Auto-Injector
Ana-Guard Epinephrine

DID YOU KNOW?   Injectable epinephrine (Adrenalin) is included in Ana-Kit, an emergency kit for treating anaphylaxis caused by an insect bite. Those individuals with a history of severe allergic reactions to bee stings or other insect bites can inject a premeasured dose of epinephrine subcutaneously at the time of the sting.

MISCELLANOUS EMERGENCY DRUGS

edetate calcium disodium (calcium EDTA) (Calcium Disodium Versenate):   Used to treat lead poisoning.

succimer (Chemet):   Used to treat arsenic, lead, and mercury poisoning.

REVIEW QUESTIONS

1. Name the drug of choice for resuscitating patients with ventricular arrhythmias.
2. List five emergency drugs that can be given via an endotracheal tube. What mnemonic device helps you remember these drugs?
3. Describe the potential hazards involved in administering an emergency drug via the intracardiac route.
4. What emergency drug is given to counteract bradycardia?
5. What is the therapeutic action of activated charcoal? What are its limitations?
6. Name four categories of drugs used to treat overdose/suicide attempts and give an example of a drug in each category.

SPELLING TIPS

EpiPen Auto-Injector, EpiPen Jr. Auto-Injector   Unusual internal capitalization.
ReVia   Unusual internal capitalization.

GET CONNECTED

Multimedia Extension Activities

   www.prenhall.com/turley

Use the above address to access the free, interactive Companion Website created for this textbook. Included in the features of this site are drug updates and additional chapter-specific exercises for further practice.

17

Anticoagulant and Thrombolytic Drugs

CHAPTER CONTENTS

Anticoagulant drugs
Thrombolytic drugs
Miscellaneous anticoagulant and thrombolytic drugs
Review questions
Spelling tips

LEARNING OBJECTIVES

After studying this chapter, you should be able to do the following:

1. Describe the therapeutic effect of anticoagulant drugs.
2. Describe the therapeutic effect of thrombolytic drugs.
3. Given the generic and trade name of an anticoagulant or thrombolytic drug, identify what drug category it belongs to or what disease it is used to treat.
4. Given an anticoagulant or thrombolytic drug category, give the generic or trade name of several drugs in that category.
5. Identify the Did You Know? section in this chapter that you found most interesting.

ANTICOAGULANT DRUGS

Blood coagulates to form a clot following a complex series of steps involving clotting factors I through XIII and platelets. Anticoagulants prevent clot formation, but cannot dissolve a clot that has already formed. Anticoagulant drugs and platelet aggregation inhibitors are used to prevent deep venous thrombosis (DVT) and pulmonary embolus; to provide anticoagulation during hemodialysis; to prevent clots from forming postoperatively after heart, valve, or vascular surgery; to decrease the risk of a stroke in patients with transient ischemic attacks; and to decrease the risk of myocardial infarction in patients with atherosclerosis.

These anticoagulant drugs prevent clot formation by inhibiting one or more of the clotting factors. All of these drugs are given subcutaneously, with the exception of heparin, which is given subcutaneously or intravenously. Hospitalized patients receiving I.V. heparin are switched to another anticoagulant before being discharged to home.

dalteparin (Fragmin)

danaparoid (Orgaran)

enoxaparin (Lovenox)

heparin

tinzaparin (Innohep)

DID YOU KNOW?   Heparin, enoxaparin, dalteparin, and danaparoid are prepared from cows' or pigs' intestines or lungs.

Note: The ending *-parin* is common to most low molecular weight heparins.

IN DEPTH: All of the aforementioned drugs (except heparin) are known as *low molecular weight heparins*. Heparin is composed of large molecules that are not easily absorbed from the tissues. About 70 to 80% of a dose of heparin is not absorbed, so it cannot exert a therapeutic effect. Low molecular weight heparin is created by treating heparin with chemicals or enzymes to fracture the heparin molecule and decrease the molecular weight by one-third. Almost 100% of a dose of low molecular weight heparin is absorbed from the tissues after subcutaneous administration.

DID YOU KNOW?   A **heparin lock** is a special type of device for intravenous access. It contains a small reservoir of heparin to keep the vein free of clots without the use of I.V. fluids. A heparin lock is used to administer drugs on an intermittent basis. Following drug administration, the reservoir is again filled with heparin.

Vitamin K is essential to the synthesis of several clotting factors. These anticoagulants inhibit the production of vitamin K in the liver. This prevents clot formation or prevents an already-formed clot from growing larger. These drugs are given orally.

anisindione (Miradon)

warfarin (Coumadin)

Platelet Aggregation Inhibitors

These drugs prevent platelets from clumping together to begin the formation of a clot. Some of these drugs block a receptor (glycoprotein IIb/IIIa) on the platelet and prevent it from binding with fibrinogen (Factor I).

> abciximab (ReoPro)
>
> aspirin (Bayer Low Adult Strength, Ecotrin, Ecotrin Adult Low Strength, Empirin, Genuine Bayer Aspirin, Halfprin 81, Heartline, St. Joseph Adult Chewable Aspirin)
>
> clopidogrel (Plavix)
>
> dipyridamole (Persantine)
>
> eptifibatide (Integrilin)
>
> ticlopidine (Ticlid)
>
> tirofiban (Aggrastat)

Abciximab, eptifibatide, and tirofiban are used to prevent blood clots in patients undergoing angioplasty or atherectomy. Aspirin is taken during a myocardial infarction (MI) to limit damage to the heart muscle. Aspirin is also taken prophylactically in low doses to prevent a second MI or stroke. Clopidogrel is used to prevent a second MI or stroke. Dipyridamole is used to prevent a blood clot after cardiac valve surgery. Ticlopidine is used to prevent a second stroke.

Direct Thrombin Inhibitor Drugs

These drugs act specifically on thrombin. They bind to receptor sites on both circulating thrombin and thrombin already in a clot. They are used to treat patients with unstable angina who are undergoing percutaneous transluminal coronary angioplasty or to prevent thrombosis in patients with heparin-induced thrombocytopenia.

> argatroban (Acova)
>
> bivalirudin (Angiomax)

Combination Anticoagulant Drugs

> Aggrenox (aspirin, dipyridamole)

THROMBOLYTIC DRUGS

Anticoagulant drugs are not effective in dissolving clots that have already formed. Instead, **thrombolytic enzymes** and **tissue plasminogen activators** are used to lyse (break apart) the thrombi that obstruct cerebral, coronary, or pulmonary arteries. Both tissue plasminogen activators and thrombolytic enzymes bind to fibrin, the elastic strands that hold a clot together. These drugs then convert plasminogen in the clot to plasmin. Plasmin (also known as *fibrinolysin*) is an enzyme that lyses fibrin. As fibrin strands break, the clot dissolves.

Thrombolytic Enzymes

Thrombolytic enzymes were the first drugs that could dissolve a clot. Their appearance revolutionized the treatment of MIs and strokes.

anistreplase (Eminase)

streptokinase (Streptase)

Tissue Plasminogen Activators

Tissue plasminogen activators (tPA) are created using recombinant DNA technology, although their action is essentially the same as that of the thrombolytic enzymes.

alteplase (Activase, Cathflo Activase)

reteplase (Retavase)

tenecteplase (TNKase)

Note: The ending *-ase* is common to both the generic and trade names of thrombolytic drugs; *-ase* is a suffix meaning *enzyme*.

MISCELLANEOUS ANTICOAGULANT AND THROMBOLYTIC DRUGS

aminocaproic acid (Amicar):   Hemostatic drug used to treat excessive bleeding in patients with certain blood-clotting abnormalities.

anagrelide (Agrylin):   Used to reduce an elevated platelet count in patients with thrombocythemia.

antithrombin III (Thrombate III):   Used to treat patients with antithrombin III deficiency.

Autoplex T: Used to treat hemophiliac patients who produce abnormal inhibitors against clotting Factor VIII.

Avitene: Topical hemostatic microfibers used to control bleeding during surgery.

Coagulin-B: This drug is the gene for coagulation Factor IX, carried on a virus vector, and used to treat hemophilia B.

cryoprecipitate: A plasma extract prepared by freezing and slow thawing of plasma, it contains concentrated amounts of various clotting factors and is used to treat hemophiliac patients.

desmopressin (DDAVP, Stimate):   Used to treat bleeding in hemophiliac patients.

folic acid (Folvite):   Used to treat megaloblastic anemia.

fondaparinux (Arixtra):   Used to prevent venous thromboembolus after orthopedic surgery.

Gelfilm, Gelfilm Ophthalmic: Topical hemostatic gelatin film used to control bleeding during surgery.

Gelfoam: Topical hemostatic gelatin sponge used to control bleeding during surgery.

Hematrol: Used to treat immune thrombocytopenic purpura.

Hemofil M: Clotting factor VIII used to treat hemophiliac patients.

hydroxyurea (Hydrea, Mylocel): Used to treat thrombocytopenia.

iron sucrose (Venofer): Used to treat iron deficiency anemia in hemodialysis patients.

Koate-HP: Used to treat clotting Factor VIII deficiency in hemophiliac patients.

Kogenate: Used to treat clotting Factor VIII deficiency in hemophiliac patients.

Konyne 80: Used to treat clotting Factor IX deficiency in hemophiliac patients.

lepirudin (Refludan): Used to treat heparin-induced thrombocytopenia.

NovoSeven: Clotting factor used to treat hemophiliac patients.

oprelvekin (Neumega): Interleukin used to prevent thrombocytopenia in patients undergoing chemotherapy.

Oxycel: Topical hemostatic pad or pledget used to control bleeding during surgery.

oxymetholone (Anadrol-50): Used to increase RBC production to treat anemia.

Proplex T: Used to treat clotting Factor IX deficiency in hemophiliac patients.

protamine sulfate: By binding with heparin to neutralize its anticoagulant effect, this drug's only therapeutic purpose is to treat heparin overdose or reverse the therapeutic effect of heparin administered during surgery using cardiopulmonary bypass.

Recombinate: Used to treat clotting Factor VIII deficiency in hemophiliac patients.

ReFacto: Used to treat clotting Factor VIII deficiency in hemophiliac patients. This is the first clotting factor product that does not come from human albumin, so there is no risk of transmission of viruses.

Surgicel: Topical hemostatic cellulose pad used to control bleeding during surgery.

thrombin (Thrombogen, Thrombostat): Topical hemostatic powder used to control oozing bleeding.

tranexamic acid (Cyklokapron): Hemostatic drug used to prevent or treat hemorrhage in hemophiliac patients; used during tooth extractions in these patients.

vitamin K (AquaMEPHYTON, Mephyton): Used to treat patients with clotting factor deficiency and restore normal blood clotting times in patients who have had an overdose of anticoagulants other than heparin. Given prophylactically to newborns to prevent hemorrhagic disease of the newborn. Newborns' blood levels of vitamin K are less than 60% of normal. A one-time dose is sufficient because vitamin K levels are normal by 6 weeks of age.

REVIEW QUESTIONS

1. Describe the difference between the therapeutic action of anticoagulants and that of thrombolytic enzymes.
2. What drug is given to reverse the effects of heparin?
3. Name several topical drugs that are used to control bleeding during surgery.
4. What ending is common to generic thrombolytic drugs?

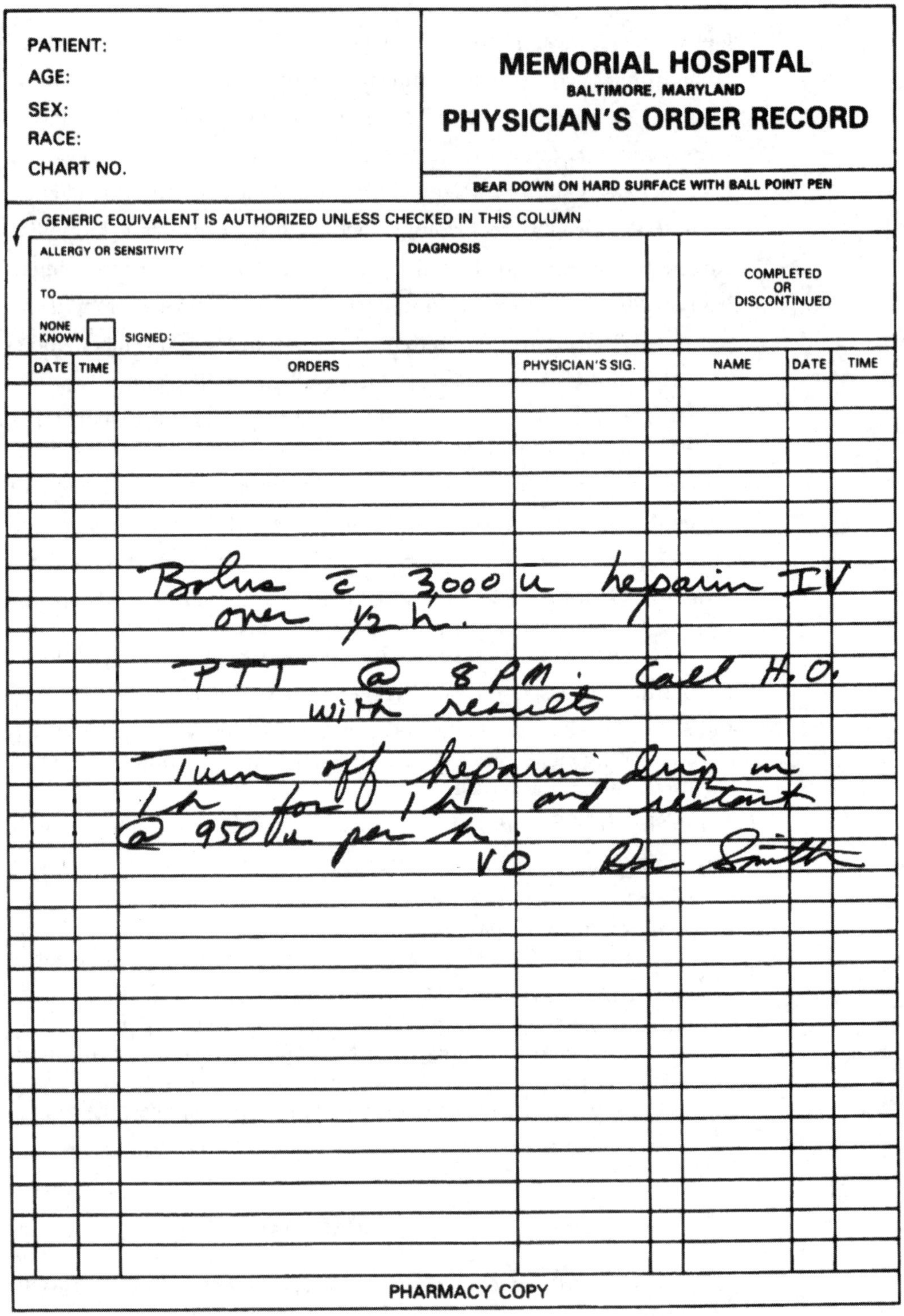

PATIENT:
AGE:
SEX:
RACE:
CHART NO.

MEMORIAL HOSPITAL
BALTIMORE, MARYLAND
PHYSICIAN'S ORDER RECORD

BEAR DOWN ON HARD SURFACE WITH BALL POINT PEN

GENERIC EQUIVALENT IS AUTHORIZED UNLESS CHECKED IN THIS COLUMN

ALLERGY OR SENSITIVITY

TO____

NONE KNOWN ☐   SIGNED:____

DIAGNOSIS

COMPLETED OR DISCONTINUED

DATE	TIME	ORDERS	PHYSICIAN'S SIG.	NAME	DATE	TIME

Bolus c̄ 3,000 u heparin IV over ½ h.

PTT @ 8 P.M. Call H.O. with results

Turn off heparin drip for 1 h and restart @ 950 u per h. V.O. Dr. Smith

PHARMACY COPY

Figure 17–1 Physician's Order Record. *Reprinted courtesy of Marvin Stoogenke,* The Pharmacy Technician, *2nd ed. (Upper Saddle River, NJ: Brady/Prentice Hall, 1998), p. 31.*

CLINICAL SCENARIO

Review this patient's Physician's Order Record (Figure 17–1) and answer the following questions. Use the Glossary/Index at the end of this textbook to verify the spelling of this drug.

What drug did the physician prescribe?

What measurement is used for this dosage?

What is the prescribed route?

What is a bolus? (See Chapter 32)

What does this abbreviation stand for: VO? (See Chapter 10)

What healthcare professional probably wrote this order? (See Chapter 10)

SPELLING TIPS

AquaMEPHYTON   Unusual internal capitalization.
Cyklokapron   Unusual spelling of syllable *cyclo-*.
Reteplase with an *e*, but Retavase with an *a*.

GET CONNECTED

Multimedia Extension Activities

 www.prenhall.com/turley

Use the above address to access the free, interactive Companion Website created for this textbook. Included in the features of this site are drug updates and additional chapter-specific exercises for further practice.

18

Pulmonary Drugs

CHAPTER CONTENTS

Bronchodilator drugs
Leukotriene receptor blockers
Corticosteroid drugs
Mast cell stabilizer drugs
Drugs used to treat tuberculosis (TB)
Drugs used to treat Legionnaire's disease
Drugs used to treat pulmonary arterial hypertension
Drugs used to treat ventilator patients
Drugs used to stop smoking
Miscellaneous pulmonary drugs
Review questions
Spelling tips

LEARNING OBJECTIVES

After studying this chapter, you should be able to do the following:

1. Name several categories of drugs used to treat pulmonary diseases.
2. Describe the therapeutic action of drugs used to treat tuberculosis, Legionnaire's disease, ventilator patients, and to help patients stop smoking.
3. Describe the therapeutic action of bronchodilators, leukotriene receptor blockers, corticosteroid drugs, and mast cell stabilizer drugs.
4. Given the generic and trade name of a pulmonary drug, identify what drug category it belongs to or what disease it is used to treat.
5. Given a pulmonary drug category, give the generic or trade name of several drugs in that category.
6. Identify the Historical Notes or Did You Know? section in this chapter that you found most interesting.

Respiratory diseases such as asthma (reversible obstructive airway disease), bronchitis, chronic obstructive pulmonary disease (COPD), and emphysema require medication to treat chronic symptoms as well as to prevent acute attacks. Aside from the antibiotics used to treat respiratory infections, there are two main classes of drugs prescribed to treat these pulmonary diseases: bronchodilators and corticosteroids. The specialized drugs used to treat tuberculosis are also discussed.

BRONCHODILATOR DRUGS

Bronchodilators are used to treat asthma, COPD, emphysema, and exercise-induced bronchospasm. Bronchodilators relax the smooth muscle that surrounds the bronchi, thereby increasing air flow. This dilatation of the bronchi is due to stimulation of beta$_2$ receptors in the smooth muscle of the bronchi; to the release of epinephrine, which itself stimulates beta$_2$ receptors; or to inhibition of acetylcholine at cholinergic receptor sites in the smooth muscle.

Bronchodilators are given orally as a tablet or liquid, via nebulizer as a liquid that is made into a fine mist, intravenously, or as a solution or powder released from an aerosol canister through a dispenser with a special mouthpiece. This devise is known as a *meter-dose inhaler (MDI)*. It automatically injects a premeasured dose into the lungs as the patient inhales through the mouth. The dosage for MDIs is given as a number of metered sprays or **puffs**. Bronchodilators can also be given as a capsule that releases a microfine powder for inhalation when used with a Rotahaler inhalation device.

> albuterol (Proventil, Proventil HFA, Proventil Repetabs, Ventolin HFA, Ventolin Nebules, Ventolin Rotacaps)
> aminophylline (Phyllocontin)
> bitolterol (Tornalate)
> dyphylline (Lufyllin, Lufyllin-400)
> ephedrine
> epinephrine (Ana-Guard, AsthmaHaler Mist, AsthmaNefrin, microNefrin, Primatene Mist)
> fenoterol (Berotec)
> formoterol (Foradil Aerolizer)
> ipratropium (Atrovent)
> isoetharine
> isoproterenol (Isuprel)
> levalbuterol (Xopenex)
> metaproterenol (Alupent)
> oxtriphylline (Choledyl SA)
> pirbuterol (Maxair Autohaler, Maxair Inhaler)
> salmeterol (Serevent, Serevent Diskus)
> terbutaline (Brethaire, Bricanyl)
> theophylline (Accurbron, Bronkodyl, Elixophyllin, Quibron-T Dividose, Quibron-T/SR Dividose, Respbid, Slo-bid Gyrocaps, Slo-Phyllin, Slo-Phyllin Gyrocaps, Sustaire, Theobid Duracaps, Theo-Dur, Theolair, Theolair-SR, Theovent, T-Phyl, Uniphyl)

DID YOU KNOW?   Proventil HFA and Ventolin HFA contain a propellant in the MDI that is not chlorofluorocarbon (CFC) as the use of CFC propellants is banned in the United States under the U.S. Clean Air Act. The new propellant is hydrofluoroalkane (HFA).

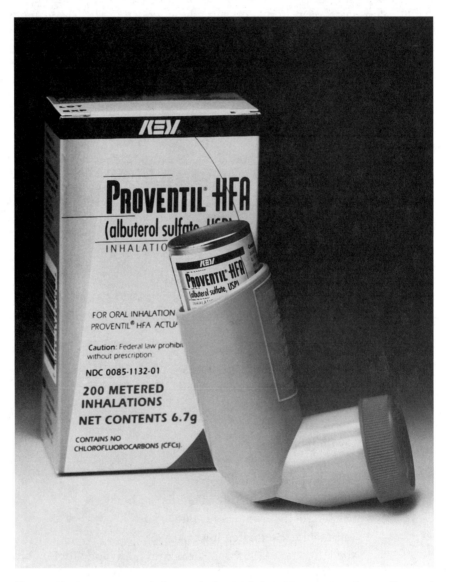

Figure 18–1   A metered-dose inhaler and the prescription drug albuterol (Proventil), an inhaled bronchodilator. *Photo reproduced with permission of Schering Corporation and Key Pharmaceuticals, Inc. All rights reserved.*

Note: The endings *-terol/-terenol* and *-phylline* are common to many generic bronchodilator drugs.

Aminophylline and theophylline are also used to prevent apnea in premature infants.

Combination Bronchodilator Drugs

The following drugs combine one or more bronchodilators with other drugs.

> Advair Diskus (salmeterol, fluticasone [corticosteroid])
> Combivent (albuterol, ipratropium)
> DuoNeb (albuterol, ipratropium)
> Elixophyllin GG, Elixophyllin-Kl (theophylline, guaifenesin or potassium iodide [expectorant])
> Lufyllin-EPG (dyphylline, ephedrine, guaifenesin [expectorant], phenobarbital [sedative])
> Lufyllin-GG (dyphylline, guaifenesin [expectorant])
> Marax (theophylline, ephedrine)
> Marax-DF (theophylline, ephedrine, hydroxyzine [antihistamine])
> Primatene Dual Action (theophylline, ephedrine, guaifenesin [expectorant])
> Quibron, Quibron-300 (theophylline, guaifenesin [expectorant])
> Slo-Phyllin GG (theophylline, guaifenesin [expectorant])

LEUKOTRIENE RECEPTOR BLOCKERS

Leukotriene receptor antagonists or blockers are used to prevent and treat asthma, but not other obstructive respiratory diseases. Leukotriene is produced in the body in response to inhaled antigens and causes airway edema, bronchial constriction, and inflammation. Leukotriene receptor blockers block the action of leukotriene at the receptor level or block the production of leukotriene.

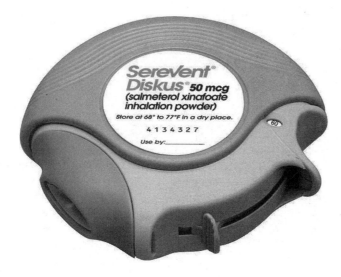

Figure 18–2 A Diskus inhalation device for the prescription drug salmeterol (Serevent Diskus), an inhaled bronchodilator. *Photo reprinted courtesy of GlaxoSmithKline, Inc.*

montelukast (Singulair)
zafirlukast (Accolate)
zileuton (Zyflo)

CORTICOSTEROID DRUGS

Corticosteroids (hydrocortisone and cortisone) are produced naturally by the adrenal glands. They suppress the inflammatory response of the immune system. Corticosteroid drugs reduce inflammation and tissue edema associated with asthma and other chronic lung diseases and prevent acute attacks. These drugs do not produce bronchodilation; therefore, they cannot be used to treat acute attacks, so the patient must also take bronchodilators. These drugs are given by inhaler, and the dosage is prescribed in numbers of puffs.

beclomethasone (Beclovent, QVAR, Vanceril, Vanceril Double Strength)
budesonide (Pulmicort Turbuhaler)
flunisolide (AeroBid, AeroBid-M)
fluticasone (Flovent, Flovent Diskus, Flovent Rotadisk)
triamcinolone (Azmacort)

MAST CELL STABILIZER DRUGS

Mast cell stabilizer drugs stabilize the cell membranes of mast cells and prevent them from releasing histamine during the immune system's response to an antigen. This prevents bronchospasm in patients with bronchial asthma due to allergies. Mast cell stabiliz-

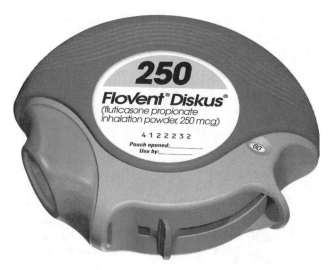

Figure 18–3　A Diskus inhalation device for the prescription drug fluticasone (Flovent Diskus), an inhaled corticosteroid. *Photo reprinted courtesy of GlaxoSmithKline, Inc.*

ers are not bronchodilators, so they are not effective in treating acute asthma attacks but only in preventing attacks.

cromolyn (Intal)
nedocromil (Tilade)

DRUGS USED TO TREAT TUBERCULOSIS (TB)

Tuberculosis (TB) is caused by *Mycobacterium tuberculosis*, a gram-positive bacterium that is resistant to antibiotics that are usually effective against gram-positive bacteria. Treatment with a combination of antituberculosis drugs is necessary.

aminosalicylic acid (Paser Granules)
aminosidine (Gabbromicina)
capreomycin (Capastat)
cycloserine (Seromycin Pulvules)
ethambutol (Myambutol)
ethionamide (Trecator-SC)
isoniazid (INH) (Nydrazid)
pyrazinamide
rifampin (Rifadin, Rimactane)
rifapentine (Priftin)
streptomycin

Combination Drugs for Tuberculosis

Rifamate (isoniazid, rifampin)
Rifater (isoniazid, pyrazinamide, rifampin)

HISTORICAL NOTES: The microbiologist Selman Waksman (who discovered the antibiotic neomycin and the chemotherapy drug actinomycin D and who coined the term *antibiotic*) was a professor at Rutgers University where he studied soil bacteria. He was looking for a drug that would be effective against tuberculosis, because the newly discovered wonder drug penicillin was not. He and his students examined 10,000 different soil samples looking for a substance that could kill the tuberculosis bacteria. They examined a clump of dirt taken from the throat of a sick chicken. On it was growing the mold that would be found to destroy the tuberculosis bacteria. They called it *streptomycin*. Just before their discovery, however, a financial officer at Rutgers suggested Waksman be fired to cut down on expenses, stating that Waksman's work was obscure and his research would never repay the money invested in it. After the discovery of streptomycin he was offered $10 million; he gave it to Rutgers, which, at his suggestion, used the money to build a microbiology laboratory.

FOCUS ON HEALTHCARE ISSUES: Tuberculosis that is resistant to multiple drugs is a serious community health problem. Resistance occurs when a strain of *Mycobacterium tuberculosis* is not sensitive to the first-line drugs (isoniazid, rifampin, ethambutol, and pyrazinamide). Resistance can also occur when the patient is not compliant and does not take the drug for the prescribed length of time. San Francisco has the hightest TB rate on the West Coast. When patients are noncompliant with the TB drug regimen, the attorney general can order them to remain in their homes (except for doctor visits) and can even send them to jail (where their treatment is continued).

DRUGS USED TO TREAT LEGIONNAIRE'S DISEASE

Legionnaire's disease, a serious and sometimes fatal pneumonia caused by *Legionnella pneumophilia*, was named for its first recognized outbreak, which occurred in 1976 at an American Legion convention in Philadelphia. The gram-negative bacteria grew in standing water in the air conditioning system and was distributed throughout the hotel through ventilation ducts. Legionnaire's disease is treated with these antibiotics.

> azithromycin (Zithromax)
> ciprofloxacin (Cipro, Cipro I.V.)
> dirithromycin (Dynabac)
> gatifloxacin (Tequin)
> levofloxacin (Levaquin)
> lomefloxacin (Maxaquin)
> norfloxacin (Noroxin)
> ofloxacin (Floxin)
> rifampin (Rifadin, Rimactane)
> trovafloxacin (Trovan)

DRUGS USED TO TREAT PULMONARY ARTERIAL HYPERTENSION

This disease is characterized by hypertension within the lungs from a variety of causes. The heart, which must pump blood into the pulmonary arteries, is forced to work against this increased pressure and often develops right-sided failure. Patients with this condition may require heart–lung transplantation. These drugs relax the smooth muscle in the arteries in the lungs and lower the blood pressure.

> beraprost
> bosentan (Tracleer)
> epoprostenol (Flolan)
> treprostinil (Remodulin)

DID YOU KNOW?   Epoprostenol (Flolan) is administered continuously by a computer-controlled pump through a catheter that is surgically implanted in a vein in the patient's chest. This drug costs about $100,000 annually. Bosentan (Tracleer) is given orally and only costs $30,000 annually.

DRUGS USED TO TREAT VENTILATOR PATIENTS

These drugs are used to relax the skeletal muscles and paralyze patients on mechanical ventilation so that they will not resist the inflow of air from the ventilator.

atracurium (Tracrium)
cisatracurium (Nimbex)
doxacurium (Nuromax)
mivacurium (Mivacron)
pancuronium (Pavulon)
rocuronium (Zemuron)
succinylcholine (Anectine, Anectine Flo-Pack, Quelicin)
vecuronium (Norcuron)

These narcotic drugs are used to sedate patients who are on the ventilator.

midazolam (Versed)
propofol (Diprivan)
sufentanil (Sufenta)

DRUGS USED TO STOP SMOKING

Smoking has been linked to lung cancer, emphysema, bronchitis, and other pulmonary diseases. The American Lung Association and other organizations offer stop smoking classes, but because nicotine is an addictive substance, some patients find a gradual withdrawal from nicotine diminishes the craving for a cigarette and helps them to successfully stop smoking. Several drugs supply decreasing amounts of nicotine in various forms: chewing gum, transdermal patch, or nasal spray.

Habitrol
Nicoderm CQ
Nicorette, Nicorette DS
Nicotrol, Nicotrol Inhaler, Nicotrol NS
ProStep

Clonidine (Catapres, Catapres-TTS-1, Catapres-TTS-2, Catapres-TTS-3), an oral and transdermal patch drug used to treat HTN, has also been used successfully to help patients stop smoking.

Bupropion (Zyban), an antidepressant that is also marketed under the trade name Wellbutrin, is used to help patients stop smoking. It is thought to inhibit norepinephrine and dopamine in the brain.

> **DID YOU KNOW?**   The Centers for Disease Control states that about 48 million Americans smoke (27% of all men and 22% of all women). Smokers are at higher risk for heart attack and stroke, and smoking kills about 400,000 Americans annually. Surveys indicate that 75% of smokers want to quit, but only about 10% who try each year actually succeed. More than 6,000 people under age 18 try smoking each day and more than 3,000 of these become daily smokers.

DRUGS USED TO TREAT PNEUMOCYSTIS CARINII PNEUMONIA IN AIDS PATIENTS

See Chapter 28, "AIDS Drugs and Antiviral Drugs."

DRUGS USED TO TREAT MYCOBACTERIUM AVIUM-INTRACELLULARE IN AIDS PATIENTS

See Chapter 28, "AIDS Drugs and Antiviral Drugs."

DRUGS USED TO TREAT INFLUENZA AND RESPIRATORY SYNCYTIAL VIRUS INFECTION

See Chapter 28, "AIDS Drugs and Antiviral Drugs."

MISCELLANEOUS PULMONARY DRUGS

acetylcysteine (Mucomyst): Mucolytic drug used to break apart very thick mucus secretions in patients with acute or chronic pulmonary disease such as pneumonia, asthmatic bronchitis, emphysema, cystic fibrosis, or tuberculosis. This drug dissolves the chemical bonds of mucoproteins and thins the mucus so that it can be expectorated.

> **DID YOU KNOW?**   Acetylcysteine (Mucomyst) is used as an antidote for acetaminophen (Tylenol) overdose.

alpha$_1$-proteinase inhibitor (Prolastin): Enzyme replacement therapy for emphysema patients with alpha$_1$-antitrypsin deficiency.

alteplase (Activase): Tissue plasminogen activator used to dissolve a pulmonary embolus.

beractant (Survanta): This natural lung surfactant derived from ground-up cows' lungs is used to supplement low levels of natural surfactant in the lungs of premature infants. It is used to prevent and treat respiratory distress syndrome (RDS), a disease that was known in the past as *hyaline membrane disease*. Surfactant maintains surface tension to prevent the lungs from collapsing with each breath. It is administered via an endotracheal tube.

bleomycin (Blenoxane): Sclerosing drug administered via a chest tube into the lung to treat malignant pleural effusion.

caffeine (Cafcit): Central nervous system stimulant used to prevent apnea in premature infants.

calfactant (Infasurf): Natural lung surfactant. See *beractant* for an explanation of its therapeutic action.

ciprofloxacin (Cipro, Cipro I.V.): Antibiotic used to treat inhaled anthrax from bioterrorism.

colfosceril (Exosurf Neonatal): Synthetic lung surfactant. See *beractant* for an explanation of its therapeutic action.

dexmedetomidine (Precedex): Nonbarbiturate drug used to sedate patients who are intubated and on the ventilator.

dextran sulfate (Uendex) Inhaled drug used to treat cystic fibrosis.

diuretics: Used specifically to treat pulmonary edema caused by left-sided congestive heart failure. See Chapter 12, "Urinary Tract Drugs."

dopamine (Intropin): Vasopressor used to treat chronic obstructive pulmonary disease; used to treat RDS in infants.

dornase alfa (Pulmozyme): This enzyme (deoxyribonuclease) breaks apart DNA strands in the sputum of patients with cystic fibrosis and thins the mucus so it can be expectorated.

DID YOU KNOW? Dornase alfa is manufactured using recombinant DNA technology and ovary cells from Chinese hamsters.

doxycycline (Doryx, Vibramycin, Vibramycin I.V., Vibra-Tabs): Antibiotic used to treat inhaled anthrax from bioterrorism.

dyclonine (Dyclone): Topical anesthetic applied to the throat prior to bronchoscopy.

FocalSeal-L: Surgical sealant used during lung surgery after the tissue has been sutured or stapled. This two-part topical drug is applied as a liquid primer to penetrate the tissue, then as a sealant. Exposure to light causes the liquids to polymerize and form a flexible gel that seals air leaks. The *L* stands for *long-term* because this drug is absorbed in about the same amount of time as long-term absorbable sutures.

Mantoux test (Aplisol, Tubersol):   Diagnostic test for tuberculosis. Purified protein derivative of *Mycobacterium tuberculosis* (PPD) solution is injected intradermally. A raised, red reaction after 48 to 72 hours is diagnostic of exposure to tuberculosis. See also *PPD*.

minocycline (Minocin):   Used to treat malignant pleural effusion.

nitric oxide (INOmax):   Inhaled gas used, along with a ventilator, to treat newborn infants in respiratory failure with persistent pulmonary hypertension. This drug dilates the pulmonary blood vessels in the least affected areas of the lung to increase the amount of oxygen in the blood.

> **DID YOU KNOW?**   Don't confuse nitric oxide (INOmax), described earlier, with nitrous oxide (N_2O), an inhaled gas used to produce general anesthesia.

pneumococcal vaccine (Pneumovax 23, Pnu-Imune 23):   Given prophylactically to protect against the 23 most prevalent strains of pneumococcal pneumonia. Given to the elderly, immunocompromised patients, persons with chronic diseases, or those in residential schools or nursing homes.

pneumococcal vaccine (Prevnar):   Given prophylactically to infants to protect against the seven most prevalent strains of *Streptococcus pneumoniae*.

poractant alfa (Curosurf):   Natural lung surfactant. See *beractant* for an explanation of its therapeutic action.

PPD (purified protein derivative of *Mycobacterium tuberculosis*):   This solution is on the tines of the tine test or injected intradermally in the Mantoux test. It will provoke a raised, red reaction in persons who have or have been exposed to tuberculosis.

Procysteine: Used to treat adults with RDS.

Pulmocare: A liquid nutritional supplement specifically formulated to meet the nutritional needs of patients with chronic pulmonary disease.

streptokinase (Streptase):   Thrombolytic enzyme used to dissolve a pulmonary embolus.

talc (Sclerosol Intrapleural Aerosol, Steritalc):   Powdered sclerosing drug administered via chest tube into the lung to treat malignant pleural effusion and pneumothorax.

telithromycin (Ketek):   A ketolide antibiotic used to treat community-acquired pneumonia.

tetracaine (Pontocaine):   Topical anesthetic applied to the throat prior to bronchoscopy.

TICE BCG: Immunization drug used to treat children who are around persons with untreated or poorly treated tuberculosis.

tine test (Aplitest, Tine Test PPD):   Screening test for tuberculosis that uses a four-pronged applicator. The tines (similar to the prongs or tines of a fork) have PPD solution on them; the tines puncture the skin and introduce the PPD. A raised, red reaction is suggestive of exposure to tuberculosis. A position tine test is followed up with a Mantoux test to confirm the diagnosis of exposure to tuberculosis.

REVIEW QUESTIONS

1. List several ways in which bronchodilator drugs can be administered.
2. Corticosteroids can be inhaled to provide relief from an acute asthma attack. True or False?
3. What is a metered-dose inhaler (MDI)?
4. What condition is a mast cell stabilizer drug used to treat?
5. What is the name of the causative agent of tuberculosis?
6. Mucomyst is used to treat patients with cystic fibrosis and acetaminophen overdose. True or False?
7. Describe the action of surfactant.
8. Name three categories of pulmonary drugs and give an example of a drug in each category.
9. What disease does Pneumovax prevent?
10. To what category of drugs does each of these drugs belong?
    aminophylline (Phyllocontin)
    cromolyn (Intal)
    isoniazid (INH, Nydrazid)
    pirbuterol (Maxair)
    triamcinolone (Azmacort)
    zileuton (Zyflo)
11. Name several drugs used to help patients to stop smoking.
12. The ending *-phylline* is common to what category of drugs?
13. Rewrite this prescription in plain English. Use the Glossary/Index at the back of this textbook to help you verify the correct spelling and dosage of this drug. (See Figure 18–4.)

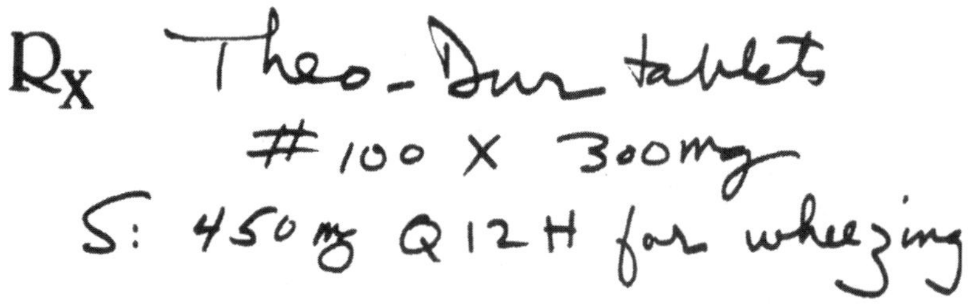

Rx Theo-Dur tablets
 # 100 X 300mg
 S: 450 mg Q12H for wheezing

Figure 18–4 A prescription. *Reprinted courtesy of Marvin Stoogenke, The Pharmacy Technician, 2nd ed. (Upper Saddle River, NJ: Brady/Prentice Hall, 1998), p. 373.*

SPELLING TIPS

AeroBid   Unusual internal capitalization.

AsthmaHaler Mist   Unusual internal capitalization.

AsthmaNefrin   Unusual internal capitalization.

Azmacort   Note the difference in spelling between the drug and the disease *asthma*.

microNefrin   No initial capital letter.

Pulmicort Turbuhaler   *Pulmi-*, not *pulmo-* as in *pulmonary. Turbu-*, not *turbo*.

Slo-Phyllin   Difficult to spell because it is alternately pronounced as "sah-LAH'-fah-lin" or "slo-fillin."

GET CONNECTED

Multimedia Extension Activities

   www.prenhall.com/turley

Use the above address to access the free, interactive Companion Website created for this textbook. Included in the features of this site are drug updates and additional chapter-specific exercises for further practice.

19

Ear, Nose, and Throat (ENT) Drugs

CHAPTER CONTENTS

Decongestant drugs
Antihistamine drugs
Mast cell stabilizer drugs
Corticosteroid drugs
Antibiotic drugs
Antitussive drugs
Expectorant drugs
Antifungal drugs
Combination ENT drugs
Miscellaneous ENT drugs
Review questions
Spelling tips

LEARNING OBJECTIVES

After studying this chapter, you should be able to do the following:

1. Name several categories of ENT drugs.
2. Describe the therapeutic action of decongestants, antihistamines, antitussive drugs, expectorant drugs, corticosteroid drugs, antibiotic drugs, and antifungal drugs.
3. Given the generic and trade name of an ENT drug, identify what drug category it belongs to or what disease it is used to treat.
4. Given an ENT drug category, identify several generic and trade name drugs in that category.
5. Identify the Did You Know? section in this chapter that you found most interesting.

ENT drugs are prescribed for various conditions of the ears, nose, and throat ranging from swimmer's ear to nasal polyps to coughs and colds to seasonal or allergic rhinitis.

ENT drugs comprise several distinct classes of drugs, including decongestants, antihistamines, antitussives, expectorants, corticosteroids, and antibiotics.

> **DID YOU KNOW?**   Most people contract two or more colds per year. There are over 120 different viruses, not to mention bacteria, that cause colds. The common cold is considered the single most expensive illness in the United States in terms of time lost from work/school. No medication is currently available to cure the common cold; available drugs merely provide temporary relief of various symptoms until the cold has run its course.

DECONGESTANT DRUGS

Decongestants act as vasoconstrictors to reduce blood flow to edematous mucous membranes in the nose, sinuses, and pharynx; they produce vasoconstriction by stimulating alpha receptors in the smooth muscle around the blood vessels. Decongestants decrease the swelling of mucous membranes, alleviate nasal stuffiness, allow secretions to drain, and help to unclog the eustachian tubes. Decongestants are commonly prescribed for colds and allergies. They can be administered topically as nose drops or nasal sprays or can be taken orally. Decongestants are often combined with antihistamines in cold remedies.

> desoxyephedrine (Vicks Inhaler)
>
> ephedrine
>
> naphazoline (Privine)
>
> oxymetazoline (Afrin Nasal Spray, Afrin Children's Nose Drops, Afrin Sinus, Allerest 12 Hour Nasal, Cheracol Nasal, Dristan 12 Hr Nasal, Duramist Plus, Duration, 4-Way Long Lasting Nasal, Nostrilla, Sinarest 12 Hour, Vicks Sinex 12-Hour)
>
> phenylephrine (Children's Nostril, Neo-Synephrine, Nostril, Rhinall, Sinex)
>
> pseudoephedrine (Afrin, Drixoral Non-Drowsy Formula, Efidac/24, PediaCare Infants' Decongestant, Sudafed, Sudafed 12 Hour, Triaminic AM Decongestant Formula, Triaminic Infant Oral Decongestant)
>
> tetrahydrozoline
>
> xylometazoline (Otrivin, Otrivin Pediatric Nasal Drops)

ANTIHISTAMINE DRUGS

Antihistamines exert their therapeutic effect by blocking **histamine (H_1) receptors** in the nose and throat. Histamine is released from mast cells in the tissues when an antibody–antigen complex is created during allergic reactions. Histamine causes vasodilation, which causes the blood vessels and mucous membranes to become engorged, swollen, and red. Histamine also irritates these tissues directly, causing pain and itching. Antihistamines block the action of histamine at the H_1 receptors to dry up secretions, shrink edematous mucous membranes, and decrease itching and redness. A significant side effect of older antihistamines was drowsiness; however, newer antihistamines have a different chemical structure that does not produce significant drowsiness.

azatadine (Optimine)

azelastine (Astelin)

brompheniramine (Dimetane Allergy)

carbinoxamine

cetirizine (Zyrtec)

chlorpheniramine (Chlor-Trimeton Allergy 4 Hour, Chlor-Trimeton Allergy 8 Hour, Chlor-Trimeton Allergy 12 Hour)

clemastine (Tavist)

cyproheptadine (Periactin)

desloratadine (Clarinex)

dexchlorpheniramine (Polaramine, Polaramine Repetabs)

diphenhydramine (AllerMax Caplets , Benadryl, Benadryl Allergy, Benadryl Allergy Kapseals, Benadryl Allergy Ultratabs, Benadryl Dye-Free Allergy Liqui Gels)

fexofenadine (Allegra)

loratadine (Claritin, Claritin Reditabs)

phenindamine (Nolahist)

promethazine (Phenergan, Phenergan Fortis, Phenergan Plain)

Antihistamines are not effective in treating the common cold. Although symptoms of allergies and colds are similar, there is no release of histamine with the common cold. Nevertheless, pharmaceutical manufacturers continue to combine antihistamines with decongestants in cold remedies. Antihistamines may have some drying effect on the mucous membranes, but probably not enough to justify any extra cost.

HISTORICAL NOTES: Astemizole (Hismanal) and terfenadine (Seldane) were hailed as superior to older antihistamines because they were nonsedating. The caveat "All drugs can cause adverse effects" became painfully clear when both of these drugs were implicated in sudden deaths due to cardiac arrest. At first, these drugs were given a new warning label that they should not be used by patients taking the antibiotic erythromycin or the antifungal drugs ketoconazole and itraconazole. Later, Hismanal and Seldane were removed from the market. The chemical structure of terfenadine (Seldane) was modified to have less cardiac side effects, and the resulting new drug was released as the antihistamine fexofenadine (Allegra).

MAST CELL STABILIZER DRUGS

Mast cell stabilizer drugs stabilize the cell membranes of mast cells and prevent them from releasing histamine during the immune system's response to an antigen. This prevents edema of the nasal mucous membranes and sneezing in patients with allergic rhinitis.

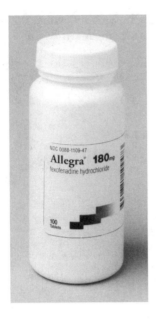

Figure 19–1   The prescription drug fexofenadine (Allegra) is an antihistamine that is used to treat allergies. Fexofenidine HCl (Allegra) 180 mg tablet. *Photo reprinted courtesy of Aventis Pharmaceuticals.*

cromolyn (Children's NasalCrom, NasalCrom)

CORTICOSTEROID DRUGS

Corticosteroids act by inhibiting the body's inflammatory response: decreasing vasodilation and edema of the mucous membranes and reducing inflammation. Corticosteroids have no antihistamine effect. Corticosteroids are not used to treat the common cold. They are administered intranasally to treat allergic and nonallergic rhinitis.

beclomethasone (Beconase, Beconase AQ, Vancenase, Vancenase AQ 84, Vancenase Pockethaler)
budesonide (Rhinocort, Rhinocort Aqua)
flunisolide (Nasalide)
fluticasone (Flonase)
mometasone (Nasonex)
triamcinolone (Nasacort, Nasacort AQ, Tri-Nasal)

Corticosteroids can be applied topically as a paste to treat mouth ulcers and inflammation.

triamcinolone (Kenalog in Orabase)

Corticosteroids and antibiotics are often combined in a single drug for topical application in the ear. See the section, "Combination ENT Drugs."

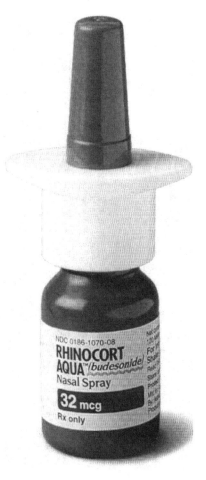

Figure 19–2 The prescription drug budesonide (Rhinocort Aqua), a topical intranasal anti-inflammatory corticosteroid drug. *Photo reprinted courtesy of AstraZeneca Pharmaceuticals LP.*

DID YOU KNOW? The trade name Rhinocort is a combination of *rhino*, the Greek word for *nose* and *cort* for *corticosteroid*. You can remember the meaning of *rhino* because a rhinocerous has a large horn on its nose!

ANTIBIOTIC DRUGS

Antibiotics are not effective in treating the common cold because it is usually caused by a virus. However, antibiotics are prescribed for colds caused by bacterial infections, particularly streptococci. Antibiotics may also be prescribed prophylactically for patients with viral colds to prevent subsequent superimposed bacterial infections, although this practice is not recommended as it contributes to the overuse of antibiotics. See Chapter 27, "Anti-Infective Drugs," for a complete discussion of oral antibiotics.

Antibiotics may be prescribed for topical application in the ears to treat external otitis media and other infections.

chloramphenicol (Chloromycetin Otic)

Note: Otic is an adjective that means *pertaining to the ear*.
Corticosteroids and antibiotics are often combined in a single solution for topical application in the ear. See the section, "Combination ENT Drugs."

ANTITUSSIVE DRUGS

Antitussives decrease coughing by suppressing the cough center in the brain or anesthetizing the stretch receptors in the respiratory tract. Their main purpose is to control nonproductive dry coughs. These drugs are not prescribed to treat a productive cough that generates sputum because it is important for the patient to cough up this sputum. Some antitussives, such as codeine and hydrocodone, are narcotics and are classified as schedule drugs.

benzonatate (Tessalon Perles)
codeine
dextromethorphan (Benylin Adult, Benylin DM, Benylin Pediatric, Drixoral Cough Liquid Caps, Pediatric Vicks 44d Dry Hacking Cough and Head Congestion, Pertussin CS, Pertussin ES, Robitussin Cough Calmers, Robitussin Pediatric, St. Joseph Cough Suppressant, Sucrets Cough Control, Sucrets 4-Hour Cough, Vicks Dry Hacking Cough)
diphenhydramine
hydrocodone (Hycodan)

EXPECTORANT DRUGS

Expectorants reduce the viscosity or thickness of sputum so that patients can more easily cough it up. Expectorants are only prescribed for productive coughs.

guaifenesin (Humibid L.A., Humibid Sprinkle, Naldecon Senior EX, Organidin NR, Robitussin)
iodinated glycerol
potassium iodide (SSKI)
terpin hydrate

ANTIFUNGAL DRUGS

Yeasts, which are closely related to fungi, grow easily in the warm, dark environment of the mouth, particularly in immunocompromised patients. *Candida albicans* yeast infections are alternatively known as *oral candidiasis, monilia,* or *thrush*. These liquid antifungal drugs are applied topically (the patient is told to "swish and swallow") or supplied as a troche (to suck on as a lozenge).

clotrimazole (Mycelex)

nystatin (Mycostatin, Mycostatin Pastilles, Nilstat)

Antifungal drugs that act systemically to treat severe oral yeast infections are discussed in Chapter 29, "Antifungal Drugs."

DRUGS USED TO TREAT MOTION SICKNESS

For drugs that control the dizziness associated with overstimulation of the inner ear, see Chapter 13, "Gastrointestinal Drugs."

COMBINATION ENT DRUGS

Combination ENT trade name drugs are used to treat colds, the flu, allergies, coughs, and infections. They contain various combinations of these drugs:

analgesics (acetaminophen, aspirin, ibuprofen)

antibiotics (ciprofloxacin, colistin, neomycin, polymyxin B)

antihistamines (azatadine, brompheniramine, carbinoxamine, cetirizine, chlorpheniramine, clemastine, dexbrompheniramine, diphenhydramine, doxylamine, fexofenadine, loratadine, pheniramine, phenyltoloxamine, promethazine, pyrilamine, triprolidine)

antitussives (caramiphen, codeine, dextromethorphan, hydrocodone, hydromorphone)

corticosteroids (hydrocortisone)

decongestants (ephedrine, naphazoline, phenylephrine, pseudoephedrine),

expectorants (guaifenesin)

HISTORICAL NOTES: Phenylpropanolamine was a popular decongestant in many trade name combination ENT drugs. It was found to cause stokes in people under age 50 so it was removed from the market. This required the reformulation of many combination ENT drugs.

This is a partial list of the many combination ENT drugs currently on the market. See the Glossary/Index at the end of this textbook for a complete list.

Actifed Cold & Allergy (pseudoephedrine, triprolidine)

Advil Cold & Sinus (pseudoephedrine, ibuprofen)

Alka-Seltzer Plus Cold & Cough Liqui-Gels (pseudoephedrine, chlorpheniramine, dextromethorphan, acetaminophen)

Allegra-D (pseudoephedrine, fexofenadine)

Allerest Sinus Pain Formula (pseudoephedrine, chlorpheniramine, acetaminophen)

Aspirin-Free Bayer Select Head & Chest Cold (pseudoephedrine, dextromethorphan, guaifenesin)

Benadryl Allergy/Cold, Benadryl Allergy/Sinus Headache (pseudoephedrine, diphenhydramine, acetaminophen)

Benylin Expectorant (dextromethorphan, guaifenesin)

Bronkaid Dual Action (ephedrine, guaifenesin)

Brontex (codeine, guaifenesin)

Cheracol Cough (codeine, guaifenesin)

Children's Cepacol (pseudoephedrine, acetaminophen)

Chlor-Trimeton 12 Hour Relief (pseudoephedrine, chlorpheniramine)

Cipro HC Otic (hydrocortisone, ciprofloxacin)

Claritin-D 24-Hour (pseudoephedrine, loratadine)

Coly-Mycin S Otic (hydrocortisone, colistin, neomycin)

Comtrex Maximum Strength Multi-Symptom Cold & Flu Relief Caplet/Tablet (pseudoephedrine, chlorpheniramine, dextromethorphan, acetaminophen)

Contac Day & Night Cold & Flu (pseudoephedrine, diphenhydramine, dextromethorphan, acetaminophen)

Coricidin, Coricidin HB (chlorpheniramine, acetaminophen)

Cortisporin-TC Otic (hydrocortisone, colistin, neomycin)

Deconamine SR (pseudoephedrine, chlorpheniramine)

Dilaudid Cough (hydromorphone, guaifenesin)

Dimetane Decongestant (phenylephrine, brompheniramine)

Dimetapp-DX Cough (pseudoephedrine, brompheniramine, dextromethorphan)

Dristan Cold Multi-Symptom Formula (phenylephrine, chlorpheniramine, acetaminophen)

Drixoral Cold & Flu, Drixoral Plus (pseudoephedrine, dexbrompheniramine, acetaminophen)

Entex PSE (pseudoephedrine, guaifenesin)

4-Way Fast Acting Original (naphazoline, phenylephrine, pyrilamine)

Humibid DM, Humibid DM Sprinkle (dextromethorphan, guaifenesin)

Hycomine Compound (phenylephrine, chlorpheniramine, hydrocodone)

Hycotuss Expectorant (hydrocodone, guaifenesin)

Medi-Flu (pseudoephedrine, pyrilamine, dextromethorphan, acetaminophen)

Naldecon Senior DX (dextromethorphan, guaifenesin)

NightTime TheraFlu (pseudoephedrine, chlorpheniramine, dextromethorphan, acetaminophen)

Novafed A (pseudoephedrine, chlorpheniramine)

Novahistine DMX (pseudoephedrine, dextromethorphan, guaifenesin)

NyQuil Hot Therapy, NyQuil Nighttime Cold/Flu Medicine (pseudoephedrine, doxylamine, dextromethorphan, acetaminophen)

Otobiotic Otic (hydrocortisone, polymyxin B)

OtiTricin (hydrocortisone, neomycin, polymyxin B)

Percogesic (phenyltoloxamine, acetaminophen)

Phenergan with Codeine (promethazine, codeine)

Primatene (ephedrine, guaifenesin)

Robitussin Cold & Cough (pseudoephedrine, dextromethorphan, guaifenesin)

Rondec-DM (pseudoephedrine, carbinoxamine, dextromethorphan)

Sinarest Extra Strength, Sinarest Sinus (pseudoephedrine, chlorpheniramine, acetaminophen)

Sine-Aid IB (pseudoephedrine, ibuprofen)

Sine-Off Sinus Medicine (pseudoephedrine, chlorpheniramine, acetaminophen)

Sinutab Maximum Strength Sinus Allergy (pseudoephedrine, chlorpheniramine, acetaminophen)

Sudafed Severe Cold (pseudoephedrine, dextromethorphan, acetaminophen)

TheraFlu Flu, Cold & Cough (pseudoephedrine, chlorpheniramine, dextromethorphan, acetaminophen)

Triaminic AM Cough & Decongestant (pseudoephedrine, dextromethorphan)

Trinalin Repetabs (pseudoephedrine, azatadine)

Tussi-Organidin NR, Tussi-Organidin-S NR (codeine, guaifenesin)

Tylenol Flu Maximum Strength (pseudoephedrine, dextromethorphan, acetaminophen)

Vicks DayQuil (pseudoephedrine, dextromethorphan, guaifenesin)

Vicks Formula 44 Cough Control Discs (dextromethorphan, benzocaine [topical anesthetic])

Vicks NyQuil, Vicks NyQuil Multi-Symptom Cold/Flu Relief (pseudoephedrine, doxylamine, dextromethorphan, acetaminophen)

Vicodin Tuss (hydrocodone, guaifenesin)

Zyrtec-D 12 Hour (cetirizine, pseudoepherine)

MISCELLANEOUS ENT DRUGS

amlexanox (Aphthasol):   Topical drug used to treat aphthous ulcers of the mouth.

benzocaine (Anbesol, Baby Anbesol, Maximum Strength Anbesol, Hurricane, Numzit Teething, Orabase-B, Orabase Baby, Orabase Gel, Orabase Lip, Zilactin-B Medicated):   Topical anesthetic for the mouth.

benzocaine (Auralgan Otic, Tympagesic):   Topical anesthetic for the ear.

benzocaine (Cepacol Anesthetic, Cepacol Maximum Strength, Mycinettes, Spec-T, Vicks Children's Chloraseptic, Vicks Chloraseptic Sore Throat):   Topical anesthetic used to treat sore throats.

Cerumenex Drops: Topical drug used to soften hardened earwax (cerumen) so it can be flushed from the ear.

Cetacaine: Combination drug with three topical anesthetics for the mouth.

cevimeline (Evoxac):   Used to treat dry mouth due to Sjögren's syndrome.

chlorhexidine (Peridex, PerioGard):   Topical drug used to treat gingivitis.

cocaine (Cocaine Viscous):   Topical anesthetic and vasoconstrictor used during ENT examinations and operations on the nose.

DID YOU KNOW?   Cocaine addicts who sniff the powder often have intranasal ulcers and can even develop a perforated nasal septum. This is due to the powerful topical vasoconstrictor action of cocaine that causes sloughing of the mucous membranes.

Debacterol: Topical chemical cautery drug that debrides necrotic tissue and kills bacteria. Used to treat canker sores and ulcerating mouth lesions.

Debrox: Topical drug used to soften hardened earwax (cerumen) so it can be flushed from the ear.

docosanol (Abreva):   Topical drug used to treat herpes simplex lesions (cold sores) on the mouth.

doxycycline (Periostat):   Used to treat periodontal disease.

dyclonine (Sucrets, Sucrets Children's Sore Throat, Sucrets Maximum Strength):   Topical anesthetic used to treat sore throats.

hydrogen peroxide (Orabase HCA, Peroxyl):   Topical antiseptic for the mouth.

ipratropium (Atrovent):   Anticholinergic drug used to treat allergic rhinitis.

lidocaine (Dentipatch, Xylocaine, Xylocaine 10% Oral, Xylocaine Viscous):   Topical anesthetic for mouth ulcers, denture pain, and for use prior to dental procedures. Viscous lidocaine is formulated as a thickened liquid that stays in contact with the mucous membranes.

minocycline (Arestin):   Topical drug used to treat periodontal disease. It consists of microspheres that are placed in the pockets between the gums and teeth.

Murine Ear: Topical drug used to soften hardened earwax (cerumen) so it can be flushed from the ear.

Optimoist: Artificial saliva used to treat dry mouth due to salivary gland dysfunction.

Otic Domeboro: Topical antibacterial Burow's solution for the ear.

pilocarpine (Salagen):   Used to treat dry mouth due to salivary gland dysfunction.

saline (Afrin Moisturizing Saline Mist, Ayr Saline, Dristan Saline Spray, Mycinaire Saline Nasal Mist, Ocean):   Moisturizing drug for the nose.

silver nitrate: Topical drug used to cauterize superficial blood vessels causing nosebleeds.

tannic acid (Zilactin Medicated): Topical gel that forms a protective covering over canker sores and cold sores in and around the mouth.

tetracycline (Actisite): Topical drug used to treat periodontitis in the mouth.

Vicks VapoRub: Topical irritant and aromatic drug used to treat the muscle aches and stuffy nose of the common cold.

> **DID YOU KNOW?** Vicks VapoRub contains cedar oil, eucalyptus oil, nutmeg oil, and spirits of turpentine.

REVIEW QUESTIONS

1. State your position as a consumer advocate on the cost-effectiveness of including an antihistamine in an OTC cold remedy.
2. Describe the difference between the therapeutic action of antitussive drugs and expectorants.
3. What are the three names commonly used to describe a yeast infection in the mouth?
4. How do antihistamines exert their therapeutic effect?
5. Contrast the therapeutic effect of antihistamines with that of mast cell stabilizers.
6. Name four categories of ENT drugs and give an example of a drug in each category.
7. To what category of drugs does each of these drugs belong?
   Beconase
   dextromethorphan
   fexofenadine (Allegra)
   Zyrtec
   guaifenesin
   Benadryl
   NasalCrom
   Rhinocort
   Claritin
   Sudafed
8. Is Coly-Mycin S Otic used to treat the ears, nose, or throat?

SPELLING TIPS

Contac not *contact*, the English word.
Dimetane versus Dimetapp (sound-alikes).
NasalCrom Unusual internal capitalization.
NyQuil Unusual internal capitalization.
PediaCare Unusual internal capitalization.
Pseudo- (pseudoephedrine) versus suda- (Sudafed).
Tessalon Perles Not *pearls.*

GET CONNECTED

Multimedia Extension Activities

 www.prenhall.com/turley

Use the above address to access the free, interactive Companion Website created for this textbook. Included in the features of this site are drug updates and additional chapter-specific exercises for further practice.

20

Ophthalmic Drugs

CHAPTER CONTENTS

Drugs used to treat ophthalmic infections
Drugs used to treat ophthalmic inflammation
Drugs used to treat ophthalmic allergy symptoms
Drugs used to treat glaucoma
Anesthetic ophthalmic drugs
Mydriatic drugs
Miscellaneous ophthalmic drugs
Review questions
Spelling tips

LEARNING OBJECTIVES

After studying this chapter, you should be able to do the following:

1. Name several categories of ophthalmic drugs.
2. Describe the therapeutic action of drugs used to treat glaucoma.
3. Describe the therapeutic action of antibiotics, antiviral drugs, corticosteroids, and topical anesthetics for the eye, as well as mydriatics.
4. Given the generic and trade name of an ophthalmic drug, identify what drug category it belongs to or what disease it is used to treat.
5. Given a category of ophthalmic drugs, give the name of several generic and trade name drugs in that category.
6. Identify the Historical Notes or Did You Know? section in this chapter that you found most interesting.

Ophthalmic drugs may be applied topically to treat superficial infections or inflammations of the cornea and surrounding tissues, treat allergy symptoms in the eye, treat glaucoma, or produce anesthesia or mydriasis to facilitate examination of the eye. Some ophthalmic drugs are taken systemically for severe infection or inflammation in the interior of the eye. All drugs intended for topical application in the eye are specially formulated in a solution that is physiologically similar to fluids in the eye so as not to damage the delicate tissues of the eye.

DRUGS USED TO TREAT OPHTHALMIC INFECTIONS

These drugs are used to treat superficial bacterial, fungal, and viral infections of the corneas, conjunctivae, eyelids, and tear ducts.

Antibiotic Drugs for Bacterial Ophthalmic Infections

Topical antibiotics disrupt the cell wall of bacteria. Antibiotics are not effective against viral infections. Topical ophthalmic antibiotics are dispensed as ointments or solutions.

bacitracin

chloramphenicol (Chloromycetin, Chloroptic)

ciprofloxacin (Ciloxan)

erythromycin (Ilotycin)

gentamicin (Garamycin, Genoptic, Genoptic S.O.P., Gentacidin, Gentak)

levofloxacin (Quixin)

norfloxacin (Chibroxin)

ofloxacin (Ocuflox)

polymyxin B

tobramycin (Defy, Tobrex)

For severe eye infections, various systemic antibiotics are prescribed. For a discussion of these drugs, see Chapter 27, "Anti-Infective Drugs."

Most states either recommend or require a topical anti-infective drug to be applied to the eyes of newborn infants to prevent infection and possible blindness from gonorrhea (contracted as the baby's head moves through the infected birth canal). Anti-infectives used for this purpose include:

erythromycin (Ilotycin)

silver nitrate

Although silver nitrate has been commonly used for years and is the least expensive of the two, it has several drawbacks: It produces conjunctival irritation/swelling that interferes with mother–child bonding. Erythromycin does not cause this side effect.

Sulfonamide Drugs for Bacterial Ophthalmic Infections

These anti-infective drugs are not classified as antibiotics, but they do inhibit the growth of bacteria and are used to treat bacterial infections of the eye.

sulfacetamide (Bleph-10, Cetamide, Ocusulf-10, Storz-Sulf, Sulster)

sulfisoxazole (Gantrisin)

Drugs for Fungal Ophthalmic Infections

These anti-infective drugs are not classified as antibiotics. They are only effective in treating fungal infections of the eye.

> natamycin (Natacyn)

Drugs for Viral Ophthalmic Infections

These anti-infective drugs are not classified as antibiotics. They are only effective in treating viral infections of the eye. Antiviral drugs act by inhibiting viral DNA reproduction.

Topical antiviral drugs for the eye that are effective against herpes simplex virus (HSV) include:

> trifluridine (Viroptic)
> vidarabine (Vira-A)

These antiviral drugs are effective against cytomegalovirus (CMV) retinitis, an infection most often seen in patients with AIDS. These drugs are administered by intraocular injection or intraocular implant.

> fomivirsen (Vitravene)
> ganciclovir (Vitrasert)

For antiviral drugs that act systemically against cytomegalovirus, see Chapter 28, "AIDS Drugs and Antiviral Drugs."

DRUGS USED TO TREAT OPHTHALMIC INFLAMMATION

Corticosteroid Ophthalmic Drugs

Corticosteroid drugs are used topically in the eye to treat the inflammation that results from trauma, surgery, contact with chemicals, or allergies.

> dexamethasone (Decadron, Maxidex)
> fluorometholone (Flarex, Fluor-Op, FML, FML Forte, FML S.O.P.)
> loteprednol (Alrex, Lotemax)
> medrysone (HMS)
> prednisolone (Econopred, Econopred Plus, Inflamase Forte, Inflamase Mild, Pred Forte, Pred Mild)
> rimexolone (Vexol)

Nonsteroidal Anti-Inflammatory Ophthalmic Drugs

Nonsteroidal anti-inflammatory drugs (NSAIDs) are used topically in the eye to treat inflammation that results from surgery or allergic reactions.

> diclofenac (Voltaren)
> ketorolac (Acular)

DRUGS USED TO TREAT OPHTHALMIC ALLERGY SYMPTOMS

Antihistamine Ophthalmic Drugs

Topical antihistamines relieve the symptoms of allergic conjunctivitis. These symptoms are caused by histamine released by the antibody–antigen complex that forms during allergic reactions. Histamine causes vasodilation and the blood vessels and tissues of the eye become engorged, swollen, and red. Histamine also irritates these tissues directly, causing pain and itching. Antihistamines exert their therapeutic effect by blocking histamine (H_1) receptors in the eye.

> azelastine (Optivar)
> emedastine (Emadine)
> levocabastine (Livostin)
> olopatadine (Patanol)

Mast Cell Stabilizer Ophthalmic Drugs

Topical mast cell stabilizers prevent the cell membranes of mast cells from releasing histamine. This prevents redness and vasodilation in the eye.

> cromolyn (Crolom)
> ketotifen (Zaditor)
> lodoxamide (Alomide)
> nedocromil (Alocril)
> pemirolast (Alamast)

Decongestant Ophthalmic Drugs

These drugs cause vasoconstriction in the eyes which reduces the redness and vasodilation caused by histamine.

> naphazoline (Albalon, Allerest Eye Drops, Nafazair, Naphcon, Naphcon Forte, VasoClear, VasoClear A Solution, Vasocon Regular)
> oxymetazoline (OcuClear, Visine L.R.)
> phenylephrine (Mydfrin, Neo-Synephrine, Prefrin Liquifilm, Relief, Zincfrin)
> tetrahydrozoline (Collyrium Fresh, Eyesine, Murine Plus, Optigene 3, Tetrasine, Tetrasine Extra, Visine Allergy Relief)

DRUGS USED TO TREAT GLAUCOMA

Glaucoma is a disease whose presenting symptom is increased intraocular pressure. If untreated, it can lead to blindness. Drugs for glaucoma act either by decreasing the amount of aqueous humor circulating in the anterior and posterior chambers (to decrease the intraocular pressure) or constricting the pupil (miosis) to open the angle of contact between the iris and the trabecular meshwork (to allow the aqueous humor to flow freely).

Direct-acting Miotic Drugs for Glaucoma

These drugs cause pupillary constriction by stimulating the iris muscle around the pupil to contract and produce miosis. These were the first drugs developed for glaucoma but are used less often now. These drugs are administered topically as eyedrops.

> carbachol (Carboptic, Isopto Carbachol)
> phenylephrine (Mydfrin, Neo-Synephrine)
> pilocarpine (Akarpine, Isopto Carpine, Pilocar, Pilopine HS)

Cholinesterase Inhibitors for Glaucoma

These drugs inhibit cholinesterase, an enzyme that normally destroys acetylcholine. As excess acetylcholine accumulates, it causes miosis.

> demecarium (Humorsol)
> echothiophate iodide (Phospholine Iodide)

Carbonic Anhydrase Inhibitors for Glaucoma

These drugs decrease the production of aqueous humor by blocking the enzyme carbonic anhydrase, which is active in the production of aqueous humor.

> acetazolamide (Diamox, Diamox Sequels)
> brinzolamide (Azopt)
> dichlorphenamide (Daranide)
> dorzolamide (Trusopt)
> methazolamide (GlaucTabs, Neptazane)

Alpha- or Beta-Receptor Blockers for Glaucoma

These drugs block alpha or beta receptors in the eye and decrease the production of aqueous humor to decrease intraocular pressure. With the exception of dapiprazole (an alpha-receptor blocker), these beta-receptor blocker drugs have no effect on pupil size and therefore do not cause the blurred vision or night blindness associated with some other glaucoma drugs.

> betaxolol (Betoptic, Betoptic S)
> carteolol (Ocupress)
> dapiprazole (Rev-Eyes)
> levobetaxolol (Betaxon)
> levobunolol (Betagan Liquifilm)
> metipranolol (OptiPranolol)
> timolol (Betimol, Timoptic, Timoptic-XE)

Note: The ending *-olol* is common to generic beta-blocker drugs.

Alpha- /Beta-Receptor Agonist Drugs for Glaucoma

These drugs have a combined action that activates alpha or alpha and beta receptors in the eye. This dilates the pupil and increases the outflow of aqueous humor, but also decreases the overall production of aqueous humor.

> apraclonidine (Iopidine)
> brimonidine (Alphagan, Alphagan P)
> dipivefrin (Propine)
> epinephrine (Epifrin, Glaucon)
> epinephryl (Epinal)

Prostaglandin F Agonist Drugs for Glaucoma

These drugs mimic the action of naturally occurring prostaglandin F by activating its receptors. This increases the outflow of aqueous humor.

> bimatoprost (Lumigan)
> latanoprost (Xalatan)
> travoprost (Travatan)
> unoprostone (Rescula)

Combination Drugs for Glaucoma

These drugs combine a miotic drug and an alpha-/beta-receptor agonist.

> E-Pilo-1, E-Pilo-2, E-Pilo-4, E-Pilo-6 (pilocarpine, epinephrine)
> P_1E_1, P_2E_1, P_4E_1, P_6E_1 (pilocarpine, epinephrine)

This drug combines a carbonic anhydrase inhibitor and a beta-blocker.

> Cosopt (dorzolamide, timolol)

ANESTHETIC OPHTHALMIC DRUGS

Topical anesthetic drugs are used in the eye to facilitate examination and for short surgical procedures such as foreign body removal or suture removal.

> proparacaine (Alcaine, Ophthaine, Ophthetic)
> tetracaine

MYDRIATIC DRUGS

These topical drugs are used to dilate the pupil (mydriasis) and paralyze the muscles of accommodation (cycloplegia) in the iris. They block the action of acetylcholine, which normally tends to constrict the pupil. Mydriatic drugs are used to prepare the eye for an internal examination and to treat inflammatory conditions of the iris and uveal tract.

atropine (Atropine Care, Atropisol, Isopto Atropine)

cyclopentolate (Cyclogyl, Pentolair)

homatropine (Isopto Homatropine)

hydroxyamphetamine (Paredrine)

phenylephrine (Neo-Synephrine, Mydfrin)

scopolamine (Isopto Hyoscine)

tropicamide (Mydriacyl)

Combination Mydriatic Drugs

These drugs combine a mydriatic with an ophthalmic decongestant.

Cyclomydril (cyclopentolate, phenylephrine)

Murocoll-2 (scopolamine, phenylephrine)

HISTORICAL NOTES: The belladonna plant was the original source of atropine and scopolamine. Belladonna means *beautiful lady* in Italian. "Sixteenth century Italian women . . . squeezed the berries of these plants into their eyes to widen and brighten them."

Michael C. Gerald, *Pharmacology: An Introduction to Drugs*, 2nd ed. (Englewood Cliffs, NJ: Prentice Hall, 1981), p. 149, out of print.

COMBINATION OPHTHALMIC DRUGS

These topical ophthalmic drugs contain a corticosteroid and one or more anti-infective drugs.

Blephamide, Blephamide Suspension (prednisolone, sulfacetamide)

Cetapred Ointment (prednisolone, sulfacetamide)

Cortisporin (bacitracin, hydrocortisone, neomycin, polymyxin B)

Cortisporin Ophthalmic Suspension (hydrocortisone, neomycin, polymyxin B)

Dexacidin, Dexacidin Ophthalmic Suspension (dexamethasone, neomycin, polymyxin B)

Isopto Cetapred Suspension (prednisolone, sulfacetamide)

Maxitrol Ophthalmic Suspension (dexamethasone, neomycin, polymyxin B)

Metimyd, Metimyd Suspension (prednisolone, sulfacetamide)

NeoDecadron Ophthalmic Solution (dexamethasone, neomycin)

Ophthocort (chloramphenicol, hydrocortisone, polymyxin B)

Poly-Pred Liquifilm Ophthalmic Suspension (prednisolone, neomycin, polymyxin B)

Pred-G Ophthalmic Suspension, Pred-G S.O.P. (gentamicin, prednisolone)

Sulster Solution (prednisolone, sulfacetamide)

TobraDex Ophthalmic Suspension (dexamethasone, tobramycin)
Vasocine Ointment (prednisolone, sulfacetamide)

These topical ophthalmic drugs contain two or more antibiotics.

Neosporin Ophthalmic Ointment (bacitracin, neomycin, polymyxin B)
Neosporin Ophthalmic Solution (gramicidin, neomycin, polymyxin B)
Polysporin Ophthalmic Ointment (bacitracin, polymyxin B)
Polytrim Ophthalmic Solution (polymyxin B, trimethoprim)

These topical ophthalmic drugs contain a decongestant and an antihistamine.

Naphcon-A Solution (naphazoline, pheniramine)
Opcon-A Solution (naphazoline, pheniramine)

This topical ophthalmic drug contains a decongestant and an anti-infective.

Vasosulf (phenylephrine, sulfacetamide)

These topical ophthalmic drugs contain an ophthalmic dye and an anesthetic.

Fluoracaine (fluorescein, proparacaine)
Flurate (benoxinate, fluorescein)

MISCELLANEOUS OPHTHALMIC DRUGS

acetylcholine (Miochol-E):   Miotic drug used only during eye surgery and given by intraocular injection.

AdatoSil 5000:   Silicone oil injected into the posterior chamber of the eyes to stop retinal detachment.

Adsorbonac: A hypertonic sodium chloride solution applied topically to help reduce corneal edema following cataract surgery and other procedures.

aminocaproic acid (Caprogel):   Used to treat traumatic hyphema.

artificial tears (Akwa Tears, AquaSite, Bion Tears, Celluvisc, Comfort Tears, Dry Eyes, GenTeal, HypoTears, HypoTears PF, Isopto Plain, Isopto Tears, Liquifilm Tears, Moisture Drops, Moisture Eyes, Murine, Murocel, Nu-Tears, Nu-Tears II, OcuCoat, OcuCoat PF, Refresh, Refresh Plus, Refresh Tears, Tears Naturale, Tears Naturale Free, Tears Naturale II, Tears Plus, Tears Renewed, Ultra Tears):   A solution of salt that is similar to tears, with other additives to increase viscosity. Used to treat dry eyes.

balanced salt solution (B-Salt Forte, BSS, BSS Plus, Iocare Balanced Salt):   Physiologic saline solution used during eye surgery to irrigate and protect the eye.

botulinum toxin type A (Botox, Dysport):   Derived from a culture of the same bacteria that cause botulism (food poisoning), this drug is injected into eye muscles to paralyze the muscle fibers and allow them to lengthen. It is used to treat blepharospasm, nystagmus, and strabismus.

brimonidine (Alphagan):   Used to treat optic neuropathy.

bromhexine (Bisolvon):   Used to treat the dry eyes of Sjögren's syndrome.

bupivacaine (Marcaine, Sensorcaine):   A local anesthetic given by retrobulbar injection to produce corneal anesthesia and akinesia (temporary paralysis) of the eye muscles before eye surgery.

carbachol (Carbastat, Miostat):   Miotic drug used only during eye surgery and given by intraocular injection.

cromolyn (Opticrom):   Used to treat keratoconjunctivitis.

cyclosporine (Optimmune):   Used to treat the dry eyes of Sjögren's syndrome.

dextran 70 (Dehydrex):   Used to treat corneal erosions.

Duratears Naturale: Lubricating ointment for the eyes.

fluorescein (Fluorescite, Ful-Glo, Fluorets):   A yellow water-based dye that shows green under fluorescent light, this drug is used to reveal corneal abrasions and ulcers caused by foreign bodies or ill-fitting contact lenses.

fluorexon (Fluoresoft):   Topical dye used to assist in fitting contact lenses.

flurbiprofen (Ocufen):   Topical NSAID used only during eye surgery to prevent miosis.

Galardin: Used to treat corneal ulcers.

gangliosides (Cronassial):   Used to treat retinitis pigmentosa.

glycerin (Ophthalgan):   Used to treat corneal edema.

Healon Yellow: Combination drug of sodium hyaluronate and fluorescein dye injected into the eye to keep the anterior chamber open during surgery and help visualize tissues.

indocyanine green (Cardio-Green):   Dye used during angiography of the eye.

interferon alfa-2a (Roferon-A):   Used to treat herpes keratoconjunctivitis.

Lacri-Lube NP, Lacri-Lube S.O.P.:   Lubricating ointment for the eyes.

Lacrisert: A pellet inserted into the conjunctival sac to continuously release artificial tears to lubricate the eye.

lidocaine (Xylocaine):   A local anesthetic given by retrobulbar injection to produce corneal anesthesia and akinesia (temporary paralysis) of the eye muscles before eye surgery.

methylcellulose (Gonak, Goniosol, OcuCoat):   Injected into the anterior chamber of the eye to replace intraocular fluid lost during surgery.

Moisture Eyes PM: Lubricating ointment for the eyes.

Muro 128:   A hypertonic sodium chloride solution applied topically to help reduce corneal edema following cataract surgery and other procedures.

Panretin: Used to prevent retinal detachment in patients with proliferative retinopathy.

pilocarpine (Salagen):   Used to treat the dry eyes of Sjögren's syndrome.

Refresh PM: Lubricating ointment for the eyes.

rose bengal (Rosets):   Dye strips used to reveal corneal abrasions.

sodium hyaluronate (AMO Vitrax, Amvisc, Amvisc Plus, Healon, Healon GV):   Injected into the eye to replace intraocular fluid lost during surgery.

suprofen (Profenal): Topical NSAID used only during eye surgery to prevent miosis.

tretinoin: Used to treat squamous metaplasia of the cornea.

tyloxapol (Enuclene): Solution to clean and wet an artificial eye.

urea (Ureaphil): Given intravenously to decrease intraocular pressure.

urogastrone: Used to promote healing after corneal transplant.

verteporfin (Visudyne): Used to treat macular degeneration. The drug is administered intravenously and then the eyes are exposed to a red laser light to activate the drug. It is also used to treat ocular histoplasmosis.

Viscoat: Combination drug of sodium hyaluronate and chondroitin injected into the eye to keep the anterior chamber expanded during eye surgery.

REVIEW QUESTIONS

1. Discuss the use of silver nitrate versus erythromycin to prevent newborns from developing eye infections due to gonorrhea.
2. What advantage do beta-blockers have over other miotic drugs used to treat glaucoma?
3. What class of ophthalmic drugs is used to prepare the eye for internal examination?
4. Contrast the therapeutic effect of antibiotic, sulfonamide, and corticosteroid ophthalmic drugs.
5. Contrast the therapeutic effect of antihistamine ophthalmic drugs with that of ophthalmic mast cell stabilizers.
6. Name three categories of ophthalmic drugs and give an example of a drug in each category.
7. To what category of drugs does each of these drugs belong?
   - cromolyn (Crolom)
   - dexamethasone (Decadron, Maxidex)
   - levobunolol (Betagan Liquifilm)
   - levofloxacin (Quixin)
   - pilocarpine (Akarpine, Isopto Carpine, Ocusert Pilo-20, Ocusert Pilo-40, Pilocar, Pilopine HS)
   - tropicamide (Mydriacyl)
8. Rewrite this prescription in plain English. Use the Glossary/Index at the back of the textbook to help you verify the spelling and dosage of this drug. (See Figure 20–1.)

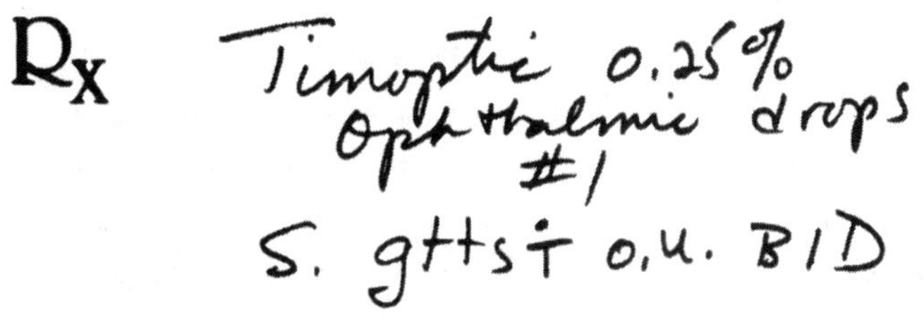

R̲x   Timoptic 0.25%
       Ophthalmic drops
       #1
    S. gtts ī o.u. BID

Figure 20–1 A prescription. *Reprinted courtesy of Marvin Stoogenke, The Pharmacy Technician, 2nd ed. (Upper Saddle River, NJ: Brady/Prentice Hall, 1998), p. 366.*

SPELLING TIPS

Akwa Tears   Phonetic spelling of *aqua*.

Alocril with an *o*, but Alamast with an *a*.

genta**mic**in (generic) but Gara**myc**in (trade).

Inflamase   *Inflammation* has two *m*'s; *Inflamase* has one *m*.

NeoDecadron   Unusual internal capitalization.

OcuClear   Unusual internal capitalization.

ophthalmic   This is correctly pronounced "of-thal-mik." However, because of the pronunciation of optic and optician, which also have to do with the eyes, ophthalmic is commonly mispronounced as "op-thal-mik." This common mispronunciation makes the first *h* silent and the word is frequently misspelled without the first *h*.

OptiPranolol   Unusual internal capitalization.

TobraDex   Unusual internal capitalization.

GET CONNECTED

Multimedia Extension Activities

 www.prenhall.com/turley

Use the above address to access the free, interactive Companion Website created for this textbook. Included in the features of this site are drug updates and additional chapter-specific exercises for further practice.

21

Endocrine Drugs

CHAPTER CONTENTS

Drugs used to treat thyroid gland dysfunction
Drugs used to treat pituitary gland dysfunction
Drugs used to treat adrenal gland dysfunction
Corticosteroids
Anabolic steroids
Miscellaneous endocrine drugs
Review questions
Spelling tips

LEARNING OBJECTIVES

After studying this chapter, you should be able to do the following:

1. Name several categories of endocrine drugs.
2. Describe the therapeutic action of drugs used to treat thyroid, pituitary, and adrenal gland dysfunction.
3. Describe the therapeutic action of corticosteroids versus anabolic steroids.
4. Given the generic and trade name of an endocrine drug, identify what drug category it belongs to or what disease it is used to treat.
5. Given an endocrine drug category, name several generic and trade name drugs in that category.
6. Identify the Historical Notes or Did You Know? section in this chapter that you found most interesting.

The endocrine system consists of many glands that secrete hormones into the bloodstream. When these glands malfunction, they release either a decreased or an increased amount of hormone. Some of these hormones are available as drugs and are used as replacement therapy to treat diseases caused by too little of the hormone; other hormone drugs are used to suppress the gland when it secretes too much hormone.

DRUGS USED TO TREAT THYROID GLAND DYSFUNCTION

Drugs for Hypothyroidism

The thyroid gland secretes the hormones triiodothyronine (T_3) and thyroxine (T_4). Decreased levels of these hormones cause hypothyroidism. Drugs used to treat hypothyroidism supplement existing levels of T_3 and/or T_4. These drugs are obtained from natural sources, such as desiccated (dried) ground beef or pork thyroid glands, or they are synthetically manufactured.

These thyroid hormone drugs contain both T_3 and T_4.

desiccated thyroid (Armour Thyroid)
liotrix (Thyrolar)

This thyroid hormone drug contains only T_3.

liothyronine (Cytomel, Triostat)

This thyroid hormone drug contains only T_4.

levothyroxine (Levo-T, Levothroid, Synthroid, Unithroid)

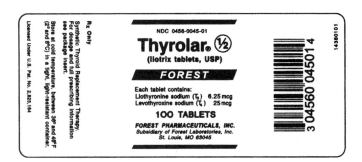

Figure 21–1   Thyroid hormone drugs are one of the few drugs in current use in which the dosage is measured in both the metric and apothecary systems. The prescription thyroid hormone liotrix (Thyrolar), showing both the metric dosage in micrograms (mcg) and the apothecary dosage (½ grain). *Photograph reprinted courtesy of Forest Pharmaceuticals, Inc.*

Drugs for Hyperthyroidism

Increased levels of T_3 and T_4 cause hyperthyroidism. Antithyroid drugs used to treat hyperthyroidism inhibit the production of T_3 and T_4 in the thyroid gland. These drugs can also be given prior to a thyroidectomy. Radioactive sodium iodide 131 is used to treat both hyperthyroidism and thyroid cancer. The low-level radiation emitted by this drug destroys both hyperactive benign thyroid tissue as well as cancerous thyroid tissue.

methimazole (Tapazole)

propylthiouracil

radioactive sodium iodide 131 (Iodotope)

This drug can be given to patients prior to a thyroidectomy in addition to other antithyroid drugs.

Lugol's Solution

This drug is used to suppress the release of thyroid-stimulating hormone (TSH) from the pituitary gland in patients with thyroid cancer.

tiratricol (Triacana)

DRUGS USED TO TREAT PITUITARY GLAND DYSFUNCTION

Growth Hormone Replacement Drugs

The anterior pituitary gland secretes growth hormone. Decreased levels of this hormone result in a lack of growth in children. Chronic renal failure as well as certain genetic abnormalities can also cause a lack of growth. Drugs used as growth hormone replacement therapy include:

sermorelin (Geref)

somatrem (Protropin)

somatropin (Genotropin, Genotropin MiniQuick, Humatrope, Norditropin, Nutropin, Nutropin AQ, Nutropin Depot, Saizen)

DID YOU KNOW?   Both somatrem and somatropin are created using recombinant DNA technology. The root word *somato* is Greek for *body*.

Drugs for Acromegaly

An increased level of growth hormone causes acromegaly in adults. These drugs are given to suppress the overproduction of growth hormone by the anterior pituitary gland.

lanreotide (Ipstyl)

octreotide (Sandostatin, Sandostatin LAR Depot)

Trovert

DID YOU KNOW? Octreotide is also used to treat severe diarrhea associated with VIPomas and AIDS-related diarrhea. This drug has a side effect of decreased peristalsis; this is used as the therapeutic drug effect in treating the diarrhea.

Drugs for Syndrome of Inappropriate Antidiuretic Hormone (SIADH)

The posterior pituitary gland secretes the hormone vasopressin to inhibit the excretion of water by the kidneys. Because of this effect, vasopressin is also known as *antidiuretic hormone (ADH)*. A tumor of the posterior pituitary gland can cause it to secrete inappropriately large amounts of ADH. Furosemide and urea act as diuretics to counteract the action of excessive amounts of ADH, but the mechanism of the therapeutic action of the other drugs in treating SIADH is not well understood.

demeclocycline (Declomycin)
furosemide (Lasix)
lithium (Eskalith, Eskalith CR, Lithobid)
urea (Ureaphil)

Drugs for Diabetes Insipidus

Insufficient levels of ADH cause diabetes insipidus. Drugs are used to treat diabetes insipidus by acting as replacement therapy for ADH.

desmopressin (DDAVP, Stimate)
vasopressin (Pitressin)

DID YOU KNOW? Desmopressin is also used to treat bed-wetting. Studies have shown that many patients who habitually bed-wet have low levels of ADH. Desmopressin (DDAVP) is administered as a nasal spray for replacement ADH therapy. Desmopressin is also used to stop bleeding following trauma in patients with hemophilia.

DRUGS USED TO TREAT ADRENAL GLAND DYSFUNCTION

Drugs for Cushing's Syndrome

The adrenal cortex secretes the glucocorticoid hormones hydrocortisone and cortisol. A benign tumor (adenoma) or malignant tumor (carcinoma) can cause the adrenal cortex to produce increased amounts of glucocorticoids, and this causes Cushing's syndrome. This drug is used to treat Cushing's syndrome; it inhibits the synthesis of glucocorticoids in the adrenal cortex.

aminoglutethimide (Cytadren)

Drugs for Addison's Disease

The adrenal cortex also secretes mineralocorticoid hormone. When the adrenal cortex mal-functions, there is a deficiency of both glucocorticoid and mineralocorticoid hormones, resulting in Addison's disease. Glucocorticoids available as drugs are known as *cortico-steroids*. Some corticosteroid drugs are used as glucocorticoid replacement therapy to treat Addison's disease. The other corticosteroid drugs are discussed in the next section.

methylprednisolone (Depo-Medrol, Depopred-40, Depopred-80)

triamcinolone (Aristocort, Kenacort)

The decreased levels of mineralocorticoid hormone in Addison's disease are treated with the following drug.

fludrocortisone (Florinef)

Sometimes the adrenal cortex itself is normal, but it does not produce enough hor-mones because it is not stimulated by ACTH from the anterior pituitary gland; this also results in Addison's disease. This drug provides replacement ACTH therapy to stimulate the adrenal cortex.

corticotropin (ACTH, Acthar)

CORTICOSTEROIDS

The adrenal cortex secretes the glucocorticoids hydrocortisone and cortisone, two powerful anti-inflammatory hormones. Both natural and synthetic glucocorticoids are available as drugs and are known as *corticosteroids* because they act like the natural hormones produced by the adrenal cortex (root word *cortico-*) and their chemical structure is that of a steroid. Some corticosteroids are used as replacement therapy to treat Addison's disease, as de-scribed earlier. Other corticosteroids are used to treat inflammatory reactions involving various areas of the body (severe psoriasis or dermatitis, severe inflammation of the eye, ul-cerative colitis and Crohn's disease, cerebral edema following head trauma, and so forth). Corticosteroids are also used to treat systemic inflammation caused by autoimmune dis-eases (rheumatoid arthritis, multiple sclerosis, lupus erythematosus, and so forth).

betamethasone (Celestone)
cortisone (Cortone)
dexamethasone (Decadron, Dexameth, Dexamethasone Intensol, Dexone, Hexadrol)
hydrocortisone (A-Hydrocort, Cortef, Hydrocortone, Solu-Cortef)
methylprednisolone (A-Methapred, Medrol, Solu-Medrol)
prednisolone (Hydeltrasol, Orapred, Pediapred, Predalone 50, Prelone)
prednisone (Deltasone, Meticorten, Orasone, Prednisone Intensol Concentrate)

triamcinolone (Aristocort, Aristocort Forte, Kenacort, Kenalog-40, Tac-40, Trilog, Trilone)

Topical and systemic corticosteroid drugs used to treat inflammation of the skin, GI system, musculoskeletal system, respiratory system, ears, nose, and eyes are further discussed in Chapters 11, 13, 14, 18, 19, and 20.

HISTORICAL NOTES: A researcher at the Mayo Clinic was attempting to identify hormones in the adrenal gland. He located five substances that he called Substances A, B, C, D, and E. To obtain only 2 ounces of Substance E, he had to grind 300,000 pounds of cattle adrenal glands. In 1941, the United States received an intelligence report that Germany was giving adrenal gland extract to its pilots to enable them to fly at high altitudes. Although this report was false, it stimulated financial backing for adrenal gland research. Substance E later became known as *cortisone*.

ANABOLIC STEROIDS

Anabolic steroids change the natural balance between anabolism (tissue building) and catabolism (tissue breakdown). These drugs increase tissue building and have been used for years by athletes to increase muscle mass, strength, and endurance. Although the use of these drugs is illegal in amateur and professional sports competitions, the use of anabolic steroids by all types of athletes and bodybuilders continues. The drugs are discontinued before a competition to avoid detection during random drug testing. The use of two or more anabolic steroids at the same time is referred to as "stacking." Often the dose taken is up to 100 times the dose that would be written for a prescription use of the drug. The use of anabolic steroids can cause decreased sperm count, shrunken testicles, baldness, and irreversible breast enlargement in men. In women, these drugs can cause baldness and excessive growth of facial hair. The serious side effects of anabolic steroids include aggressive behavior, atherosclerosis, and even liver cancer. All anabolic steroids are classified as Schedule III controlled substances because of their high potential for addiction and abuse.

FOCUS ON HEALTHCARE ISSUES: Anabolic steroids have been used by athletes since the 1950s. A recent study by the National Institute of Drug Abuse found that there was a 50% increase in the use of anabolic steroids by children in grades 8 to 10 over the 9 years since the previous study.

For AIDS patients, anabolic steroids are legally prescribed to counteract the loss of muscle mass and strength that occurs with AIDS wasting syndrome. These drugs may also be legally prescribed to promote weight gain following extensive surgery or trauma, to increase the RBC count and treat anemia, or to treat metastatic breast cancer. Oxandrolone is also used to treat lack of growth in patients with Turner's syndrome.

> nandrolone (Deca-Durabolin)
> oxandrolone (Oxandrin)
> oxymetholone (Anadrol-50)
> stanozolol (Winstrol)

MISCELLANEOUS ENDOCRINE DRUGS

Acthrel: Used to help diagnose whether Cushing's syndrome is due to a pituitary gland malfunction or another cause.

cosyntropin (Cortrosyn):   Used during diagnostic testing to determine adrenal cortex function.

cyproterone (Androcur):   Used to treat severe hirsutism.

dacarbazine (DTIC-Dome):   Chemotherapy drug used to treat pheochromocytoma, a tumor of the adrenal cortex.

danazol (Danocrine):   Used to treat precocious puberty and gynecomastia in males.

deslorelin (Somagard):   Used to treat precocious puberty.

dexamethasone (Decadron, Dexameth, Dexamethasone Intensol, Dexone, Hexadrol):   Used during diagnostic testing (dexamethasone suppression test) to diagnose Cushing's syndrome.

fluoxymesterone (Halotestin):   Male sex hormone used to treat decreased testosterone due to absence, injury, or dysfunction of the testes or dysfunction of the pituitary gland; used to treat delayed puberty in boys.

follitropin alfa (Gonal-F):   Anterior pituitary gland follicle-stimulating hormone replacement used to increase sperm count and treat infertility in men.

flutamide (Eulexin):   Hormonal chemotherapy drug also used to treat hirsutism.

histrelin (Supprelin):   Used to treat precocious puberty.

labetalol (Normodyne, Trandate):   Beta-blocker antihypertensive drug used to treat the hypertension caused by a pheochromocytoma, a benign tumor of the adrenal medulla.

leuprolide (Lupron Depot-Ped):   Hormonal chemotherapy drug used to treat precocious puberty.

mecasermin (Myotrophin):   Used to treat growth hormone insufficiency syndrome.

methyltestosterone (Android, Methitest, Testred, Virilon, Virilon M):   Male sex hormone used to treat decreased testosterone due to absence, injury, or dysfunction of the testes or dysfunction of the pituitary gland; used to treat delayed puberty in boys.

metyrosine (Demser):   Inhibits the enzyme that helps produce epinephrine and norepinephrine. Used to treat hypertension caused by excessive epinephrine and norepinephrine produced by a pheochromocytoma of the adrenal medulla.

nafarelin (Synarel):   Used to treat precocious puberty in boys and girls.

phentolamine (Regitine):   Alpha-adrenergic blocker drug used to treat hypertension caused by a pheochromocytoma of the adrenal medulla.

propranolol (Inderal, Inderal LA):   Beta-blocker antihypertensive drug used to treat hypertension caused by a pheochromocytoma of the adrenal medulla.

Somatrel: Used to diagnose lack of growth hormone due to pituitary gland dysfunction.

tamoxifen (Nolvadex):   Hormonal chemotherapy drug also used to treat gynecomastia in men.

testosterone (Androderm, AndroGel, Delatestryl, Depo-Testosterone, Testoderm, Testoderm TTS, Testopel):   Male sex hormone used to treat decreased testosterone due to absence, injury, or dysfunction of the testes or dysfunction of the pituitary gland; used to treat delayed puberty in boys.

urofollitropin (Fertinex):   Used to treat low sperm count and infertility in men with pituitary gland dysfunction.

REVIEW QUESTIONS

1. What are two sources for the manufacture of thyroid hormone drugs?
2. What two powerful natural anti-inflammatory hormones are secreted by the adrenal cortex?
3. Name three categories of endocrine drugs and give an example of a drug from each category.
4. Name one detrimental effect and one therapeutic effect of anabolic steroids.

SPELLING TIPS

Synthroid   Although *thyroid* has a *y*, the *y* has been deleted from this drug.
Unithroid   Although thyroid has a *y*, the *y* has been deleted from this drug.

GET CONNECTED

Multimedia Extension Activities

   www.prenhall.com/turley

Use the above address to access the free, interactive Companion Website created for this textbook. Included in the features of this site are drug updates and additional chapter-specific exercises for further practice.

22

Antidiabetic Drugs

CHAPTER CONTENTS

Insulin
Oral antidiabetic drugs
Drugs used to treat diabetic neuropathy
Miscellaneous diabetic drugs
Review questions
Spelling tips

LEARNING OBJECTIVES

After studying this chapter, you should be able to do the following:

1. Describe the therapeutic action of insulin and oral antidiabetic drugs.
2. Given the generic and trade name of a drug used to treat diabetes, identify what drug category it belongs to.
3. Given a drug category, name several drugs that belong to that category.

Diabetes mellitus results when the pancreas fails to produce any insulin (type I diabetes mellitus), when the pancreas produces too little insulin (type II diabetes mellitus), or when the number or sensitivity of insulin receptors on body cells decreases (type II diabetes mellitus). **Type I diabetes mellitus** is also known as *insulin-dependent diabetes mellitus (IDDM)* or *juvenile-onset diabetes mellitus.* **Type II diabetes mellitus** is also known as *non-insulin-dependent diabetes mellitus (NIDDM)* or *adult-onset diabetes mellitus.* Type I must always be treated with subcutaneously injected insulin; type II may be treated with insulin or, more commonly, with oral antidiabetic drugs, or both. A diet with controlled amounts of calories from carbohydrates and fats, exercise, and antidiabetic drugs are all important components of diabetic management.

INSULIN

Insulin is secreted by beta cells in the islets of Langerhans in the pancreas. This hormone plays an essential role in sugar metabolism. Insulin lowers blood sugar levels by enabling cells to utilize glucose, particularly skeletal muscle cells.

HISTORICAL NOTES: Insulin was first isolated in the 1920s. Until that time, diabetic patients were kept on an extremely low-calorie diet (often to the point of starvation)—the only treatment known. The term *insulin* is from the Latin word *insula* meaning *island*, a reference to the islets of Langerhans. Insulin is broken down by digestive enzymes and so it can never be given orally. The first insulin injections were thick and muddy brown in color due to impurities from their source: ground-up beef and pork pancreas.

Traditionally, insulin has been derived from beef or pork pancreas. Human insulin drugs are not actually insulin from the human body, as the name would imply. These drugs are synthetic insulins (as opposed to animal-product insulins) that are created using recombinant DNA technology. Human insulin drugs are so named because their chemical structure more closely resembles that of natural human insulin than of animal-product insulins. The natural insulin molecule consists of two chains of amino acids; the A chain contains 21 amino acids and the B chain contains 30 amino acids. In the drug human insulin aspart, aspartic acid is inserted at site B28 in place of the amino acid proline. In the drug human insulin lispro, the amino acids are reversed at sites B28 and B29 when compared to a molecule of natural human insulin. The term *lispro insulin* was derived from the two reversed amino acids: **lys**ine and **pro**line. As a group, human insulin drugs are also known as *human insulin analog drugs*. An analog is structurally similar to the original molecule but is not entirely the same. Human insulin drugs can be recognized by trade names that contain the words *Humulin, Humalog, Novolin,* or *Novolog*.

DID YOU KNOW? Humulin insulin was the first recombinant DNA technology drug of any type to be marketed. The trade name Humalog is derived from the phrase *human insulin analog*.

The drugs human insulin aspart, human insulin lispro, and human insulin glargine were created using recombinant DNA technology to modify a bacterium or yeast to produce the drug molecule. Many recombinant DNA technology products are created using bacteria because they multiply quickly and produce large quantities of the desired drug. The yeast used to make human insulin aspart is the same as baker's yeast used in the kitchen!

Regardless of the source or how the drug is manufactured, all insulins are classified according to how quickly they act in the body to lower the blood glucose level (this depends on the size of the insulin crystal) and how many hours their therapeutic action continues (this depends on the amount of added protamine and zinc).

Rapid-acting Insulins

This type of insulin is known as *regular insulin*.

> Iletin II Regular
> Humulin R
> insulin aspart (NovoLog)
> insulin lispro (Humalog)
> Novolin R, Novolin R PenFill
> Velosulin BR

DID YOU KNOW?   NovoLog was the first insulin to be approved by the FDA specifically for use with an external insulin pump.

Intermediate-acting Insulins

This type of insulin is combined with protamine and zinc and is known as *NPH insulin*.

> NPH Iletin II
> Humulin N
> Novolin N, Novolin N PenFill

This type of insulin has two different sizes of insulin crystals and is known as *lente insulin*.

> Lente Iletin II
> Humulin L
> Novolin L

Long-acting Insulins

This type of insulin has large crystals and contains zinc. It is known as *ultralente insulin*.

> Humulin U Ultralente
> insulin glargine (Lantus)

> **DID YOU KNOW?**   Insulin glargine (Lantus) is the only insulin that can lower the blood glucose for a full 24 hours after just one dose. It is absorbed more slowly than other types of insulin so it continues to work for a longer period of time.

Concentrated Insulins

Most type I diabetic patients require no more than 60 units of insulin per day. However, some type I diabetics are resistant or unresponsive to the effects of insulin and require much larger dosages. This drug is a concentrated insulin that contains 500 units/mL rather than the usual 100 units/mL.

>   Humulin R Regular U-500

Combination Insulins

These drugs contain various mixtures of NPH and regular insulin.

>   Humalog Mix 75/25
>   Humulin 50/50
>   Humulin 70/30
>   Novolin 70/30, Novolin 70/30 PenFill

Insulin dosages are always measured in units. Insulin comes as a standard 100 units/mL, also known as U-100. Concentrated insulin comes as 500 units/mL or U-500. Insulin is administered with special insulin syringes calibrated in units.

Insulin is given subcutaneously once or twice a day at various sites on the arms, thighs, and abdomen. It can also be administered directly into the bloodstream by a portable insulin pump that is attached to a belt or carried in a pocket. This pump weighs less than 4 ounces and uses watch batteries. It can deliver as little as 0.1 unit of insulin and has alarms to alert the patient when the tubing is blocked or the reservoir is nearly empty. A totally implantable computerized insulin pump is also available for patients who have poorly controlled diabetes or who wish to avoid injections. The pump is implanted in the abdomen and the patient programs how much insulin to give via a remote controller.

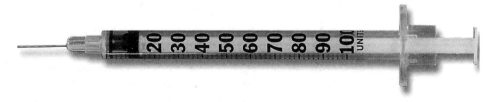

Figure 22–1   Insulin syringe calibrated in units. This syringe holds a total of 1 mL. *Photo reprinted courtesy of BD (Becton, Dickinson, and Company).*

FOCUS ON HEALTHCARE ISSUES: Beef and beef/pork insulins have been withdrawn from the market in the United States because bovine spongiform encephalopathy (a fatal disease in cattle) has been linked to outbreaks of an incurable neurological condition in humans known as Creutzfeldt–Jakob disease. Some diabetics who have tried to switch to other types of insulin have found that they have poorly controlled blood sugar levels. Some diabetics have tried to obtain beef/pork insulin from other countries and have petitioned the U.S. government to allow them continued access to beef and beef/pork insulin.

ORAL ANTIDIABETIC DRUGS

Patients with type II diabetes mellitus have pancreases that are still producing limited amounts of insulin. With diet control, exercise, and weight loss, the amount of available insulin may be sufficient to keep blood glucose levels within a normal range. If not, an oral antidiabetic drug will be prescribed. Contrary to popular opinion, these drugs are not insulin and are not effective in treating patients with type I diabetes mellitus. Oral antidiabetic drugs stimulate the beta cells of the pancreas to produce more insulin; these drugs also increase the number of insulin receptors.

> acetohexamide
> chlorpropamide (Diabinese)
> glimepiride (Amaryl)
> glipizide (Glucotrol, Glucotrol XL)
> glyburide (DiaBeta, Glynase PresTab, Micronase)
> nateglinide (Starlix)
> pioglitazone (Actos)
> repaglinide (Prandin)
> rosiglitazone (Avandia)
> tolazamide (Tolinase)
> tolbutamide (Orinase)

DID YOU KNOW?   The trade name DiaBeta is a combination of *diabetes* and *beta* for the beta cells of the islets of Langerhans of the pancreas that produce insulin.

Other antidiabetic drugs inhibit an enzyme in the intestine that digests glucose. This causes delayed digestion of glucose, which prevents a sharp rise in blood sugar from occurring after a meal. This is of particular importance in the long-term management of diabetes because elevated blood sugar levels contribute to an increased incidence of diabetic complications: arteriosclerosis, diabetic neuropathy, diabetic nephropathy, and so forth. These drugs do not stimulate the pancreas to produce more insulin.

acarbose (Precose)

metformin (Glucophage, Glucophage XR)

miglitol (Glyset)

Combination Oral Antidiabetic Drugs

Glucovance (glyburide, metformin)

> **DID YOU KNOW?**   The cost of antidiabetic oral drugs varies widely from $3/month to $70/month, depending on the individual drug and dosage prescribed. In 2001, about $1.8 billion of Glucophage was sold.

DRUGS USED TO TREAT DIABETIC NEUROPATHY

Diabetic neuropathy is a chronic complication of diabetes mellitus that is characterized by degenerative changes in the nerves of the lower extremities, pain, and altered sensation (paresthesias).

Most of the drugs used to treat this disease are antidepressants. Although antidepressants do not have a direct analgesic effect, they are effective in treating various types of pain syndromes. Lamotrigine is an anticonvulsant drug, but it also affects opioid receptors and is effective in treating chronic pain syndrome.

amitriptyline (Elavil)

amoxapine

desipramine (Norpramin)

doxepin (Sinequan, Sinequan Concentrate)

imipramine (Tofranil, Tofranil-PM)

lamotrigine (Lamictal)

nortriptyline (Aventyl, Pamelor)

protriptyline (Vivactil)

This investigational drug is used to treat both diabetic neuropathy and diabetic retinopathy.

tolrestat (Alredase)

MISCELLANEOUS ANTIDIABETIC DRUGS

BetaRx: Encapsulated islet cells from pigs, used to treat type I diabetics who are on immunosuppression.

Choice dm: Liquid nutritional supplement specifically formulated to meet the nutritional needs of patients with diabetes mellitus.

diazoxide (Proglycem):   Used to treat hypoglycemia.

glucagon: Used to treat hypoglycemia.

Glucerna: Liquid nutritional supplement specifically formulated to meet the nutritional needs of patients with diabetes mellitus.

glucose (B-D Glucose, Insta-Glucose):   Used to treat hypoglycemia.

Innovo Dial-a-Dose: Computerized insulin injection device.

pramlintide (Symlin):   Investigational drug given subcutaneously to patients with type I and type II diabetes mellitus to delay gastric emptying and control postprandial blood glucose elevation.

REVIEW QUESTIONS

1. Oral antidiabetic drugs contain a special type of insulin that can be taken orally. True or False?
2. What are some trade names for recombinant DNA technology-produced insulin?
3. List some of the differences between diabetics with type I and type II diabetes.
4. How are doses of insulin measured?
5. Name two categories of drugs used to treat diabetes and give examples of drugs in each category.
6. Why was beef/pork insulin removed from the market? What is the significance of this to diabetic patients?

SPELLING TIPS

BetaRx   Unusual internal capitalization.
Choice dm   Lack of capitalization.
DiaBeta   Unusual internal capitalization.

GET CONNECTED

Multimedia Extension Activities

 www.prenhall.com/turley

Use the above address to access the free, interactive Companion Website created for this textbook. Included in the features of this site are drug updates and additional chapter-specific exercises for further practice.

23

Obstetric/ Gynecologic Drugs

CHAPTER CONTENTS

Drugs used to treat infertility

Drugs used during pregnancy

Drugs used to treat premature labor

Drugs used to induce labor

Drugs used to treat postpartum bleeding

Drugs used to treat endometriosis

Oral contraceptives

Drugs used to treat menopause

Drugs used to treat abnormal menstruation

Drugs used to treat premenstrual syndrome (PMS) and premenstrual dysphoric disorder (PMDD)

Drugs used to treat dysmenorrhea

Drugs used to produce abortion

Drugs used to treat vaginal infections

Drugs used to treat sexually transmitted diseases (STDs)

Miscellaneous OB/GYN drugs

Review questions

Spelling tips

LEARNING OBJECTIVES

After studying this chapter, you should be able to do the following:

1. Name several categories of obstetric and gynecologic (OB/GYN) drugs.
2. Describe the therapeutic action of drugs used to treat infertility, premature labor, endometriosis, amenorrhea, dysmenorrhea, postpartum bleeding, vaginal infections, and sexually transmitted diseases (STDs).

3. Describe the therapeutic action of oral contraceptives, hormone replacement therapy (HRT), drugs used to produce abortion, and drugs used to induce labor.

4. Given the generic and trade name of an OB/GYN drug, identify what drug category it belongs to or what disease it is used to treat.

5. Given an OB/GYN drug category, give an example of several generic and trade name drugs in that category.

6. Identify the Did You Know? section of the chapter that you found most interesting.

Drugs used to treat women with obstetric and gynecologic (OB/GYN) problems include drugs for infertility, drugs that stimulate or suppress labor contractions, drugs that correct menstrual disorders and endometriosis, prophylactically prescribed birth control drugs, estrogen hormone replacement therapy, and drugs used to treat OB/GYN infections.

DRUGS USED TO TREAT INFERTILITY

Ovulation-stimulating Drugs for Infertility

Ovulation-stimulating drugs block estrogen receptors on the ovary so estrogen cannot enter. The ovary responds to the lack of estrogen by signaling the pituitary gland that estrogen levels are low, and then the pituitary gland secretes luteinizing hormone (LH) and follicle-stimulating hormone (FSH). These hormones stimulate a nonovulating ovary to develop an ovarian follicle and release mature eggs. These drugs also aid in the formation of the corpus luteum, which secretes progesterone to maintain the pregnancy if the egg is fertilized. Ovulation-stimulating drugs are appropriate for patients with anovulation (failure to ovulate), but are not appropriate for patients with infertility due to blocked fallopian tubes or other mechanical problems that require surgical intervention.

> sermorelin (Geref)
> choriogonadotropin alfa (Ovidrel)
> clomiphene (Clomid, Serophene)
> follitropin alfa (Gonal-F)
> follitropin beta (Follistim)
> human chorionic gonadotropin (HCG) (A.P.L., Pregnyl, Profasi)
> menotropins (Humegon, Pergonal, Repronex)
> somatropin (Norditropin)
> urofollitropin (Fertinex, Metrodin)

Note: Follitropin alfa, follitropin beta, menotropins, and urofollitropin must be given concurrently with HCG to achieve a complete therapeutic effect.

DID YOU KNOW?   Urofollitropin is extracted from the urine of postmenopausal women. Follitropin alfa and follitropin beta are manufactured using recombinant DNA technology. HCG is a hormone normally produced by the placenta in pregnant women.

FOCUS ON HEALTHCARE ISSUES: Ovulation-stimulating drugs may cause several mature eggs to be released at the same time. This is beneficial for patients undergoing *in vitro* fertilization in which the mature eggs are removed and combined in a test tube with sperm. The more eggs that are released, the better the chances for a successful harvesting and subsequent implantation of a fertilized egg. However, the use of only one or two of the fertilized eggs, while the rest of them are frozen (or possibly used in research), creates ethical and moral issues. Patients who become pregnant while on ovulation-stimulating drugs can have a pregnancy with multiple babies. This can endanger the life of the mother and the babies. Some obstetricians recommend elective removal of one or more of the growing fetuses, but this too creates ethical and moral issues.

Bobbi McCaughey, age 29, of Carlisle, Iowa, took Pergonal before she became pregnant, carried, and gave birth to the world's only surviving set of septuplets on November 20, 1997. The four boys and three girls were born at 30 weeks' gestation and each weighed from 2 pounds, 5 ounces, to 3 pounds, 4 ounces.

Progesterone Drugs for Infertility

This drug is used in conjunction with other treatments for infertility in women with progesterone deficiency.

progesterone (Crinone, Prometrium)

Other Drugs for Infertility

These drugs decrease excessive amounts of gonadotropin-releasing hormone that may be released from the pituitary gland in response to ovulation-stimulating drugs.

cetrorelix (Cetrotide)
ganirelix (Antagon)

DRUGS USED DURING PREGNANCY

Few drugs are prescribed during pregnancy, particularly during the first trimester, because of the increased risk of birth defects in the developing fetus. However, antibiotics to treat infections; drugs necessary to maintain health (such as insulin or heart medications); as well as prenatal vitamins, iron, and folic acid are given to pregnant women.

DID YOU KNOW? The U.S. Public Health Service recommends the use of folic acid supplements for all women of childbearing age. Folic acid significantly decreases the incidence of babies with neural tube defects (spina bifida, myelomeningocele). Since 1988, some breads, cereals, and pastas have had additional folic acid added to them.

DRUGS USED TO TREAT PREMATURE LABOR

Premature or preterm labor and delivery greatly increase morbidity and mortality in newborn infants. Premature labor contractions can be inhibited by using uterine-relaxing drugs. These drugs act on beta$_2$ receptors in the smooth muscle of the uterus to decrease both the frequency and strength of uterine contractions. These drugs are known as *tocolytics* (from the Greek words *toco-*, which means *childbirth*, and *–lysis*, which means *to dissolve or reduce*).

ritodrine (Yutopar)

DID YOU KNOW?   Terbutaline (Bricanyl), a drug used to treat asthma, had been used unofficially in the past (not approved by the FDA) to relax the smooth muscle of the uterus and treat preterm labor. This use was discontinued when one pregnant woman died and others experienced chest pain, tachycardia, and pulmonary edema.

Misoprostol (Cytotec), a drug approved by the FDA to prevent gastric ulcers in patients taking NSAIDs or aspirin, has been unofficially used in the past to induce labor. Patients do not know they are being given a drug that has not been approved by the FDA to induce labor. In some women who had had a previous cesarean section, this drug caused the uterus to rupture.

DRUGS USED TO INDUCE LABOR

Women in labor may be given a uterine stimulant if their uterine contractions are too weak to effect delivery (uterine inertia) or if complications such as preeclampsia or diabetes necessitate induction of labor. Normally, oxytocin (produced by the pituitary gland) stimulates the uterus by binding to special oxytocin receptors on the smooth muscle cells of the uterus. The drug oxytocin increases both the frequency and strength of uterine contractions. Oxytocin is not indicated when prolonged labor is due to cephalopelvic disproportion—the baby's skull is too large to fit through the mother's pelvic outlet.

hexoprenaline (Delaprem)
oxytocin (Pitocin, Syntocinon)

DID YOU KNOW?   Skeletons of prehistoric women have been discovered with the skull of the baby wedged into the mother's pelvic bones (cephalopelvic disproportion).

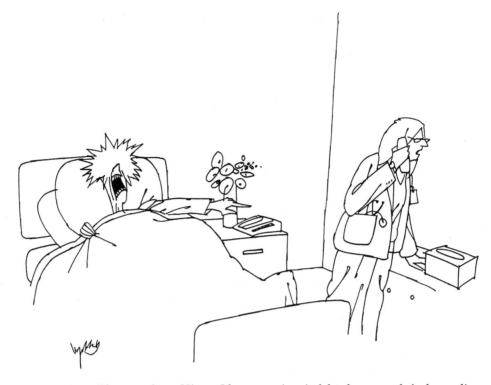

Figure 23–1   *Pharmacy? . . . Hi, . . . I have a patient in labor here, . . . she's demanding your entire inventory of narcotics.*—David W. Harbaugh. *Reprinted with permission.*

Labor consists of uterine contractions as well as cervical dilatation (widening) and effacement (thinning). When the cervix does not dilate and thin, these drugs may be applied topically to the cervix to ripen it.

dinoprostone (Cervidil, Prepidil)

> **IN DEPTH:**   Dinoprostone is the drug form of prostagladin E_2. This substance is secreted by the placenta and helps prepare or ripen the cervix as labor begins. Cervical ripening occurs when smooth muscle fibers in the cervix relax and collagen fibers in the cervix break down. This allows the cervical opening to dilate and the cervix itself to thin or efface.

DRUGS USED TO TREAT POSTPARTUM BLEEDING

Normally, after delivery, the uterus contracts strongly. Postpartum bleeding is due to uterine relaxation or atony, which results in increased bleeding at the site of placental separation. Drugs used to treat postpartum bleeding include:

carboprost (Hemabate)
oxytocin (Pitocin, Syntocinon)
ergonovine (Ergotrate)
methylergonovine (Methergine)

DRUGS USED TO TREAT POSTPARTUM DEPRESSION

See Chapter 25, "Psychiatric Drugs."

DRUGS USED TO TREAT ENDOMETRIOSIS

Endometriosis develops when tissue from the uterus implants within the pelvic cavity and on the ovaries and other organs. It remains sensitive to hormonal influences, secreting blood when the uterus begins menstruation. Endometriosis causes pelvic pain, inflammation, and cyst formation. After hormonal drugs suppress the menstrual cycle for several months, endometrial implants may atrophy. Hormonal drugs used to treat endometriosis include:

abarelix depot
danazol (Danocrine)
goserelin (Zoladex)
leuprolide (Lupron Depot)
nafarelin (Synarel)
norethindrone (Aygestin)

DID YOU KNOW?   Danazol is also used to treat fibrocystic breast disease, precocious puberty, and gynecomastia. Leuprolide is also used to treat uterine leiomyomata.

ORAL CONTRACEPTIVES

Oral contraceptives or **birth control pills** exert a hormonal influence to prevent pregnancy and are 95% effective if taken as directed. Most oral contraceptives contain a combination of estrogen and progestins (a group name for progesterone and progesterone derivatives) that is taken for 21 days. During the final 7 days of the 28-day menstrual cycle, the patient may take no tablets, 7 sugar-filled tablets, or 7 sugar tablets with iron (Fe). Other oral contraceptives contain only progestins.

IN DEPTH: Estrogen is normally secreted by the ovaries and causes the endometrium to proliferate. Estrogen also causes follicles to grow on the ovary and mature eggs to be released during ovulation. Progesterone is first secreted by the corpus luteum in the middle of the menstrual cycle. If an egg is fertilized, the corpus luteum continues to secrete progesterone to prepare the endometrium to accept the fertilized egg. If the ovum is not fertilized, the corpus luteum disintegrates, and progesterone production stops. When this happens, the uterine lining sloughs off in the process of menstruation.

Combination oral contraceptives that contain both estrogen and progestins are divided into three basic groups according to the relative amounts of progestins and estrogen provided during each day of the menstrual cycle. These three groups are known as *monophasic, biphasic,* and *triphasic oral contraceptives.*

Monophasic Oral Contraceptives

Monophasic oral contraceptives provide fixed amounts of progestins and estrogen in each tablet for each day of the 21-day period. The amounts of progestins and estrogen are designated by two numbers in the trade name of the drug. Example: Norinyl 1+50 contains l mg of progestins and 50 mg of estrogen in each tablet. Because an increased incidence of side effects (particularly thrombophlebitis) has been associated with higher estrogen dosages, a physician may elect to prescribe Norinyl 1+35, which contains l mg of progestins and just 35 mg of estrogen in each tablet.

Alesse
Apri
Brevicon
Demulen 1/35, Demulen 1/50
Desogen
Levlen
Levlite
Loestrin Fe 1/20, Loestrin Fe 1.5/30, Loestrin 21 1/20, Loestrin 21 1.5/30
Lo/Ovral
Modicon
Necon 0.5/35, Necon 1/35, Necon 1/50
Nelova 1/35E, Nelova 1/50M
Nordette
Norinyl 1+35, Norinyl 1+50
Ortho-Cept
Ortho-Cyclen
Ortho-Novum 1/35, Ortho-Novum 1/50

Ovcon-35, Ovcon-50
Ovral-28
Zovia 1/35E, Zovia 1/50E

This drug provides a fixed amount of progestins and estrogen in a once-monthly injection.

Lunelle

This transdermal patch drug provides a fixed amount of progestins and estrogen.

Ortho Evra

This drug provides a fixed amount of progestins and estrogen in a vaginal ring.

NuvaRing

> **DID YOU KNOW?**   Ortho Evra, introduced in 2001, is the first transdermal patch contraceptive. It was introduced by the drug manufacturer that introduced the first prescription oral contraceptive in 1931. The patch is worn for 3 weeks out of every month. NuvaRing, introduced in 2001, is the first contraceptive vaginal ring. It is a flexible, clear, 3-inch polymer ring that is inserted into the vagina for 3 weeks of every month.

Biphasic Oral Contraceptives

Biphasic oral contraceptives provide a fixed amount of estrogen in every tablet for each day of the 21-day time period; the amount of progestins is fixed in the first half but then increases in the second half of this time period. This change is designated by two numbers following the trade name of the drug. Example: Ortho-Novum 10/11 provides 0.5 mg of progestins and 35 mg of estrogen in each tablet for the first 10 days, and 1 mg of progestins and 35 mg of estrogen in each tablet for the next 11 days.

Jenest-28
Mircette
Necon 10/11
Ortho-Novum 10/11

Triphasic Oral Contraceptives

Triphasic oral contraceptives provide a fixed amount or slightly varying amount of estrogen for each day of the 21-day time period, while the amount of progestins increases or varies throughout that time. These progestins dose changes are designated in the case of Ortho-Novum by the numbers 7/7/7. Other drugs in this category have the prefix *tri-* in their trade names to indicate the three phases of different dosages of progestins in the 21 days.

Cyclessa
Estrostep Fe, Estrostep 21
Ortho-Novum 7/7/7
Ortho Tri-Cyclen
Tri-Levlen
Tri-Norinyl
Triphasil
Trivora-28

Progestins-only Contraceptives

Contraceptives that contain only progestins are slightly less effective in preventing pregnancy than combination contraceptives, particularly if the patient forgets to take even one daily tablet. However, the risks of thrombophlebitis and other side effects of estrogen therapy are avoided. Progestins-only contraceptives are taken orally, given by injection, implanted under the skin, or inserted into the uterus.

medroxyprogesterone (Depo-Provera)
Micronor
Mirena
Nor-Q.D.
Ovrette
Norplant System
Progestasert

DID YOU KNOW?   Progestasert is a T-shaped device containing progesterone and silicone; it is inserted into the uterine cavity and is effective for 1 year. Mirena is similar to Progestasert but is effective for 5 years. Norplant consists of six small silicone capsules that are implanted under the skin of the upper arm; Norplant is an effective contraceptive for 5 years.

These progestins-only drugs are taken in two doses after intercourse to prevent pregnancy.

Plan B
Preven

DID YOU KNOW?   The herb St. John's wort can cause serum hormone levels to decrease in patients taking oral contraceptives and this increases the chance of pregnancy.

DRUGS USED TO TREAT MENOPAUSE

As women enter menopause, the ovaries secrete decreasing amounts of estrogen. This causes symptoms of vaginal dryness, hot flashes, and fatigue. Estrogen hormone replacement therapy corrects the deficiency of estrogen and eliminates these symptoms. The long-term use of estrogen replacement therapy may reduce the risk of osteoporosis (after menopause, a woman can lose up to one-third of the bone mass in the spine) and keep cholesterol levels low; however, estrogen replacement therapy has been associated with an increased risk of endometrial cancer and thrombophlebitis.

Estrogen Hormone Replacement Therapy (HRT) for Menopause

> conjugated estrogens (Cenestin, Premarin, Premarin Intravenous, Premarin Vaginal Cream)
>
> dienestrol (Ortho Dienestrol Vaginal Cream)
>
> esterified estrogens (Estratab, Menest)
>
> estradiol (Alora, Climara, Esclim, Estrace, Estrace Vaginal Cream, Estraderm, Estring, FemPatch, Vivelle, Vivelle-Dot)
>
> estradiol cypionate (Depo-Estradiol Cypionate, depGynogen, DepoGen)
>
> estradiol hemihydrate (Vagifem)
>
> estradiol valerate (Delestrogen, Gynogen L.A. 20, Valergen 20, Valergen 40)
>
> estrone (Kestrone 5)
>
> estropipate (Ogen, Ortho-Est)
>
> ethinyl estradiol (Estinyl)

DID YOU KNOW?   Over 40 billion Premarin tablets have been sold. The trade name shows the drug's source: **pre**gnant **mar**es' **ur**ine. Animal rights activists claim that the horse is treated inhumanely by being confined to a stall with a catheter in its bladder to collect the urine. Other HRT drugs are derived from yams or soybeans (Climara, Estrace, Estraderm, Estratab, Menest, Ogen, Ortho-Est, and Vivelle). Other HRT drugs are synthetic.

The trade name Climera refers to *climacteric*, the physiologic and psychological changes that occur as a woman enters menopause. *Climacteric* is from a Greek word that means *the rungs of a ladder*, because menopause represents moving toward a different stage of life.

The estrogen replacement drugs estradiol cypionate and estradiol valerate are given by injection and provide a slow release of estrogen over 2 to 4 weeks. Castor oil, sesame seed oil, or cottonseed oil is used as the base for these drugs because it slows their rate of absorption.

Other Drugs for Menopause

This drug is a steroid that stimulates estrogen, progesterone, and androgen receptors. It is given to women who cannot or will not take estrogen HRT.

tibolone (Livial, Xyvion)

Combination Drugs for Menopause

These drugs are used to treat the symptoms of menopause as well as to prevent or treat osteoporosis in menopause. They combine estrogens (conjugated estrogens, ethinyl estradiol, or estradiol) with progestins (medroxyprogesterone, norethindrone, or norgestimate).

Activella
Combipatch
Femhrt
Ortho-Prefest
Premphase
Prempro

These drugs combine estrogens (esterified estrogens or estradiol cypionate) with androgens (methyltestosterone or testosterone cypionate). They are indicated for the treatment of menopausal symptoms, but not for the prevention or treatment of osteoporosis.

Depo-Testadiol
Estratest, Estratest H.S.

DRUGS USED TO TREAT POSTMENOPAUSAL OSTEOPOROSIS

For drugs that specifically inhibit bone resorption and are used to treat osteoporosis, see Chapter 14, "Musculoskeletal Drugs."

DRUGS USED TO TREAT ABNORMAL MENSTRUATION

Primary hypothalamic amenorrhea—the absence of menstruation due to decreased levels of gonadotropin-releasing hormone (GnRH)—may be treated with a drug that mimics GnRH and stimulates the release of the gonadotropins LH and FSH from the pituitary gland. A special pump is needed to administer this drug intravenously so that it can be given in pulses that mimic the natural release of GnRH from the pituitary gland.

gonadorelin (Lutrepulse)

Amenorrhea and abnormal uterine bleeding are treated with progesterone hormone drugs that act directly on the tissues of the endometrium to restore a normal menstrual cycle.

hydroxyprogesterone (Hylutin)
medroxyprogesterone (Amen, Cycrin, Provera)

norethindrone (Aygestin)

progesterone (Crinone, Prometrium)

This estrogen drug is used to correct hormonal imbalance and treat abnormal uterine bleeding.

conjugated estrogens (Premarin Intravenous)

DRUGS USED TO TREAT PREMENSTRUAL SYNDROME (PMS) AND PREMENSTRUAL DYSPHORIC DISORDER (PMDD)

Premenstrual syndrome (PMS) is characterized by breast tenderness, fluid retention ("bloating"), and mild mood changes. It is treated with various analgesics (aspirin, acetaminophen, NSAIDs). Other drugs used to treat PMS combine an analgesic to relieve pain and a diuretic to treat fluid retention.

Midol Maximum Strength PMS (acetaminophen, pamabrom)

Midol Teen Maximum Strength (acetaminophen, pamabrom)

Pamprin Maximum Pain Relief (magnesium salicylate, pamabrom)

Pamprin Multi-Symptom Maximum Strength (acetaminophen, pamabrom)

Premsyn PMS (acetaminophen, pamabrom)

Women's Tylenol Multi-Symptom Menstrual Relief (acetaminophen, pamabrom)

This drug combines an analgesic to relieve pain and an antihistamine for sedation.

Midol Maximum Strength Menstrual (acetaminophen, pyrilamine)

Premenstrual dysphoric disorder (PMDD) includes physical and emotional symptoms like PMS, but to a much greater degree. During the time between ovulation and menstruation, PMDD causes increasing symptoms of depression, feelings of hopelessness and anxiety, mood shifts, tearfulness, difficulty concentrating, tiredness, sleep disturbances, eating disturbances, as well as breast tenderness, joint pains, muscle pains, and fluid retention ("bloating") that significantly interfere with life. PMDD is considered a mood disorder caused by an alteration in the level of brain neurotransmitters. It is treated with psychiatric drugs that are used to treat depression and anxiety, sedatives, as well as NSAIDs for pain relief.

acecarbromal (Paxarel)

alprazolam (Xanax)

buspirone (Buspar)

citalopram (Celexa)

clomipramine (Anafranil)

desipramine (Norpramin)

fluoxetine (Sarafem)

fluvoxamine (Luvox)

nortriptyline (Aventyl, Pamelor)

paroxetine (Paxil)

sertraline (Zoloft)

DRUGS USED TO TREAT DYSMENORRHEA

Dysmenorrhea, or painful menstrual cramps, is caused by an increase in prostaglandins that causes the uterus to contract painfully. Some of the NSAID and COX-2 inhibitor drugs that inhibit the action of prostaglandins are specifically used to treat dysmenorrhea.

diclofenac (Cataflam, Voltaren, Voltaren-XR)

ibuprofen (Advil, Haltran, Midol Maximum Strength Cramp Formula, Motrin, Motrin IB)

ketoprofen (Orudis, Orudis KT, Oruvail)

meclofenamate

mefenamic acid (Ponstel)

naproxen (Aleve, Anaprox, Anaprox DS, EC-Naprosyn, Naprosyn)

piroxicam (Feldene)

rofecoxib (Vioxx)

valdecoxib (Bextra)

DRUGS USED TO PRODUCE ABORTION

When injected or given by suppository, large doses of certain prostaglandins can cause the uterus to contract strongly enough to spontaneously abort a fetus. Other abortion drugs inhibit progesterone from the corpus luteum that is necessary for the fertilized egg to develop. Most of these drugs are used for the sole purpose of terminating a pregnancy.

carboprost (Hemabate)

dinoprostone (Prostin E2)

mifepristone (Mifeprex)

misoprostol (Cytotec)

urea (Ureaphil)

DID YOU KNOW?   Mifepristone is actually RU-486, the drug that right-to-life activists protested prior to its approval by the FDA in 2000.

Dinoprostone, under the trade name Prostin E2, is used to produce abortion, while the same drug under the trade names Cervidil and Prepidil is used to cause the cervix to dilate and efface in preparation for delivery of a baby.

> While prostaglandin E_2 (Prostin E2) is used to abort a fetus, prostaglandin E_1 (Prostin VR) is used to save the lives of infants born with congenital heart defects. Prostin VR keeps open the ductus arteriosus that normally closes at birth so that these infants can maintain adequate oxygenation in spite of their heart anomalies until surgical correction can be performed.

DRUGS USED TO TREAT VAGINAL INFECTIONS

Many drugs used to treat vaginal infections are applied topically and are manufactured in the form of creams/ointments, suppositories, or vaginal tablets.

Candidal vaginal infections are caused by *Candida albicans*, a yeast. Topical drugs used to treat this infection include:

butoconazole (Femstat 3, Gynazole-1, Mycelex-3)

clotrimazole (Gyne-Lotrimin 3, Gyne-Lotrimin 7, Mycelex-7)

miconazole (Monistat, Monistat 3, Monistat 7)

nystatin

terconazole (Terazol 3, Terazol 7)

tioconazole (Monistat 1, Vagistat-1)

Note: Many drugs used to treat candidal infections end in -*azole*. Many antifungal drugs also have this ending. This is because yeast and fungi are closely related, and drugs that are effective against one often are effective against the other.

DID YOU KNOW?   Nystatin was discovered in 1950 by two physicians who named the drug for their employer—the New York State Department of Health.

Bacterial vaginal infections (bacterial vaginosis) are caused by several different bacteria, including *Haemophilus vaginalis* (also known as *Gardnerella vaginalis*) and *Trichomonas vaginalis*. Drugs used to treat bacterial vaginal infections include:

clindamycin (Cleocin, Cleocin Vaginal Ovules)

metronidazole (MetroGel-Vaginal)

DID YOU KNOW?   Metronidazole is both an antibacterial and an antiprotozoal drug. It is taken orally to treat *Trichomonas* vaginal infection, a sexually transmitted disease (STD). Metronidazole, in combination with other anti-infective drugs, is taken orally to treat peptic ulcers caused by *Helicobacter pylori*. Metronidazole (MetroGel) is applied topically to treat acne rosacea.

DRUGS USED TO TREAT SEXUALLY TRANSMITTED DISEASES (STDs)

Common sexually transmitted diseases (STDs) include gonorrhea, syphilis, chlamydia, HIV/AIDS, herpes simplex, and condyloma acuminatum. Gonorrhea, syphilis, and *Chlamydia* can cause widespread inflammation and scarring known as *pelvic inflammatory disease* (PID). The patient and any sexual partners are treated with antibiotics or antiviral drugs for these infections.

This section discusses oral antibiotic drugs used to treat gonorrhea, syphilis, and chlamydial infections. Topical antiviral drugs used to treat herpes simplex and condyloma acuminatum are discussed in Chapter 11, "Dermatologic Drugs." Oral drugs used to treat AIDS/HIV, herpes simplex, and condyloma acuminatum are discussed in Chapter 28, "AIDS Drugs and Antiviral Drugs."

Drugs for Gonorrhea

Gonorrhea is caused by the gram-negative coccus *Neisseria gonorrhoeae*. Drugs used systemically to treat gonorrhea include antibiotics from several different categories (penicillins, cephalosporins, tetracyclines, fluoroquinolones, and so forth).

amoxicillin (Amoxil, Trimox, Wymox)
ampicillin (Principen, Totacillin)
penicillin G (Pfizerpen)
penicillin G benzathine (Bicillin L-A, Permapen)
penicillin G procaine (Wycillin)
piperacillin (Pipracil)

cefixime (Suprax)
cefoperazone (Cefobid)
cefotetan (Cefotan)
cefoxitin (Mefoxin)
cefpodoxime (Vantin)
ceftizoxime (Cefizox)
ceftriaxone (Rocephin)
cefuroxime (Ceftin, Kefurox, Zinacef)

doxycycline (Doryx, Vibramycin, Vibramycin IV, Vibra-Tabs)
minocycline (Dynacin, Minocin, Minocin IV, Vectrin)
tetracycline (Panmycin, Sumycin, Tetracyn, Tetralan)
ciprofloxacin (Cipro, Cipro I.V.)
enoxacin (Penetrex)
gatifloxacin (Tequin)
levofloxacin (Levaquin)
norfloxacin (Noroxin)
ofloxacin (Floxin)

azithromycin (Zithromax)

erythromycin (E.E.S. 200, E.E.S. 400, E-Mycin, Eryc, EryPed, EryPed 200, EryPed 400, Ery-Tab, Erythrocin, Ilotycin, PCE Dispertab)

spectinomycin (Trobicin)

Drugs for Syphilis

Syphilis is caused by the gram-negative spirochete *Treponema pallidum*. Drugs used systemically to treat syphilis include:

penicillin G (Pfizerpen)

penicillin G procaine (Wycillin)

doxycycline (Doryx, Vibramycin, Vibramycin IV, Vibra-Tabs)

erythromycin (E.E.S. 200, E.E.S. 400, E-Mycin, Eryc, EryPed, EryPed 200, EryPed 400, Ery-Tab, Erythrocin, Ilotycin, PCE Dispertab)

minocycline (Dynacin, Minocin, Minocin IV, Vectrin)

tetracycline (Panmycin, Sumycin, Tetracyn, Tetralan)

Drugs for Chlamydial Infections

Chlamydial vaginal infections are caused by *Chlamydia trachomatis*, a gram-negative coccus. Drugs used systemically to treat chlamydial vaginal infections include:

amoxicillin (Amoxil, Trimox, Wymox)

azithromycin (Zithromax)

clindamycin (Cleocin)

doxycycline (Doryx, Vibramycin, Vibramycin IV, Vibra-Tabs)

erythromycin (E.E.S. 200, E.E.S. 400, E-Mycin, Eryc, EryPed, EryPed 200, EryPed 400, Ery-Tab, Erythrocin, Ilotycin, PCE Dispertab)

minocycline (Dynacin, Minocin, Minocin IV, Vectrin)

ofloxacin (Floxin)

sulfisoxazole

tetracycline (Panmycin, Sumycin, Tetracyn, Tetralan)

Women with STDs can transmit them to their newborn infants *in utero* or via the infected birth canal. Therefore, most states either recommend or require that a topical anti-infective drug be applied to the eyes of newborn infants to prevent infection and possible blindness caused by gonorrhea. Topical solutions and ointments specially prepared for ophthalmic use include:

silver nitrate

erythromycin (Ilotycin)

Erythromycin is also used to prevent eye infections due to *Chlamydia*.

Topical Drugs for Genital Herpes

Herpes simplex virus type 2 infection in the genital area is called *genital herpes* and is an STD. (Herpes simplex virus type 1 infections involve other areas of the body, particularly the mouth, and are known as *cold sores.*) Genital herpes lesions are treated topically with the drug listed here.

    acyclovir (Zovirax)

Oral drugs used systemically to treat genital herpes are discussed in Chapter 28, "AIDS Drugs and Antiviral Drugs."

Drugs for Genital Warts

The human papilloma virus causes both common warts (verrucae) and genital or venereal warts (condyloma acuminatum). Drugs used to treat common warts are discussed in Chapter 11, "Dermatology Drugs."
Topical and locally injected drugs used to treat genital warts are listed here.

    imiquimod (Aldara)
    interferon alfa-2b (Intron A)
    interferon alfa-n3 (Alferon N)
    podofilox (Condylox)
    podophyllum (Podocon-25)

DID YOU KNOW?   Podophyllum contains powdered May apple, and podofilox is derived from juniper evergreens.

Oral drugs used systemically to treat genital warts are discussed in Chapter 28, "AIDS Drugs and Antiviral Drugs."

DRUGS USED TO TREAT BREAST, OVARIAN, OR UTERINE CANCER

See Chapter 30, "Chemotherapy Drugs."

MISCELLANEOUS OB/GYN DRUGS

BayRho-D Full Dose: Immunoglobulin used after delivery to treat an Rh-negative mother with an Rh-positive baby. See *RhoGAM.*

BayRho-D Mini Dose: Immunoglobulin given after abortion, amniocentesis, or chorionic villus sampling to treat an Rh-negative mother with an Rh-positive baby. See *RhoGAM.*

Betadine Medicated Douche: Antibacterial povidone-iodine vaginal douche.

guaifenesin (Humibid L.A., Humibid Sprinkle, Robitussin):   This drug, an antitussive used to thin mucus in the throat and lungs, is also given to thin cervical mucus to treat infertility when the sperm have difficulty reaching the egg.

Hyskon: Dextran and water solution used intraoperatively to distend the uterine cavity and facilitate visualization with a hysteroscope.

magnesium sulfate: Anticonvulsant drug used to prevent and control seizures associated with preeclampsia and eclampsia.

DID YOU KNOW?   Magnesium sulfate is also manufactured in a nonsterile crystalline form that is mixed with water and drunk as a laxative. Its trade name is Epsom Salt.

Massengill Medicated Douche: Antibacterial povidone-iodine vaginal douche.

metformin (Glucophage):   Oral antidiabetic drug used to treat the elevated insulin levels seen in polycystic ovary disease.

MICRhoGAM: Immunoglobulin given after abortion, amniocentesis, or chorionic villus sampling to treat an Rh-negative mother with an Rh-positive baby. See *RhoGAM*.

pioglitazone (Actos):   Oral antidiabetic drug used to treat the elevated insulin levels seen in polycystic ovary disease.

RhoGAM: Immunoglobulin given after delivery to an Rh-negative woman with an Rh-positive baby to prevent hemorrhagic disease of the newborn in a subsequent pregnancy.

IN DEPTH: In hemorrhagic disease of the newborn, some of the baby's Rh-positive red blood cells enter the mother's bloodstream during pregnancy. The Rh-negative mother then develops antibodies against Rh-positive RBCs. This does not affect the first infant while it is in the uterus, but the RBCs of Rh-positive babies in subsequent pregnancies will be attacked by the maternal antibodies. These babies can develop hemolytic disease of the newborn. RhoGAM is given to Rh-negative mothers whose babies, when blood typing is performed after birth, are Rh positive. In cases where the baby's blood type cannot be determined (as during amniocentesis), RhoGAM is given prophylactically. RhoGAM is never given to the infant. For women who have had a miscarriage, spontaneous or induced abortion, amniocentesis, or chorionic villus sampling, a smaller dose of this drug is given.

rosiglitazone (Avandia):   Oral antidiabetic drug used to treat the elevated insulin levels seen in polycystic ovary disease.

Summer's Eve Medicated Douche: Antibacterial povidone-iodine vaginal douche.

Vagisil: Combination local anesthetic and lanolin cream for the perineal area.

WinRho SDF: Immunoglobulin used to treat an Rh-negative mother with an Rh-positive baby. See *RhoGAM*.

REVIEW QUESTIONS

1. Describe how the drug ritodrine acts to prevent premature labor.
2. Describe how a cervical ripening drug works.
3. What physiologic action do hormonal drugs exert to treat endometriosis?
4. Name the three categories of oral contraceptives (birth control pills). Describe the difference between the categories and give generic and trade name drugs for each category.
5. What are the benefits and drawbacks of estrogen replacement therapy?
6. Name three STDs and at least one drug used to treat each STD.
7. Define these abbreviations: HRT, STD.
8. What is the therapeutic action of RhoGAM?
9. Name several categories of OB/GYN drugs and give an example of a drug in each category.
10. Describe the difference between PMS and PMDD and the drugs used to treat them.
11. To what category of drugs does each of these drugs belong?
    clomiphene (Clomid, Serophene)
    Demulen
    Norplant System
    oxytocin (Pitocin, Syntocinon)
    metronidazole (MetroGel-Vaginal)
    Triphasil
    valacyclovir (Valtrex)

SPELLING TIPS

Amen   Refers to the drug's use in treating **amen**orrhea.
depGynogen, DepoGen   Unusual internal capitalization.
Fem**hrt**   Refers to the drug's use as HRT.
Gyn**a**zole-1   Most GYN terms are spelled with a gyn**e**-.
MICRhoGAM, RhoGAM, WinRho SDF   Unusual internal capitalization.
MetroGel-Vaginal   Unusual internal capitalization.

GET CONNECTED

Multimedia Extension Activities

 www.prenhall.com/turley

Use the above address to access the free, interactive Companion Website created for this textbook. Included in the features of this site are drug updates and additional chapter-specific exercises for further practice.

24

Neurological Drugs

CHAPTER CONTENTS

Drugs used to treat epilepsy
Drugs used to treat Parkinson's disease
Drugs used to treat Alzheimer's disease
Drugs used to treat myasthenia gravis
Drugs used to treat insomnia
Drugs used to treat narcolepsy
Miscellaneous neurological drugs
Review questions
Spelling tips

LEARNING OBJECTIVES

After studying this chapter, you should be able to do the following:

1. Name several categories of neurological drugs.
2. Describe the therapeutic action of drugs used to treat epilepsy, Parkinson's disease, myasthenia gravis, Alzheimer's disease, insomnia, and narcolepsy.
3. Given the generic and trade name of a neurological drug, identify the category it belongs to or the disease it is used to treat.
4. Given a neurological drug category, give the generic and trade names of drugs in that category.
5. Identify the Historical Notes or Did You Know? section in this chapter that you found most interesting.

Various disease conditions of the central nervous system benefit from pharmacologic therapy. These include epilepsy, Parkinson's disease, myasthenia gravis, Alzheimer's disease, insomnia, and narcolepsy.

DRUGS USED TO TREAT EPILEPSY

An epileptic seizure originates in the brain when a group of neurons spontaneously begins to send out impulses in an abnormal, uncontrolled way. These impulses are spread from neuron to neuron by neurotransmitter hormones. Symptoms of epilepsy range from barely noticeable staring or a lack of attention to a full tonic-clonic seizure with unconsciousness, muscle jerking, tongue biting, and incontinence. The type of symptoms depends on the number and location of the affected neurons. Drugs used to treat epilepsy are known as *anticonvulsants* because epilepsy is characterized by seizures or convulsions.

HISTORICAL NOTES: Efforts to control epilepsy were largely in vain for centuries. The cause was attributed to supernatural forces, poison, and so forth. The treatment could involve trephining (boring a hole in the skull), prayers, or herbal remedies. Phenobarbital (Luminal), the first drug found to be effective for epilepsy (tonic-clonic seizures only), was introduced in 1912.

> In 1923, young Tracy Putnam was a resident in neurology. . . . He became intrigued with the possibility that epilepsy might be caused by a chemical abnormality in the brain. He noted, for example, that patients who "rebreathed" their own carbon dioxide by putting a bag over their heads got some relief [from seizures]. He asked himself, "Might an institution for the treatment of epilepsy be established adjacent to a brewery, and the content of carbon dioxide in the atmosphere metered so as to be tolerable and yet sufficient to prevent attacks?"
>
> Putnam later abandoned this idea and instead began searching for drugs that might be effective for epilepsy.
>
> "I combed the catalog," Putnam later wrote, "for suitable compounds that were not obviously poisonous." He was looking for drugs in particular containing a benzene ring because among the barbitals, only phenobarbital, which also had a benzene ring, possessed the ability to suppress epilepsy. "Parke-Davis . . . wrote back to me that it had on hand samples of 19 different compounds analogous to phenobarbital and that I was welcome to them."
>
> Edward Shorter, *The Health Century* (New York, NY: Doubleday, 1987), pp. 110–111.

Of the 19 compounds in the shipment, all were inactive and ineffective against epilepsy except one—phenytoin (Dilantin), which was introduced in 1938 and is still the drug of choice for treating adult tonic-clonic seizures.

The following categories of drugs are used to treat epilepsy.

Barbiturate Drugs for Epilepsy

Barbiturates are sedative drugs, but some of them also possess an anticonvulsant action. Barbiturates are controlled substance drugs (Schedule IV) that inhibit conduction of nerve impulses coming into the cortex of the brain and depress neurons in the motor areas of the brain.

mephobarbital (Mebaral)

phenobarbital (Luminal, Solfoton)

DID YOU KNOW?   Phenobarbital is also used to treat trigeminal neuralgia/tic douloureux. It is also used to treat the seizures that occur with eclampsia in pregnancy.

Hydantoin Drugs for Epilepsy

Hydantoins act on the cell membrane of neurons in the cortex of the brain. These drugs affect the flow of sodium in and out of the cell, thereby preventing the neuron from depolarizing and repolarizing (i.e., sending out an impulse) too rapidly or repeatedly.

ethotoin (Peganone)

mephenytoin (Mesantoin)

phenytoin (Dilantin Infatabs, Dilantin Kapseals, Dilantin-125)

Succinimide Drugs for Epilepsy

Succinimides depress the cortex of the brain and raise the seizure threshold.

ethosuximide (Zarontin)

methsuximide (Celontin Kapseals)

phensuximide (Milontin Kapseals)

Benzodiazepine Drugs for Epilepsy

The benzodiazepine drugs act on several different types of receptors throughout the body to affect memory, emotion, and muscles. This makes them useful drugs in treating a variety of psychiatric and muscular disorders. In addition, they exert an anticonvulsant effect on receptors in the brainstem. All of these are controlled substance drugs (Schedule IV).

clonazepam (Klonopin)

clorazepate (Tranxene, Tranxene-SD, Tranxene-SD Half Strength, Tranxene-T)

diazepam (Diazepam Intensol, Valium)

DID YOU KNOW?   Clonazepam is also used to treat Lennox–Gastaut syndrome (an autoimmune disorder with symptoms similar to myasthenia gravis), the muscular symptoms of Parkinson's disease, neuralgia, and the hyperactive reflexes of startle disease. It is also used to treat schizophrenia and the manic phase of manic-depressive disorder.

In the trade name of clorazepate, the *SD* in Tranxene-SD stands for *single dose*. The *T* in Tranxene-T refers to the actual shape of the tablet.

Other Drugs for Epilepsy

The mechanism of action of these antiepileptic drugs varies.

acetazolamide (Diamox)
carbamazepine (Atretol, Carbatrol, Epitol, Tegretol, Tegretol-XR)
clobazam (Frisium)
felbamate (Felbatol)
fosphenytoin (Cerebyx)
gabapentin (Neurontin)
lamotrigine (Lamictal, Lamictal Chewable Dispersible Tablet)
levetiracetam (Keppra)
nitrazepam (Mogadon)
oxcarbazepine (Trileptal)
primidone (Mysoline)
tiagabine (Gabitril Filmtabs)
topiramate (Topamax)
trimethadione (Tridione)
valproic acid (Depacon, Depakene, Depakote, Depakote ER)
vigabatrin (Sabril)
zonisamide (Zonegran)

No one drug has a therapeutic effect against all types of seizures. Some drugs that are effective for controlling one type of seizure may actually provoke another type. Each type of epilepsy displays a specific EEG pattern during a seizure. The choice of drug therapy is dependent on proper classification of the type of seizure based on the patient's clinical symptoms and EEG pattern. In patients with poorly controlled seizures, the physician will try different **antiepileptic drugs** to find the one that best controls the patient's seizures. If a patient's seizures were under control but then returned, the physician would order a blood test to check that there was a therapeutic level of the drug in the bloodstream. If the drug level was therapeutic during the seizures, the physician would prescribe a different anticonvulsant drug.

There are four common types of seizures: (1) **tonic-clonic** (also known as *grand mal*), (2) **absence** (also known as *petit mal*), (3) **complex partial** (also known as *psychomotor*), and (4) *simple partial* (also known as *focal motor*).

Drugs for Tonic-Clonic/Grand Mal Seizures

carbamazepine (Atretol, Carbatrol, Epitol, Tegretol, Tegretol-XR)
ethotoin (Peganone)
mephenytoin (Mesantoin)
mephobarbital (Mebaral)
phenobarbital (Luminal, Solfoton)
phenytoin (Dilantin Infatabs, Dilantin Kapseals, Dilantin-125)
primidone (Mysoline)
topiramate (Topamax)

Note: Phenytoin is the drug of choice for treating adults with tonic-clonic seizures, whereas phenobarbital is the drug of choice for treating children with tonic-clonic seizures.

Tonic-clonic seizures resistant to other drugs are treated with this orphan drug.

antiepilepsirine

Drugs for Absence/Petit Mal Seizures

acetazolamide (Diamox)

clonazepam (Klonopin)

ethosuximide (Zarontin)

mephobarbital (Mebaral)

methsuximide (Celontin Kapseals)

phensuximide (Milontin Kapseals)

trimethadione (Tridione)

valproic acid (Depacon, Depakene, Depakote, Depakote ER)

Drugs for Complex Partial/Psychomotor Seizures

carbamazepine (Atretol, Carbatrol, Epitol, Tegretol, Tegretol-XR)

clorazepate (Tranxene, Tranxene-SD, Tranxene-SD Half Strength, Tranxene-T)

ethotoin (Peganone)

felbamate (Felbatol)

gabapentin (Neurontin)

lamotrigine (Lamictal, Lamictal Chewable Dispersible Tablet)

levetiracetam (Keppra)

mephenytoin (Mesantoin)

oxcarbazepine (Trileptal)

phenytoin (Dilantin Infatabs, Dilantin Kapseals, Dilantin-125)

primidone (Mysoline)

tiagabine (Gabitril Filmtabs)

topiramate (Topamax)

valproic acid (Depacon, Depakene, Depakote, Depakote ER)

zonisamide (Zonegran)

Drugs for Simple Partial/Focal Motor Seizures

carbamazepine (Atretol, Carbatrol, Epitol, Tegretol, Tegretol-XR)

clorazepate (Tranxene, Tranxene-SD, Tranxene-SD Half Strength, Tranxene-T)

felbamate (Felbatol)

gabapentin (Neurontin)

lamotrigine (Lamictal, Lamictal Chewable Dispersible Tablet)

levetiracetam (Keppra)

mephenytoin (Mesantoin)

oxcarbazepine (Trileptal)
phenobarbital (Luminal, Solfoton)
primidone (Mysoline)
tiagabine (Gabitril Filmtabs)
topiramate (Topamax)
zonisamide (Zonegran)

Drugs for Other Types of Seizures

These drugs are used to treat Lennox–Gastaut syndrome, a variant of petit mal seizures that occurs in children and adults and may be accompanied by mental retardation.

felbamate (Felbatol)
lamotrigine (Lamictal, Lamictal Chewable Dispersible Tablet)
topiramate (Topamax)

This drug is prescribed to prevent seizures during alcoholic detoxification.

chlordiazepoxide (Librium)

This drug is used to treat seizures associated with preeclampsia/eclampsia in pregnancy.

magnesium sulfate

Drugs for Status Epilepticus

Status epilepticus is a state of prolonged continuous seizure activity or frequently repeated individual seizures that occur without the patient regaining consciousness. Before 1960, up to 50% of persons with status epilepticus died. Seizures lasting over 30 seconds can cause brain damage. Therefore, status epilepticus is a medical emergency. It is treated with one or more of the following drugs.

diazepam (Diastat)
fosphenytoin (Cerebyx)
lorazepam (Ativan)
phenobarbital (Luminal, Solfoton)
phenytoin (Dilantin)

DRUGS USED TO TREAT PARKINSON'S DISEASE

The symptoms of Parkinson's disease were first described in 1817 by the English physician James Parkinson. Parkinson's disease is a chronic, degenerative condition affecting the brain. Its early symptoms, first appearing usually in adults of late middle age, include muscle rigidity, tremors, and a slowing of voluntary movements. Parkinson's disease follows a progressively downhill clinical course. Later symptoms include a mask-like facial expression, drooling from rigidity of the facial muscles, resting tremor, and loss of ability to ambulate.

The symptoms of Parkinson's disease may be attributed to a disturbance in the balance of dopamine and acetylcholine, two neurotransmitters in the brain. These two substances normally exert opposing, balancing effects. It is a lack of dopamine in the brain that upsets this delicate balance, leading to the symptoms of Parkinson's disease.

IN DEPTH: Early attempts to replenish the diminished supply of dopamine in the brain were unsuccessful because dopamine given orally or circulating in the blood cannot cross the blood–brain barrier. It was discovered, however, that the metabolic precursor of dopamine, levodopa, could not only penetrate the blood–brain barrier, but could actually increase brain levels of dopamine. Once in the brain, levodopa (or L-dopa) is converted into dopamine by the action of the enzyme dopa decarboxylase. Unfortunately, this same enzyme is also present in the bloodstream.

After oral administration of levodopa, dopa decarboxylase immediately begins to change levodopa in the bloodstream into dopamine, which then cannot cross the blood–brain barrier. This results in two problems:

1. A very large oral dose of levodopa must be given because a substantial amount (97 to 99%) of the levodopa in the blood is converted into dopamine and does not reach the brain.

2. The extra dopamine in the bloodstream causes side effects that are undesirable.

To avoid both of these problems, levodopa is given orally along with another drug, carbidopa. Carbidopa inhibits the enzyme dopa decarboxylase; this allows a greater amount of levodopa to cross the blood–brain barrier. The use of carbidopa allows the dose of levodopa to be decreased by 75%. Fortunately, oral carbidopa cannot cross the blood–brain barrier to inhibit the enzyme dopa decarboxylase in the brain where it is needed to change levodopa into dopamine.

Drug therapy for Parkinson's disease is divided into two main categories: drugs that increase or enhance the action of dopamine in the brain and drugs that inhibit the action of acetylcholine. All of these drugs restore the natural balance between dopamine and acetylcholine.

Drugs that increase the amount of dopamine, enhance its action in the brain, or directly stimulate dopamine receptors include:

amantadine (Symmetrel)
bromocriptine (Parlodel, Parlodel Snap Tabs)
carbidopa (Lodosyn)
levodopa (L-dopa) (Larodopa)
pergolide (Permax)
pramipexole (Mirapex)

ropinirole (Requip)

selegiline (Carbex, Eldepryl)

> **DID YOU KNOW?**   Amantadine (under the trade name Symmetrel) was originally used as an antiviral drug to prevent the Asian flu. It was given for this reason to a patient at Harvard Medical School who also had Parkinson's disease. By coincidence, it was noted that his Parkinson's disease improved. Today, amantadine (Symmetrel) is still given to high-risk patients to prevent influenza A virus respiratory infections.

Drugs that inhibit the action of acetylcholine in the brain are called *anticholinergic drugs* and include:

benztropine (Cogentin)

biperiden (Akineton)

diphenhydramine (Benadryl)

procyclidine (Kemadrin)

trihexyphenidyl (Artane, Artane Sequels)

> **DID YOU KNOW?**   Diphenhydramine (Benadryl) is a popular antihistamine. It has an antihistamine action as well as another action that inhibits the action of acetylcholine; it is this latter action that is therapeutic in treating Parkinson's disease.

Other Drugs for Parkinson's Disease

Catechol-O-methyltransferase (COMT) is the main enzyme that metabolizes the drug levodopa in the bloodstream. Drugs known as *COMT inhibitors* inhibit COMT and allow more levodopa in the bloodstream to cross the blood–brain barrier.

entacapone (Comtan)

tolcapone (Tasmar)

These drugs are specifically used to treat the tremors of Parkinson's disease.

nadolol (Corgard)

propranolol (Inderal, Inderal LA)

These drugs are used to treat the abnormal muscle movements that characterize Parkinson's disease or are a side effect of levodopa therapy.

clonazepam (Klonopin)
fluoxetine (Prozac, Prozac Weekly)

The FDA has approved the use of these orphan drugs to treat Parkinson's disease.

apomorphine
NeuroCell-PD
Spheramine

DID YOU KNOW?   NeuroCell-PD contains fetal pig neuron cells. The *PD* stands for *Parkinson's disease*. Approximately 12 million cells are surgically implanted within the patient's cerebrum to replace nerve cells lost because of Parkinson's disease. This treatment helps to delay the progression of parkinsonian symptoms such as tremors, muscle rigidity, and difficulty speaking.

This is an investigational drug used to treat Parkinson's disease.

ritanserin

Combination Drugs for Parkinson's Disease

Duodopa (carbidopa, levodopa)
Sinemet-10/100 (carbidopa, levodopa)
Sinemet-25/100 (carbidopa, levodopa)
Sinemet-25/250 (carbidopa, levodopa)
Sinemet CR (carbidopa, levodopa)

None of the drugs prescribed for Parkinson's disease can cure the disease. In fact, over time tolerance to the drugs' therapeutic effects can develop. Larger drug doses are then required to maintain control of parkinsonian symptoms; however, these larger doses also produce more side effects. When doses can no longer be increased or side effects become intolerable, the physician will gradually withdraw all medication, placing the patient on a **drug holiday** for a few days. When drug therapy is again initiated, the patient will respond to lower doses of antiparkinsonian drugs.

DRUGS USED TO TREAT ALZHEIMER'S DISEASE

The dementia of Alzheimer's disease is caused by low levels of the neurotransmitter acetylcholine in the cortex of the brain. This is associated with the destruction of neurons. The more neurons that are destroyed, the greater the degree of cognitive impairment. As the disease progresses, the loss of neurons causes memory difficulties and eventually dementia.

Cholinesterase Inhibitor Drugs for Alzheimer's Disease

Drugs that inhibit the enzyme cholinesterase (which breaks down acetylcholine) effectively raise the acetylcholine level in the brain and help the available acetylcholine continue to function without being broken down. These drugs cannot, however, stop or reverse the underlying destruction of neurons.

donepezil (Aricept)
galantamine (Reminyl)
rivastigmine (Exelon)
tacrine (Cognex)
velnacrine (Mentane)

DID YOU KNOW?   Galantamine is derived from daffodil bulbs.

Other Drugs for Alzheimer's Disease

By increasing brain metabolism and cerebral blood flow, this drug (which is a combination of several ergot alkaloids) can improve cognitive skills and mental capacity.

ergoloid mesylates (Gerimal, Hydergine, Hydergine LC)

This drug is an antipsychotic drug used to treat the dementia associated with Alzheimer's disease.

olanzapine (Zyprexa, Zyprexa Zydis)

DRUGS USED TO TREAT MYASTHENIA GRAVIS

Myasthenia gravis is characterized by excessive fatigue of the voluntary muscles. On a cellular level, patients produce antibodies against their own acetylcholine receptors that are on the cell membranes of voluntary muscle cells. These antibodies destroy many of the receptors. There are normal levels of acetylcholine, but too few receptors on the muscles to produce a contraction. Normally, acetylcholine is released, briefly acts on a receptor, and is then broken down by the enzyme cholinesterase. Drugs used to treat myasthenia gravis block cholinesterase so that the acetylcholine is not broken down and can activate the remaining receptors for a longer period of time. These anticholinesterase drugs are used to treat myasthenia gravis.

ambenonium (Mytelase)
neostigmine (Prostigmin)
pyridostigmine (Mestinon, Regonol)

DRUGS USED TO TREAT INSOMNIA

Drugs used to induce sleep are termed *hypnotics* after *hypnos*, the Greek word for *sleep*. **Hypnotics** include nonbarbiturates, which have a low risk of addiction, or barbiturates (Schedule II or III drugs), which are more addictive and are not the drugs of choice for treating simple insomnia.

Nonbarbiturate Hypnotic Drugs for Insomnia

Nonbarbiturate hypnotics nonselectively depress the central nervous system to produce sedation and sleep. Nonbarbiturate hypnotics include both benzodiazepine antianxiety drugs and other types of nonbarbiturate drugs.

> acecarbromal (Paxarel)
> chloral hydrate (Aquachloral Supprettes)
> estazolam (ProSom)
> flurazepam (Dalmane)
> glutethimide
> lorazepam (Ativan)
> quazepam (Doral)
> temazepam (Restoril)
> triazolam (Halcion)
> zaleplon (Sonata)
> zolpidem (Ambien)

> *Note:* The ending *-azepam* is common to generic benzodiazepines.

Barbiturate Hypnotic Drugs for Insomnia

Some barbiturates are useful in preventing epileptic seizures, but other barbiturates have no anticonvulsant activity and are only used to treat insomnia. These drugs exert a general depressing action on the central nervous system and cause sedation. Barbiturate hypnotics are Schedule II, III, and IV drugs and, because of their greater capacity to cause addiction, are not preferred over nonbarbiturate hypnotics. They also appear to lose their therapeutic effect when used for more than a few weeks.

> amobarbital (Amytal)
> butabarbital (Butisol)
> pentobarbital (Nembutal)
> phenobarbital (Luminal, Solfoton)
> secobarbital (Seconal Sodium Pulvules)

Combination Barbiturate Hypnotic Drugs for Insomnia

> Tuinal Pulvules (amobarbital, secobarbital)

> *Note:* The ending *-barbital* is common to many generic barbiturates.

Other Drugs for Insomnia

OTC sleep aids commonly contain the antihistamine diphenhydramine. These sleep aids use the antihistamine's side effect of drowsiness as the therapeutic effect to induce sleep. Melatonin is a dietary supplement that helps the body adjust to jet lag and different time zones.

Bayer Select Maximum Strength Night Time Pain Relief
Bufferin AF Nite Time
Compoz Nighttime Sleep Aid
Excedrin P.M., Excedrin P.M. Liquigels
Extra Strength Doan's P.M.
Extra Strength Tylenol PM, Extra Strength Tylenol PM Gelcaps
Melagesic PM
Midol PM
Miles Nervine
Nighttime Pamprin
Nytol, Maximum Strength Nytol
Sleep-eze 3
Sominex, Sominex Pain Relief

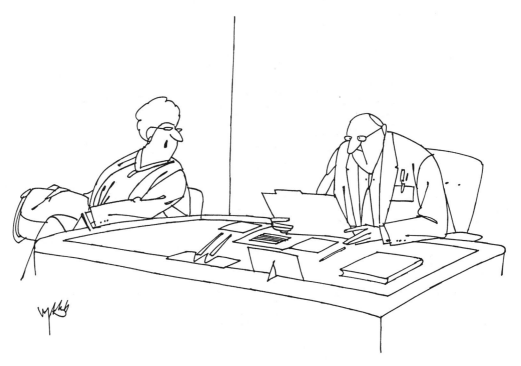

Figure 24–1 *I feel much better because I* didn't *take what you prescribed.*—David W. Harbaugh. *Reprinted with permission.*

Unisom Nighttime Sleep-Aid, Unisom with Pain Relief, Maximum Strength Unisom SleepGels

DRUGS USED TO TREAT NARCOLEPSY

Narcolepsy is characterized by brief, involuntary episodes of falling asleep and extreme daytime sleepiness. Patients with narcolepsy often fall asleep at work or at school, or while driving. There is an underlying abnormality in REM sleep. There is also an hereditary component to narcolepsy and it may be related to some form of autoimmune disorder. Narcolepsy and the related disorder cataplexy are treated with drugs from many different categories. Some drugs are Schedule II central nervous system stimulants; some are prescription, nonschedule antidepressants; others are orphan drugs.

> amphetamine
> dextroamphetamine (Dexedrine, Dexedrine Spansules, Dextrostat)
> fluoxetine (Prozac, Prozac Weekly)
> gamma hydroxybutyrate (GHB)
> methamphetamine (Desoxyn, Desoxyn Gradumet)
> methylphenidate (Concerta, Metadate CD, Metadate ER, Methylin ER, Ritalin, Ritalin-SR)
> modafinil (Provigil)
> pemoline (Cylert, PemADD, PemADD CT)
> oxybate (Xyrem)
> viloxazine (Catatrol)

DID YOU KNOW?   GHB is now a Schedule I orphan drug used to treat narcolepsy. Previously, this drug was illegal because of its use as a date-rape drug. It is now classified as an orphan drug.

Some central nervous system stimulants used to treat narcolepsy are also used, paradoxically, to treat attention-deficit/hyperactivity disorder!

Combination Drugs for Narcolepsy

Adderall, Adderall XR (amphetamine, dextroamphetamine)

DRUGS USED TO TREAT MIGRAINE HEADACHES

See Chapter 26, "Analgesic Drugs."

MISCELLANEOUS NEUROLOGICAL DRUGS

Acthar Gel: ACTH hormonal drug used to treat multiple sclerosis.

agalsidase alfa (Replagal):   Used to replace a missing enzyme and improve cerebral blood flow in Fabry's disease.

Aggrenox: Combination dipyridamole and aspirin drug given to decrease the risk of stroke.

alteplase (Activase, Cathflo Activase):   Tissue plasminogen activator used to dissolve blood clots from a stroke.

amitriptyline (Elavil):   Tricyclic antidepressant used to treat neuralgia caused by a herpes zoster infection (shingles).

amoxapine: Tricyclic antidepressant used to treat neuralgia caused by a herpes zoster infection (shingles).

amphotericin B (AmBisome):   Used to treat cryptococcal meningitis in AIDS patients.

baclofen (Lioresal):   Skeletal muscle relaxant used to treat trigeminal neuralgia; used to treat severe muscle spasticity associated with multiple sclerosis, cerebral palsy, stroke, or spinal cord injury.

botulinum toxin type A (Botox, Dysport):   Used to treat muscle contractures in patients with cerebral palsy.

Ceresine: Used to treat severe head injury.

ciliary neurotrophic factor: Used to treat amyotrophic lateral sclerosis.

cladribine (Mylinax):   Used to treat multiple sclerosis.

clopidogrel (Plavix):   Platelet aggregation inhibitor used to reduce the risk of stroke in patients with atherosclerosis and prior history of stroke.

colchicine: Used to treat multiple sclerosis.

corticotropin-releasing factor (Xerecept):   Used to treat edema associated with a brain tumor.

desipramine (Norpramin):   Tricyclic antidepressant used to treat neuralgia caused by a herpes zoster infection (shingles).

dexamethasone (Dalalone, Decadron, Hexadrol):   Corticosteroid used to treat cerebral edema.

doxepin (Sinequan, Sinequan Concentrate):   Tricyclic antidepressant used to treat neuralgia caused by a herpes zoster infection (shingles).

edetate calcium disodium (calcium EDTA) (Calcium Disodium Versenate):   Used to treat lead poisoning and lead encephalopathy.

edrophonium (Enlon, Reversol, Tensilon):   Anticholinesterase drug used to diagnose (not treat) myasthenia gravis.

fampridine (Neurelan):   Used to treat multiple sclerosis.

Flocor: Used to treat subarachnoid hemorrhage and ruptured cerebral aneurysm.

flunarizine (Sibelium):   Used to treat alternating hemiplegia.

FocalSeal-S: Surgical sealant used during neurosurgery to seal the dura. This two-part topical drug is applied as a liquid primer to penetrate the tissue, then as a sealant. Exposure to light causes the liquids to polymerize and form a flexible gel that seals air leaks. The *S* stands for *short-term* because this drug is absorbed in about the same amount of time as short-term absorbable sutures.

folic acid (Folvite):   The U.S. Public Health Service recommends the use of folic acid supplements for all women of childbearing age. Folic acid significantly decreases the incidence of babies with neural tube defects (spina bifida, myelomeningocele). Since 1998, some breads, cereals, and pastas have additional folic acid added to them.

gabapentin (Neurontin):   Used to treat multiple sclerosis and amyotrophic lateral sclerosis.

glatiramer (Copaxone):   Immunosuppressant drug used to treat multiple sclerosis.

guanethidine (Ismelin):   Used to treat sympathetic dystrophy and causalgia.

guanidine: Anticholinesterase drug used to treat Eaton–Lambert syndrome, an autoimmune disease with symptoms similar to myasthenia gravis.

imipramine (Tofranil):   Tricyclic antidepressant used to treat neuralgia caused by a herpes zoster infection (shingles).

interferon beta-1a (Avonex):   Interferon is produced in the body in response to a viral infection. This drug is used to treat multiple sclerosis (which may be triggered by a virus, although its exact cause is unknown).

interferon beta-1b (Betaseron):   Interferon is produced in the body in response to a viral infection. This drug is used to treat multiple sclerosis (which may be triggered by a virus, although its mechanism of action is unknown).

inosine pranobex (Isoprinosine):   Used to treat sclerosing panencephalitis.

lidocaine (Lidoderm):   Transdermal patch used to treat postherpetic neuralgia.

L-baclofen (Neuralgon):   Skeletal muscle relaxant used to treat trigeminal neuralgia; used to treat severe muscle spasticity associated with multiple sclerosis, cerebral palsy, stroke, or spinal cord injury.

L-threonine (Threostat):   Used to treat spasticity associated with amyotrophic lateral sclerosis (Lou Gehrig's disease).

mannitol (Osmitrol):   Diuretic used to relieve cerebral edema and decrease intracranial pressure.

mecasermin (Myotrophin):   Used to treat amyotrophic lateral sclerosis.

meropenem (Merrem IV):   Cephalosporin antibiotic used to treat bacterial meningitis.

mitoxantrone (Novantrone):   Chemotherapy drug used to treat multiple sclerosis.

NeuroCell-HD: Fetal pig nerve cells are surgically implanted in the cerebrum to produce GABA, one of the chemical compounds lacking in patients with Huntington's chorea. This fatal, genetically transmitted disease is characterized by involuntary muscle movements, rigidity, and dementia.

nimodipine (Nimotop):   Calcium channel blocker used to relax arterial spasms, increase blood flow, and improve neurological deficits after subarachnoid hemorrhage.

nortriptyline (Aventyl, Pamelor):   Tricyclic antidepressant used to treat neuralgia caused by a herpes zoster infection (shingles).

oxycodone (Endocodone, M-oxy, OxyContin, OxyFast, OxyIR, Percolone, Roxicodone, Roxicodone Intensol):   Used to treat neuralgia from herpes zoster infection (shingles).

physostigmine (Antilirium): Used to treat ataxia.

pralidoxime (Protopam): Used to reverse an overdose of an anticholinergic drug used to treat myasthenia gravis.

prednisolone (Hydeltrasol, Orapred, Predalone 50, Prelone): Corticosteroid anti-inflammatory drug used to treat acute exacerbations of multiple sclerosis.

Procysteine: Used to treat multiple sclerosis.

protirelin: Used to treat amyotrophic lateral sclerosis.

protriptyline (Vivactil): Tricyclic antidepressant used to treat obstructive sleep apnea; used to treat neuralgia caused by a herpes zoster infection (shingles).

rifaximin (Normix): Used to treat hepatic encephalopathy.

riluzole (Rilutek): Used to treat amyotrophic lateral sclerosis by blocking excess glutamate that causes nerve cells to die; also used to treat Huntington's chorea.

succimer (Chemet): Used to treat lead poisoning and lead encephalopathy.

tetrabenazine: Used to treat Huntington's chorea.

ticlopidine (Ticlid): Platelet aggregation inhibitor used to reduce the risk of stroke in patients with atherosclerosis and prior history of stroke.

tirilazad: Antioxidant that helps tissue survive after a central nervous system injury.

tizanidine (Zanaflex): Used to treat muscle spasticity in multiple sclerosis and spinal cord injury.

Trufill n-BCA: A cyanoacrylate compound used to block a cerebral arteriovenous malformation prior to surgery.

urea (Ureaphil): Used to decrease intracranial pressure.

REVIEW QUESTIONS

1. Explain why levodopa is administered with carbidopa for patients with Parkinson's disease.
2. The choice of a drug for treating epilepsy in a specific patient is based on what two clinical criteria?
3. Explain the meaning of the phrase *drug holiday*.
4. Why are barbiturates not the drugs of choice for treating insomnia?
5. What vitamin supplement is recommended during pregnancy to avoid neural tube defects in the baby?
6. Drugs prescribed for Alzheimer's disease have what two different ways of improving patient's symptoms?
7. To what category of drugs does each of these drugs belong?
    carbamazine (Atretol, Carbatrol, Epitol, Tegretol, Tegretol-XR)
    estazolam (ProSom)
    pemoline (Cylert, PemADD, PemADD CT)
    Sinemet-10/100
    tacrine (Cognex)
    valproic acid (Depacon, Depakene, Depakote, Depakote ER)
    zolpidem (Ambien)

SPELLING TIPS

carbamazepine (Atretol, Carbatrol, Epitol, Tegretol, Tegretol-XR) All of the trade names of this drug end in *–tol*, except Carbatrol which ends in *-trol*.

Cerebyx This is easily confused with the sound-alike drug Celebrex (used to treat osteoarthritis).

Comtan The drug name reflects its action; it inhibits the COMT enzyme that metabolizes levodopa.

phenytoin The drug is easily misspelled because the *y* is not usually pronounced.

ProSom Unusual internal capitalization.

GET CONNECTED

Multimedia Extension Activities

 www.prenhall.com/turley

Use the above address to access the free, interactive Companion Website created for this textbook. Included in the features of this site are drug updates and additional chapter-specific exercises for further practice.

25

Psychiatric Drugs

CHAPTER CONTENTS

Drugs used to treat anxiety and neurosis
Drugs used to treat psychosis
Drugs used to treat depression
Drugs used to treat manic-depressive disorder
Drugs used to treat obsessive-compulsive disorder (OCD)
Drugs used to treat panic disorder
Drugs used to treat social anxiety disorder
Drugs used to treat posttraumatic stress disorder (PTSD)
Drugs used to treat anorexia nervosa and bulimia nervosa
Drugs used to treat attention-deficit/hyperactivity disorder (ADHD)
Miscellaneous drugs used to treat psychiatric disorders
Review questions
Spelling tips

LEARNING OBJECTIVES

After studying this chapter, you should be able to do the following:

1. Name several categories of psychiatric drugs.
2. Describe the therapeutic action of tranquilizers, antipsychotic drugs, and antidepressant drugs.
3. Describe the therapeutic action of drugs used to treat OCD, panic disorder, social anxiety, PTSD, anorexia nervosa, bulimia nervosa, and ADHD.
4. Given a generic and trade name psychiatric drug, identify the drug category it belongs to or the disease it is used to treat.
5. Given a category of psychiatric drugs, name several generic and trade name drugs that belong to that category.
6. Identify the Historical Notes or Did You Know? section in this chapter that you found most interesting.

The term *mental illness* encompasses a variety of emotional disorders that involve abnormalities of personality, mood, or behavior. It is estimated that nearly 50% of all hospital admissions are in some way related to a mental health problem such as anxiety, depression, suicide, postpartum depression, psychosis, psychosomatic illness, attention-deficit/hyperactivity disorder (ADHD), panic attacks, social phobias, obsessive-compulsive disorder (OCD), posttraumatic stress disorder (PTSD), drug addiction, or alcoholism. Drugs, as well as psychotherapy, behavior modification, or educational programs, are used to treat these diseases.

HISTORICAL NOTES: During the 1800s, the treatment for mental illness could include the use of the drugs digitalis, ipecac, alcohol, or opium. In 1903, barbiturates were synthesized and used effectively as sedative drugs for agitated mentally ill patients. Barbiturates now have only limited use in treating insomnia. Before World War II, schizophrenic patients were treated in several ways: they were exposed to malaria to produce a high fever and delirium, injected with enough insulin to cause convulsions and coma, or given electroshock therapy. Amphetamines were used to alleviate depression.

However, beginning in the early 1950s, advances were made in the treatment of mental illness with the introduction of new drugs to treat neurosis, psychosis, and depression.

DRUGS USED TO TREAT ANXIETY AND NEUROSIS

The symptoms of neurosis include anxiety, anxiousness, and tension—all at a more intense level than normal—and a feeling of apprehension with vague, unsubstantiated fears. The neurotic patient, however, never experiences any loss of touch with reality.

The treatment of neurosis involves the use of **antianxiety drugs**, also known as *anxiolytic drugs* or *minor tranquilizers*. The term *minor tranquilizer* is somewhat of a misnomer in that it carries the connotation that this class of drugs is somehow less effective than the major tranquilizers (used to treat psychosis) or that the minor tranquilizers are only major tranquilizers given at a lower dose. In fact, minor tranquilizers are completely unrelated chemically to major tranquilizers. They are extremely effective drugs with a specific therapeutic action for treating neurosis.

HISTORICAL NOTES: In 1945, researchers were looking for a new antibiotic to use against bacteria that were already becoming resistant to penicillin. One drug tested was found to produce muscle relaxation and exert a calming effect in animals. From this parent molecule, the first minor tranquilizer was developed in 1955 and marketed as meprobamate (Equanil, Miltown).

In 1955, a researcher at Hoffmann–La Roche laboratories was searching for a compound to make a commercial dye, but the chemicals he tested were not useful as dyes. A year and a half of research yielded no usable products. As he was doing his final clean up of the project, he noted a single sample that he had forgotten to send for testing. He noted, "We were under great pressure by this time because my boss told us to stop these foolish things and go back to more useful work. I submitted it [the sample] for animal testing. . . . I thought myself that it was just to finish up." That last sample, which was nearly forgotten, turned out to be chlordiazepoxide (Librium). It was released for sale in 1960 and became the first of the benzodiazepine class of minor tranquilizers that would come to dominate the treatment of neurosis.

The same researcher continued to work with the basic molecular structure of chlordiazepoxide (Librium), and in 1959, even before marketing of Librium had begun, he had synthesized the new drug diazepam (Valium) (see Figure 25–1). The trade name *Valium* is derived from the Latin word *valere*, which means *to be healthy*. The wild European plant valerian has been known since the time of Hippocrates to calm the nerves. In 1970, Valium became the number one prescription drug in the United States. Even 10 years later, Hoffman–La Roche was still manufacturing 30 million Valium tablets every day.

Edward Shorter, *The Health Century* (New York, NY: Doubleday, 1987), p. 127.

Benzodiazepine Drugs for Anxiety and Neurosis

The benzodiazepines are by far the most commonly prescribed drugs for the treatment of anxiety and neurosis. They bind to several specific types of receptor sites in the brain to provide sedation. They affect thought processes; they affect emotional behavior by their action in the limbic area of the brain. They also decrease the muscle tension that comes with anxiety. All of the benzodiazepines are Schedule IV controlled substance drugs.

alprazolam (Xanax)

chlordiazepoxide (Librium, Mitran, Reposans-10)

clorazepate (Tranxene, Tranxene Half Strength, Tranxene-SD, Tranxene-T)

diazepam (Valium)

lorazepam (Ativan)

oxazepam (Serax)

Note: The ending -*azepam* is common to generic benzodiazepine drugs used to treat anxiety and neurosis.

DID YOU KNOW?   The *SD* in Tranxene-SD stands for *single dose*. The *T* in Tranxene-T refers to the actual shape of the tablet.

Other Drugs for Anxiety and Neurosis

Some of these drugs are antidepressants whose therapeutic effect is described in the next section. The exact mechanism of action of the other antianxiety drugs varies or is not well

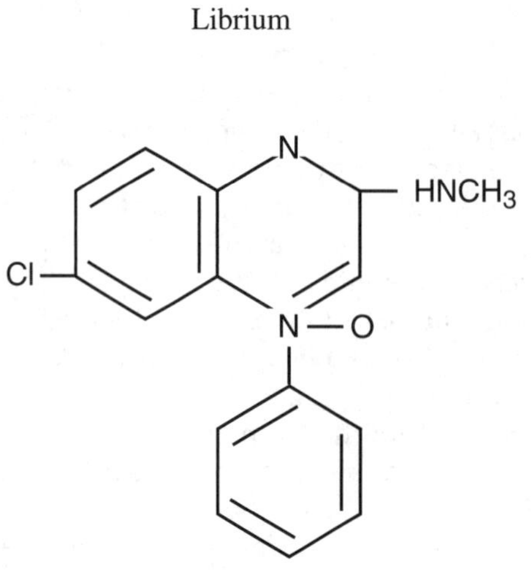

Librium   Valium

Figure 25–1   The similar chemical structures of chlordiazepoxide (Librium) and diazepam (Valium), the first two benzodiazepine antianxiety drugs.

understood. Of these drugs, only meprobamate is a controlled substance drug (Schedule IV).

acecarbromal (Paxarel)
buspirone (BuSpar)
clobazam (Frisium)
doxepin (Sinequan, Sinequan Concentrate)
fluvoxamine (Luvox)
gepirone
hydroxyzine (Atarax, Atarax 100, Vistaril)
meprobamate (Equanil, Miltown)
paroxetine (Paxil)
prochlorperazine (Compazine)
ritanserin
trifluoperazine (Stelazine)
venlafaxine (Effexor, Effexor XR)

DID YOU KNOW?   Hydroxyzine has many actions: It depresses areas of the central nervous system; relaxes skeletal muscle; and acts as an analgesic, antihistamine/antipruritic, and antiemetic. It is used as a preoperative sedative under the trade name Vistaril. It is given postoperatively to control nausea. Under the trade names Atarax and Atarax 100, it is also used to control severe itching (antipruritic action).

DRUGS USED TO TREAT PSYCHOSIS

The symptoms of psychosis include a loss of touch with reality resulting in delusions, hallucinations, inappropriate mood, and bizarre behaviors. Psychotic symptomatology may be based, in part, on overactivity of the neurotransmitter dopamine in the brain either from overproduction of dopamine or from hypersensitivity of dopamine receptors. Imbalances in the neurotransmitters serotonin, acetylcholine, and norepinephrine, and the chemical histamine are also thought to play a role in psychosis. Schizophrenia is the most common form of psychosis.

The treatment of psychosis involves the use of **antipsychotic drugs**, which are also known as *neuroleptics* or *major tranquilizers*. These drugs block dopamine receptors in many areas of the brain including the limbic system, which controls emotions. Antipsychotic drugs decrease psychotic symptoms of hostility, agitation, and paranoia without causing confusion or sedation. Some of these drugs are specifically used to treat schizophrenia. Unlike antianxiety drugs, none of the antipsychotic drugs are addictive; they are not schedule drugs or controlled substances.

> **HISTORICAL NOTES:** Prior to the introduction of modern antipsychotic drugs, barbiturates were used to sedate agitated psychotic patients. These drugs have been replaced by the phenothiazine group of drugs. Phenothiazine was the original parent drug for this group. It was first manufactured in 1883 as a wormer for livestock. Some minor changes in its chemical structure resulted in the creation of chlorpromazine (Thorazine), the first of the modern antipsychotic drugs; it is still one of the most widely used antipsychotic drugs.

Phenothiazine Drugs for Psychosis

      chlorpromazine (Thorazine, Thorazine Spansules)
      fluphenazine (Permitil, Prolixin)
      mesoridazine (Serentil)
      perphenazine (Trilafon)
      prochlorperazine (Compazine)
      thioridazine (Mellaril, Mellaril-S)
      trifluoperazine (Stelazine)

Note: The ending *-azine* is common to generic phenothiazine antipsychotic drugs.

Other Drugs for Psychosis

These drugs have various actions. For some of them, the exact mechanism of the antipsychotic therapeutic effect is not well understood.

      carbamazepine (Atretol, Carbatrol, Epitol, Tegretol, Tegretol-XR)
      clonazepam (Klonopin)

clonidine (Catapres, Catapres-TTS-1, Catapres-TTS-2, Catapres-TTS-3)

clozapine (Clozaril)

fluoxetine (Prozac, Prozac Weekly)

haloperidol (Haldol, Haldol Decanoate 50, Haldol Decanoate 100)

loxapine (Loxitane, Loxitane C, Loxitane IM)

molindone (Moban)

olanzapine (Zyprexa, Zyprexa Zydis)

quetiapine (Seroquel)

remoxipride (Roxiam)

risperidone (Risperdal)

ritanserin

sertindole (Serlect)

thiothixene (Navane)

ziprasidone (Geodon)

DID YOU KNOW?   Haloperidol is also used to treat the symptoms of Tourette's syndrome, which include involuntary muscle tics (shrugging, winking, twisting), hyperactivity, obsessive-compulsive disorder, and involuntary spontaneous cursing.

Zyprexa Zydis is the trade name for a special tablet form of Zyprexa that dissolves in the mouth within 5 to 15 seconds. Because of their mental illness, many psychotic patients are noncompliant with their medications as they do not understand the importance of the drugs or they feel someone is trying to poison them. Psychotic patients commonly refuse medication or hide a tablet between their cheek and teeth and later discard it. This new drug form helps assure patient compliance. Antipsychotic drugs are available in a liquid form, but this must be refrigerated. Zyprex Zydis does not need refrigeration because it does not become a liquid until it is in the mouth.

IN DEPTH: The antipsychotic drugs, particularly the phenothiazines, cause a distinctive group of side effects known collectively as *tardive dyskinesia*. Symptoms of tardive dyskinesia include involuntary, repetitive movements of the face (grimacing, smacking the lips, blinking the eyes, sticking out the tongue), but can also include movements of the arms, legs, and fingers. The term *tardive dyskinesia* was introduced in 1964. The word *tardive* means *late* and refers to the fact that these symptoms appear late in the course of therapy with antipsychotic drugs. The physician may recommend that the patient take a short "drug holiday" from his or her antipsychotic medication to lessen the symptoms of tardive dyskinesia. These drugs are used to treat tardive dyskinesia.

baclofen (Lioresal)

lithium (Eskalith, Eskalith CR, Lithobid)

tetrabenazine

DRUGS USED TO TREAT DEPRESSION

The term *affect* refers to an emotional feeling or mood expressed by a patient's outward appearance. **Affective disorders** center on two major emotions: **depression** and **mania**.

The depressed patient experiences insomnia; crying; lack of pleasure in any activity; increased or decreased appetite; lack of ability to act or concentrate; feelings of guilt, helplessness, hopelessness, or worthlessness; and thoughts of suicide and death. These symptoms occur daily, interfere with life activities, and last longer than 2 weeks. Depression is caused by decreased levels of the neurotransmitters norepinephrine and serotonin in the brain. The treatment for depression involves the use of antidepressant drugs.

Antidepressants, or **mood-elevating drugs**, not only alleviate the symptoms of depression, but they also increase mental alertness, normalize sleep patterns, normalize the appetite, and decrease suicidal ideation. There are four main categories of antidepressant drugs: tricyclic antidepressants, tetracyclic antidepressants, selective serotonin reuptake inhibitors (SSRIs), and monoamine oxidase (MAO) inhibitors.

HISTORICAL NOTES: Originally, amphetamines were used to treat depression; they acted to stimulate the central nervous system and mask the patient's depressive symptoms. Amphetamines have a high potential for abuse and do not correct the underlying chemical imbalance causing depression. Therefore, they are no longer used to treat depression.

In 1951, while evaluating a drug for its effectiveness in treating tuberculosis, researchers noted that even seriously ill and dying patients developed a happy, optimistic attitude despite the lack of clinical improvement in their tuberculosis. This drug was identified as an MAO inhibitor, the first of the MAO inhibitor class of antidepressants.

In 1958, a drug being tested as an antipsychotic showed significant antidepressant effects. That drug was imipramine (Tofranil), and it was the first of the tricyclic antidepressant drugs.

Tricyclic Antidepressant (TCA) Drugs

Tricyclic antidepressants (TCA) inhibit the reuptake of and prolong the action of norepinephrine or serotonin released by neurons in the brain. This helps to correct the low levels of these neurotransmitters that are found in patients with depression. Also, tricyclic antidepressants increase the sensitivity of receptors on the neurons to available norepinephrine and serotonin. Thus, these drugs act to both prolong and enhance the effect of norepinephrine and serotonin. The tricyclic antidepressants are so named because of the triple-ring configuration of their chemical structure (see Figure 25–2).

amitriptyline (Elavil)
amoxapine
desipramine (Norpramin)
dothiepin (Prothiaden)
doxepin (Sinequan, Sinequan Concentrate)

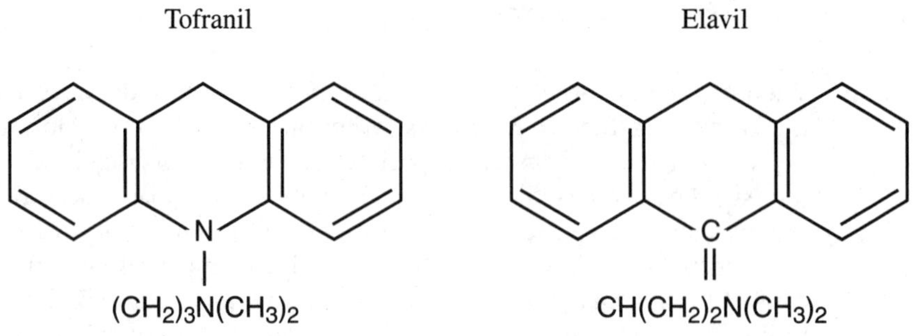

Tofranil   Elavil

(CH$_2$)$_3$N(CH$_3$)$_2$ CH(CH$_2$)$_2$N(CH$_3$)$_2$

Figure 25–2   The chemical structures of the tricyclic antidepressants imipramine (Tofranil) and amitriptyline (Elavil), showing the three-ring structure from which the drug category derives its name.

imipramine (Tofranil, Tofranil-PM)
nortriptyline (Aventyl, Aventyl Pulvules, Pamelor)
protriptyline (Vivactil)
trimipramine (Surmontil)

Note: The endings *-triptyline* and *-ipramine* are common to many tricyclic antidepressants.

DID YOU KNOW?   Desipramine is also used to treat the symptoms of cocaine withdrawal.

Tetracyclic Antidepressant Drugs

Although slightly different in chemical structure, tetracyclic antidepressants have essentially the same therapeutic effect as the tricyclic antidepressants described previously.

maprotiline
mirtazapine (Remeron, Remeron SolTab)

Note: SolTab is the trade name for a special tablet that can swallowed, chewed, or allowed to disintegrate in the mouth.

Selective Serotonin Reuptake Inhibitors (SSRIs) for Depression

Selective serotonin reuptake inhibitors (SSRIs) block the normal reuptake of free serotonin by nerve cells. When serotonin levels are low (in patients with depression), these drugs allow the available serotonin to bind with more receptors for a longer period of time.

citalopram (Celexa)

fluoxetine (Prozac, Prozac Weekly)

fluvoxamine (Luvox)

paroxetine (Paxil)

sertraline (Zoloft)

DID YOU KNOW?   Fluoxetine is also used to treat alcoholism, narcolepsy, kleptomania, attention-deficit/hyperactivity disorder, social anxiety disorder, panic disorder, schizophrenia, autism, bulimia nervosa, anorexia nervosa, premenstrual dysphoric disorder, migraine pain, and diabetic peripheral neuropathy.

Fluoxetine is also used to treat seasonal affective disorder (SAD). This disorder, which occurs during the fall and winter when there are fewer hours of daylight, is characterized by depression, fatigue, increased sleep, and weight gain. Treatment also includes increased exposure to natural or artifical light.

Paroxetine is also used to treat SAD, premature ejaculation, fibromyalgia, and diabetic peripheral neuropathy. During 2001, approximately $1.7 billion dollars worth of paroxetine (Paxil) was prescribed.

DID YOU KNOW?   A new class of antidepressant drugs may soon be on the market. **Selective norepinephrine reuptake inhibitors (SNRIs)** are said to have a faster onset and fewer side effects than current antidepressant drugs. The first drug in this class is reboxetine (Vestra).

Another new class of antidepressant drugs is also under investigation: **bicyclic antidepressants**. The first drug in this class is viloxazine (Catatrol).

Monoamine Oxidase (MAO) Inhibitors for Depression

The neurotransmitters epinephrine, norepinephrine, dopamine, and serotonin are known as *monoamines* because of their chemical structure. Monoamine oxidase (MAO) is an enzyme in the body that breaks down these monoamines. MAO inhibitors prevent the enzyme monoamine oxidase from breaking down the neurotransmitters norepinephrine and serotonin in the brain. MAO inhibitor drugs are an older group of antidepressant drugs that are prescribed less frequently than other antidepressants because of the possibility of severe side effects from drug–food interactions.

IN DEPTH: The enzyme monoamine oxidase normally breaks down norepinephrine and serotonin in the brain; in the intestine, it also breaks down tyramine in the foods we eat. Because this enzyme is blocked when a person takes an MAO inhibitor, tyramine is not broken down, but is absorbed directly into the bloodstream.

The tyramine in the blood stimulates the release of large amounts of stored norepinephrine, and this causes violent headaches, severe hypertension, and possible stroke. This can occur quickly if a patient taking MAO inhibitors for depression ingests foods that contain high levels of tyramine. These foods include aged cheese, red wine, beer, chicken liver, bananas, bologna, salami, sausage, avocados, sauerkraut, raspberries, dried fruits, anchovies, caviar, meat tenderizer, soy sauce, ginseng, coffee, tea, colas, and chocolate.

MAO inhibitors are usually not the drug of choice for initiating treatment for depression, but they are often prescribed for patients who do not respond to other antidepressants.

> isocarboxazid (Marplan)
> phenelzine (Nardil)
> tranylcypromine (Parnate)

Other Drugs for Depression

The mechanism of action of these drugs is not clearly understood.

> bupropion (Wellbutrin, Wellbutrin SR)
> nefazodone (Serzone)
> trazodone (Desyrel, Desyrel Dividose)
> venlafaxine (Effexor, Effexor XR)

DRUGS USED TO TREAT MANIC-DEPRESSIVE DISORDER

The second emotion of affective disorders is that of **mania**. The manic patient exhibits hyperactivity, agitation, and euphoria; thinks and talks rapidly; and devises many grandiose plans, but shows poor judgment. Mania is associated with increased levels of norepinephrine in the brain. Drugs used to treat mania have varied actions. Clonazepam is a benzodiazepine that acts on receptors in the limbic system that affect emotion. Olanzapine inhibits the action of the excess norepinephrine and may also increase the action of serotonin. The therapeutic action of the other drugs in treating mania is not well understood.

> clonazepam (Klonopin)
> clonidine (Catapres, Catapres-TTS-1, Catapres-TTS-2, Catapres-TTS-3)
> lithium (Eskalith, Eskalith CR, Lithobid)
> olanzapine (Zyprexa, Zyprexa Zydis)
> valproic acid (Depacon, Depakene, Depakote, Depakote ER)

Mania coupled with depression is known as *manic-depressive disorder* or *bipolar disorder* because the patient's mood swings between the two opposite poles of emotion. The drugs used to treat manic-depressive disorder lessen the severity of mood swings from depression to mania and decrease the frequency with which these cycles occur. These drugs include both antipsychotic drugs and antidepressant drugs that may be given in conjunction with lithium.

> carbamazepine (Atretol, Carbatrol, Epitol, Tegretol, Tegretol-XR)
> chlorpromazine (Thorazine, Thorazine Spansules)
> fluoxetine (Prozac, Prozac Weekly)
> paroxetine (Paxil)
> risperidone (Risperdal)

DRUGS USED TO TREAT OBSESSIVE-COMPULSIVE DISORDER (OCD)

Obsessive-compulsive disorder (OCD) is characterized by thoughts that cause anxiety, followed by repetitive actions to relieve or escape the anxiety of a perceived threatening situation. These repetitive actions typically occupy hours of each day and involve repetitive cleaning, checking, hoarding, arranging, labeling, or even praying. Although the person knows the behavior is excessive and unreasonable, he or she is unable to stop. This disorder is treated with antidepressants.

> clomipramine (Anafranil)
> fluoxetine (Prozac, Prozac Weekly)
> fluvoxamine (Luvox)
> paroxetine (Paxil)
> sertraline (Zoloft)

DRUGS USED TO TREAT PANIC DISORDER

Panic disorder, also known as *panic attacks*, is characterized by a sudden, overwhelming sense of great fear in the absense of any situation or reason that would create anxiety or fear. The physical symptoms are intense and can even mimic a heart attack. This disorder is treated with various types of antianxiety and antidepressant drugs.

> alprazolam (Xanax)
> citalopram (Celexa)
> clomipramine (Anafranil)
> desipramine (Norpramin)
> fluoxetine (Prozac, Prozac Weekly)
> fluvoxamine (Luvox)
> imipramine (Tofranil, Tofranil-PM)
> nortriptyline (Aventyl, Aventyl Pulvules, Pamelor)
> paroxetine (Paxil)
> sertraline (Zoloft)
> trazodone (Desyrel, Desyrel Dividose)

DRUGS USED TO TREAT SOCIAL ANXIETY DISORDER

Social anxiety disorder, also known as *social phobia*, is characterized by fear in social situations: in crowds, stores, meetings, parties, and even on the telephone. There is also a fear of speaking to strangers or authority figures or speaking in front of a group. Physical symptoms include extreme nervousness, sweating, blushing, tremors, nausea, stammering, inability to think clearly, and the fear that everyone is looking at you. The person with social anxiety disorder knows that the fear is out of proportion to the situation, but cannot control the anxiety. This disorder is treated with SSRI antidepressant drugs.

citalopram (Celexa)

fluoxetine (Prozac, Prozac Weekly)

fluvoxamine (Luvox)

paroxetine (Paxil)

sertraline (Zoloft}

Professional actors, musicians, singers, and others in the public eye can experience temporary **performance anxiety** that is limited to that occasion. Instead of taking daily SSRI antidepressant drugs, these individuals usually take the following drug just prior to the performance to block the physical effects of the excess epinephrine released in response to anxiety.

propranolol (Inderal, Inderal LA)

DRUGS USED TO TREAT POSTTRAUMATIC STRESS DISORDER (PTSD)

Posttraumatic stress disorder (PTSD) is caused by exposure to a real life-threatening event or trauma, such as war, natural disasters, rape, or physical/mental abuse. This disorder is characterized by both physical and mental changes. Brainwave activity is altered. There are increased levels of epinephrine and norepinephrine and decreased levels of cortisol. Sleep abnormalities, headaches, nausea, dizziness, and chest pain are common. These symptoms may be mild or severe, constant or intermittent. This disorder also impairs personal and family relationships, activities of daily living, and employment. This disorder is treated with SSRI antidepressant drugs.

fluoxetine (Prozac, Prozac Weekly)

fluvoxamine (Luvox)

paroxetine (Paxil)

sertraline (Zoloft)

DRUGS USED TO TREAT ANOREXIA NERVOSA AND BULIMIA NERVOSA

Anorexia nervosa is a psychiatric illness in which the patient weighs much less than expected for his or her age and height, but cannot recognize this. The patient continues to diet, eats poorly, denies being thin, and actually feels fat. Bulimia nervosa, on the other hand, is a psychiatric illness in which the patient is of normal weight, but wishes to be thinner. The patient diets, vomits, and uses laxatives to lose weight. Alternatively, the patient binges or eats large quantities of food. Bulimia nervosa is treated with tricyclic and SSRI antidepressant drugs, as well as lithium, a drug also used to treat mania. Only imipramine is used to treat anorexia nervosa.

> amitriptyline (Elavil)
> desipramine (Norpramin)
> fluoxetine (Prozac, Prozac Weekly)
> imipramine (Tofranil, Tofranil-PM)
> lithium (Eskalith, Eskalith CR, Lithobid)

DRUGS USED TO TREAT ATTENTION-DEFICIT/HYPERACTIVITY DISORDER (ADHD)

Hyperactive children exhibit extreme symptoms of restlessness, short attention span, distractibility, emotional lability, and impulsive or disruptive behavior. This complex of symptoms was previously known as *minimal brain dysfunction* and *attention deficit disorder* (ADD); it is now known as *attention-deficit/hyperactivity disorder (ADHD)*. The cause of ADHD may be brain damage at birth, genetic factors, or other abnormalities. It is five times more common in boys than in girls. Most children outgrow the symptoms of ADHD in late childhood. Drugs used to treat ADHD include amphetamines and other related CNS-stimulating drugs. These drugs exert a paradoxical effect in that they do not overstimulate but actually reduce impulsive behavior and lengthen the attention span. Drug therapy for ADHD is accompanied by psychological counseling as well as special educational intervention.

Amphetamines for ADHD

These are classified as Schedule II drugs. They have the highest potential for abuse and addiction of any drugs used medically.

> amphetamine
> dextroamphetamine (Dexedrine, Dexedrine Spansules, Dextrostat)
> methamphetamine (Desoxyn, Desoxyn Gradumet)

DID YOU KNOW?   Amphetamine was synthesized in the late 1920s. It became a drug of abuse during World War II when it helped soldiers keep alert and avoid battle fatigue. During the 1960s, methamphetamine ("speed") became a popular drug of abuse. In 1972, amphetamines were classified as Schedule II drugs with a high potential for abuse.

Other Drugs for ADHD

These drugs stimulate the CNS but are not schedule drugs and are not addictive.

chlorpromazine (Thorazine, Thorazine Spansules)
clonidine (Catapres, Catapres-TTS-1, Catapres-TTS-2, Catapres-TTS-3)
dexmethylphenidate (Focalin)
fluoxetine (Prozac, Prozac Weekly)
methylphenidate (Concerta, Metadate CD, Metadate ER, Methylin ER, Ritalin, Ritalin-SR)
pemoline (Cylert, PemADD, PemADD CT)
thioridazine (Mellaril, Mellaril-S)

DID YOU KNOW?   Focalin contains only the dextro isomer, the more active isomer, of the chemical molecule of Ritalin.

Each capsule of Metadate CD contains tiny beads. Each bead acts as a drug reservoir that slowly releases the drug over time. The *CD* stands for *controlled dosage*. The *ER* in Metadate ER and Methylin ER stands for *extended release*. The *SR* in Ritalin-SR stands for *slow release*.

Combination Drugs for ADHD

Adderall, Adderall XR (amphetamine, dextroamphetamine)

Note: The spelling of the name of the combination drug Adderall alludes to the previous disease name of ADD.

FOCUS ON HEALTHCARE ISSUES: The American Academy of Pediatrics reports that between 1991 and 1995 prescriptions for the drugs Ritalin and Prozac doubled in number for preschool children with ADHD in the United States. They attribute this to managed care wanting a quick diagnosis, the low cost of these drugs, and the fact that so many working parents do not have time to enforce a behavioral modification program. Other sources report a 500% increase in prescriptions for Ritalin since 1996.

COMBINATION DRUGS USED TO TREAT PSYCHIATRIC CONDITIONS

The following drug contains an antidepressant and an antianxiety drug.

Limbitrol DS 10-25 (amitriptyline, chlordiazepoxide)

The following drugs contain an antidepressant and an antipsychotic drug.

Etrafon, Etrafon-A, Etrafon-Forte, Etrafon 2-10 (amitriptyline, perphenazine)
Triavil 2-10, Triavil 2-25, Triavil 4-10, Triavil 4-25 (amitriptyline, perphenazine)

The following drugs contain an antianxiety drug and another drug.

Equagesic (meprobamate, aspirin)
Librax (chlordiazepoxide, clidinium [GI antispasmodic drug])

MISCELLANEOUS DRUGS USED TO TREAT PSYCHIATRIC DISORDERS

buprenorphine (Subutex):   Used to treat narcotic addiction.

dantrolene (Dantrium):   Used to treat neuroleptic malignant syndrome caused by an adverse reaction to antipsychotic drugs.

disulfiram (Antabuse):   Given to alcoholics who want to remain sober, to prevent them from consuming alcohol. This drug inhibits an enzyme that normally metabolizes acetaldehyde in the bloodstream (one of the breakdown products of alcohol). If the patient drinks while taking disulfiram, the alcohol is oxidized to acetaldehyde but cannot be metabolized further. Acetaldehyde levels greatly increase, causing symptoms of flushing, headache, dizziness, nausea, and even severe hypotension and arrhythmias. These adverse reactions are supposed to keep alcoholic patients from taking a drink. However, patients cannot be placed on disulfiram without first giving consent, expressing a desire to remain sober, and being thoroughly forewarned of the dangerous complications that could result from alcohol consumption. Compliance with this drug regimen is strictly voluntary. Patients must also be warned to avoid cough syrups, mouthwashes, and aftershaves that contain alcohol.

HISTORICAL NOTES: Disulfiram (Antabuse) was originally used in the commercial production of rubber. In 1948, two Danish researchers began testing this drug for its possible effectiveness in treating intestinal worms. To study its safety in humans, they both took the drug. When each became ill after consuming alcohol, they concluded that the alcohol–disulfiram combination had produced the reaction. Antabuse was first prescribed for the prevention of alcoholism that same year.

flumazenil (Romazicon):   Benzodiazepine antagonist drug used as an antidote to reverse an overdose of a benzodiazepine antianxiety drug.

flunitrazepam (Rohypnol):   Illegal drug not approved for use in the United States. So-called "date-rape drug."

guanfacine (Tenex):   Alpha$_2$-receptor blocker used to treat withdrawal from heroin.

mecamylamine (Inversine):   Used to treat Tourette's syndrome, which is characterized by involuntary muscle tics, spontaneous cursing, obsessions, compulsions, and hyperactivity.

metoprolol (Lopressor, Toprol-XL): Antihypertensive beta-receptor blocker used to treat the side effects of muscle restlessness caused by antipsychotic drugs.

nicotine patch (Habitrol, Nicoderm CQ): Used to treat Tourette's syndrome.

paraldehyde (Paral): Used to provide sedation during alcohol withdrawal.

pergolide (Permax): Used to treat Tourette's syndrome.

physostigmine (Antilirium): Tricyclic antidepressant antagonist drug used as an antidote to reverse an overdose of a tricyclic antidepressant.

DID YOU KNOW? Physostigmine is derived from the calabar bean (*Physostigma venenosum*), a vine in Nigeria that grows 50 feet long.

pimozide (Orap): This drug belongs to the class of antipsychotic drugs, but it is only used to treat Tourette's syndrome, not psychosis.

pramiracetam: Used to treat symptoms of mental dysfunction following electroshock therapy.

propranolol (Inderal, Inderal LA): Antihypertensive beta-receptor blocker used to treat the side effects of muscle restlessness caused by antipsychotic drugs.

ritanserin: Used to treat anxiety, depression, schizophrenia, alcoholism, and drug abuse.

secretin: Used to treat pediatric autism.

Suboxone: Combination narcotic and narcotic antagonist drug used to treat narcotic addiction.

tiapride: Used to treat Tourette's syndrome.

REVIEW QUESTIONS

1. Minor tranquilizers are the same drugs as major tranquilizers but are given at a lower dosage. True or False?
2. Give three names assigned to the class of drugs used to treat psychosis.
3. The terms *tricyclic* and *tetracyclic* bring to mind what class of drugs? Why?
4. Name a drug used to treat each of these conditions.

alcoholism (to prevent drinking)	drug: _____
manic-depressive disorder	drug: _____
OCD	drug: _____
social anxiety disorder	drug:_____
depression	drug:_____
ADHD	drug:_____

5. Describe several ways in which benzodiazepines exert their antianxiety therapeutic effect.
6. What are the two major emotions of affective disorder?
7. Describe the symptoms of psychosis.

8. Why must certain foods be avoided when taking an MAO inhibitor?

9. Name three categories of psychiatric drugs and give an example of a drug in each category.

10. To what category of drugs does each of these drugs belong?

> alprazolam (Xanax)
> amitriptyline (Elavil)
> doxepin (Sinequan)
> fluoxetine (Prozac)
> fluvoxamine (Luvox)
> risperidone (Risperdal)
> sertraline (Zoloft)
> thiothixene (Navane)
> trimipramine (Surmontil)

11. Rewrite this prescription in plain English. Use the Glossary/Index at the back of the textbook to help you verify the spelling and dosage of this drug. (See Figure 25–3.)

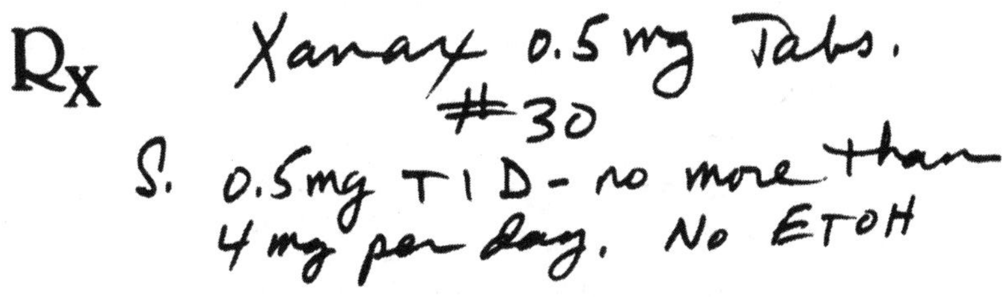

R_X Xanax 0.5 mg Tabs.
#30
S. 0.5 mg TID - no more than
4 mg per day. No ETOH

Figure 25–3   A prescription. *Reprinted courtesy of Marvin Stoogenke,* The Pharmacy Technician, *2nd ed. (Upper Saddle River, NJ: Brady/Prentice Hall, 1998), p. 370.*

SPELLING TIPS

Antabuse   Not *Antiabuse*; there is no *i*.

BuSpar   Unusual internal capitalization.

Remeron SolTab   Unusual internal capitalization.

trifluoperazine versus **triflupromazine**   These antipsychotic drugs have a very similar sound and spelling.

GET CONNECTED

Multimedia Extension Activities

 www.prenhall.com/turley

Use the above address to access the free, interactive Companion Website created for this textbook. Included in the features of this site are drug updates and additional chapter-specific exercises for further practice.

26

Analgesic Drugs

CHAPTER CONTENTS

Narcotic analgesic drugs
Nonnarcotic analgesic drugs
Combination nonnarcotic analgesic drugs
Combination narcotic and nonnarcotic drugs
Nonsteroidal anti-inflammatory drugs (NSAIDs)
Drugs used to treat migraine headaches
Drugs used to treat narcotic addiction and overdose
Miscellaneous analgesic drugs
Review questions
Spelling tips

LEARNING OBJECTIVES

After studying this chapter, you should be able to do the following:

1. Name several categories of analgesic drugs.
2. Describe the therapeutic effect of drugs used to treat migraines, narcotic addiction, and narcotic overdose.
3. Describe the therapeutic effect of narcotic analgesics, nonnarcotic analgesics, and nonsteroidal anti-inflammatory drugs.
4. Given the generic and trade name of an analgesic drug, identify what drug category it belongs to or what disease it is used to treat.
5. Given an analgesic drug category, name several generic and trade name drugs in that category.
6. Identify the Historical Notes or Did You Know? section in the chapter that you found most interesting.

Drugs for pain can be divided into three large categories: narcotics, nonnarcotics, and nonsteroidal anti-inflammatory drugs (NSAIDs).

The ideal analgesic drug would (1) provide maximum pain relief, (2) produce no side effects, and (3) cause no dependence or addiction. Unfortunately, the ideal analgesic drug does not exist! Drugs that effectively relieve severe pain are usually addictive (narcotics), whereas nonnarcotic drugs and NSAIDs are only effective for mild-to-moderate pain.

NARCOTIC ANALGESIC DRUGS

The term *narcotic* is derived from the Greek word *narke* which means *numbness*. Narcotic drugs relieve pain by binding with opiate receptor sites in the brain; they block pain impulses coming to the brain from ascending neural pathways. Natural opiate-like substances in the body (**endorphins**) normally occupy these receptors and produce a natural pain relief. There are several different types of opiate receptors; this accounts for the stronger addicting quality of some narcotic drugs compared with others and the different classifications of schedule drugs. The existence of different opiate receptors also accounts for the different kinds of side effects seen with various narcotic drugs.

Common side effects of narcotics include constipation, respiratory depression, sedation, and euphoria. It is the presence of significant euphoria that causes some narcotic drugs to be more psychologically addicting than others. One common narcotic side effect, suppression of the cough center (antitussive effect), is used as a therapeutic effect by including certain narcotic drugs in cough syrups (e.g., Hycodan). For a discussion of antitussive drugs, see Chapter 19, "Ear, Nose, and Throat (ENT) Drugs." For narcotic drugs that use the side effect of constipation as a therapeutic effect to treat diarrhea, see Chapter 13, "Gastrointestinal Drugs."

Narcotic drugs may be directly derived from opium or may be synthetically manufactured. Narcotic drugs are used to treat moderate-to-severe pain; provide preoperative and postoperative pain relief, sedation, and a feeling of well-being (euphoria); and maintain general anesthesia. Narcotic analgesic drugs are controlled substances (Schedule II to IV drugs).

buprenorphine (Buprenex)

butorphanol (Stadol, Stadol NS)

codeine

fentanyl (Actiq, Duragesic-25, Duragesic-50, Duragesic-75, Duragesic-100)

hydromorphone (Dilaudid, Dilaudid-5, Dilaudid HP)

levorphanol (Levo-Dromoran)

meperidine (Demerol)

methadone (Dolophine, Methadone Intensol, Methadose)

morphine sulfate (Astramorph PF, Duramorph, Duramorph PF, Infumorph, Kadian, MS Contin, MSIR, OMS Concentrate, Oramorph SR, RMS, Roxanol, Roxanol 100, Roxanol Rescudose, Roxanol T)

nalbuphine (Nubain)

opium (paregoric)

oxycodone (Endocodone, M-oxy, OxyContin, OxyFast, OxyIR, Percolone, Roxicodone, Roxicodone Intensol) oxymorphone (Numorphan)

pentazocine (Talwin)

propoxyphene (Darvon-N, Darvon Pulvules)

sufentanil (Sufenta)

DID YOU KNOW?　　Fentanyl (Actiq) is used to treat breakthrough pain in cancer patients. The drug comes as a lozenge on a stick. Informally, it is known as the *Actiq lollipop*.

FOCUS ON HEALTHCARE ISSUES:　　Oxycodone (OxyContin) has launched an epidemic of drug abuse that some law enforcement officials compare to the crack epidemic of the 1980s. One U.S. detoxification treatment clinic reported that 75% of its patients were recovering OxyContin addicts. Pharmacies that carry OxyContin have been the target of armed robberies, and this drug can be obtained more easily than illegal drugs by writing forged prescriptions or stealing from hospital supplies. Unlike heroin and other illegal drugs, OxyContin was introduced in 1995 as a legal Schedule II drug for treating moderate-to-severe pain. Today, OxyContin is the best-selling narcotic in the United States. Physicians wrote almost 7 million prescriptions for OxyContin in 2001. Oxycodone is available under several other trade names besides OxyContin, but addicts use OxyContin because it is a time-release formula that contains up to 10 times more narcotic than other forms of oxycodone. The time-release formula is meant to control pain for 12 hours; however, addicts chew the tablet, crush the tablet and snort the powder, or dissolve the tablet and inject it so the time-release mechanism is circumvented and the full narcotic dose is received immediately. There are many lawsuits pending against Purdue Pharma, the makers of OxyContin. The manufacturer, in cooperation with the FDA, has put new warning labels on OxyContin; however, it is the illegal sale and use of the drug that have been responsible for multiple deaths and an epidemic of addiction.

HISTORICAL NOTES:　　Did you know that opium is obtained from the dried seeds of the poppy? Morphine was first isolated from opium in 1815. Morphine was named for the Greek god of dreams, Morpheus, who was the son of Hypnos, the Greek god of sleep. Morphine was used extensively during the Civil War, resulting in a very high rate of addiction among veterans. Heroin, a semisynthetic narcotic, was introduced in 1898 as a nonaddicting substitute for morphine. It proved to be more addicting and, at the present time, is classified as a Schedule I drug with no medical uses because of its high potential for physical and psychological addiction. In 1939, meperidine (Demerol), the first synthetic narcotic drug, was introduced.

NONNARCOTIC ANALGESIC DRUGS

Nonnarcotic analgesic drugs are used to treat moderate-to-severe pain but are not addicting and are not schedule drugs. These drugs activate narcotic receptors in the brain or spinal cord. They also act on the neurotransmitters norepinephrine and serotonin.

clonidine (Duraclon)

tramadol (Ultram)

DID YOU KNOW?   Clonidine is best known as an antihypertensive drug (trade name Catapres). It blocks alpha receptors in the brain, decreases the release of norepinephrine, and allows blood vessels to dilate. When given epidurally by continuous infusion, clonidine (Duraclon) blocks receptors in the spinal cord and prevents pain signals from reaching the brain.

Nonnarcotic analgesics are also used to treat mild-to-moderate pain. These nonnarcotic analgesics are the first step in pain control and have the advantage over narcotic analgesics in that they are nonaddicting and less expensive. In fact, most nonnarcotic analgesics are available OTC unless they are offered in combination with a narcotic drug. However, nonnarcotic analgesics are not as effective as narcotics for the relief of sharp or moderate-to-severe pain.

Salicylate Analgesic Drugs

Salicylate is a general term that includes aspirin and other chemically related compounds. Salicylate drugs have three distinct therapeutic actions.

- **Analgesic.** They provide relief of mild-to-moderate pain by inhibiting the release of prostaglandins from damaged tissue.
- **Anti-inflammatory.** They decrease inflammation by inhibiting the release of prostaglandins from damaged tissue.
- **Antipyretic.** They reduce fever by acting on the hypothalamus, to cause vasodilation and sweating, which increase heat loss from the skin.

Of all the salicylate analgesic drugs, only aspirin has a fourth therapeutic action.

- **Anticoagulant.** It prolongs the clotting time by inhibiting thromboxane, which normally causes platelets to aggregate. One low-dose tablet of aspirin daily is used to treat an evolving current heart attack and decrease the risk of a second heart attack. Aspirin is also used prophylactically as an anticoagulant in patients with a history of transient ischemic attacks (small, recurring strokes).

aspirin (Arthritis Foundation Pain Reliever, Aspergum, Bayer Children's Aspirin, Bayer Low Adult Strength, Ecotrin, Ecotrin Adult Low Strength, Ecotrin Maximum Strength, Empirin, Extended Release Bayer 8-Hour, Extra Strength Bayer Enteric 500, Genuine Bayer Aspirin, ½ Halfprin, Halfprin 81, Heartline, Maximum Bayer Aspirin, Norwich Extra-Strength, St. Joseph Adult Chewable Aspirin, ZORprin)

choline salicylate (Arthropan)

diflunisal (Dolobid)

magnesium salicylate (Backache Maximum Strength Relief, Bayer Select Maximum Strength Backache Formula, Extra Strength Doan's)

salsalate (Disalcid)

DID YOU KNOW?   Prostaglandins, which are present throughout the body and exert various effects, were so named because they were originally isolated from semen from the prostate gland.

Prostaglandins play a role in causing pain. When body tissue is damaged, cells are destroyed. The contents of the cells spill into the interstitial fluid. There, the cyclooxygenase (COX) enzyme converts one of the intracellular chemicals into prostaglandins. The prostaglandins then stimulate pain receptors in that area. The greater the amount of tissue damage, the more prostaglandins are produced and the greater the sensation of pain.

HISTORICAL NOTES: Aspirin was first introduced in 1899, although for many years prior to that it was used for pain relief in its natural form from willow bark. Aspirin is also known as *acetylsalicylic acid* (ASA), from the word *salix*, which means *willow* in Latin.

Because aspirin is an acid (acetylsalicylic acid) and is irritating to the stomach, long-term therapy may produce stomach ulcers. To reduce this irritation, aspirin is manufactured as an enteric-coated tablet (Ecotrin) that dissolves only in the higher pH environment of the duodenum. Aspirin may also be combined with antacids such as magnesium or aluminum to protect the stomach.

Note: The use of aspirin to treat the aches and pains of a viral illness has been linked to the occurrence of Reye's syndrome. Reye's syndrome can cause liver damage, increased serum levels of ammonia, and encephalitis. Therefore, treating the symptoms of viral illnesses (colds, flu, chickenpox) with aspirin is no longer recommended.

Nonsalicylate Analgesic Drugs

Acetaminophen has two distinct therapeutic actions.

- **Analgesic.** The mechanism by which it relieves pain is unclear.
- **Antipyretic.** It reduces fever by acting on the hypothalamus to cause vasodilation and sweating, which increase heat loss from the skin.

Unlike aspirin, acetaminophen has no anti-inflammatory properties and is not effective in treating inflammation. It has no anticoagulant effect and therefore is not given to prevent second heart attacks or transient ischemic attacks.

acetaminophen (Aspirin Free Anacin Maximum Strength, Children's Feverall, Children's Panadol, Children's Tylenol, Children's Tylenol Soft Chews, Infant Feverall, Infants' Drops Panadol, Infants' Drops Tylenol, Junior Strength Feverall, Junior Strength Panadol, Neopap, Panadol, Tempra 1, Tempra 2, Tempra 3, Tylenol, Tylenol Arthritis, Tylenol Extended Relief, Tylenol Extra Strength, Tylenol Junior Strength, Tylenol Regular Strength)

HISTORICAL NOTE: During just a few days in the fall of 1982, seven people in the Chicago area died after having taken Extra Strength Tylenol capsules laced with cyanide. The first death was that of a 12-year-old girl who had taken the drug for cold symptoms. Several other deaths were from a single family who shared the same contaminated bottle of Tylenol capsules. Each capsule contained 10,000 times the amount of cyanide needed to kill a person. Chicago police drove through the neighborhoods with loudspeakers and all the television networks broadcast warnings about taking Tylenol. Tylenol's manufacturer, Johnson & Johnson, immediately had all 31 million bottles of Tylenol capsules removed from store shelves and offered to replace already-purchased Tylenol capsules with Tylenol tablets. The FDA set a deadline for drug manufacturers to convert to tamper-resistant packaging. The legacy of the Tylenol murders is still with us today in the form of tamper-resistant packaging. No one has ever been charged with the Tylenol murders.

COMBINATION NONNARCOTIC ANALGESIC DRUGS

These drugs contain the salicylate aspirin and one or more antacids (aluminum, calcium, magnesium, or sodium bicarbonate) to minimize stomach irritation from the aspirin.

Adprin-B
Alka-Seltzer with Aspirin, Alka-Seltzer Extra Strength with Aspirin
Arthritis Pain Formula
Ascriptin, Ascriptin A/D, Ascriptin Extra Strength
Asprimox, Asprimox Extra Protection for Arthritis Pain
Bayer Buffered Aspirin, Bayer Plus Extra Strength
Bufferin, Tri-Buffered Bufferin
Cama Arthritis Pain Reliever

These drugs contain a nonnarcotic analgesic and a sedative or two nonnarcotic analgesics.

Mobigesic (magnesium salicylate, phenyltoloxamine [sedative])

Trilisate (choline salicylate, magnesium salicylate)
Ultracet (tramadol, acetaminophen)

These drugs contain a variety of combinations of the salicylate aspirin or aceta-minophen, as well as other drugs.

Anacin, Anacin Maximum Strength (aspirin, caffeine)
Bayer PM Extra Strength Aspirin Plus Sleep Aid (aspirin, diphenhydramine)
Equagesic (aspirin, meprobamate [for anxiety])
Excedrin Aspirin Free (acetaminophen, caffeine)
Excedrin Extra Strength, Excedrin Migraine (aspirin, acetaminophen, caffeine)
Fioricet (acetaminophen, caffeine, barbiturate sedative)
Fiorinal (aspirin, caffeine, barbiturate sedative)
Vanquish (aspirin, acetaminophen, caffeine)

COMBINATION NARCOTIC AND NONNARCOTIC DRUGS

Narcotic and nonnarcotic drugs are often given in combination with each other for two reasons.

1. The nonnarcotic drug provides a foundation of pain relief upon which the narcotic drug can build; therefore, less narcotic is needed.
2. This combination of drugs acts against the two components of pain—pain that re-sults from actual stimulation of nerve endings and pain that is initiated and height-ened by anxiety.

These drugs contain aspirin and a narcotic.

Darvon Compound-65 (aspirin, propoxyphene)
Empirin with Codeine No. 3 (aspirin, 30 mg codeine)
Empirin with Codeine No. 4 (aspirin, 60 mg codeine)
Lortab ASA (aspirin, hydrocodone)
Percodan, Percodan-Demi (aspirin, oxycodone)
Roxiprin (aspirin, oxycodone)
Talwin Compound (aspirin, pentazocine)
Synalgos-DC (aspirin, dihydrocodeine)

These drugs contain acetaminophen and a narcotic.

Anexsia 5/500, Anexsia 7.5/650, Anexsia 10/660 (acetaminophen, hydrocodone)
Darvocet-N 50, Darvocet-N 100 (acetaminophen, propoxyphene)
Lorcet-HD, Lorcet Plus (acetaminophen, hydrocodone)

Lortab, Lortab 2.5/500, Lortab 5/500, Lortab 7.5/500, Lortab 10/500, Lortab 10/650 (acetaminophen, hydrocodone)

Percocet (acetaminophen, oxycodone)

Phenaphen with Codeine No. 3 (acetaminophen, 30 mg codeine)

Phenaphen with Codeine No. 4 (acetaminophen, 60 mg codeine)

Roxicet, Roxicet 5/500 (acetaminophen, oxycodone)

Roxilox (acetaminophen, oxycodone)

Talacen (acetaminophen, pentazocine)

Tylenol with Codeine (acetaminophen, 12 mg codeine)

Tylenol with Codeine No. 2 (acetaminophen, 15 mg codeine)

Tylenol with Codeine No. 3 (acetaminophen, 30 mg codeine)

Tylenol with Codeine No. 4 (acetaminophen, 60 mg codeine)

Tylox (acetaminophen, oxycodone)

Vicodin, Vicodin ES, Vicodin HP (acetaminophen, hydrocodone)

Wygesic (acetaminophen, propoxyphene)

Zydone (acetaminophen, hydrocodone)

This drug contains a narcotic and an NSAID.

Vicoprofen (hydrocodone, ibuprofen)

This drug contains a narcotic and an antihistamine drug for sedation.

Mepergan Fortis (meperidine, promethazine)

These drugs contain a narcotic, a nonnarcotic analgesic, and a barbiturate sedative.

Fioricet with Codeine (codeine, acetaminophen, butalbital)

Fiorinal with Codeine (codeine, aspirin, butalbital)

This drug contains a narcotic and an antispasmodic drug.

B&O Supprettes No. 15A, B&O Supprettes No. 16A (opium, belladonna)

This drug contain a narcotic and other ingredients.

Talwin NX (naloxone, pentazocine)

DID YOU KNOW?   The sound-alike drugs Fioricet and Fiorinol as well as Percocet and Percodan can be easily confused. One has acetaminophen and the other has aspirin as the nonnarcotic analgesic. You can remember which is which by associating **ac**etaminophen with Fiori**cet** and Per**cocet**.

NONSTEROIDAL ANTI-INFLAMMATORY DRUGS (NSAIDs)

NSAIDs have analgesic effects and also inhibit the production of prostaglandins. They have less of a tendency than salicylates to cause GI side effects and ulcers. They are structurally similar enough to aspirin that patients who are allergic to aspirin should not take NSAIDs. They are used to treat mild-to-moderate pain from arthritis, migraine, menstruation, and a variety of other causes.

carprofen (Rimadyl)

diclofenac (Cataflam, Voltaren, Voltaren-XR)

etodolac (Lodine, Lodine XL)

fenoprofen (Nalfon Pulvules)

flurbiprofen (Ansaid)

ibuprofen (Advil, Advil Migraine, Children's Advil, Children's Motrin, Haltran, Infants' Motrin, Junior Strength Advil, Junior Strength Motrin, Midol Maximum Strength Cramp Formula, Motrin, Motrin IB, Motrin Migraine Pain, Pediatric Advil Drops, PediaCare Fever)

indomethacin (Indocin, Indocin SR)

ketoprofen (Orudis, Orudis KT, Oruvail)

ketorolac (Toradol)

meclofenamate

mefenamic acid (Ponstel)

meloxicam (Mobic)

nabumetone (Relafen)

naproxen (Aleve, Anaprox, Anaprox DS, EC-Naprosyn, Naprosyn)

oxaprozin (Daypro)

piroxicam (Feldene)

sulindac (Clinoril)

tolmetin (Tolectin 200, Tolectin 600, Tolectin DS)

Note: The ending *-profen* is common to generic nonsteroidal anti-inflammatory drugs.

DID YOU KNOW?   Carprofen (Rimadyl) is an investigational drug for humans, but it has already been approved for use in cats and dogs.

COX-2 Inhibitors

These drugs, which also belong to the larger category of NSAIDs, selectively inhibit the COX-2 enzyme to decrease the production of prostaglandins and relieve pain.

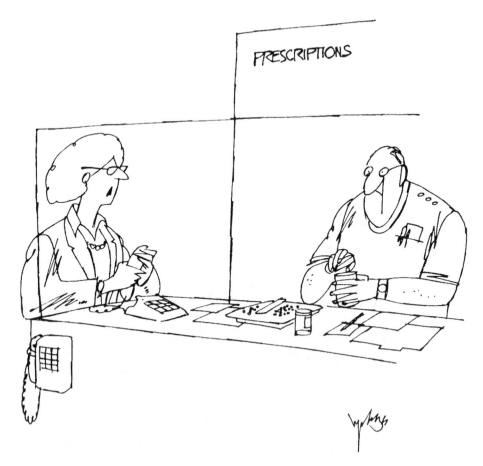

Figure 26–1 *This customer thinks he needs I Boo Propane.*—David W. Harbaugh. *Reprinted with permission.*

celecoxib (Celebrex)
rofecoxib (Vioxx)
valdecoxib (Bextra)

Combination NSAID Drugs

This drug combines an NSAID with a GI protectant drug.

Arthrotec (diclofenac, misoprostol)

DRUGS USED TO TREAT MIGRAINE HEADACHES

The pain of migraine headaches is caused by vasodilation of arteries in the brain and the release of neuropeptides by the trigeminal nerve (which travels from deep within the skull outward to the jaw, cheeks, eyes, and forehead). Drugs that prevent or treat this pain act in several different ways.

Serotonin Receptor Agonist Drugs for Migraines

Serotonin is a neurotransmitter that normally causes vasoconstriction of the arteries in the brain. Prior to the occurrence of a migraine, there are elevated levels of serotonin. The serotonin levels then decrease, and this causes vasodilation of the cerebral arteries and pain. These drugs stimulate serotonin receptor sites on the arteries to keep the blood vessels constricted during a migraine attack.

> almotriptan (Axert)
> frovatriptan (Frova)
> naratriptan (Amerge)
> rizatriptan (Maxalt, Maxalt-MLT)
> sumatriptan (Imitrex)
> zolmitriptan (Zomig, Zomig ZMT)

DID YOU KNOW?   Ergotamine (Ergostat) for migraines, ergonovine (Ergotrate) for postpartum bleeding, and ergoloid mesylates (Gerimal, Hydergine) for Alzheimer's disease are all chemically related drugs that are derived from ergot, a fungus that affects rye grass.

Beta-Receptor Blocker Drugs for Migraines

The exact mechanism of action of these drugs in treating migraines is not known.

> atenolol (Tenormin)
> metoprolol (Lopressor, Toprol-XL)
> nadolol (Corgard)
> propranolol (Inderal, Inderal LA, Propranolol Intensol)
> timolol (Blocadren)

Calcium Channel Blocker Drugs for Migraines

The exact mechanism of action of these drugs in treating migraines is not known.

> nifedipine (Adalat, Procardia)
> nimodipine (Nimotop)
> verapamil (Calan, Verelan)

Other Drugs for Migraines

Some of these drugs are primarily used to treat anxiety and depression. The exact mechanism of action of these drugs in treating migraines is not known.

> amitriptyline (Elavil)
> amoxapine

desipramine (Norpramin)

dihydroergotamine (D.H.E. 45, Migranal)

doxepin (Sinequan, Sinequan Concentrate)

ergotamine (Ergomar)

fluoxetine (Prozac, Prozac Weekly)

imipramine (Tofranil)

methysergide (Sansert)

nortriptyline (Aventyl, Aventyl Pulvules, Pamelor)

protriptyline (Vivactil)

valproic acid (Depacon, Depakene, Depakote, Depakote ER)

These drugs are NSAIDs; their therapeutic action was discussed previously in this chapter.

fenoprofen (Nalfon Pulvules)

flurbiprofen (Ansaid)

ibuprofen (Advil, Advil Migraine, Motrin, Motrin Migraine Pain)

ketoprofen (Orudis, Orudis KT, Oruvail)

ketorolac (Toradol)

meclofenamate

mefenamic acid (Ponstel)

naproxen (Aleve, Anaprox, Anaprox DS, EC-Naprosyn, Naprosyn)

Combination Drugs for Migraines

These drugs include vasoconstrictors (including caffeine), acetaminophen, and dichloralphenazone, a sedative.

Cafergot (ergotamine, caffeine)

Duradrin (isometheptene, dichloralphenazone, acetaminophen)

Midrin (isometheptene, dichloralphenazone, acetaminophen)

Wigraine (ergotamine, caffeine)

DID YOU KNOW? Lithium, the drug used to treat the manic phase of manic-depressive disorder, is also used to treat cluster headaches.

DRUGS USED TO TREAT NARCOTIC ADDICTION AND OVERDOSE

Narcotic antagonists are used to treat narcotic addiction. Narcotic antagonists compete for the same receptor sites as narcotics. Because they are not schedule drugs, they have no potential for abuse or physical or psychological addiction. These drugs are used to manage the withdrawal or ongoing treatment of former heroin and narcotic-dependent patients. On these drugs, the addict remains mentally alert and able to participate in counseling. These drugs are given at an outpatient clinic every other day, and the dosage is gradually tapered and finally discontinued.

buprenorphine (Subutex)
clonidine (Catapres)
levomethadyl (Orlaam)
lofexidine
methadone (Dolophine, Methadone Intensol, Methadose)
naltrexone (ReVia, Trexan)
Suboxone

These narcotic antagonists are used to reverse the effects of narcotic overdose, particularly life-threatening respiratory depression.

nalmefene (Revex)
naloxone (Narcan)

FOCUS ON HEALTHCARE ISSUES: Methadone was developed in the 1960s and levomethadyl was approved in 1993. Currently, there are about 200,000 addicts being treated with methadone in the United States. Methadone costs about $3 per week and is used more frequently by treatment clinics than levomethadyl, which costs $13 per week. In late 2000, then-President Clinton signed a law that made it legal for narcotic and heroin addicts to receive buprenorphine from a physician instead of a clinic. This drug is considered safe enough for patients to take without supervision at home because, unlike levomethadyl or methadone, it does not cause toxicity even when taken as an overdose. An additional benefit is the fact that an addict can be treated privately by a physician rather than having to visit a treatment clinic every day (for methadone) or every other day (for levomethadyl). The social stigma of visiting a public treatment clinic keeps many addicts from pursuing treatment. In addition, the shortage of openings for new patients at treatment clinics could be remedied by the availability of buprenorphine from private physicians.

ANALGESIC DRUGS USED TO TREAT DYSMENORRHEA

See Chapter 23, "Obstetric/Gynecologic Drugs."

MISCELLANEOUS ANALGESIC DRUGS

acetylcysteine (Mucomyst): Used as an antidote for acetaminophen overdose, this drug acts to protect the liver, the main site of acetaminophen toxicity.

> **DID YOU KNOW?**   Acetylcysteine (Mucomyst) is also used to thin the thick mucus secretions associated with cystic fibrosis.

elcatonin: Given intrathecally for severe pain.

flupirtine: Investigational nonnarcotic analgesic.

misoprostol (Cytotec):   Given to patients on long-term aspirin or NSAIDs to prevent the common side effect of stomach ulcer. Aspirin and NSAIDs inhibit the formation of prostaglandins that cause pain and inflammation. However, prostaglandins also normally act to protect the integrity of the stomach lining. Misoprostol is a synthetic prostaglandin that protects the stomach when natural prostaglandin is inhibited by taking aspirin or NSAIDs.

ziconotide: Investigational drug used to treat intractable pain.

REVIEW QUESTIONS

1. Describe the four therapeutic effects of aspirin.
2. Describe the two therapeutic effects of acetaminophen.
3. What are three advantages and one disadvantage of nonnarcotic analgesics compared to narcotic analgesics.
4. What is the therapeutic action of buffered aspirin?
5. Explain why nonnarcotic and narcotic analgesic drugs are often given in combination with each other.
6. Describe how narcotic addiction can be treated with drugs.
7. Name three categories of drugs used to treat migraine headaches and give an example of a drug in each category.
8. To what category of drugs does each of these drugs belong?
   acetylcysteine (Mucomyst)
   Cama
   diclofenac (Cataflam, Voltaren, Voltaren-XR)
   Fiorinal
   meperidine (Demerol)
   methadone (Dolophine)
   nabumetone (Relafen)
   oxaprozin (Daypro)
   Roxicet
9. Define these abbreviations: *NSAIDs, ASA.*

SPELLING TIPS

Ansaid versus NSAID (sound-alikes).
MS Contin   Unusual double capital.
OxyContin, OxyFast, OxyIR   Unusual internal capitalization.

ReVia   Unusual internal capitalization.

Roxanol with an *a*, but Roxicodone with an *i*.

Vioxx   Unusual for two *x*'s.

ZORprin   Unusual internal capitalization.

GET CONNECTED

Multimedia Extension Activities

   www.prenhall.com/turley

Use the above address to access the free, interactive Companion Website created for this textbook. Included in the features of this site are drug updates and additional chapter-specific exercises for further practice.

27

Anti-Infective Drugs

CHAPTER CONTENTS

Sulfonamide anti-infective drugs
Penicillin antibiotic drugs
Cephalosporin antibiotic drugs
Aminoglycoside antibiotic drugs
Tetracycline antibiotic drugs
Carbapenem antibiotic drugs
Monobactam antibiotic drugs
Quinolone antibiotic drugs
Fluoroquinolone antibiotic drugs
Macrolide antibiotic drugs
Miscellaneous anti-infective drugs
Review questions
Spelling tips

LEARNING OBJECTIVES

After studying this chapter, you should be able to do the following:

1. Name several categories of anti-infective drugs.
2. Describe the therapeutic action of sulfonamides, penicillins, cephalosporins, aminoglycosides, tetracyclines, and other antibiotics.
3. Given the generic and trade name of an anti-infective drug, identify what drug category it belongs to and what disease it is used to treat.
4. Given an anti-infective drug category, name several generic and trade name drugs in that category.
5. Identify the Historical Notes or Did You Know? section in this chapter that you found most interesting.

Systemic anti-infective drugs are used to treat infections in all the body systems: the eyes, brain, ears, nose, heart, lungs, abdominal organs, and so forth. Anti-infective drugs include sulfonamides as well as all groups of antibiotics (penicillins, cephalosporins, aminoglycosides, tetracyclines, etc.). These drugs are effective against gram-positive and gram-negative bacteria to varying degrees. Those antibiotics that are effective against both gram-positive and gram-negative bacteria are known as *broad-spectrum antibiotics*. Anti-infective drugs and antibiotics are not effective against viruses, yeasts, or fungi.

SULFONAMIDE ANTI-INFECTIVE DRUGS

These anti-infective drugs are not classified as antibiotics, but they do inhibit the growth of bacteria. Some bacteria must manufacture folic acid because it is essential to their metabolism. Sulfonamides interfere with this process and cause these bacteria to die. Human cells (as well as some bacteria) that can utilize folic acid from outside the cell are not affected by sulfonamide drugs. Sulfonamides are effective against many gram-negative and gram-positive bacteria. Sulfonamides are often called *sulfa drugs*.

sulfadiazine
sulfamethoxazole (Gantanol)
sulfisoxazole (Gantrisin Pediatric)

DID YOU KNOW?   The sulfa drug sulfasalazine (Azulfidine) is used for its anti-inflammatory effect (not as an anti-infective drug) to treat ulcerative colitis, Crohn's disease, and rheumatoid arthritis.

HISTORICAL NOTES: In 1934, a German researcher was screening chemicals for possible medicinal use. A red dye used to color cloth was tested. It seemed to cure streptococcal infections in mice. The researcher's own daughter was dying of streptococcal septicemia from pricking her finger. In desperation, he injected her with the dye and she recovered. The red dye was converted in the body into the anti-infective drug sulfanilamide. For the discovery of the first anti-infective drug, he won the Nobel Prize.

PENICILLIN ANTIBIOTIC DRUGS

The penicillins comprise a group of antibiotics that can kill bacteria. This group of drugs includes both natural and semisynthetic drugs that share the common molecular structure of a **beta-lactam ring** (see Figure 27–1). All penicillins interfere with the structure of the cell wall that surrounds each bacterium, causing disruption of the intracellular contents and cell death. Human cells have a cell membrane but no cell wall and so are not adversely affected by penicillin drugs.

amoxicillin (Amoxil, Trimox, Wymox)
ampicillin (Principen, Totacillin)
carbenicillin (Geocillin)
cloxacillin (Cloxapen)
dicloxacillin (Dycill, Dynapen, Pathocil)
nafcillin (Unipen)
oxacillin
penicillin G (Pfizerpen)
penicillin G benzathine (Bicillin L-A, Permapen)
penicillin G procaine (Wycillin)
penicillin V (Beepen-VK, Penicillin VK, Pen-Vee K, Veetids)
piperacillin (Pipracil)
ticarcillin (Ticar)

The various drugs in the penicillin group differ among themselves in the following ways:

- Inactivated by gastric acid (only penicillin G).
- Inactivated by **penicillinase** (an enzyme produced by penicillin-resistant bacteria). This enzyme is also known as **beta lactamase** because it inactivates penicillins by breaking their chemical structure at the site of the beta-lactam ring. All of the penicillins are inactivated by penicillinase except methicillin, nafcillin, oxacillin, cloxacillin, dicloxacillin, Augmentin, Timentin, Unasyn, and Zosyn. Penicillins inactivated by penicillinase are combined with a beta-lactamase inhibitor drug so that they are effective against penicillin-resistant bacteria.
- Little antibiotic activity against gram-negative bacteria. Extended spectrum penicillins such as carbenicillin, ticarcillin, mezlocillin, and piperacillin are active against gram-negative bacteria as well as gram-positive bacteria like other penicillins.

Note: The ending *-cillin* is common to generic penicillins.

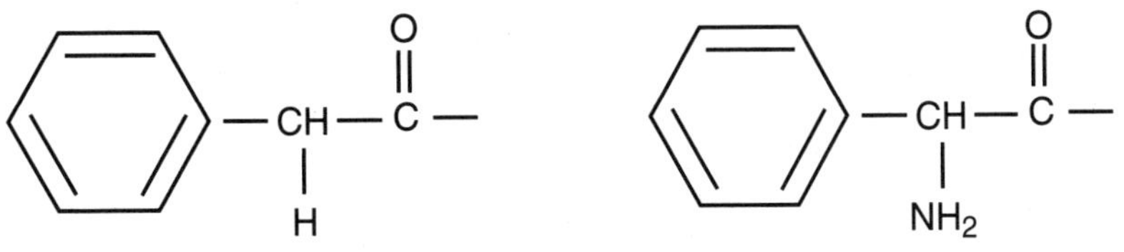

penicillin G   ampicillin

Figure 27–1 The chemical structures of penicillin G and ampicillin, showing the beta-lactam ring that is common to all drugs in the penicillin class of antibiotics.

HISTORICAL NOTES: In 1928, the Scottish bacteriologist, Alexander Fleming, concluded experiments in which he was looking for drugs that would inhibit the growth of staphylococcus. He left for a vacation and instructed an assistant to wash the culture plates that were soaking in the sink. When Fleming returned from vacation, the plates had not been washed. One culture plate had remained above the water and on it had grown a blue-green mold with a ring around it where the staphylococcus had been killed. Fleming identified this mold as *Penicillium notatum*; however, he was unable to extract a drug from this. (The mold itself contained only 1 part penicillin per 2 million parts mold.) He wrote a paper about his findings, which remained generally unknown to the scientific world.

Work halted on penicillin until the 1940s. In the meantime, the sulfonamide anti-infective drugs were discovered. During World War II, two researchers in England who were working with penicillin were afraid all of the supply would be destroyed in the bombing of London. Therefore, they smeared some of the mold inside their coat jackets and brought penicillin to the United States to be produced.

A 43-year-old policeman was the first person to be injected with penicillin. He was dying of septicemia, which had begun as an abscess when he scratched his face on a rosebush. Penicillin was in such short supply that his urine was saved each day and the penicillin in it was extracted to provide the next day's dose. He was given the world's entire supply of penicillin. He responded well to the treatment, but on the fifth day the supply of penicillin ran out and he relapsed and died.

Because *Penicillium notatum* only grew on the surface of a culture medium, it had to be produced in many shallow bottles and the yield was very small. Later, researchers found the strain *Penicillium chrysogenum* on a moldy cantaloupe in Peoria, Illinois. It was approximately 20 times more potent than the original mold and could be grown in larger quantities (see Figure 27–2).

The first small amounts of commercially produced penicillin became available in 1942. By the end of that year, 100 patients had been treated with it.

On Wednesday, July 26, 1943, the *Pittsburgh Press* ran an article entitled, "Penicillin Drug Hailed as Boon to Mankind." The article stated:

> Penicillin takes its place along side the sulfonamides as a deadly enemy of infection and disease. When the United States entered the war in December of 1941, the government took immediate control of the supplies and production of penicillin to date, and advised the Committee on Medical Research to distribute the drug carefully for medical investigation. The details of this investigation are still secret, [but] enormous interest has been stimulated by the discovery of the drug Penicillin [sic] (pronounced peni sillin), which provides an example of how war may affect medicine.

By 1945, *penicillin* had become a household word, and the term *antibiotic* was coined as well.

CEPHALOSPORIN ANTIBIOTIC DRUGS

The cephalosporins are a group of antibiotics that can kill bacteria. They interfere with the structure of the cell wall that surrounds each bacterium, causing disruption of the intracellular contents and cell death. This group of antibiotics is further divided into first-,

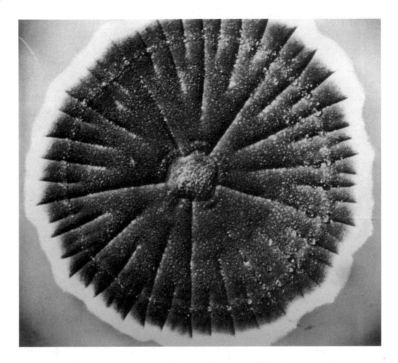

Figure 27–2   A culture of *Penicillium* mold. *Photo reprinted courtesy of Pfizer Inc, New York.*

second-, and third-generation cephalosporins. This designation has nothing to do with when these antibiotics were discovered or first marketed, but instead divides them according to their therapeutic antibiotic properties. First-generation cephalosporins are generally inactivated by bacteria that produce penicillinase, whereas third-generation cephalosporins show the greatest activity against resistant bacteria. In addition, third-generation cephalosporins show greater activity against gram-negative bacteria in general; however, the cost of these drugs is greater. Cephalosporins and penicillins are structurally similar, and patients who are allergic to penicillin may have an allergic reaction if given cephalosporin antibiotics.

First-generation Cephalosporins

cefadroxil (Duricef)
cefazolin (Ancef, Kefzol, Zolicef)
cephalexin (Biocef, Keflex, Keftab)
cephapirin (Cefadyl)
cephradine (Velosef)

Second-generation Cephalosporins

cefaclor (Ceclor, Ceclor CD, Ceclor Pulvules)
cefamandole (Mandol)
cefditoren (Spectracef)

cefmetazole (Zefazone)

cefonicid (Monocid)

cefotetan (Cefotan)

cefoxitin (Mefoxin)

cefprozil (Cefzil)

cefuroxime (Ceftin, Kefurox, Zinacef)

loracarbef (Lorabid)

Third-generation Cephalosporins

cefdinir (Omnicef)

cefepime (Maxipime)

cefixime (Suprax)

cefoperazone (Cefobid)

cefotaxime (Claforan)

cefpodoxime (Vantin)

ceftazidime (Ceptaz, Fortaz, Tazicef, Tazidime)

ceftibuten (Cedax)

ceftizoxime (Cefizox)

ceftriaxone (Rocephin)

Note: Generic antibiotics beginning with *cefa-* or *cepha-* commonly belong to the cephalosporin group.

DID YOU KNOW?   The fungus *Cephalosporium*, from which the first cephalosporins were produced, was discovered in a sewer outlet near Sardinia (an island off the coast of Italy) in 1948.

AMINOGLYCOSIDE ANTIBIOTIC DRUGS

The aminoglycosides comprise a group of antibiotics that kill bacteria by interfering with the synthesis of protein in the bacterial wall. This disrupts the intracellular contents and causes cell death. Aminoglycosides are primarily effective against gram-negative bacteria. Some aminoglycosides (kanamycin, neomycin) are given orally as a bowel prep to inhibit intestinal bacteria prior to surgery because they are not absorbed from the intestine into the bloodstream.

amikacin (Amikin)

gentamicin (Garamycin)

kanamycin (Kantrex)

neomycin

netilmicin (Netromycin)

paromomycin (Humatin)

tobramycin (Nebcin, Nebcin Pediatric, TOBI)

All aminoglycoside antibiotics have the potential to cause toxic effects to the auditory nerve (**ototoxicity**) and kidneys (**nephrotoxicity**). Patients on aminoglycosides are carefully monitored with hearing tests and blood tests to avoid these toxicities.

TETRACYCLINE ANTIBIOTIC DRUGS

This group of antibiotics inhibits the growth of bacteria. Tetracyclines inhibit protein synthesis in the cell wall of bacteria. Tetracyclines are effective against both gram-positive and gram-negative bacteria.

demeclocycline (Declomycin)

doxycycline (Doryx, Vibramycin, Vibramycin IV, Vibra-Tabs)

minocycline (Dynacin, Minocin, Minocin IV, Vectrin)

oxytetracycline (Terramycin IM)

tetracycline (Panmycin, Sumycin, Sumycin 250, Sumycin 500, Tetracyn, Tetracyn 500, Tetralan)

Note: The ending *-cycline* is common to generic tetracycline antibiotics.

DID YOU KNOW?   Tetracyclines can cause permanent discoloration of the teeth; therefore, they are not prescribed for pregnant women (to protect the fetus's developing teeth) or for children under age 8.

CARBAPENEM ANTIBIOTIC DRUGS

This group of antibiotics kills bacteria by interfering with the structure of the cell wall. These drugs are effective against most gram-negative and gram-positive bacteria.

ertapenem (Invanz)

meropenem (Merrem IV)

MONOBACTAM ANTIBIOTIC DRUGS

This group of antibiotics kills bacteria by interfering with the structure of the cell wall. This drug is effective against gram-negative bacteria.

aztreonam (Azactam)

QUINOLONE ANTIBIOTIC DRUGS

This group of drugs inhibits DNA replication in bacterial cells. These drugs are effective against gram-negative bacteria.

cinoxacin (Cinobac)
nalidixic acid (NegGram)

FLUOROQUINOLONE ANTIBIOTIC DRUGS

This group of antibiotics kills bacteria by interfering with an enzyme the bacteria need to synthesize their DNA. These drugs are effective against gram-negative and gram-positive bacteria.

ciprofloxacin (Cipro, Cipro I.V.)
enoxacin (Penetrex)
gatifloxacin (Tequin)
levofloxacin (Levaquin)
lomefloxacin (Maxaquin)
moxifloxacin (Avelox)
norfloxacin (Noroxin)
ofloxacin (Floxin)
sparfloxacin (Zagam)
trovafloxacin (Trovan)

DID YOU KNOW? Ciprofloxacin (Cipro) was the first drug used to treat cutaneous and inhaled anthrax during the 2001 bioterrorism attack in the United States. Many people demanded that their physicians give them Cipro prophylactically. Because of the sudden widespread demand, the Centers for Disease Control (CDC) asked physicians to first prescribe doxycycline, an older antibiotic with a more narrow spectrum of antibacterial action. Then, if doxycycline was ineffective, the second line of treatment would be the newer antibiotic Cipro with its broader spectrum of antibacterial action. Doxycycline (Doryx, Vibramycin, Vibramycin IV, Vibra-Tabs) and penicillin G procaine (Wycillin) are approved for the treatment of cutaneous and inhaled anthrax infections.

MACROLIDE ANTIBIOTIC DRUGS

This group of antibiotics inhibits or kills bacteria by interfering with RNA and protein synthesis within the bacteria. These drugs are effective against most gram-negative and gram-positive bacteria. Note: Troleandomycin is only effective against steptococcal infections.

azithromycin (Zithromax)

clarithromycin (Biaxin, Biaxin XL)

dirithromycin (Dynabac)

erythromycin (E.E.S. 200, E.E.S. 400, E-Mycin, ERYC, EryPed, EryPed 200, EryPed 400, Ery-Tab, Erythrocin, Ilotycin, PCE Dispertab)

troleandomycin (Tao)

DID YOU KNOW? Azithromycin, erythromycin, and dirithromycin are used to treat Legionnaire's disease. Azithromycin, clarithromycin, and gentamicin are used to treat *Mycobacterium avium-intracellulare* infection in AIDS patients.

OTHER ANTIBIOTIC DRUGS

bacitracin

chloramphenicol (Chloromycetin)

clindamycin (Cleocin, Cleocin Pediatric)

colistimethate (Coly-Mycin M)

furazolidone (Furoxone)

iodoquinol (Yodoxin)

lincomycin (Lincocin)

linezolid (Zyvox)

methenamine (Hiprex, Urex)

nitrofurantoin (Furadantin, Macrobid, Macrodantin)

polymyxin B

spectinomycin (Trobicin)

telithromycin (Ketek)

vancomycin (Vancocin, Vancoled)

Methicillin-resistant *Staphylococcus aureus* (MRSA) (pronounced "MEHR-sah") is a serious problem in hospitals and nursing homes. This resistant bacteria is treated with linezolid or vancomycin.

FOCUS ON HEALTHCARE ISSUES: *Staphylococcus aureus* infections can be very serious. For years, this bacterium could be killed by penicillin drugs. Then it became resistant to penicillins and only vancomycin was effective against it. In 1996, the first case of vancomycin-resistant staphylococcal infection was reported in Japan, and a second case was reported in the United States in 1997. Whenever antibiotics are used indiscriminately, mildly resistant bacteria survive and breed, creating increasingly resistant bacteria. Pharmaceutical companies are racing to create new antibiotics that can replace vancomycin.

Each year, nearly 2 million Americans acquire an infection while they are in the hospital, and about 14,000 die because the infections were caused by antibiotic-resistant bacteria.

A 2001 report found that livestock are fed approximately 25 million pounds of antibiotics each year to prevent disease and promote growth. Overuse of antibiotics gives rise to resistant strains of bacteria in meat that can then infect people who eat the meat. In addition, patients take about 3 million pounds of antibiotics each year. Antibiotics are the fourth most commonly prescribed drug, and the CDC estimates that 50% of all prescriptions for antibiotics are not necessary.

Christine Gorman, "Germ Warfare," *Time*, September 2, 1997, p. 65.

COMBINATION ANTI-INFECTIVE DRUGS

Penicillin antibiotics that are inactivated by penicillinase are combined with clavulanic acid, sulbactam, or tazobactam, which can inactivate penicillinase. These drugs are used to treat infections caused by penicillin-resistant bacteria.

Augmentin, Augmentin ES-600 (amoxicillin, clavulanic acid)
Timentin (ticarcillin, clavulanic acid)
Unasyn (ampicillin, sulbactam)
Zosyn (piperacillin, tazobactam)

These drugs combine an antibiotic with a sulfonamide drug.

Bactrim (trimethoprim, sulfamethoxazole)
Pediazole (erythromycin, sulfisoxazole)
Septra, Septra DS, Septra IV (trimethoprim, sulfamethoxazole)

DID YOU KNOW?   Bactrim and Septra are also used to treat *Pneumocystis carinii* infection in AIDS patients.

This drug combines a carbapenem antibiotic with a drug that inhibits an enzyme in the kidneys that normally breaks down the carbapenem.

Primaxin I.M., Primaxin I.V. (imipenem, cilastatin)

This drug combines two antibiotics that do not belong to any particular class of antibiotics and are not used individually as antibiotic drugs but are chemically related to each other.

Synercid (dalfopristin, quinupristin)

TOPICAL ANTIBIOTIC DRUGS

See Chapter 11, "Dermatologic Drugs."

DRUGS USED TO TREAT URINARY TRACT INFECTIONS

See Chapter 12, "Urinary Tract Drugs."

DRUGS USED TO TREAT TUBERCULOSIS

See Chapter 18, "Pulmonary Drugs."

DRUGS USED TO TREAT SEXUALLY TRANSMITTED DISEASES

See Chapter 23, "Obstetric/Gynecologic Drugs."

DRUGS USED TO TREAT AIDS AND VIRAL INFECTIONS

See Chapter 28, "AIDS Drugs and Antiviral Drugs."

DRUGS USED TO TREAT FUNGAL AND YEAST INFECTIONS

See Chapter 29, "Antifungal Drugs."

MISCELLANEOUS ANTI-INFECTIVE DRUGS

anthrax vaccine: During the anthrax pubic health scare of 2001, it became known that there was not enough anthrax vaccine to vaccinate the civilian population of the United States against anthrax. Only one drug company manufactures anthrax vaccine, and it sells its supplies to the military. For civilians, anthrax exposure is treated after the fact with the antibiotics ciprofloxacin or doxycyline.

chloroquine (Aralen):   Antiprotozoal drug used to treat intestinal amebiasis.

drotrecogin alfa (Xigris):   Used to treat severe sepsis.

nebacumab (Centoxin):   Used to treat gram-negative bacteremia and shock.

probenecid: Used to prolong the therapeutic blood levels of ampicillin and cephalosporins by inhibiting their excretion into the urine.

teicoplanin (Targocid):   Investigational antibiotic similar to vancomycin.

trospectomycin (Spexil):   Investigational antibiotic similar to spectinomycin.

REVIEW QUESTIONS

1. Describe how sulfonamides exert their therapeutic effect.
2. Describe how some penicillin-resistant bacteria inactivate penicillin.
3. Name at least four different classes of antibiotics.
4. Why are tetracycline antibiotics not given to pregnant women or to children under 8 years of age?
5. What are two potentially toxic effects of aminoglycosides?
6. The ending *-cycline* is common to what group of antibiotics?
7. What are *broad spectrum antibiotics*? What is *penicillinase*?
8. What is the consequence of overprescription of antibiotics and the use of antibiotics in animal feed?
9. To what category of drugs does each of these drugs belong?
   amoxicillin (Amoxil, Trimox, Wymox)
   Augmentin, Augmentin ES-600
   azithromycin (Zithromax)
   Bactrim
   cefaclor (Ceclor, Ceclor CD, Ceclor Pulvules)
   cefixime (Suprax)
   ciprofloxacin (Cipro, Cipro IV)
   doxycycline (Doryx, Vibramycin, Vibramycin IV, Vibra-Tabs)
   gatifloxacin (Tequin)

SPELLING TIPS

sulfisoxazole   All other generic sulfa drugs begin with *sulfa-*.

cephalosporins   This group of drugs may start with *ceph-* (as does *cephalosporin*) or with *cef-*.

cephalosporins   There are many sound-alike drugs in this class (e.g., cefixime versus cefoxitin or cefotaxime versus ceftizoxime).

aminoglycosides   This group of drugs may end with *-micin* or with *-mycin*.

Coly-Mycin M   Unusual in that the *-mycin* ending is usually part of the drug name, not separated by a hyphen.

Pfizerpen   Drug is named for the manufacturer, Pfizer.

TOBI   Unusual for all capital letters.

GET CONNECTED

Multimedia Extension Activities

 www.prenhall.com/turley

Use the above address to access the free, interactive Companion Website created for this textbook. Included in the features of this site are drug updates and additional chapter-specific exercises for further practice.

28

AIDS Drugs and Antiviral Drugs

CHAPTER CONTENTS

Drugs used to treat AIDS
Drugs used to treat AIDS wasting syndrome
Drugs used to treat AIDS-related diarrhea
Drugs used to treat *Pneumocystis carinii* pneumonia (PCP)
Drugs used to treat *Mycobacterium avium-intracellulare* complex (MAC) infection
Drugs used to treat other viral infections
Miscellaneous AIDS drugs and antiviral drugs
Review questions
Spelling tips

LEARNING OBJECTIVES

After studying this chapter, you should be able to do the following:

1. Name several categories of antiviral drugs.
2. Describe the therapeutic effect of drugs used to treat AIDS.
3. Given the generic and trade name of an antiviral drug, identify what drug category it belongs to or what disease it is used to treat.
4. Given an antiviral drug category, give several examples of drugs in that category.
5. Identify the Historical Notes or Did You Know? section of this chapter that you found most interesting.

DRUGS USED TO TREAT AIDS

Acquired immunodeficiency syndrome (AIDS) is an almost-universally fatal disease in which the human immunodeficiency virus (HIV) attaches to CD4 receptors on helper T lymphocytes (a specific type of white blood cell in the immune system) and directs the lymphocyte to produce more HIV using the lymphocyte's own DNA. Once this is accomplished, the WBC is destroyed and newly produced viruses from within it are released into the bloodstream to infect more helper T lymphocytes and further weaken the immune system. Although the body does produce antibodies against HIV, the immune system is never able to control or eradicate the virus.

HIV is transmitted through contact with an infected individual, contaminated blood, or used needles, or when an infected mother transmits the virus to the fetus or a breastfeeding infant.

A person infected with HIV usually remains without symptoms for 4 to 5 years, but with the progressive decrease in the number of T lymphocytes, the symptoms of AIDS eventually appear. A person with an HIV infection is also unable to defend against malignancies such as Kaposi's sarcoma and against infections from opportunistic organisms such as *Pneumocystis carinii*, herpes simplex virus, and *Candida albicans*, to name a few. Because these pathogens produce infection most often in patients whose immune systems are already compromised, they are termed *opportunistic infections.*

The dividing line between a diagnosis of HIV infection and a diagnosis of AIDS is determined by the presence or absence of the following indicators:

CD4 lymphocytes of <200 cells/mm^3

The presence of any of the following opportunistic infections/diseases:

candidiasis, coccidioidomycosis, CMV retinitis, histoplasmosis, toxoplasmosis, *Salmonella* septicemia, *Mycobacterium avium-intracellulare* infection, *Pneumocystis carinii* pneumonia, Kaposi's sarcoma, Burkitt's lymphoma, or AIDS wasting syndrome.

Drug therapy for AIDS currently focuses on the use of several types of drugs to suppress the virus as well as drugs to treat the secondary opportunistic illnesses mentioned earlier. Drugs used to treat HIV inhibit the growth of this retrovirus but are unable to kill it. They are, however, able to decrease the viral load and delay the onset of symptoms of AIDS and clinical complications from opportunistic infections. The goal of drug therapy is to suppress HIV replication as much as possible for as long as possible.

Nucleoside and Nucleotide Reverse Transcriptase Inhibitor Drugs for HIV/AIDS

These drugs inhibit reverse transcriptase, an enzyme needed to reproduce viral DNA. They also become part of the virus DNA chain, which causes it to break.

abacavir (Ziagen)
adefovir dipivoxil
didanosine (ddI) (Videx, Videx EC)
emtricitabine (FTC) (Coviracil)
lamivudine (3TC) (Epivir)
stavudine (d4T) (Zerit)
tenofovir (Viread)
zalcitabine (ddC) (Hivid)
zidovudine (AZT) (Aztec, Retrovir)

> **DID YOU KNOW?** Tenofovir (Viread) is the first in a new class of AIDS drugs known as *nucleotide reverse transcriptase inhibitors*. Nucleotide reverse transcriptase inhibitors are very much like nucleoside reverse transcriptase inhibitors except that they are chemically preactivated and can act more quickly in the body.

Nonnucleoside Reverse Transcriptase Inhibitor Drugs for HIV/AIDS

These drugs bind directly to reverse transcriptase, an enzyme needed to reproduce viral DNA, and disrupt its activity.

> delavirdine (Rescriptor)
> efavirenz (Sustiva)
> nevirapine (Viramune)

Protease Inhibitor Drugs for HIV/AIDS

These drugs inhibit the enzyme protease, and this prevents certain proteins in the virus from being broken down, an important last step that must happen for the virus to reproduce. The virus fails to reproduce and so is unable to infect other lymphocytes.

> amprenavir (Agenerase)
> indinavir (Crixivan)
> nelfinavir (Viracept)
> ritonavir (Novir)
> saquinavir (Fortovase, Invirase)

Combination Drugs for HIV/AIDS

This drug combines two protease inhibitor drugs. One of these drugs (lopinavir) is not available as an individual drug.

> Kaletra (lopinavir, ritonavir)

This drug combines two or three nucleoside reverse transcriptase inhibitor drugs.

> Combivir (lamivudine/zidovudine)
> Scriptene (didanosine, zidovudine)
> Trizivir (abacavir, lamivudine, zidovudine)

Other Drugs for HIV/AIDS

> aldesleukin (Proleukin)
> Ampligen
> atevirdine mesylate
> AZDU
> calanolide A

carbovir

CD4 human immunoglobulin

cytolin

dextran sulfate

diethyldithiocarbamate (Imuthiol)

foscarnet (Foscavir)

Gamimune N immunoglobulin

HIV immunoglobulin (Hivig)

hydroxyurea (Hydrea, Mylocel)

immune globulin (Gamimune N)

Immupath

interferon alfa-n3 (Alferon LDO)

interferon beta-1a (Avonex, Rebif)

interferon beta-1b (Betaseron)

interleukin-10 (Tenovil)

Lidakol

Multikine

probucol (Panavir)

recombinant human CD4 (Receptin)

soluble T4

thymopentin (Timunox)

trichosanthin

tumor necrosis factor

VaxSyn HIV-1

Zintevir

Originally, HIV-positive patients were not begun on drug therapy until they started to exhibit symptoms. Later, the standard treatment was to treat patients with one drug as soon as a diagnosis of HIV was made. However, the first study of combined therapy using indinavir, zidovudine, and lamivudine showed that these drugs increased the CD4 cell count so significantly that combination therapy became the standard treatment.

Current drug therapy uses two or three antiviral drugs in combination; this is more effective than one drug and also decreases the risk of developing resistant strains of HIV.

DID YOU KNOW?   The first antiretroviral drug, zidovudine, is no longer given by itself; it loses its effectiveness against HIV over time.

HISTORICAL NOTES: Azidothymidine (AZT, zidovudine, Retrovir) was originally synthesized in 1974. It was tested as a treatment for cancer but was not effective. Other uses for it were not investigated and it was simply "shelved."

In 1984, although there were only 3,000 reported cases of AIDS in the United States, researchers at the National Cancer Institute, including the codiscoverer of the AIDS virus, Dr. Robert Gallo, approached Burroughs Wellcome pharmaceutical company to develop a drug to treat AIDS. Although other pharmaceutical companies were also approached, their concern about working with the deadly virus as well as the apparently limited use for the drug at that time resulted in an unenthusiastic response. Burroughs Wellcome, however, responded to the request and tested many different drugs, one of which was AZT.

In 1986, clinical testing of AZT was begun using a double-blind study in which severely ill AIDS patients were divided into two groups: one group received AZT while the control group received a placebo. Shortly after the study was begun, it was ended when it was found that those in the control group had a 40% mortality rate while those receiving AZT had only a 6% mortality rate. In March 1988, just four months after a new drug application was filed, the FDA approved AZT.

Burroughs Wellcome chose the generic name zidovudine for this new AIDS drug and the trade name Retrovir. The trade name refers to the fact that the AIDS virus belongs to a class of viruses known as *retroviruses*.

HIV/AIDS Vaccine

In 1988, the National Institutes of Health began efforts to develop an AIDS vaccine. This vaccine, which consists of purified protein derived from genetic material from the AIDS virus, is reproduced using recombinant DNA technology. The purpose of the vaccine is to stimulate the body to produce antibodies against HIV. Because the vaccine only contains pieces of the virus, it cannot cause AIDS. However, because the virus continues to mutate, no vaccine has yet been approved by the FDA. Several pharmaceutical companies have AIDS vaccines undergoing clinical testing.

AIDSVAX
Genevax-HIV
Remune

DRUGS USED TO TREAT AIDS WASTING SYNDROME

These drugs stimulate the appetite of AIDS patients.

Cachexon
cyproheptadine (Periactin)
dihydrotestosterone (Androgel-DHT)
dronabinol (Marinol)
marijuana
megestrol (Megace)
oxandrolone (Oxandrin)
sermorelin (Geref)

somatropin (BioTropin, Serostim)

testosterone (AndroGel, Theraderm Testosterone Transdermal System)

thalidomide (Synovir, Thalomid)

HISTORICAL NOTE: In the late 1950s, the drug thalidomide was developed in West Germany and used extensively to treat morning sickness in women early in pregnancy. The FDA refused to approve it for use in the United States without further studies. Before these additional studies by the manufacturer could be completed, evidence against the safety of the drug began to accumulate. Over 8,000 babies in Europe were born with deformed limbs ("seal limbs" or phocomelia). In 1997, thalidomide was discovered to be useful in treating AIDS, cancer, and leprosy. The potential side effects are so great that it is only being considered a viable treatment option because all of these are life-threatening diseases. Still, the FDA regulates the use of thalidomide in two ways: (1) by limiting the number of physicians who can prescribe it and (2) by requiring women taking the drug not to have sex or to use two forms of birth control if they have sex.

DRUGS USED TO TREAT AIDS-RELATED DIARRHEA

These drugs slow intestinal transit time and are used to treat AIDS-related diarrhea.

bovine colostrum

lactobin

letrazuril

octreotide (Sandostatin, Sandostatin LAR Depot)

SYNSORB Cd

DRUGS USED TO TREAT PNEUMOCYSTIS CARINII PNEUMONIA (PCP)

Pneumocystis carinii pneumonia (PCP) is the most common serious complication in AIDS patients and eventually affects about three-fourths of all AIDS patients. *Pneumocystis carinii* is a protozoan that seldom causes symptoms in normal individuals.

atovaquone (Mepron)

clindamycin (Cleocin)

dapsone

eflornithine (Ornidyl)

pentamidine (NebuPent, Pentam 300, Pneumopent)

piritrexim

primaquine

trimetrexate (NeuTrexin)

Combination Drugs for Pneumocystis carinii Pneumonia

Bactrim (trimethoprim, sulfamethoxazole)

Septra (trimethoprim, sulfamethoxazole)

DRUGS USED TO TREAT MYCOBACTERIUM AVIUM-INTRACELLULARE COMPLEX (MAC) INFECTION

Mycobacterium avium-intracellulare complex (MAC) infection is a common late-stage complication of AIDS.

aminosidine (Gabbromicina)

clarithromycin (Biaxin, Biaxin XL)

gentamicin liposomal (Maitec)

piritrexim

rifabutin (Mycobutin)

rifalazil

rifapentine (Priftin)

streptomycin

DRUGS USED TO TREAT KAPOSI'S SARCOMA

See Chapter 30, "Chemotherapy Drugs."

DRUGS USED TO TREAT OTHER VIRAL INFECTIONS

Other antiviral drugs act systemically to prevent or treat severe viral infections.

Drugs for Cytomegalovirus (CMV) Infections and Retinitis

These antiviral drugs are effective against cytomegalovirus (CMV) retinitis. These drugs are administered by intraocular injection or intraocular implant.

benzimidavir

fomivirsen (Vitravene)

foscarnet (Foscavir)

ganciclovir (Vitrasert)

These antiviral drugs are given systemically to treat CMV retinitis.

Centovir

cidofovir (Vistide)

foscarnet (Foscavir)

ganciclovir (Cytovene)

valganciclovir (Cymeval, Valcyte)

For antiviral drugs that act topically to treat cytomegalovirus, see Chapter 20, "Ophthalmic Drugs."

Drugs for Herpes Simplex Infections

These oral drugs act systemically to treat both type 1 and type 2 herpes simplex virus infections in AIDS patients. For topical drugs used to treat herpes simplex type 1 lesions (cold sores), see Chapter 11, "Dermatologic Drugs." For topical drugs used to treat herpes simplex type 2 lesions (genital herpes), see Chapter 23, "Obstetric/Gynecologic Drugs."

acyclovir (Zovirax)

cidofovir (Forvade)

famciclovir (Famvir)

foscarnet (Foscavir)

interferon alfa-2a (Roferon-A)

interferon beta-1a (Avonex)

interferon beta-1b (Betaseron)

valacyclovir (Valtrex)

Drugs for Herpes Zoster Infections

Herpes zoster virus infections, also known as *shingles*, are due to a reemergence of the same virus that first caused chickenpox in the patient. Drugs used to treat herpes zoster infections interfere with DNA synthesis to keep the virus from reproducing.

acyclovir (Zovirax)

famciclovir (Famvir)

sorivudine (Bravavir)

valacyclovir (Valtrex)

Topical drugs used to treat herpes zoster infections are discussed in Chapter 11, "Dermatologic Drugs."

Drugs for Influenza A Virus Infection

amantadine (Symmetrel)

rimantadine (Flumadine)

oseltamivir (Tamiflu)

zanamivir (Relenza)

Drugs to Prevent Influenza A Virus Infection

influenza virus vaccine ("flu shot") (FluShield, Fluvirin, Fluzone)

oseltamivir (Tamiflu)

> **DID YOU KNOW?** Flu shots are given prophylactically to prevent influenza. They use either the whole virus, a part of the virus, or a surface antigen from the virus to provoke the body's immune response and create temporary immunity. Annual revaccination is necessary to provide protection against the most current strains of the influenza A virus.

Drugs Used to Treat Respiratory Syncytial Virus (RSV) Infection

palivizumab (Synagis)
respiratory syncytial virus immunoglobulin (Hypermune RSV, RespiGam)
ribavirin (Virazole)

MISCELLANEOUS AIDS DRUGS AND ANTIVIRAL DRUGS

amphotericin B (AmBisome): Used to treat cryptococcal meningitis in AIDS patients.

bovine immunoglobulin (Immuno-C, Sporidin-G): Cow immunoglobulin used to treat *Cryptosporidium parvum* GI tract infection in AIDS patients.

clindamycin (Cleocin): Used to treat CNS toxoplasmosis in AIDS patients.

CytoGam: Used to prevent CMV infection in organ transplant patients.

epoetin alfa (Epogen, Procrit): Erythropoietin-type drug that stimulates RBC production in AIDS patients.

filgrastim (Neupogen): Granulocyte colony-stimulating factor used to treat severe neutropenia in AIDS patients.

fluconazole (Diflucan): Used to treat cryptococcal meningitis in AIDS patients.

lactic acid (Aphthaid): Used to treat aphthous stomatitis in AIDS patients.

levocarnitine (Carnitor): Used to protect against toxicity from zidovudine drug therapy.

lithium (Eskalith, Eskalith CR, Lithobid): An antipsychotic drug used to treat the mania of manic-depressive disorder, lithium has the known side effect of causing leukocytosis (increased WBC count). This becomes a desirable therapeutic effect in AIDS patients who have a low WBC count because of zidovudine.

memantine: Investigational drug used to treat AIDS dementia.

molgramostim (Leucomax): Granulocyte macrophage-colony stimulating factor used to treat neutropenia in AIDS patients; used to treat neutropenia in patients taking ganciclovir.

nitazoxanide (NTZ) (Cryptaz): Used to treat *Cryptosporidium parvum* diarrhea in AIDS patients.

nystatin (Mycostatin, Mycostatin Pastilles, Nilstat): An antifungal/antiyeast drug used to treat *Candida albicans* yeast infections in the mouth/esophagus of AIDS patients. This oral infection is also known as *oral candidiasis* or *thrush*. The drug is given topically as a solution (the patient is told to "swish and swallow") or as a troche (the patient sucks on it).

piritrexim: Used to treat *Toxoplasma gondii* in AIDS patients.

poloxamer 331 (Protox):   Used to treat toxoplasmosis in AIDS patients.

sargramostim (Leukine):   Granulocyte macrophage colony-stimulating factor used to increase WBC count in patients receiving zidovudine.

spiramycin (Rovamycine):   Used to treat *Cryptosporidium parvum* infection in AIDS patients.

sulfadiazine: Used to treat *Toxoplasma gondii* encephalitis in AIDS patients.

Trugene test: Used to tell which AIDS drugs are no longer effective for an individual patient because the virus has undergone mutation while in that patient's body.

REVIEW QUESTIONS

1. Define these abbreviations: *AIDS, HIV, RSV, CMV*.
2. How does the HIV virus reproduce in the body?
3. Describe the therapeutic action of the various drug categories used to treat AIDS.
4. Why is an AIDS vaccine difficult to develop?
5. What two distinct and very different medical uses does the drug lithium have?
6. What is the history of the drug thalidomide?
7. What is an opportunistic infection?
8. Name three opportunistic infections that affect AIDS patients.
9. How is nystatin used to treat candidal infections in AIDS patients?
10. What is the name of the category to which each of these drugs belongs?
   amantadine (Symmetrel)
   Combivir
   didanosine (Videx, Videx EC)
   efavirenz (Sustiva)
   indinavir (Crixivan)
   octreotide (Sandostatin, Sandostatin LAR Depot)
   pentamidine (NebuPent, Pentam 300, Pneumopent)
   somatropin (BioTropin, Serostim)
   thalidomide (Synovir, Thalomid)
   zidovudine (Aztec, Retrovir)

SPELLING TIPS

Hivid   *HIV* appears in the name to show the drug's use.

Many trade name drugs for AIDS are spelled with *vir* to show they are antiviral drugs: Invirase, Viramune, Epivir, Norvir, Retrovir, Viracept, Combivir, Trizivir, Viread.

Many trade name drugs for other viral infections are spelled with *vir* to show they are antiviral drugs: Foscavir, Zovirax, Famvir, Bravavir, Virazole.

Many trade name drugs used to prevent or treat influenza are spelled with *flu:* Flumadine, Tamiflu, FluShield, Fluvirin, Fluzone.

Gamimune   Not *immune* with two *m*'s, as in *the immune system*.

FluShield   Unusual internal capitalization.

RespiGam   Unusual internal capitalization.

GET CONNECTED

Multimedia Extension Activities

 www.prenhall.com/turley

Use the above address to access the free, interactive Companion Website created for this textbook. Included in the features of this site are drug updates and additional chapter-specific exercises for further practice.

29

Antifungal Drugs

CHAPTER CONTENTS

Antifungal drugs
Review questions

LEARNING OBJECTIVES

After studying this chapter, you should be able to do the following:

1. Name several diseases caused by fungi.
2. Name several generic/trade name drugs used to treat fungal infections.

Fungi can cause disease topically or systemically. Fungi are related to yeasts and both these organisms are treated with many of the same drugs. Antifungal drugs act by binding to a specific receptor on the cell membrane of the fungus, changing the permeability of the membrane, and causing the cellular contents to leak out.

Topical fungal infections of the skin include ringworm, athlete's foot, and jock itch, all of which are caused by the fungus *Tinea*. Topical drugs used to treat these fungal infections are discussed in Chapter 11, "Dermatologic Drugs." A *Tinea* infection of the nails (onychomycosis) is very difficult to treat topically because the infection is embedded in the nail and nailbed. This type of topical fungal infection is often treated with oral antifungal drugs that act systemically.

> griseofulvin (Fulvicin P/G, Fulvicin U/F, Grisactin 250, Grisactin 500, Grisactin Ultra, Griseofulvin Ultramicrosize)
>
> itraconazole (Sporanox)
>
> ketoconazole (Nizoral)
>
> terbinafine (Lamisil)

Topical fungal infections can occur in the eye. The topical antifungal drugs used to treat these infections are discussed in Chapter 20, "Ophthalmic Drugs."

Topical yeast infections caused by *Candida* can occur in the mouth. The topical anti-fungal drugs used to treat these infections are discussed in Chapter 19, "Ear, Nose, and Throat (ENT) Drugs."

Severe oral infections and infections that extend into the esophagus and stomach are treated with antifungal drugs that act systemically.

fluconazole (Diflucan)

itraconazole (Sporanox)

ketoconazole (Nizoral)

Both fungi and yeasts are **opportunistic organisms** that grow most successfully when the patient's immune system is already under stress. In immunocompromised patients like those with cancer or AIDS, fungal infections can become widespread and extremely serious. Systemic infections with yeast (*Candida albicans*, candidiasis); fungi (*Aspergillus*, aspergillosis), (*Blastomyces*, blastomycosis), (*Coccidioides*, coccidioidomycosis), (*Histoplasma*, histoplasmosis); yeast-like fungi (*Cryptococcus*); and the parasitic protozoa (*Leishmania*, leishmaniasis) are treated with oral or intravenous antifungal drugs. These drugs may also be given prophylactically to prevent a fungal infection from developing in cancer patients who have had a bone marrow transplant.

amphotericin B (Abelcet, AmBisome, Amphocin, Amphotec, Fungizone Intravenous)

caspofungin (Cancidas)

fluconazole (Diflucan)

flucytosine (Ancobon)

itraconazole (Sporanox)

ketoconazole (Nizoral)

nystatin (Nyotran)

DID YOU KNOW?   The antifungal drug fluconazole (Diflucan) costs more than $4 per tablet.

Drugs used to treat vaginal yeast infections are discussed in Chapter 23, "Obstetric/Gynecologic Drugs."

REVIEW QUESTIONS

1. What is the medical name for a fungal infection of the nails?
2. Name two oral drugs that are used to treat fungal infections of the nails.
3. Name two drugs that are used to treat yeast infections of the mouth.
4. What is an opportunistic organism?
5. Name four drugs used to treat serious systemic fungal infections.

GET CONNECTED

Multimedia Extension Activities

 www.prenhall.com/turley

Use the above address to access the free, interactive Companion Website created for this textbook. Included in the features of this site are drug updates and additional chapter-specific exercises for further practice.

30

Chemotherapy Drugs

CHAPTER CONTENTS

Antimetabolite chemotherapy drugs
Alkylating chemotherapy drugs
Chemotherapy antibiotic drugs
Hormonal chemotherapy drugs
Mitosis inhibitor chemotherapy drugs
Platinum chemotherapy drugs
Chemotherapy enzyme drugs
Interferon chemotherapy drugs
Monoclonal antibodies
Cancer vaccines
Chemotherapy protocols
Drugs used to protect against chemotherapy toxicity
Corticosteroid drugs
Drugs used to treat specific cancers
Miscellaneous chemotherapy drugs
Review questions
Spelling tips

LEARNING OBJECTIVES

After studying this chapter, you should be able to do the following:

1. Name several categories of chemotherapy drugs.
2. Describe the therapeutic action of the various categories of chemotherapy drugs.
3. Given the generic and trade name of a chemotherapy drug, identify the drug category to which it belongs.
4. Given a chemotherapy drug category, name several examples of drugs in that category.

5. Identify the Historical Notes or Did You Know? section in this chapter that you found most interesting.

A **neoplasm** is a new growth of cells that may be benign or malignant. All malignant neoplasms are called *cancers*, a Latin word meaning *crab*, because cancer metastasizes or spreads outward from the original site like the legs of a crab. Uncontrolled cell division and metastasis are identifying characteristics of cancerous cells.

DID YOU KNOW?   Cancer cells are the anarchists of the body, for they know no law, pay no regard for the commonwealth, serve no useful function, and cause disharmony and death in their surrounds.

Michael Gerald, *Pharmacology: An Introduction to Drugs*, 2nd ed. (Englewood Cliffs, NJ: Prentice Hall, 1981), p. 574, out of print.

As cancerous cells invade tissues and organs, normal function is compromised and sometimes impaired to the point of death unless treatment with surgery, radiation, or chemotherapy drugs is begun.

To properly treat any type of cancer, the physician must determine two things: the type of cancer and its stage. To determine the type of cancer, a biopsy is taken from the tumor site or a blood specimen is drawn to examine cells. In addition to the type of cancer, the physician must also know the extent of the cancer before beginning treatment. The extent of cancer progression is referred to as the **stage;** this indicates whether or not the cancer has spread beyond the primary site and metastasized to regional lymph nodes. The selection of chemotherapy drugs and protocols is based on the pathologic diagnosis and also the stage of the cancer. A treatment that is appropriate for one type of cancer might not be appropriate for the same type of cancer that is at a more advanced stage. Only when the exact type of cancer and its stage can be specified by the pathologist will the physician select an appropriate drug treatment regimen.

Drugs used to treat cancers or malignant neoplasms are known as *antineoplastic drugs* or *chemotherapy drugs*. Chemotherapy drugs are most effective when initiated during the early stages of cancer when there are fewer cancer cells present in the body.

DID YOU KNOW?   At the time of diagnosis of acute leukemia, 1 trillion cancer cells are generally present and widely distributed throughout the body of the patient. If an antileukemic drug were able to kill 99.9% of those cells, the patient would show symptomatic improvement even though he or she would still harbor 1 billion cancer cells.

Michael Gerald, *Pharmacology: An Introduction to Drugs*, 2nd ed. (Englewood Cliffs, NJ: Prentice Hall, 1981), p. 574, out of print.

Chemotherapy drugs exert their action against rapidly dividing cancer cells. However, some normal cells in the body also divide rapidly—cells lining the GI tract, hair cells, and blood cells. These normal cells are greatly affected by chemotherapy, with resulting inflammation of the mouth and GI tract, loss of hair, and decreased numbers of RBCs and WBCs.

The term *adjuvant therapy* is taken from a Latin word meaning *aiding*. Adjuvant therapy refers to chemotherapy (or radiation therapy) that is given to cancer patients after they have had surgery to remove a tumor. The purpose of adjuvant therapy is to irradicate any remaining tumor cells.

A **remission** occurs when cancerous cells stop actively reproducing. Some cancer patients experience a complete remission following chemotherapy, others have a partial remission, but some patients actually experience tumor growth while being treated with chemotherapy. When tumor size increases or new metastatic lesions appear despite chemotherapy, the patient is said to have failed chemotherapy. A new combination of chemotherapy drugs may then be tried.

There are many types of chemotherapy drugs: antimetabolite chemotherapy drugs, alkylating chemotherapy drugs, chemotherapy antibiotic drugs, hormonal chemotherapy drugs, mitosis inhibitor chemotherapy drugs, platinum chemotherapy drugs, chemotherapy enzyme drugs, interferon chemotherapy drugs, and monoclonal antibodies, as well as many chemotherapy drugs that do not fit into specific categories.

ANTIMETABOLITE CHEMOTHERAPY DRUGS

As a group, antimetabolites compete with certain chemicals that are necessary for cell metabolism and DNA synthesis. Acting as antagonists, antimetabolites take the place of these necessary chemicals within a cell while also blocking more of the chemical from entering the cell. Cell metabolism is disrupted and the cell dies. Antimetabolite chemotherapy drugs target rapidly dividing cells like cancer cells that use the chemical more often.

Purine Antagonist Chemotherapy Drugs

Purines is a general term that includes several of the amino acids in DNA as well as other chemicals. Purine antagonists block DNA from using purines; this prevents cell division.

cladribine (Leustatin)
fludarabine (Fludara)
mercaptopurine (Purinethol)
pentostatin (Nipent)
thioguanine (Tabloid)

Pyrimidine Antagonist Chemotherapy Drugs

Pyrimidines is a general term that includes several of the amino acids in DNA as well as other chemicals. Pyrimidine antagonists block DNA from using pyrimidines; this prevents cell division.

capecitabine (Xeloda)

cytarabine (Cytosar-U, Tarabine PFS)
floxuridine (FUDR)
fluorouracil (5-FU, Adrucil)
gemcitabine (Gemzar)

DID YOU KNOW?   Cytarabine was developed from a substance found in Caribbean sea sponges.

Folic Acid Antagonist Chemotherapy Drugs

The B vitamin folic acid is required for the synthesis of both purines and pyrimidines, which in turn are used to form DNA and RNA. Folic acid antagonists block the uptake of folic acid by cells.

methotrexate (Methotrexate LPF, Rheumatrex Dose Pack)

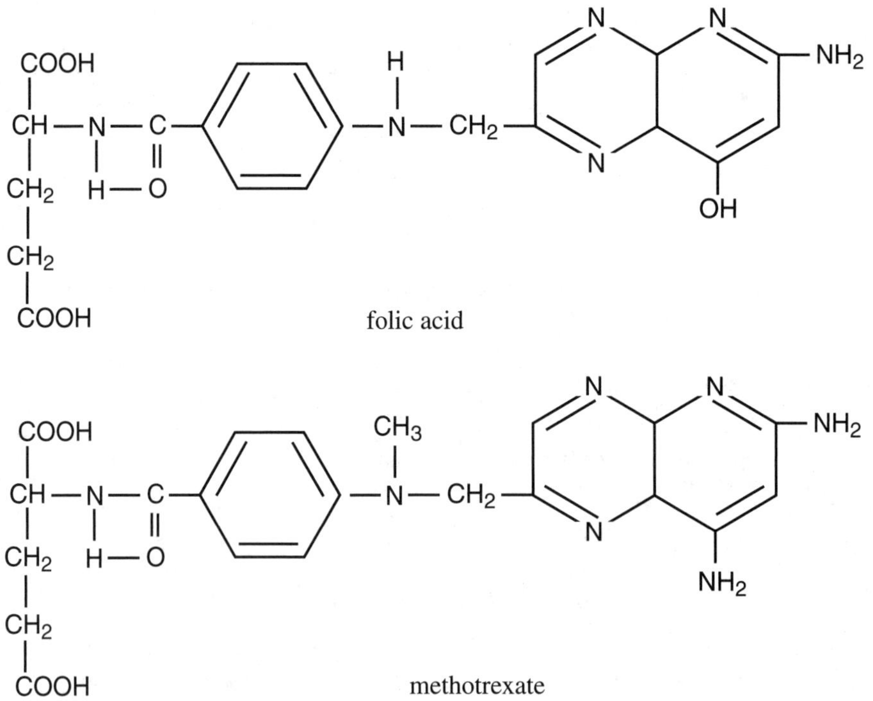

Figure 30–1 The chemical structure of folic acid and the similar chemical structure of the folic acid antagonist chemotherapy drug methotrexate (Methotrexate LPF, Rheumatrex Dose Pack).

Other Antimetabolite Drugs

This drug inhibits DNA synthesis, possibly by blocking the uptake of the pyrimidine thymidine by DNA.

hydroxyurea (Hydrea, Mylocel)

ALKYLATING CHEMOTHERAPY DRUGS

Alkylation is a chemical reaction in which an alkyl group from the chemotherapy drug is substituted for a hydrogen molecule on a DNA strand. This causes the DNA strand to break apart. The cell is then unable to divide properly. Although some normal cells are unable to divide after alkylation, these drugs exert their greatest effect on rapidly dividing cancer cells. Many alkylating drugs are derivatives of nitrogen mustard.

altretamine (Hexalen)
busulfan (Busulfex, Myleran, Spartaject)
carmustine (BiCNU, Gliadel)
cyclophosphamide (Cytoxan, Cytoxan Lyophilized, Neosar)
dacarbazine (DTIC-Dome)
estramustine (Emcyt)
ifosfamide (Ifex)
lomustine (CeeNu)
mechlorethamine (Mustargen)
melphalan (Alkeran)
mitoxantrone (Novantrone)
streptozocin (Zanosar)
thiotepa (Thioplex)

HISTORICAL NOTES: In the early 1900s, the only treatments available for tumorous cancers were surgical excision and radiation therapy. The discovery of the first chemotherapy drug came about serendipitously. During the 1940s, researchers reviewing records from World War I noticed that Allied soldiers who were exposed to the chemical weapon nitrogen mustard gas had a decreased level of WBCs. It was thought that this could be used as a therapeutic effect in leukemia patients whose WBC counts were elevated. Nitrogen mustard and its derivatives are still used to treat leukemia today.

CHEMOTHERAPY ANTIBIOTIC DRUGS

Antibiotics that are used to treat infections act only on the cell walls of bacteria. Human cells, which do not have a cell wall (they only have a cell membrane), are not affected by antibiotics used to treat infections. However, there is a special class of antibiotics that are not used to treat infections, but are only used as chemotherapy drugs. Unlike regular antibiotic drugs, these chemotherapy antibiotic drugs do affect human cells. Some of these drugs bind to DNA strands and inhibit the enzyme that splits each DNA strand into two strands prior to cell division. These drugs affect cancer cells more than other types of cells.

bleomycin (Blenoxane)

dactinomycin (Cosmegen)

daunorubicin (Cerubidine, DaunoXome)

doxorubicin (Adriamycin PFS, Adriamycin RDF, Doxil, Rubex)

doxorubicin (MTC-DOX)

epirubicin (Ellence)

idarubicin (Idamycin, Idamycin PFS)

mitomycin (Mutamycin)

plicamycin (Mithracin)

valrubicin (Valstar)

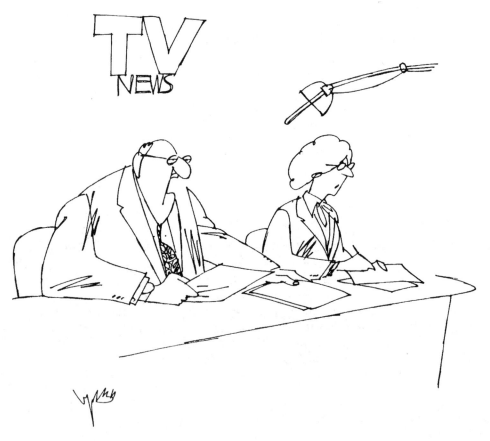

Figure 30–2 *Six white mice were ordered to appear today before a Senate investigating committee concerning their alleged reaction to a new drug.*—David W. Harbaugh. *Reprinted with permission.*

HORMONAL CHEMOTHERAPY DRUGS

Certain tumors, specifically those arising from tissues influenced by the sex hormones estrogen and progesterone/androgen, show regression when treated with a drug that produces the opposite hormonal effect/environment. For example, estrogen given to a patient with testicular cancer changes the naturally favorable hormonal environment provided by endogenous androgens (male hormones) and causes the tumor cells to die.

Hormonal Drugs for Breast, Endometrial, or Ovarian Cancer

Hormonal drugs used to treat breast, endometrial, or ovarian cancer include androgens/progestins as well as estrogen-blocking drugs. In addition, drugs that act like pituitary gland gonadotropin hormones cause normal pituitary gland secretion to decrease and this in turn decreases serum estradiol (estrogen).

> anastrozole (Arimidex)
>
> exemestane (Aromasin)
>
> fluoxymesterone (Halotestin)
>
> letrozole (Femara)
>
> medroxyprogesterone (Depo-Provera)
>
> megestrol (Megace)
>
> methyltestosterone (Testred, Virilon, Virilon IM)
>
> tamoxifen (Nolvadex)
>
> testolactone (Teslac)
>
> testosterone (Delatestryl)
>
> toremifene (Fareston)
>
> triptorelin (Decapeptyl)

Hormonal Drugs for Prostate Cancer

Hormonal drugs used to treat prostate cancer include estrogen or androgen-blocking drugs. In addition, drugs that act like pituitary gland hormones cause normal pituitary gland secretion to decrease and this in turn decreases serum testosterone.

> abarelix-depot-M
>
> bicalutamide (Casodex)
>
> conjugated estrogens (Premarin, Premarin Intravenous)
>
> esterified estrogens (Estratab, Menest)
>
> estradiol/estradiolvalerate (Delestrogen, Estrace, Gynogen L.A. 20)
>
> estramustine (Emcyt)
>
> estrone (Kestrone 5)
>
> ethinyl estradiol (Estinyl)
>
> flutamide (Eulexin)
>
> goserelin (Zoladex)
>
> leuprolide (Eligard, Lupron, Lupron Depot-Ped, Lupron Depot-4 Month, Lupron Depot-3 Month, Viadur)

nilutamide (Nilandron)

triptorelin (Trelstar Depot)

MITOSIS INHIBITOR CHEMOTHERAPY DRUGS

Mitosis inhibitor drugs act at very specific times during the early stages of cell division. Mitosis inhibitor drugs cause DNA strands to break; this prevents any of the subsequent steps of cell division from taking place. These drugs target rapidly dividing cells, so their effect is felt more on cancer cells than on normal cells.

docetaxel (Taxotere)

etoposide (Etopophos, Toposar, VePesid)

irinotecan (Camptosar)

paclitaxel (Onxol, Taxol)

teniposide (Vumon)

topotecan (Hycamtin)

vinblastine (Velban)

vincristine (Vincasar PFS)

vindesine (Eldisine)

vinorelbine (Navelbine)

DID YOU KNOW?   Paclitaxel was originally derived from an extract of the bark of the Pacific yew tree (*Taxus brevifolia*). However, this yew tree is small and grows slowly, and collection of the bark kills the tree. The yew is only found in old-growth forests in the Pacific Northwest. An outcry by environmentalists led to the discovery that the needles of the European and Himalayan yews contain 10 times more paclitaxel and harvesting of the needles does not kill the trees.

M. Suffness and S. Arbuck, "Paclitaxel: Cancer Treatment from Nature," *Pharmacy and Therapeutics*, 1994, pp. 937–938.

DID YOU KNOW?   Vincristine, vinblastine, and vindesine are derived from the periwinkle plant. Another common name for this evergreen ground cover is *vinca* (see Figure 30–3). It takes over 6 tons of periwinkle leaves to produce 1 ounce of these drugs. Etoposide is a semisynthetic derivative of the May apple plant.

PLATINUM CHEMOTHERAPY DRUGS

These drugs use the precious metal platinum, which creates crosslinks in DNA strands and prevents cancer cells from dividing properly.

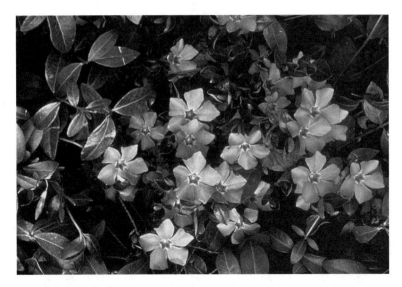

Figure 30–3 Vinca (periwinkle) is the original source of the chemotherapy drugs vinblastine (Velban), vincristine (Vincasar), and vindesine (Eldisine). *Photo reprinted courtesy of W. Atlee Burpee Company, Warminster, PA.*

carboplatin (Paraplatin)
cisplatin (Platinol-AQ)
oxaliplatin (Eloxatin)

CHEMOTHERAPY ENZYME DRUGS

These drugs are enzymes, as indicated by the suffix *-ase*. As enzymes, they break down the amino acid asparagine. Asparagine is not one of the eight essential amino acids needed by the human body to produce protein. Normal human cells can synthesize their own supply of asparagine. Leukemic cells, however, cannot synthesize asparagine. By eliminating asparagine, this drug selectively kills leukemic cells.

asparaginase (Elspar)
erwinia L-asparaginase (Erwinase)
pegaspargase (Oncaspar)

DID YOU KNOW? Asparaginase is derived from the common intestinal bacteria *Escherichia coli* (*E. coli*) that causes most urinary tract infections. Cancer patients who are hypersensitive to asparaginase can be treated with pegaspargase, a modified form of asparaginase that contains polyethylene glycol (PEG).

INTERFERON CHEMOTHERAPY DRUGS

Interferon is a chemical that is released when a cell is invaded by a virus. Interferon then stimulates surrounding cells to produce certain proteins that prevent the virus from spreading. Interferon drugs are manufactured by recombinant DNA technology and are used to treat many different types of viral diseases and cancers.

interferon alfa-2a (Roferon-A)

interferon alfa-2b (Intron A)

interferon beta-1a (Avonex)

interferon gamma-1b (Actimmune)

peginterferon alfa-2a (Pegasys)

peginterferon alfa-2b (PEG-Intron)

DID YOU KNOW?   In the 1960s, in an episode of the then-popular adventure series *Flash Gordon*, a spaceman infected with an extraterrestrial virus was saved by injections of interferon. At one point, it was hoped that interferon would be the magic cure for common colds caused by viruses, but its cost was prohibitively expensive.

"Interferon: Trying to Live Up to Its Press," *FDA Consumer* (Rockville, MD: Department of Health and Human Services, 1981), p. 1.

MONOCLONAL ANTIBODIES

Monoclonal antibodies are created using recombinant DNA technology. The process takes human antibodies and modifies them so that they selectively bind to specific antigens on the surface of a cancer cell. As a monoclonal antibody combines with an antigen, it destroys the antigen and in the process kills the cancer cell.

alemtuzumab (Campath)

cetuximab

LymphoCide

Oncolym

OvaRex

Panorex

rituximab (Rituxan)

Theragyn

trastuzumab (Herceptin)

Note: The ending *-mab* is common to generic monoclonal antibodies and represents the abbreviation for *monoclonal antibodies* (MAB).

OTHER CHEMOTHERAPY DRUGS

These drugs exert a therapeutic effect through various mechanisms or their action is not well understood. Interleukins are proteins released by T lymphocytes in response to contact with an antigen. Aldesleukin is an interleukin-2 drug that is produced by recombinant DNA technology. BCG is a specially prepared weakened live strain (bacille Calmette–Guerin) of the bacterium that causes tuberculosis in cows (*Mycobacterium bovis*). In third-world countries where human tuberculosis is common, BCG is given as a vaccine to stimulate the body to make antibodies against human tuberculosis (*Mycobacterium tuberculosis*). Denileukin is a recombinant DNA drug that combines interleukin-2 and diphtheria toxin. The interleukin-2 attaches the drug to malignant T lymphocytes, and the diphtheria toxin kills those cells. Porfimer sensitizes tumor cells to light. Laser light is then applied to the cells, which causes a chemical reaction and a release of free radicals that destroy the tumor cells. Tretinoin is chemically related to vitamin A.

adenosine
aldesleukin (Proleukin)
Allovectin-7
Ampligen
amsacrine (Amsidyl)
arsenic trioxide (Atrivex, Trisenox)
BCG (Pacis, TheraCys, TICE BCG)
Betathine
bexarotene (Targretin)
Borocell
coumarin (Onkolox)
Cytoimplant
decitabine
denileukin (Ontak)
diaziquone
ECCO11
Endostatin
exisulind (Aptosyn)

DID YOU KNOW?   Exisulind is the first of a new class of chemotherapy drugs known as *selective apoptotic antineoplastic drugs*.

fenretinide
Genasense
Hepacid
hypericin

imatinib (Gleevec)

Imuvert

Leuvectin

levamisole (Ergamisol)

Melanocid

mitoguazone (Zyrkamine)

mitolactol

mitotane (Lysodren)

nolatrexed (Thymitaq)

Normosang

O-Vax

Panretin

Panzem

phenylbutyrate

porfimer (Photofrin)

porfiromycin (Pormycin)

procarbazine (Matulane)

Revimid

suramin (Metaret)

temoporfin (Foscan)

temozolomide (Temodal, Temodar)

thalidomide (Thalomid)

thymalfasin (Zadaxin)

tiazofurin (Tiazole)

treosulfan (Ovastat)

tretinoin (Atragen, Vesanoid)

DID YOU KNOW?   Tretinoin (Retin-A) is a topical drug that is used to treat acne vulgaris and wrinkles.

trimetrexate (NeuTrexin)

Xomazyme-791

COMBINATION CHEMOTHERAPY DRUGS

These drugs combine a monoclonal antibody with a radioactive isotope.

Bexxar (monoclonal antibody, iodine 131)
CEA-Cide Y-90 (monoclonal antibody, yttrium 90)
Melimmune (monoclonal antibody, indium 111)

CANCER VACCINES

Unlike flu vaccines that are given prior to the flu season to prevent patients from getting influenza, cancer vaccines are given after a person has cancer. Cancer vaccines stimulate the immune system to attack cancer cells. The vaccine targets a specific type of cancer by including a fragment of protein that is unique to that type of cancer. CancerVax, Melacine, and M-Vax are used to treat malignant melanoma. Provenge is used to treat prostate cancer. Oncophage is used to treat kidney cancer. Theratope-STn is used to treat breast cancer. Many other vaccines are in the initial stages of testing.

CancerVax
Melacine
M-Vax
Provenge
Oncophage
Theratope-STn

CHEMOTHERAPY PROTOCOLS

Chemotherapy protocols were introduced in the late 1960s to combine the effectiveness of several chemotherapy drugs and direct it against one specific type of cancer. Prior to this, only single-agent chemotherapy drugs were used. In selecting drugs for a chemotherapy protocol, the success of each drug in treating a certain type of cancer is compared with that of other drugs. The most successful drugs are combined into one protocol. The various mechanisms of action maximize the effectiveness of therapy while minimizing the side effects caused by large doses of just one drug. Today, chemotherapy protocols are used to treat nearly every type of cancer. Protocols are designated by acronyms that combine the first letter of either the generic drug name, trade drug name, or drug abbreviation in the protocol. For example,

Protocol Name	Drug
MACC	**m**ethotrexate
	Adriamycin (doxorubicin)
	cyclophosphamide
	CeeNu (lomustine)

DRUGS USED TO PROTECT AGAINST CHEMOTHERAPY TOXICITY

Chemotherapy drugs target rapidly dividing cancer cells. However, their effects are also felt in other areas where cells normally divide rapidly, such as in the mucous membranes lining the mouth and intestines. These drugs are used to treat oral mucositis and dry mouth caused by chemotherapy drugs or radiation therapy.

> benzydamine (Tantum)
>
> chlorhexidine (Peridex)
>
> pilocarpine (Salagen)
>
> sucralfate (Carafate)

Antiemetic drugs that specifically treat the nausea and vomiting caused by chemotherapy drugs are discussed in Chapter 13, "Gastrointestinal Drugs."

In addition, some chemotherapy drugs are known to be toxic to particular organs of the body like the bladder, kidneys, or heart. When a patient receives a chemotherapy drug that is known to be toxic to a particular organ, the patient is also given a drug to protect that organ from toxicity. This drug exerts a cytoprotective effect to spare normal cells and organs. Each of these drugs is targeted to provide protection against the toxic side effects of a specific chemotherapy drug. Amifostine protects against cisplatin toxicity. Dexrazoxane protects against doxorubicin toxicity. Ethiofos protects against cisplatin and cyclophosphamide toxicity. Leucovorin protects against methotrexate toxicity. L-leucovorin protects against methotrexate and fluorouracil toxicity. Mesna protects against ifosfamide toxicity.

> amifostine (Ethyol)
>
> dexrazoxane (Zinecard)
>
> ethiofos
>
> leucovorin (Wellcovorin)
>
> L-leucovorin (Isovorin)
>
> mesna (Mesnex)

DID YOU KNOW?   Leucovorin is a derivative of the vitamin folic acid. Administration of leucovorin after methotrexate chemotherapy is known as *leucovorin rescue*. This drug is also known as *citrovorum factor* and *folinic acid*.

CORTICOSTEROID DRUGS

Corticosteroids are given to decrease the tissue inflammation caused by chemotherapy drugs. Corticosteroids may be given alone or in a fixed combination with chemotherapy drugs in a chemotherapy protocol. Corticosteroid drugs also suppress the production of abnormal WBCs in patients with leukemia or lymphoma. They are also used to treat the anemia caused by chemotherapy drugs.

aminoglutethimide (Cytadren)

dexamethasone (Decadron, Dexameth, Dexamethasone Intensol, Dexone, Hexadrol)

oxymetholone (Anadrol-50)

prednisone (Deltasone, Meticorten, Orasone, Prednisone Intensol Concentrate)

triamcinolone (Aristocort, Kenacort)

DRUGS USED TO TREAT SPECIFIC CANCERS

Because cancer is a life-threatening disease, the most effective chemotherapy drugs are selected to treat specific types of carcinoma. Sometimes single drugs are used, but most often a combination of chemotherapy drugs improves the chance for success. Old as well as new chemotherapy drugs are constantly being evaluated for effectiveness against various types of cancer.

Drugs for Malignant Melanoma

Allovectin-7

Ampligen

CancerVax

dacarbazine (DTIC-Dome)

docetaxel (Taxotere)

Genasense

interferon alfa-2b (Intron A)

interferon beta-1a (Avonex)

interferon beta-1b (Betaseron)

interleukin-2 (teceleukin)

IntraDose

Melacine

Melanocid

melphalan (Alkeran)

M-Vax

Revimid

temozolomide (Temodal)

Drugs for Brain Cancer

adenosine

Borocell

busulfan (Busulfex, Myleran, Spartaject)

carmustine (Gliadel)

cyclophosphamide (Cytoxan, Cytoxan Lyophilized, Neosar)

fluorouracil (5-FU)

diaziquone

hypericin

Imuvert

interferon beta-1a (Avonex)

lomustine (CeeNu)

mitolactol

thalidomide (Thalomid)

temozolomide (Temodar)

Drugs for Eye Cancer

cyclophosphamide (Cytoxan, Cytoxan Lyophilized, Neosar)

Drugs for Head and Neck Cancer

bleomycin (Blenoxane)

cetuximab

docetaxel (Taxotere)

fenretinide

hydroxyurea (Hydrea, Mylocel)

IntraDose

methotrexate (Methotrexate LPF)

nolatrexed (Thymitaq)

paclitaxel (Taxol)

porfiromycin (Pormycin)

temoporfin (Foscan)

trimetrexate (NeuTrexin)

Drugs for Thyroid Cancer

doxorubicin (Adriamycin PFS, Adriamycin RDF, Rubex)

Drugs for Lung Cancer

CEA-Cide

docetaxel (Taxotere)

doxorubicin (Adriamycin PFS, Adriamycin RDF, Rubex)

ECCO11

etoposide (Etopophos, VePesid)

exisulind (Aptosyn)

gemcitabine (Gemzar)

ifosfamide (Ifex)

mechlorethamine (Mustargen)

methotrexate (Methotrexate LPF)

nolatrexed (Thymitaq)

paclitaxel (Taxol)

porfimer (Photofrin)

topotecan (Hycamtin)

trimetrexate (NeuTrexin)

vinorelbine (Navelbine)

Drugs for Esophageal, Gastric, or Liver Cancer

docetaxel (Taxotere)

doxorubicin (Adriamycin PFS, Adriamycin RDF, Rubex)

doxorubicin (MTC-DOX)

etoposide (Etopophos, VePesid)

floxuridine (FUDR)

fluorouracil (Adrucil)

Hepacid

ifosfamide (Ifex)

mitomycin (Mutamycin)

MTC-DOX

nolatrexed (Thymitaq)

paclitaxel (Taxol)

porfimer (Photofrin)

thymalfasin (Zadaxin)

Drugs for Pancreatic Cancer

bleomycin (Blenoxane)

CEA-Cide

docetaxel (Taxotere)

Endostatin

fluorouracil (Adrucil)

ifosfamide (Ifex)

mitomycin (Mutamycin)

nolatrexed (Thymitaq)

paclitaxel (Taxol)

Panorex

streptozocin (Zanosar)

trastuzumab (Herceptin)

trimetrexate (Neutrexin)

Drugs for Colon or Rectal Cancer

aldesleukin (Proleukin)

capecitabine (Xeloda)

fluorouracil (Adrucil)

irinotecan (Camptosar)

levamisole (Ergamisol)

nolatrexed (Thymitaq)

oxaliplatin (Eloxatin)

trimetrexate (NeuTrexin)

Xomazyme-791

Drugs for Breast Cancer

anastrozole (Arimidex)

capecitabine (Xeloda)

cyclophosphamide (Cytoxan, Cytoxan Lyophilized, Neosar)

docetaxel (Taxotere)

doxorubicin (Adriamycin PFS, Adriamycin RDF, Rubex)

epirubicin (Ellence)

etoposide (Etopophos, VePesid)

exemestane (Aromasin)

exisulind (Aptosyn)

fenretinide

fluorouracil (Adrucil)

fluoxymesterone (Halotestin)

goserelin (Zoladex)

ifosfamide (Ifex)

letrozole (Femara)

medroxyprogesterone (Depo-Provera)

megestrol (Megace)

methotrexate (Methotrexate LPF)

methyltestosterone (Testred, Virilon, Virilon IM)

paclitaxel (Taxol)

tamoxifen (Nolvadex)

testolactone (Teslac)

testosterone (Delatestryl)

Theratope-STn

thiotepa

toremifene (Fareston)

trastuzumab (Herceptin)

vincristine (Vincasar PFS)

vinorelbine (Navelbine)

Drugs for Cervical, Uterine, or Ovarian Cancer

altretamine (Hexalen)

bleomycin (Blenoxane)

carboplatin (Paraplatin)

CEA-Cide Y-90

cisplatin (Platinol-AQ)

cyclophosphamide (Cytoxan, Cytoxan Lyophilized, Neosar)

dactinomycin (Cosmegen)

docetaxel (Taxotere)

doxorubicin (Adriamycin PFS, Adriamycin RDF, Rubex)

doxorubicin (Doxil)

etoposide (Etopophos, VePesid)

ifosfamide (Ifex)

medroxyprogesterone (Depo-Provera)

megestrol (Megace)

melphalan (Alkeran)

mitolactol

OvaRex

O-Vax

oxaliplatin (Eloxatin)

paclitaxel (Taxol)

porfiromycin (Pormycin)

TA-HPV

Theragyn

thiotepa

topotecan (Hycamtin)

treosulfan (Ovastat)

triptorelin (Decapeptyl)

vinorelbine (Navelbine)

Drugs for Penile or Testicular Cancer

bleomycin (Blenoxane)

cisplatin (Platinol-AQ)

dactinomycin (Cosmegen)

etoposide (Etopophos, VePesid)

ifosfamide (Ifex)

plicamycin (Mithracin)

vinblastine (Velban)

Drugs for Prostate Cancer

abarelix-depot-M

bicalutamide (Casodex)

docetaxel (Taxotere)

conjugated estrogens (Premarin, Premarin Intravenous)

esterified estrogens (Estratab, Menest)

estradiol (Delestrogen, Estrace, Gynogen L.A. 20)

estramustine (Emcyt)

estrone (Kestrone 5)

ethinyl estradiol (Estinyl)

exisulind (Aptosyn)

flutamide (Eulexin)

goserelin (Zoladex)

leuprolide (Eligard, Lupron, Viadur)

mitoxantrone (Novantrone)

nilutamide (Nilandron)

paclitaxel (Taxol)

Provenge

suramin (Metaret)

triptorelin (Trelstar Depot)

Drugs for Adrenal Cortex Cancer or Pheochromocytoma

dacarbazine (DTIC-Dome)

mitotane (Lysodren)

Drugs for Kidney Cancer or Wilm's Tumor

aldesleukin (Proleukin)

Ampligen

coumarin (Onkolox)

dactinomycin (Cosmegen)

doxorubicin (Adriamycin PFS, Adriamycin RDF, Rubex)

interferon gamma-1b (Actimmune)

interleukin-2 (teceleukin)

Leuvectin

medroxyprogesterone (Depo-Provera)

Oncophage

peginterferon alfa-2a (Pegasys)

peginterferon alfa-2b (PEG-Intron)

vincristine (Vincasar PFS)

Drugs for Bladder Cancer

BCG (Pacis, TICE BCG, TheraCys)

cisplatin (Platinol-AQ)

docetaxel (Taxotere)

doxorubicin (Adriamycin PFS, Adriamycin RDF, Rubex)
fenretinide
interferon alfa-2a (Roferon-A)
interferon alfa-2b (Intron A)
mitomycin (Mutamycin)
valrubicin (Valstar)
vincristine (Vincasar PFS)

Drugs for Bone or Muscle Cancer

dactinomycin (Cosmegen)
doxorubicin (Adriamycin PFS, Adriamycin RDF, Rubex)
etoposide (Etopophos, VePesid)
trimetrexate (NeuTrexin)
vincristine (Vincasar PFS)

Drugs for Leukemia

alemtuzumab (Campath)
arsenic trioxide (Atrivex, Trisenox)
asparaginase (Elspar)
busulfan (Busulfex, Myleran, Spartaject)
cladribine (Leustatin)
cyclophosphamide (Cytoxan, Cytoxan Lyophilized, Neosar)
cytarabine (Cytosar-U, Tarabine PFS)
daunorubicin (Cerubidine)
decitabine
doxorubicin (Adriamycin PFS, Adriamycin RDF, Rubex)
erwinia L-asparaginase (Erwinase)
etoposide (Etopophos, VePesid)
fludarabine (Fludara)
Genasense
idarubicin (Idamycin, Idamycin PFS)
ifosfamide (Ifex)
imatinib (Gleevec)
interferon alfa-2a (Roferon-A)
interferon alfa-2b (Intron A)
mercaptopurine (Purinethol)
mechlorethamine (Mustargen)
methotrexate (Methotrexate LPF)
mitoxantrone (Novantrone)
Mylotarg

Normosang

Panretin

pegaspargase (Oncaspar)

peginterferon alfa-2a (Pegasys)

pentostatin (Nipent)

phenylbutyrate

teniposide (Vumon)

thioguanine

tiazofurin (Tiazole)

tretinoin (Atragen, Vesanoid)

triamcinolone (Aristocort, Kenacort)

IN DEPTH: There are many types of leukemia. Until 2001, chronic myeloid leukemia (CML) had no treatment available except bone marrow transplant. This type of leukemia occurs when there is a mistake during bone marrow cell division. Genetic material is mistakenly transferred between chromosomes 9 and 22, creating an abnormal chromosome known as the *Philadelphia chromosome*. This abnormal chromosome then produces an abnormal enzyme (Ber-Abl). Normally, this enzyme directs the body to replace all of the WBCs that die each day. However, the abnormal enzyme directs the body to continually make too many WBCs, the main symptom of leukemia.

Imatinib (Gleevec) binds with the abnormal enzyme so that it can't use ATP, a cellular energy source. Without energy, the enzyme ceases to function. This drug costs $2400 per month, and the patient must take it for life.

Drugs for Multiple Myeloma

arsenic trioxide (Atrivex, Trisenox)

Betathine

carmustine (BiCNU)

cyclophosphamide (Cytoxan, Cytoxan Lyophilized, Neosar)

melphalan (Alkeran)

Panzem

thalidomide (Thalomid)

Drugs for Hodgkin's Disease

aldesleukin (Proleukin)

bleomycin (Blenoxane)

carmustine (BiCNU)

cyclophosphamide (Cytoxan, Cytoxan Lyophilized, Neosar)

dacarbazine (DTIC-Dome)
doxorubicin (Adriamycin PFS, Adriamycin RDF, Rubex)
etoposide (Etopophos, VePesid)
fludarabine (Fludara)
lomustine (CeeNu)
mechlorethamine (Mustargen)
procarbazine (Matulane)
thiotepa
vinblastine (Velban)
vincristine (Vincasar PFS)

Drugs for Non-Hodgkin's Lymphoma

aldesleukin (Proleukin)
Bexxar
bleomycin (Blenoxane)
cladribine (Leustatin)
cyclophosphamide (Cytoxan, Cytoxan Lyophilized, Neosar)
docetaxel (Taxotere)
doxorubicin (Adriamycin PFS, Adriamycin RDF, Rubex)
etoposide (Etopophos, VePesid)
fludarabine (Fludara)
gallium nitrate
ifosfamide (Ifex)
interferon alfa-2a (Roferon-A)
interferon alfa-2b (Intron A)
LymphoCide
Melimmune
methotrexate (Methotrexate LPF)
mitoguazone (Zyrkamine)
Oncolym
paclitaxel (Taxol)
pentostatin (Nipent)
prednimustine (Sterecyt)
rituximab (Rituxan)
tretinoin (Atragen)
vincristine (Vincasar PFS)

Drugs for T-Cell Lymphoma (Mycosis Fungoides)

bexarotene (Targretin)
carmustine (BiCNU)

cladribine (Leustatin)

cyclophosphamide (Cytoxan, Cytoxan Lyophilized, Neosar)

denileukin (Ontak)

fludarabine (Fludara)

hypericin

interferon alfa-2a (Roferon-A)

interferon alfa-2b (Intron A)

interferon beta-1a (Avonex)

interferon beta-1b (Betaseron)

mechlorethamine (Mustargen)

methotrexate (Methotrexate LPF)

pentostatin (Nipent)

vinblastine (Velban)

Drugs for Kaposi's Sarcoma

aldesleukin (Proleukin)

cidofovir

daunorubicin liposomal (DaunoXome)

doxorubicin liposomal (Doxil)

DID YOU KNOW?　　The liposomal form of a drug is one in which the drug is encased in microscopic spheres, known as *liposomes*. Liposomes have a phospholipid membrane that releases the drug slowly. The liposomal form of the drug has a significantly longer half-life in the body than that of the regular drug.

etoposide (Etopophos, VePesid)

interferon alfa-2a (Roferon-A)

interferon alfa-2b (Intron A)

interferon beta-1a (Avonex)

interferon beta-1b (Betaseron)

paclitaxel (Taxol)

thalidomide (Thalomid)

tretinoin (Atragen)

vinblastine (Velban)

vincristine (Vincasar PFS)

vinorelbine (Navelbine)

virulizin

This drug is used to treat the skin lesions of Kaposi's sarcoma.

alitretinoin (Panretin)

MISCELLANEOUS CHEMOTHERAPY DRUGS

ABX-CBL: Monoclonal antibody used to treat graft-versus-host disease following bone marrow transplantation.

allopurinol (Zyloprim): Used to treat increased serum uric acid in patients receiving certain chemotherapy drugs that cause this side effect.

ancestim (Stemgen): Used to increase the number of blood progenitor cells collected during pheresis prior to chemotherapy or bone marrow transplant.

beclomethasone (orBec): Used to prevent graft-versus-host disease.

Bonefos: Used to treat increased bone resorption in patients with cancer.

broxuridine (Broxine, Neomark): Radiation sensitizer drug used to treat brain tumors.

Colomed: Used to treat radiation proctitis.

cytarabine (DepoCyt): Liposomal form of pyrimidine antagonist chemotherapy drug used to treat malignant meningitis.

Elliott's B Solution: Diluent used when methotrexate or cytarabine are administered intrathecally.

epoetin alfa (Epogen, Procrit): Stimulates RBC production to treat anemia caused by chemotherapy drugs.

etidronate (Didronel, Didronel IV): Inhibits the breakdown of bone; used to treat hypercalcemia of malignancy.

filgrastim (Neupogen): Used to reverse bone marrow depression and low neutrophil count caused by chemotherapy; used in conjunction with bone marrow transplants. This drug is a type of granulocyte-colony stimulating factor (G-CSF), a substance that is produced in the body to stimulate the production of neutrophils (a type of granulocyte). The drug is produced by inserting the human G-CSF gene into rapidly dividing *Escherichia coli* bacteria.

gallium nitrate (Ganite): Used to treat the hypercalcemia of malignancy.

histamine (Maxamine): Used to treat leukemia and malignant melanoma.

ImmTher: Used to treat metastases in patients with colorectal carcinoma.

interleukin-1 (Antril): Used to prevent or treat graft-versus-host disease following bone marrow transplantation.

interleukin-2 (teceleukin): Used to treat kidney cancer and malignant melanoma.

IntraDose: Combination cisplatin chemotherapy drug and epinephrine used to treat head and neck cancer; used to treat malignant melanoma.

L-asparaginase: See *asparaginase.*

Leucomax: Used to increase the granulocyte count in patients with leukemia.

lithium (Eskalith, Eskalith CR, Lithobid): The drug of choice for treating manic-depressive disorders, lithium has the known side effect of causing leukocytosis (increased WBC count). This becomes a desirable therapeutic effect in patients with chemotherapy-induced neutropenia.

Metastron: Radioactive strontium 89 isotope used to treat bone pain in cancer patients with bone metastases. There is preferential uptake of the drug by sites of active osteogenesis, which are metastatic bone lesions.

minocycline (Minocin): Used to treat malignant pleural effusion.

MTC-DOX: Combination of doxorubicin and iron particles used to treat liver cancer.

> **IN DEPTH:**   MTC stands for *magnetic targeted carrier.* Iron particles are coated with the drug and then injected into the femoral artery. They travel directly to the hepatic artery where they are pulled into the liver tissue by a strong magnet positioned above the abdomen outside the body. The iron particles lodge in the liver and the doxorubicin acts directly on the liver cancer.

oprelvekin (Neumega): Used to prevent thrombocytopenia caused by chemotherapy.

pamidronate (Aredia): Inhibits the breakdown of bone; used to treat hypercalcemia of malignancy; used to treat metastatic bone lesions of breast cancer and multiple myeloma.

Quadramet: Radioactive samarium 153 isotope used to treat bone pain in cancer patients with bone metastases. There is preferential uptake of the drug by sites of active osteogenesis, which are metastatic bone lesions.

roquinimex (Linomide): Used to treat leukemia patients who have undergone bone marrow transplantation.

sargramostim (Leukine): Used to stimulate the WBC count after chemotherapy or with bone marrow transplant. This drug belongs to the category of granulocyte-macrophage colony stimulating factor (GM-CSF). It is produced naturally in the body to stimulate the production of granulocytes and macrophages. Sargramostim is produced using recombinant DNA technology in which the gene for GM-CSF is inserted into rapidly dividing yeast cells.

TA-HPV: Recombinant DNA human papillomavirus drug used to treat cervical cancer.

talc (Steritalc): Used to treat malignant pleural effusion.

thalidomide (Thalomid): Used to treat graft-versus-host disease following bone marrow transplantation.

Thymoglobulin: Used to treat myelodysplastic syndrome.

Xomazyme-H65: Immunosuppressant used to prevent rejection after bone marrow transplant.

Zenapax: Used to prevent rejection after bone marrow transplant.

zoledronic acid (Zometa):   Bone resorption inhibitor used to treat hypercalcemia caused by malignancy.

Zurase: Used to prevent hyperuricemia and tumor lysis syndrome in patients receiving chemotherapy.

REVIEW QUESTIONS

1. What two steps does the physician need to take before selecting an appropriate chemotherapy drug treatment regimen for a particular patient?
2. Define these terms: *neoplasm, adjuvant therapy, remission, chemotherapy protocol, leucovorin rescue, liposomal drugs.*
3. List the nine categories of chemotherapy drugs and name one drug from each category.
4. How do hormonal chemotherapy drugs treat breast cancer?
5. Why do many chemotherapy drugs cause a side effect of nausea and vomiting?
6. To what category of drugs does each of these drugs belong?
   asparaginase (Elspar)
   bleomycin (Blenoxane)
   cisplatin (Platinol-AQ)
   fluorouracil (Adrucil)
   goserelin (Zoladex)
   megestrol (Megace)
   methotrexate (Methotrexate LPF, Rheumatrex Dose Pack)
   pentostatin (Nipent)
   plicamycin (Mithracin)
   trastuzumab (Herceptin)
   vinblastine (Velban)

SPELLING TIPS

Bexxar   Unusual double *x*.

BiCNU   Unusual internal capitalization.

CeeNu   Unusual internal capitalization.

coumarin is a chemotherapy drug; coumadin is an anticoagulant.

DaunoXome   Unusual internal capitalization.

DepoCyt   Unusual internal capitalization.

DTIC-Dome   Unusual internal capitalization.

epoetin alfa   Unusual spelling of the Greek letter *alpha*.

interferon alfa   Unusual spelling of the Greek letter *alpha*.

LymphoCide   Unusual internal capitalization.

orBec   No initial capital letter for this trade name drug.

pacli**taxel** (generic) versus **Taxol** (trade).

TheraCys   Unusual internal capitalization.

TICE BCG   Unusual capitalization.

VePesid   Unusual internal capitalization.

GET CONNECTED

Multimedia Extension Activities

 www.prenhall.com/turley

Use the above address to access the free, interactive Companion Website created for this textbook. Included in the features of this site are drug updates and additional chapter-specific exercises for further practice.

31

Anesthetics

CHAPTER CONTENTS

Local, nerve block, spinal, and epidural anesthetic drugs
Drugs for general anesthesia
Miscellaneous anesthetic drugs
Review questions
Spelling tips

LEARNING OBJECTIVES

After studying this chapter, you should be able to do the following:

1. Describe some historical milestones in the discovery of anesthetic drugs.
2. Name several categories of anesthetic drugs.
3. Describe the therapeutic actions of various categories of anesthetic drugs and types of anesthesia.
4. Given the generic and trade names of an anesthetic drug, identify the drug category to which it belongs.
5. Given an anesthetic drug category, name several examples of drugs in that category.
6. Identify the Historical Notes or Did You Know? section in this chapter that you found most interesting.

Anesthesia may be defined as the absence of feeling, sensation, or pain. Anesthesia may be obtained on the skin (by topical application of anesthetic drugs), in the skin and deeper tissues (by subcutaneous local injection), in one body part (by regional nerve block), in the trunk and lower extremities (by epidural or spinal anesthesia), or in the entire body (by inducing unconsciousness and general anesthesia).

Topical, local, regional, epidural, and spinal anesthesias are all obtained by blocking the flow of sodium ions across the membranes of nerve cells, thereby blocking the production of nerve impulses that convey the message of pain.

General anesthesia, on the other hand, involves a loss of pain sensation through deep sedation of the central nervous system and unconsciousness. This results in the total body anesthesia that is needed for most surgical procedures.

HISTORICAL NOTES: The first mention of general anesthesia was in the book of Genesis when God caused a deep sleep to fall on Adam prior to creating Eve.

For many centuries, the only pain relief available was from the use of alcohol or opium. These drugs failed to produce complete anesthesia, and surgeries were performed as quickly as possible, with assistants holding down the patient.

In 1772, **nitrous oxide** (N_2O) was discovered. Rather than being administered as an anesthetic, it was used at social parties to produce euphoria and was commonly known as *laughing gas*. Nitrous oxide was not recognized as a general anesthetic until the 1860s.

During the first half of the 1800s, surgery was still performed without the benefit of general anesthesia. During the PBS television series *Treasure Houses of Great Britain*, the story was told of the Marquis de Angelcy, whose leg was destroyed by cannon shot during the battle of Waterloo (1815). His leg was sawed off. The surgeon wrote afterward that he was amazed that the patient's pulse did not vary during the operation. The Marquis' only recorded comment was, "I do not think the saw was very sharp."

In 1846, William Morton, a Boston dentist, recognized that **ether** could produce general anesthesia. He gave the first public demonstration of surgery performed under ether anesthesia at Massachusetts General Hospital. The term *anesthesia* was coined at that time to describe the effects of ether. A monument at Morton's grave reads:

Inventor and Revealer of Anaesthetic Inhalation.
Before Whom, in All Time, Surgery was Agony.
By Whom, Pain in Surgery Was Averted and Annulled.
Since Whom, Science Has Control of Pain.

Alfred Gilman, Louis Goodman, et al., *The Pharmacologic Basis of Therapeutics*, 7th ed. (New York, NY: Macmillan Publishing Company, 1985), p. 261.

From its first use in 1846, ether enjoyed great popularity as a general anesthetic. However, it had an extremely unpleasant odor when inhaled, was highly explosive, and frequently produced severe postoperative vomiting. Its use was discontinued in the 1960s.

At approximately the same time that ether was discovered, the Scottish obstetrician James Simpson introduced the general anesthetic **chloroform**. Chloroform had two advantages over ether: It had a more pleasant odor and it was not explosive. However, it was much more toxic, and its use was associated with a higher mortality rate. It was used little after World War I.

Thus, within the scope of 17 years, the first three general anesthetics—ether, chloroform, and nitrous oxide—were introduced. Today, only nitrous oxide is still in use.

For centuries, the South American Indians chewed the leaves of the coca bush for their euphoric effect. **Cocaine** was derived from these leaves. It was recognized as a topical anesthetic in 1880 and still has limited use as such. For many years, synthetic substitutes for cocaine were sought. This resulted in the production of **procaine (Novocain),** the prototype of local anesthetics.

In 1920, the technique of endotracheal intubation was perfected. This allowed greater control of patient ventilation and anesthetic administration.

In 1929, the fourth general anesthetic, **cyclopropane,** was discovered by accident during research on another chemical. It was used widely until the late 1950s when its use was curtailed due to the danger of explosion in operating rooms that contained more and more electrical equipment.

In 1935, **thiopental (Pentothal),** a barbiturate, was found to rapidly induce general anesthesia when given intravenously. It is still used today.

For centuries, the South American Indians had used arrows dipped in curare for hunting animals and in battle. This drug causes death by muscle paralysis. It was unknown to the rest of the world until 1595 when Sir Walter Raleigh brought it to England. Not until the 1940s, however, was **curare** introduced as the first neuromuscular blocking drug to be used with general anesthesia. Until that time, abdominal surgery presented a challenge to both the surgeon and the anesthesiologist because the abdominal muscles remained taut and unyielding except under the deepest level of general anesthesia. With curare, the anesthesiologist could maintain a lighter level of anesthesia while still obtaining complete abdominal wall relaxation. Other neuromuscular blocking drugs were developed later.

In 1948, **lidocaine (Xylocaine),** the most widely used topical, local, regional, and spinal anesthetic, was introduced.

No further advances were made in anesthetics until 1956 when **halothane** was developed from technology that arose from research with fluorine (conducted during World War II to produce the atomic bomb). Halothane marked the beginning of a new category of inhaled general anesthetic drugs that are still used today.

TOPICAL ANESTHETIC DRUGS FOR THE SKIN

Anesthetic drugs in the form of creams, gels, ointments, and sprays are applied to the skin to produce topical anesthesia. See Chapter 11, "Dermatologic Drugs."

TOPICAL ANESTHETIC DRUGS FOR THE NOSE AND MOUTH

Anesthetic drugs in the form of gels and liquids are used to produce topical anesthesia in the nose and mouth. In addition, some anesthetic drugs are injected to provide a local nerve block prior to dental procedures. See Chapter 19, "Ear, Nose, and Throat (ENT) Drugs."

ANESTHETIC DRUGS FOR OB/GYN

Anesthetic drugs are given by injection to produce regional anesthesia during labor and delivery. See Chapter 23, "Obstetric/Gynecologic Drugs."

LOCAL, NERVE BLOCK, SPINAL, AND EPIDURAL ANESTHETIC DRUGS

Anesthetic drugs can be administered subcutaneously to provide **local anesthesia** in small, localized areas of the skin and adjacent tissues. Local anesthesia is used for minor surgical procedures, such as biopsies.

Anesthetic drugs given via the subcutaneous route are injected near a nerve plexus (group of nerves) and its branches to directly block all nerve impulses. This is known as **regional anesthesia** or **nerve block anesthesia**. For example, the brachial plexus can be injected to provide anesthesia of the upper extremity for surgery in that region.

Spinal anesthesia involves the injection of an anesthetic drug into the subarachnoid space between the vertebrae of the lumbar region. **Epidural anesthesia** involves the injection of an anesthetic drug into the epidural space; the drug then moves into the subarachnoid space to produce anesthesia.

> bupivacaine (Marcaine, Sensorcaine, Sensorcaine MPF, Sensorcaine MPF Spinal)
>
> chloroprocaine (Nesacaine, Nesacaine MPF)
>
> etidocaine (Duranest, Duranest MPF)
>
> lidocaine (Xylocaine, Xylocaine MPF)
>
> mepivacaine (Carbocaine, Polocaine, Polocaine MPF)
>
> procaine (Novocain)
>
> ropivacaine (Naropin)
>
> tetracaine (Pontocaine)

Note: etidocaine (Duranest, Duranest MPF) is not used as a local anesthetic drug. Tetracaine (Pontocaine) is not used as a local or nerve block anesthetic drug.

Note: MPF stands for *methylparaben free.* Methylparaben is a preservative with antibiotic and antifungal properties; it is often present in solutions of anesthetic drugs that are in vials or ampules. Some people have an immediate and severe allergic reaction to methylparaben. Those anesthetics that do not contain methylparaben are labeled *MPF.*

The local anesthetic **lidocaine (Xylocaine)** is available with or without **epinephrine (Adrenalin)** in the solution. Epinephrine (Adrenalin) is a powerful vasoconstrictor that decreases blood flow to the tissue where it is injected. This therapeutic action controls bleeding and prolongs the anesthetic action of lidocaine. The use of locally injected epinephrine (Adrenalin) is contraindicated in certain areas of the body, such as the tip of the nose, fingers, toes, or ears, because the blood supply is limited and excessive local vasoconstriction would lead to necrosis and skin sloughing. In these areas, lidocaine (Xylocaine) without epinephrine is used for local anesthesia.

Note: The ending *-caine* is common to most generic anesthetic drugs, with the exception of those used to produce general anesthesia.

DRUGS FOR GENERAL ANESTHESIA

General anesthesia involves the loss of consciousness to produce anesthesia, a technique that distinguishes it from all other types of anesthesia. In the operating room, the patient is first given a drug to induce general anesthesia. Once the patient is unconscious and intubated, other anesthetic drugs are given to maintain general anesthesia. Drugs for the **induction of anesthesia** are generally given intravenously; drugs used to maintain general anesthesia may be given intravenously or by inhalation.

Intravenous Drugs for the Induction and Maintenance of General Anesthesia

These intravenous drugs provide a rapid loss of consciousness. This helps the anesthesiologist to quickly initiate anesthesia while minimizing patient anxiety. These drugs include ultrashort-acting barbiturates, narcotics, and other nonbarbiturate/nonnarcotic drugs. Barbiturates depress the central nervous system and produce sedation and, in higher doses, unconsciousness, but have no analgesic action. Narcotics bind with opiate receptors in the brain to block pain and, in higher doses, produce unconsciousness. Often a combination of these drugs, as well as an anesthetic gas, is used to provide balanced and sustained general anesthesia. Some of these drugs are used by themselves to provide light sedation during short procedures like endoscopies.

All of these barbiturates and narcotics are classified as Schedule II, III, or IV drugs, but the short duration of their use eliminates the possibility of addiction.

Ultrashort-acting barbiturates include:

methohexital (Brevital)
thiopental (Pentothal)

Narcotic drugs include:

alfentanil (Alfenta)
fentanyl (Sublimaze)
remifentanil (Ultiva)
sufentanil (Sufenta)

Other drugs include:

droperidol (Inapsine)
etomidate (Amidate)
ketamine (Ketalar)
midazolam (Versed)
propofol (Diprivan)

Inhaled Anesthetic Drugs for the Induction and Maintenance of General Anesthesia

Anesthetic drugs in the form of a gas may be inhaled to induce or maintain general anesthesia. These drugs are used in conjunction with one or more of the intravenous anesthetic drugs listed earlier.

> desflurane (Suprane)
> enflurane (Ethrane)
> halothane
> isoflurane (Forane)
> methoxyflurane (Penthrane)
> nitrous oxide (N_2O)
> sevoflurane (Ultane)

Neuromuscular Blocking Drugs Used During General Anesthesia

Neuromuscular blocking drugs are given intravenously to block nerve transmissions throughout the body to induce skeletal muscle relaxation. This is particularly important during abdominal surgery when the abdominal muscles must relax to provide adequate visualization of the operative field.

> atracurium (Tracrium)
> cisatracurium (Nimbex)
> doxacurium (Nuromax)
> metocurine
> mivacurium (Mivacron)
> pancuronium (Pavulon)
> pipecuronium (Arduan)
> rapacuronium (Raplon)
> rocuronium (Zemuron)
> succinylcholine (Anectine, Quelicin)
> tubocurarine
> vecuronium (Norcuron)

MISCELLANEOUS ANESTHETIC DRUGS

acecarbromal (Paxarel):   Nonbarbiturate used to provide preoperative sedation.

amobarbital (Amytal):   Barbiturate given preoperatively to produce sedation.

atropine: Given preoperatively, this anticholinergic drug blocks the action of acetylcholine. This produces the desirable effects of decreased mouth and upper airway secretions as well as relaxation of the smooth muscle of the larynx—both of which facilitate endotracheal intubation.

butabarbital (Butisol):   Nonbarbiturate used to provide preoperative sedation.

dantrolene (Dantrium): This drug is used to treat malignant hyperthermia, a rare but life-threatening systemic reaction that occurs in some patients undergoing general anesthesia. It is due to a genetic defect that, in the presence of certain general anesthetic drugs, causes the release of massive amounts of calcium from muscle cells. This reaction can be fatal. Dantrolene keeps the muscles from releasing calcium.

dexmedetomidine (Precedex): Nonbarbiturate used to provide preoperative sedation.

diazepam (Valium): Antianxiety drug given preoperatively to decrease anxiety and provide sedation. A sufficient dosage will also produce amnesia during minor surgical/dental procedures and endoscopies; the patient is still able to respond to commands to facilitate the procedure but has little memory of events upon awakening.

Enlon-Plus: Combination of anticholinesterase drug edrophonium and atropine used to reverse the effects of neuromuscular blocking drugs used during general anesthesia.

hydroxyzine (Vistaril): An antihistamine given preoperatively to produce sedation, relieve anxiety, and decrease nausea and vomiting.

levorphanol (Levo-Dromoran): Narcotic used as a preoperative drug for sedation.

lorazepam (Ativan): Benzodiazepine used to treat preoperative anxiety.

meperidine (Demerol): A narcotic given preoperatively to decrease the sensation of pain and provide sedation.

mephentermine (Wyamine): A vasopressor used specifically to treat the hypotension that can occur during spinal anesthesia.

metaraminol (Aramine): A vasopressor used specifically to treat the hypotension that can occur during spinal anesthesia.

methoxamine (Vasoxyl): A vasopressor used specifically to treat the hypotension that can occur during spinal anesthesia.

oxymorphone (Numorphan): Narcotic used as preoperative drug for sedation.

pentazocine (Talwin): Narcotic used as a preoperative drug for sedation.

pentobarbital (Nembutal): A barbiturate given preoperatively for sedation.

pyridostigmine (Mestinon, Regonol): Used to reverse the effects of neuromuscular blocking drugs used during general anesthesia.

secobarbital (Seconal): A barbiturate given preoperatively for sedation.

Septocaine: Anesthetic (generic *articaine*) with epinephrine used in infiltration and nerve block anesthesia in dentistry.

REVIEW QUESTIONS

1. Describe some historical milestones in the discovery of anesthetic drugs.
2. Define these terms: *anesthesia, epidural anesthesia, general anesthesia, induction of anesthesia, nerve block anesthesia.*
3. Name several categories of anesthetic drugs and the generic and trade names of drugs in that category.
4. Why is epinephrine not added to lidocaine for anesthesia during procedures on the fingers?

5. If a Schedule III barbiturate is used to induce general anesthesia, why does the patient not become addicted?
6. What is the therapeutic effect of neuromuscular blocking drugs?

SPELLING TIPS

fentanyl with a *y*, but remifentanil with an *i*.

Novocain   Does not have an *e* on the end of the word, unlike most other anesthetic drugs.

GET CONNECTED

Multimedia Extension Activities

 www.prenhall.com/turley

Use the above address to access the free, interactive Companion Website created for this textbook. Included in the features of this site are drug updates and additional chapter-specific exercises for further practice.

32

Intravenous Fluids and Blood Products

CHAPTER CONTENTS

Intravenous (I.V.) fluid and drug therapy
Intravenous (I.V.) fluid products
Blood and blood cellular products
Plasma and plasma volume expanders
Review questions
Spelling tips

LEARNING OBJECTIVES

After studying this chapter, you should be able to do the following:

1. Describe the process of intravenous (I.V.) fluid and drug therapy.
2. Name several categories of intravenous (I.V.) fluids.
3. Name several categories of blood products.
4. Describe the therapeutic action of various intravenous (I.V.) fluids.
5. Describe the therapeutic action of various blood products.
6. Given the generic and trade names of an intravenous (I.V.) fluid or blood product, identify the category to which it belongs.
7. Given an intravenous (I.V.) fluid or blood product category, name several examples of products in that category.
8. Discuss the purpose of umbilical cord blood transfusions.
9. Identify the Historical Notes or Did You Know? section in this chapter that you found most interesting.

INTRAVENOUS FLUID AND DRUG THERAPY

Intravenous (I.V.) fluids may be prescribed and administered for one of several reasons:

To correct decreased levels of body fluid volume

To correct decreased levels of electrolytes or glucose

To administer drugs

To administer blood or blood products

To provide nutritional support to patients who are NPO or who are unable to take sufficient nutrients or fluids to meet their body's needs

To maintain venous access between drug doses

I.V. fluid therapy and drugs to be given intravenously may be administered in various ways.

Continuous Infusion

The I.V. fluid is allowed to flow continuously into the vein at a predetermined rate. This rate is ordered by the physician and calculated on the basis of the patient's weight, fluid volume needs, and heart/kidney function. An **I.V. line** includes a bag or bottle containing I.V. fluid, connecting tubing, and a needle or flexible catheter inserted in the vein. Additional equipment may include a machine to automatically infuse a set amount of fluid (mL/hour or drops/minute).

I.V. Drip

A drug is injected into the fluid in an I.V. bag or bottle and administered continuously over several hours along with the I.V. fluid at the same rate of flow prescribed for the I.V. fluid. A label stating the name of the drug, the dosage, and the date and time is placed on the I.V. bag or bottle.

I.V. Piggyback

A drug may be mixed in a very small I.V. bag or bottle that is connected into the I.V. tubing and hung next to the main I.V. bag or bottle. Because the drug is mixed with the smaller amount of I.V. fluid, it is administered in an hour or less, even as the main I.V. continues at the prescribed rate of flow.

I.V. Push

When the drug needs to reach the bloodstream more quickly, the solution is injected all at one time (a **bolus**) through a **port** (rubber stopper) near the bottom of the I.V. tubing.

Keep Vein Open (KVO)

If the patient does not need the volume of I.V. fluid, but does need to have access maintained via the I.V. route, the physician can order the I.V. fluid to infuse at a very slow rate to just keep the vein open (KVO) and patent.

Heparin Lock

As a more convenient alternative to a KVO I.V., the physician may order a heparin lock. This is a special type of device that allows permanent I.V. access without the need for simultaneously infusing I.V. fluids. The heparin lock contains a small reservoir that holds heparin and keeps the vein free of clots. A heparin lock is a convenient way to administer I.V. drugs on an intermittent basis. Following drug administration, the heparin lock is flushed with normal saline, and the reservoir is again filled with heparin.

I.V. fluids are ordered as a volume per hour (e.g., 100 cc/hour). Any I.V. fluids (as well as any P.O. intake) are counted as "intake" when the patient has an order for I&O (strict measurements of intake and output).

INTRAVENOUS (I.V.) FLUID PRODUCTS

The most commonly used I.V. fluids contain dextrose, electrolytes, or a combination of both.

> **DID YOU KNOW?**   Glucose, a simple sugar, is the only form of carbohydrate that cells can use as a source of energy. Although the food we eat contains sugars such as sucrose (table sugar) and complex carbohydrates (starches), the body must metabolize them into glucose before they can be utilized. The glucose is then absorbed through the intestinal wall and into the bloodstream. Because I.V. fluid administration bypasses the digestive process, I.V. fluids must contain a glucose-type sugar (dextrose) rather than the types of sugars found in foods.
>
> I.V. solutions actually contain dextrose. Dextrose has the same chemical structure as glucose, but the molecule is rotated in a right-handed direction (*dextro-* means *right* in Latin) when compared to the glucose molecule. However, the action of dextrose in the body is identical to that of glucose.

Dextrose Solutions

There are many different concentrations of dextrose and water solutions.

dextrose 2.5% in water (D-2.5-W)
dextrose 5% in water (D-5-W)
dextrose 10% in water (D-10-W)

Dextrose also comes in concentrations of 20%, 25%, 40%, 50%, 60%, and 70%. These more concentrated solutions have a special use. They are administered as a bolus injection through an existing I.V. line to patients who have severely low blood sugar levels, including diabetic patients and premature infants.

Sodium Solutions

If the patient does not need dextrose, an I.V. solution consisting of just sodium and water can be administered. Sodium is an important electrolyte in both the intracellular and extracellular fluids in the body. The I.V. solution contains sodium and water in proportions that parallel those in tissue fluids. This concentration is known as a *physiologic salt solution* or *normal saline* (NS). Normal saline actually equals a 0.9% solution of sodium chloride and water. Sometimes an I.V. solution of **half normal saline** is ordered. This is written as 0.45% NaCl (not 0.5%), because 0.45% is one-half of 0.9%.

normal saline (NS) (0.9% NaCl)
half normal saline (0.45% NaCl)

Frequently, dextrose and normal saline are combined into a single solution, with 5% or 10% dextrose and normal saline or half normal saline (e.g., D5/NS, D10/0.45 NaCl).

Lactated Ringer's Solution

This combination I.V. fluid contains fixed amounts of dextrose, sodium, potassium, calcium, chloride, and lactate. It was named for the English physiologist, Sidney Ringer.

lactated Ringer's (LR)
Ringer's lactate (RL)
dextrose 5% in lactated Ringer's (D5/LR)

Crystalloid

This is a general term used to describe I.V. solutions that provide normal saline with or without other electrolytes.

Total Parenteral Nutrition (TPN)

Dextrose and electrolyte I.V. fluids are used to maintain fluid and electrolyte balance and supply calories, but they are unable to completely meet long-term nutritional needs. Specifically, they lack protein, fat, and vitamins. Patients whose nutritional needs cannot be met with dextrose and electrolyte fluids may be given a specially prepared I.V. solution known as *total parenteral nutrition (TPN).* This is prepared in the hospital pharmacy and is individually tailored to each patient's needs, according to the physician's orders. It contains specific amounts of essential amino acids (protein), as well as electrolytes, vitamins, and minerals (see Figure 32–1).

Commercially prepared I.V. TPN solutions are available; they contain specific fixed percentages of amino acids as well as electrolytes and may contain varying concentrations of dextrose. TPN is also known as *hyperalimentation solution.*

Aminess 5.2%
Aminosyn 3.5%, Aminosyn II 3.5%, Aminosyn 3.5% M, Aminosyn II 3.5% M
Aminosyn II 4.25%, Aminosyn II 4.25% M
Aminosyn 5%, Aminosyn II 5%
Aminosyn-RF 5.2%
Aminosyn 7%, Aminosyn II 7%, Aminosyn-HBC 7%, Aminosyn-PF 7%
Aminosyn 8.5%, Aminosyn II 8.5%
Aminosyn 10%, Aminosyn II 10%, Aminosyn-PF 10%
Aminosyn II 15%
BranchAmin 4%
FreAmine III 3%, FreAmine III 8.5%, FreAmine HBC 6.9%, FreAmine III 10%

TPN ORDER FORM
TOTAL PARENTERAL NUTRITION

ORDERING GUIDELINES: To order standard TPN solution, check appropriate box(s). To change a standard additive in a TPN solution, re-write ALL additives in the OTHER column. Electrolytes are ordered per LITER and drug additives are ordered per KILOGRAM.

FOR INFORMATIONAL PURPOSES ONLY:

Electrolytes

Ca = _____
phos = _____
Mg = _____

Fluid Limit _____ ml / kg. / day		Cal _____ kcal / kg. / day	
TPN _____ ml / kg. / day		Pro _____ gm / kg. / day	
Lipid _____ ml / kg. / day		Lipid _____ gm / kg. / day	
Other _____ ml / kg. / day		Na _____ mEq / kg. / day	
Other _____ ml / kg. / day		K _____ mEq / kg. / day	

Comments _____

Weight _____ kg.

TPN Solution _____ ml / kg. / day

Rate _____ ml / hour over _____ hours.

Chronological age _____ months _____ yr.

Diagnosis _____

Bag number _____

☐ PERIPHERAL SOLUTION

* AMINO ACID	DEXTROSE
☐ 1%	☐ 10%
☐ 2%	☐ 12.5%
☐ 2.5%	☐ ____ %
☐ ____ %	

☐ CENTRAL SOLUTION

* AMINO ACID	DEXTROSE
☐ 1%	☐ 15%
☐ 2%	☐ 20%
☐ 2.5%	☐ ____ %
☐ 3%	
☐ 5%	
☐ ____ %	

ADDITIVE PROFILE
Check appropriate box. To change standard, re-write all additives in OTHER column.

ADDITIVE	☐ STANDARD per liter	☐ OTHER per liter
Sodium chloride	15 mEq	mEq
Sodium acetate	15 mEq	mEq
Sodium phosphate	None	mEq
Potassium chloride	5 mEq	mEq
Potassium phosphate	15 mEq (10.2 mMol)	mEq
Potassium acetate	None	mEq
Calcium gluconate	20 mEq > 2.5 kg	
	30 mEq ≤ 2.5 kg	mEq
Magnesium sulfate	4 mEq	mEq
Heparin	500 units	units
Standard multivitamins	Standard	
† Standard trace elements	Standard	

INTRAVENOUS LIPIDS 20%

Total volume of _____ ml over _____ hours at _____ ml / hour. Infuse over 22 - 24 hours.

Maximum infusion rate for 20% lipid is 0.8 ml / kg. / hour for infants ≤ 33 wks gestation.

* AMINO ACIDS

Children ≤ 1 year receive Trophamine ® + 40 mg. L-cysteine / gm. protein delivered.
Children > 1 year receive standard amino acids.

OTHER
† Infants ≤ 2.5 kg. will receive a total of 400 µg / kg. / day Zinc.

Physician's Signature _____ Date / Time Written _____

Figure 32–1 A preprinted form for ordering customized TPN intravenous solutions.

HepatAmine

NephrAmine 5.4%

Novamine, Novamine 15%

ProcalAmine

RenAmin

Travasol 2.75%, Travasol 3.5%, Travasol 4.25%, Travasol 5.5%, Travasol 8.5%, Travasol 10%

TrophAmine 6%, TrophAmine 10%

I.V. Lipids

To meet fat requirements, a separate I.V. solution of lipids may also be given. This contains fat in the form of soybean or safflower oil along with water, glycerin, and egg yolk. Lipids are a more concentrated source of calories than dextrose and also contain essential fatty acids.

Intralipid 10%, Intralipid 20%

Liposyn II 10%, Liposyn II 20%, Liposyn III 10%, Liposyn III 20%

I.V. Multivitamins

There is a specially formulated combination of 12 vitamins for I.V. administration. It contains 9 water-soluble vitamins and 3 fat-soluble vitamins.

Berocca Parenteral Nutrition

Cernevit-12

M.V.I.-12

TPN, as well as I.V. lipids and vitamins, must be administered through a special long-term I.V. line (Broviac or Hickman catheter) that is inserted into the subclavian vein or superior vena cava.

BLOOD AND BLOOD CELLULAR PRODUCTS

HISTORICAL NOTES: Dr. Karl Landsteiner, a Viennese pathologist, categorized blood into four types: A, B, AB, and O. He won a Nobel Prize for this in 1930. In 1937, the first blood bank opened at Cook County Hospital in Chicago. In 1940, Dr. Landsteiner also discovered the Rh factor.

Whole Blood, Citrated

Whole blood contains cellular components (red blood cells [RBCs], white blood cells [WBCs], and platelets), as well as plasma and its constituents (albumin, globulins, clotting factors, and electrolytes). Whole blood provides complete correction of blood loss by supplying both plasma and cellular components in the correct proportions. It also provides the RBCs needed to support oxygenation until the patient's own body is able to produce replacement cells. Whole blood must be crossmatched with the recipient's blood type to avoid a transfusion reaction (hemolysis of RBCs due to incompatibility of blood types).

Citrated refers to the anticoagulant (citrate) that is commonly used to preserve whole blood and prolong its refrigerated shelf life to 35 days.

> **DID YOU KNOW?** A unit of whole blood contains 500 mL. The common phrase "a pint of blood" is fairly accurate and easy for laypersons to remember. One pint is equivalent to 473.17 mL, or nearly 1 unit of blood. Each year, Americans donate 12 million units of blood; about 3.6 million Americans receive a transfusion of blood or blood products each year.

Packed Red Blood Cells (PRBCs)

Packed red blood cells (PRBCs) are a concentrated preparation of RBCs (the preparation also contains WBCs and platelets) with most of the plasma removed. This product lacks plasma proteins and clotting factors. PRBCs have an advantage over whole blood in that they can be given without causing fluid overload. This is of special importance in patients

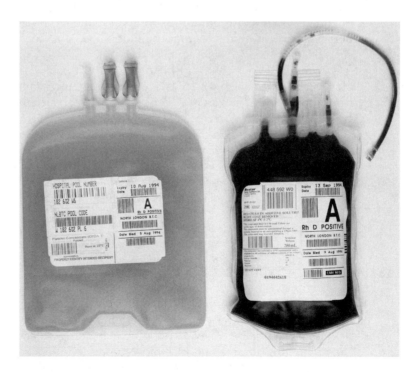

Figure 32–2 Blood and blood cellular products include whole blood, PRBCs, and platelets. These are given intravenously. *Photo reprinted courtesy of Dorling Kindersley.*

with congestive heart failure and in premature infants who need the benefits of whole blood but cannot tolerate the increased blood volume. PRBCs must be crossmatched.

Platelets

Platelets are extracted from whole blood and suspended in a small amount of plasma. Platelets are crossmatched for best results, but in an emergency (and because platelets have a shelf life of only 5 days and supplies are limited) unmatched platelets may be given. Unmatched platelets do not provoke a transfusion reaction, but the body's antibodies quickly destroy them and they are less effective than matched platelets.

Polymerized Hemoglobin (PolyHeme)

The product is made from donor whole blood from which the hemoglobin is extracted and chemically modified. The polymerized hemoglobin is then put in a unit of solution so that it contains as much hemoglobin as a unit of whole blood. This product is used for transfusion when no other blood products are available.

FOCUS ON HEALTHCARE ISSUES: Leukemia is a cancer of the WBCs. The treatment for leukemia is chemotherapy and a bone marrow transplant with normal cells from a donor. Bone marrow transplant recipients and potential donors are matched by tissue type, but this is still not a guarantee of the success of the transplant. Although there are 4 million bone marrow donors registered with the National Marrow Donor Program, only about 60% of leukemia patients can find a suitable match to their tissue type.

Umbilical cord blood contains stem cells, the blood cells from which all other blood cells originate. Stem cells are very immature. Patients given the stem cells from matched umbilical cord blood have a greater chance of survival than those who received bone marrow transplants.

The number of potential umbilical cord blood donors is high because every birth in the United States results in the availability (with the parents' permission) of a placenta and umbilical cord and the stem cell-rich blood they contain. Minorities who have less of a chance of finding a match in the National Marrow Donor Program have a greater pool of donors to pick from if umbilical cord blood is used.

PLASMA AND PLASMA VOLUME EXPANDERS

Plasma is derived from whole blood that has undergone plasmapheresis to remove the cellular components. Plasma volume expanders are manufactured from complex carbohydrates and normal saline. They do not need to be refrigerated and they retain their potency for many months. Plasma and plasma volume expanders have an advantage over blood products in that they do not need to be typed or crossmatched. Plasma and plasma volume expanders are given intravenously to restore blood volume to normal levels. Because they do not contain the cellular components of whole blood, they do not raise the patient's hematocrit or contribute to the oxygen-carrying capacity of the blood. However, they are particularly useful in restoring fluid volume, albumin, and electrolytes lost through severe, extensive burns.

Fresh Frozen Plasma

This consists of plasma containing all of the plasma proteins and clotting factors. It is frozen to prolong its shelf life and then thawed to room temperature before being administered intravenously.

Plasma Protein Fraction

Plasma protein fraction is derived from plasma. It contains 5% plasma proteins mixed with normal saline. It contains no clotting factors.

> Plasmanate
> Plasma-Plex
> Plasmatein
> Protenate

Albumin

This solution, derived from plasma, contains only the plasma protein albumin and has no clotting factors. It is prepared in 5% and 25% solutions; the 5% solution approximates the concentration of normal blood plasma.

> Albuminar-5
> Albuminar-25
> Albunex
> Albutein 5%
> Albutein 25%
> Buminate 5%
> Buminate 25%
> Plasbumin-5
> Plasbumin-25

Cryoprecipitate

This is a plasma extract prepared by freezing and then slowly thawing plasma. It contains concentrated amounts of factor VIII, von Willebrand's factor, and fibrinogen. It is used to treat hemophiliacs and patients with von Willebrand's disease.

HISTORICAL NOTES: In 1964, while watching a bag of plasma thaw, Dr. Judith Pool, a Stanford University researcher, noticed stringy flakes settling to the bottom; these subsequently turned out to be factor VIII and other clotting factors. Dr. Pool developed a method for separating the clotting factors from frozen plasma. The product was termed *cryoprecipitate*. *Cryo* means *frozen*, and *precipitate* means *something that separates out from a solution.*

Cyropreciptate and clotting factors were made available for home injection in the 1970s. Cryopreciptate was frozen, and factor concentrates were available as powder in a sterile vial for reconstitution.

Each lot of clotting factor is made from the pooled plasma of 15,000 to 60,000 donors. There are never enough volunteer donors, so companies pay plasma donors. These companies often establish their operations in poverty-stricken areas and in areas populated by I.V. drug abusers who are more than willing to sell their plasma twice a week for a few dollars. The process of blood donation, separation of blood cells from plasma, and return of the blood cells to the donor is known as **plasmapheresis**.

Plasma, albumin, and cryoprecipitate are all prepared from pooled units of donor plasma. These are tested for hepatitis and HIV and heat-treated for 10 hours to reduce the risk of transmitting these diseases. However, these precautions are not totally effective in eliminating the viruses, particularly HIV. Because of this, many hemophiliacs who were treated with clotting factors developed hepatitis and AIDS.

Although the United States has the safest blood supply in the world, there is still a small risk of transfused blood being contaminated with either hepatitis or HIV. The FDA is responsible for the safety of blood products in the United States. This agency registers and inspects more than 1,000 donor centers in the United States that collect blood. The Blood Products Advisory Committee advises the FDA on the standards for blood collection and processing that are used by donor centers, the American Red Cross, and other organizations.

Elaine DePrince, *Cry Bloody Murder: A Tail of Tainted Blood* (New York, NY: Random House), 1997, pp. 27, 31, 37.

Dextran

Dextran is a manufactured plasma volume expander that consists of synthetic complex carbohydrates with repeating three-dimensional structural units. Normal saline is able to enter these three-dimensional structures to form a viscous fluid that can be used as a substitute for plasma. Dextran is available in three different preparations based on molecular weight.

dextran 40 (Gentran 40, Rheomacrodex)
dextran 70 (Gentran 70, Macrodex)
dextran 75 (Gendex 75)

> **DID YOU KNOW?** The combination of the bacteria *Streptococcus mutans* (present in the mouth) and sucrose (table sugar) produces dextran. The viscous and sticky dextran absorbs lactic acid produced by other bacteria in the mouth and holds it in contact with the teeth, producing tooth decay.

Some patients have antibodies to dextran and can have an anaphylactic reaction when the dextran is given. This drug is given a few minutes before the patient receives a dextran infusion; it binds with the patient's antibodies and prevents an anaphylactic reaction from developing.

dextran 1 (Promit)

Hetastarch

This is a manufactured plasma volume expander derived from a waxy starch commonly found in potatoes, wheat, and corn. When hetastarch is mixed with normal saline and administered intravenously, it forms a solution similar in viscosity to normal plasma.

REVIEW QUESTIONS

1. Define these terms: *I.V. push, bolus, I.V. piggyback, I.V. drip, heparin lock.*
2. Describe the contents and use of TPN.
3. What is lacking in intravenous dextrose and saline solutions?
4. Name five plasma volume expanders.
5. Describe the controversy surrounding hemophiliac patients and I.V. administration of clotting factor from pooled blood.
6. Name three types of blood and blood cellular products.
7. Describe why the use of umbilical cord blood is more effective than the use of bone marrow transplants in treating patients who have leukemia.
8. What federal agency is responsible for the safety of blood products in the United States?
9. Review this patient's Physician's Order Record and answer the questions. Use the Glossary/ Index at the end of this textbook to help you decipher the meaning of the medical and drug abbreviations (see Figure 32–3.)
   These orders were written after the patient had surgery. True or False?
   Is the patient allowed to eat?
   What I.V. fluid is the patient to receive?
   What is added to the I.V. fluid?
   What drug is the patient to receive?
   Write the instructions for the drug route and administration in plain English.

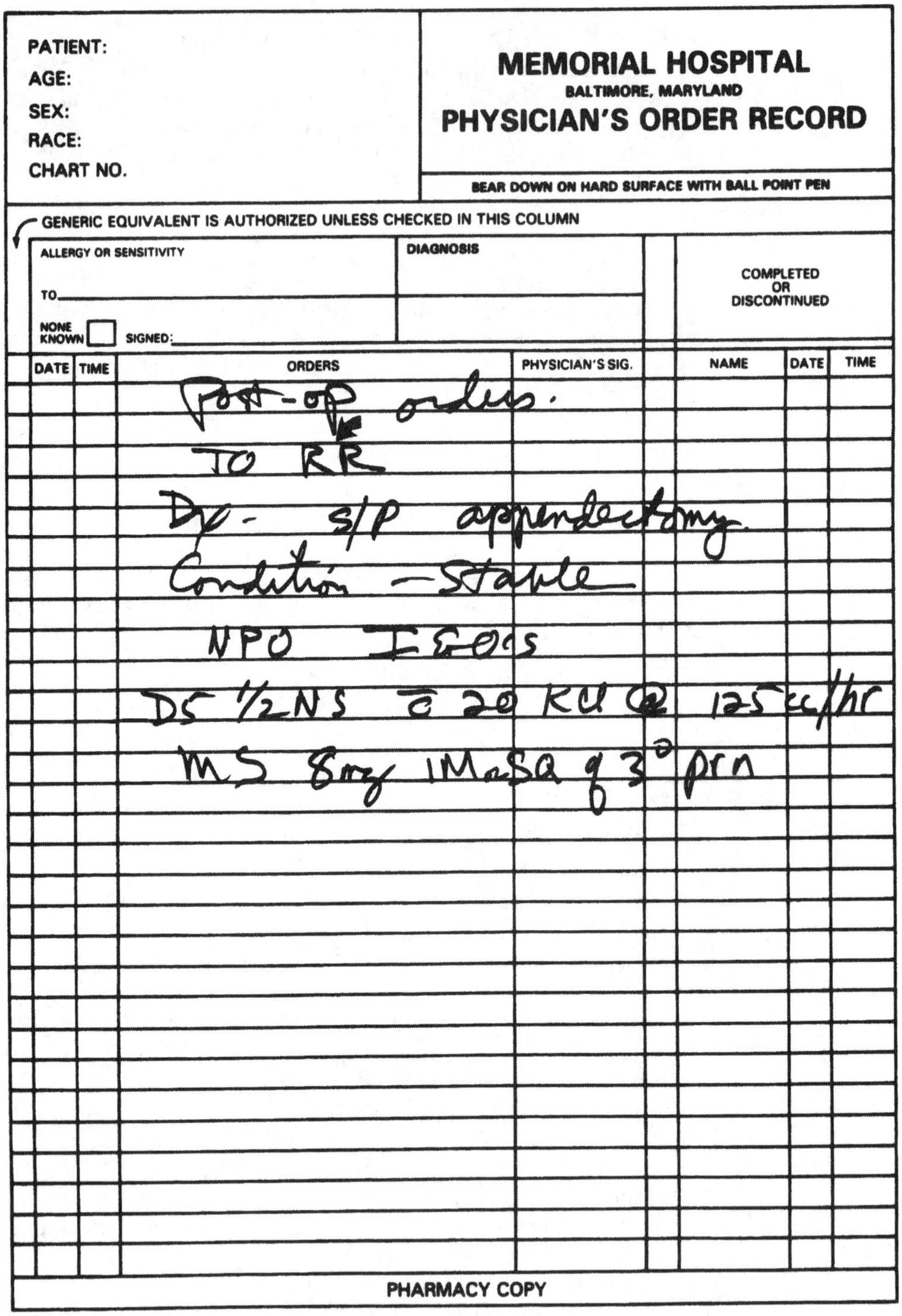

PATIENT:		MEMORIAL HOSPITAL
AGE:		BALTIMORE, MARYLAND
SEX:		**PHYSICIAN'S ORDER RECORD**
RACE:		
CHART NO.		BEAR DOWN ON HARD SURFACE WITH BALL POINT PEN

GENERIC EQUIVALENT IS AUTHORIZED UNLESS CHECKED IN THIS COLUMN

ALLERGY OR SENSITIVITY	DIAGNOSIS	COMPLETED OR DISCONTINUED
TO_____		
NONE KNOWN ☐ SIGNED:_____		

DATE	TIME	ORDERS	PHYSICIAN'S SIG.	NAME	DATE	TIME
		Post-op orders.				
		TO RR				
		Dx - s/p appendectomy				
		Condition — Stable				
		NPO I&Os				
		D5 ½NS c̄ 20 KCl @ 125cc/hr				
		M.S 8mg IM or SQ q 3° prn				

PHARMACY COPY

Figure 32–3   Physician's Order Record. *Reprinted courtesy of Marvin Stoogenke,* The Pharmacy Technician, *2nd ed. (Upper Saddle River, NJ: Brady/Prentice Hall, 1998), p. 29.*

SPELLING TIPS

FreAmine, HepatAmine, NephrAmine, and TrophAmine, but BranchAmin and RenAmin with no *e*.
intravenous   *Intra* means within (the vein). Often misspelled as *intervenous*.
parenteral   Not *parental*.

GET CONNECTED

Multimedia Extension Activities

 www.prenhall.com/turley

Use the above address to access the free, interactive Companion Website created for this textbook. Included in the features of this site are drug updates and additional chapter-specific exercises for further practice.

Glossary and Index

A and D (Derm) (generic *vitamin A, vitamin D*). Combination topical drug to promote skin healing. Ointment.

abacavir (Ziagen) (Antivir). Nucleoside reverse transcriptase inhibitor drug used to treat AIDS. Tablet: 300 mg. Liquid: 20 mg/mL. [eh-BEH-kaw-veer]. 324

abarelix-depot-M (Chemo, OB/GYN). Hormone drug used to treat prostate cancer; also used to treat endometriosis. Investigational drug. 248, 343

(Abbokinase, Abbokinase Open-Cath) (Cardio, Hem, Resp). No longer on the market. (Generic name *urokinase;* thrombolytic enzyme).

abciximab (ReoPro) (Cardio, Hem). Platelet aggregation inhibitor used to prevent blood clots in patients with unstable angina or myocardial infarction, or who are undergoing angioplasty or atherectomy. Intravenous: 2 mg/mL. (ehb-SIHK-seh-mab). 172, 187

Abelcet (Antifung). Liposomal form of amphotericin B. Used to treat severe systemic fungal and yeast infections. For dosage, see *amphotericin B*. (eh-BEHL-seht). 335

abortion, drugs used to produce. 255

Abreva (Antivir, Derm, ENT) (generic *docosanol*). Topical drug for herpes simplex type 1 infections (cold sores). Cream: 10%. [ah-BREE-vah]. 91

absorbents (Emerg). Class of drugs used to absorb toxic substances.

Absorbine Athlete's Foot Cream, Absorbine Footcare (Derm) (generic *tolnaftate*). Topical antifungal drug. Cream: 1%. Spray: 1%.

Absorbine Power Gel (Ortho). Topical irritant drug used to mask the pain of arthritis and muscular aches. Gel: 4%.

absorption, drug. 46

ABX-CBL (Chemo). Monoclonal antibody used to treat graft-versus-host disease following bone marrow transplantation. Orphan drug. 361

a.c. (abbreviation meaning *before meals*).

acarbose (Precose) (Diab). Oral antidiabetic drug. Tablet: 50 mg, 100 mg. [aa-KAWR-bohs]. 241

Accolate (Resp). Leukotriene receptor blocker used to prevent and treat asthma. For dosage, see *zafirlukast*. [EH-koh-layt]. 196

Accupril (Cardio). Angiotensin-converting enzyme inhibitor used to treat congestive heart failure and hypertension. For dosage, see *quinapril*. [EH-kyoo-prihl]. 154, 158, 164

Accurbron (Resp). Bronchodilator. For dosage, see *theophylline*. [EH-kyoor-brawn]. 193

Accuretic (Cardio) (generic *quinapril, hydrochlorothiazide*). Combination angiotensin-converting enzyme inhibitor antihypertensive and diuretic drug. Tablet: 10 mg/12.5 mg, 20 mg/12.5 mg, 20 mg/25 mg. [eh-kyoo-REH-tihk]. 166

Accutane (Derm). Oral vitamin A-type drug used to treat severe cystic acne vulgaris. For dosage, see *isotretinoin*. [EH-kyoo-tayn]. 84

Accutane and suicide attempts. Focus on Healthcare Issues feature. 53, 85

Accuzyme (Derm) (generic *papain*). Topical enzyme drug used to debride burns and wounds. Ointment. {EH-kyoo-zime]. 96

ACE (abbreviation for *angiotensin-converting enzyme*).

ACE inhibitors. In Depth feature. 163

ACE inhibitors (Cardio, Uro). Class of drugs used to treat hypertension and congestive heart failure; used to improve survival rate after myocardial infarction; used to treat nephropathy in patients with diabetes. 111, 154, 158, 163

acebutolol (Sectral) (Cardio).   Cardioselective beta-blocker drug used to treat hypertension and ventricular arrhythmias. Capsule: 200 mg, 400 mg. [aas-BYOO-toh-lawl]. 160, 162

acecarbromal (Paxarel) (Anes, OB/GYN, Neuro, Psych).   Nonbarbiturate sedative/hypnotic drug used for preoperative sedation; used to treat premenstrual dysphoric disorder; used to treat insomnia; used to treat anxiety. Tablet: 250 mg. [ah-see-tuhl-KAR-broh-mawl]. 254, 272, 282, 370

acemannan hydrogel (Ultrex) (Derm).   Topical drug used to absorb exudate from draining burns and ulcers; also moisturizes dry wounds. Gel.

Aceon (Cardio).   Angiotensin-converting enzyme inhibitor used to treat hypertension.   For dosage, see *perindopril*. [AA-see-awn]. 163

acetaminophen (Aspirin Free Anacin Maximum Strength, Children's Feverall, Children's Panadol, Children's Tylenol, Children's Tylenol Soft Chews, Infants' Feverall, Infants' Drops Panadol, Infants' Drops Tylenol, Junior Strength Feverall, Junior Strength Panadol, Neopap, Panadol, Tempra 1, Tempra 2, Tempra 3, Tylenol, Tylenol Arthritis, Tylenol Extended Relief, Tylenol Extra Strength, Tylenol Junior Strength, Tylenol Regular Strength) (Analges, Ortho).   Non-narcotic nonaspirin analgesic drug used to treat fever and pain in children and adults; used to treat the pain of osteoarthritis. Caplet: 160 mg, 500 mg, 650 mg. Capsule: 325 mg, 500 mg. Sprinkle capsule: 80 mg, 160 mg. Chewable tablet: 80 mg. Gelcap: 500 mg. Tablet: 160 mg, 325 mg, 500 mg, 650 mg. Drops: 80 mg/0.8 mL. Liquid: 80 mg/2.5 mL, 80 mg/5 mL, 100 mg/mL, 120 mg/5 mL, 160 mg/5 mL, 500 mg/15 mL. Suppository: 80 mg, 120 mg, 125 mg, 300 mg, 325 mg, 650 mg. [ah-see-tah-MIH-noh-fehn]. 139, 300, 301

acetaminophen overdose. 308

acetazolamide (Diamox, Diamox Sequels) (Cardio, Neuro, Oph).   Carbonic anhydrase inhibitor used to treat edema in congestive heart failure; used to treat absence seizures; used to treat glaucoma. Capsule: 500 mg. Tablet: 125 mg, 250 mg. Intramuscular or intravenous (powder to be reconstituted): 500 mg. [ah-see-tah-ZOH-lah-mide]. 172, 221, 265

acetohexamide (Diab).   Oral antidiabetic drug. Tablet: 250 mg, 500 mg. [ah-see-toh-HEHK-sah-mide].240

acetohydroxamic acid (Lithostat) (Uro).   Used to treat urinary tract infections caused by urea-splitting bacteria. Tablet: 250 mg. 106

(acetophenazine) (Psych).   No longer on the market. (Trade name *Tindal*; phenothiazine antipsychotic drug).

acetylcholine (Miochol-E) (Oph).   Miotic drug only used during eye surgery. Intraocular injection: 1:100 solution. [ah-see-tuhl-KOH-leen].

acetylcholine (neurotransmitter). 60

acetylcysteine (Mucomyst) (Analges, Emerg).   Used to treat acetaminophen overdose. Liquid (oral or by nasogastric tube): 10%, 20%. [ah-see-tuhl-SIHS-teen].

acetylcysteine (Mucomyst) (Resp).   Mucolytic drug used to break apart thick mucus secretions in patients with pulmonary disease and cystic fibrosis. Liquid for nebulization: 10%, 20%. [ah-see-tuhl-SIHS-teen].

acetylsalicylic acid (ASA).   See *aspirin*.

Achromycin (Derm) (generic *tetracycline*).   Topical antibiotic used to treat acne vulgaris. Ointment: 3%. [eh-kroh-MY-sihn]. 84

(Achromycin V) (Antibio).   No longer on the market. (Generic name *tetracycline*; antibiotic).

(Acidulin) (GI).   No longer on the market. (Generic name *glutamic acid*; replacement therapy for gastric acid).

Aciphex (GI).   Proton pump inhibitor used to treat peptic ulcers and gastroesophageal reflux disease. For dosage, see *rabeprazole*. [EH-seh-fehks]. 119, 121

acitretin (Soriatane) (Derm).   Oral vitamin A-type drug used to treat psoriasis. Capsule: 10 mg, 25 mg. [eh-seh-TREE-tihn]. 87

Aclovate (Derm) (generic *alclometasone*).   Topical corticosteroid anti-inflammatory drug. Cream: 0.05%. Ointment: 0.05%. [EH-kloh-vayt]. 92

acne rosacea, drugs used to treat. 85

acne vulgaris, drugs used to treat. 83

Acova (Hem).   Direct thrombin inhibitor used to prevent and treat heparin-induced thrombocytopenia. For dosage, see *argatroban*.

acromegaly, drugs used to treat. 230

ACTH (abbreviation for *adrenocorticotropic hormone*). See *corticotropin*.

Acthar (Endo).   Adrenocorticotropic hormone replacement therapy used to treat Addison's disease; used during diagnostic testing to determine adrenal cortex function.   For dosage, see *corticotropin*. [ACK-thawr]. 232

Acthar Gel (Neuro, Ortho) (generic *adrenocorticotropic hormone*).   Hormone drug used to treat multiple sclerosis and rheumatoid arthritis. Subcutaneous and intramuscular: 80 IU/mL. [ACK-thawr].

Acthrel (Endo).   Used to help diagnose whether Cushing's syndrome is due to a pituitary gland malfunction or another cause. Orphan drug.

Acticin (Derm) (generic *permethrin*).   Topical drug used to treat scabies (mites) and pediculosis (lice). Cream: 5%. [ACK-tih-sihn]. 95

(Actidil) (ENT). No longer on the market. (Generic name *triprolidine*; antihistamine).

Actifed (ENT) (generic *pseudoephedrine, triprolidine*). Combination decongestant and antihistamine drug. Syrup: 30 mg/1.25 mg.

Actifed Allergy (ENT) (generic *pseudoephedrine, diphenhydramine*). Combination decongestant and antihistamine drug. Tablet: 30 mg/25 mg.

Actifed Cold & Allergy (ENT) (generic *pseudoephedrine, triprolidine*). Combination decongestant and antihistamine drug. Tablet: 60 mg/2.5 mg.

Actifed Plus (ENT) (generic *pseudoephedrine, triprolidine, acetaminophen*). Combination decongestant, antihistamine, and analgesic drug. Caplet: 30 mg/1.25 mg/500 mg. Tablet: 30 mg/1.25 mg/500 mg.

Actifed Sinus Daytime/Nighttime (ENT) (generic *pseudoephedrine, diphenhydramine, acetaminophen*). Caplet: 30 mg/25 mg/500 mg. Tablet: 30 mg/25 mg/500 mg.

Actifed with Codeine (ENT) (generic *pseudoephedrine, triprolidine, codeine*). Combination decongestant, antihistamine, and narcotic antitussive drug. Syrup: 30 mg/1.25 mg/10 mg.

Actigall (GI). Used to dissolve gallstones. For dosage, see *ursodiol*. [ACK-tih-gawl]. 129

Actimmune (Derm). Used to treat the skin infections of chronic granulomatous disease; orphan drug used to treat renal cancer. For dosage, see *interferon gamma-1b*. [ACK-tih-myoon]. 99, 346

(Actinex) (Derm). No longer on the market. (Generic name *masoprocol*; topical drug used to treat keratoses and basal cell carcinoma).

actinomycin D. See *dactinomycin*.

Actiq (Analges). Narcotic analgesic drug used to treat breakthrough pain in patients already on other narcotics. (Schedule II drug). For dosage, see *fentanyl*. [ack-TEEK]. 297

Actisite (ENT) (generic *tetracycline*). Topical drug used to treat periodontitis in the mouth. Fiber packing.

Activase (Cardio, Hem, Neuro). Tissue plasminogen activator used to dissolve blood clots from a myocardial infarction, pulmonary embolus, or stroke. For dosage, see *alteplase*. [ACK-tih-vays]. 172, 188, 275

activated charcoal (Emerg, GI). Used to absorb drugs or toxic substances from the gastrointestinal tract after accidental ingestion or suicide attempt. Granules: 15 g. Liquid: 208 mg/mL. Suspension: 15 g, 30 g, 50 g. Powder (to be reconstituted). 132, 182

Activella (OB/GYN, Ortho) (generic *norethindrone, estradiol*). Combination progestins and estrogen drug used to treat symptoms of menopause; used to prevent or treat postmenopausal osteoporosis. Tablet: 1 mg/0.5 mg. [EHK-tih-veh-lah]. 253

Actonel (OB/GYN, Ortho). Inhibits the breakdown of bone; used to prevent and treat postmenopausal osteoporosis; used to treat Paget's disease. For dosage, see *risedronate*. [ACK-toh-nehl]. 144

Actos (Endo, OB/GYN). Oral antidiabetic drug; used to treat the elevated insulin levels caused by polycystic ovary syndrome. For dosage, see *pioglitazone*. [ACK-tohs]. 240

ACU-dyne (Derm, OB/GYN) (generic *povidone iodine*). Topical iodine-containing anti-infective drug used as a hand wash and preoperative surgical skin scrub; also used as a perineal wash. Liquid. Ointment: 10%. Perineal wash: 1%. [ACK-yoo-dine]. 97

Acular (Oph). Topical nonsteroidal anti-inflammatory drug used to treat inflammation of the eyes. For dosage, see *ketorolac*. [ACK-yoo-lahr]. 219

(Acutrim) (GI). No longer on the market. (Generic name *phenylpropanolamine*; appetite suppressant).

acyclovir (Zovirax) (Antivir, Derm, OB/GYN). Oral antiviral drug used to treat herpes simplex virus and herpes zoster virus infections; also used to treat AIDS. Capsule: 200 mg. Liquid: 200 mg/5mL. Tablet: 400 mg, 800 mg. Intravenous: 50 mg/mL. [aa-SY-kloh-veer]. 91, 330

acyclovir (Zovirax) (OB/GYN). Topical antiviral drug used to treat herpes simplex type 2 virus lesions (genital herpes). Ointment: 5%. [aa-SY-kloh-veer]. 259

A.D. or AD (abbreviation meaning *right ear*).

Adagen (Misc). Replacement therapy used to treat adenosine deaminase (ADA) deficiency. For dosage, see *pegademase bovine*. [EH-deh-jehn].

Adalat (Analges). Calcium channel blocking drug used to treat migraine headaches. For dosage, see *nifedipine*. [EH-deh-laht]. 306

Adalat, Adalat CC (Cardio). Calcium channel blocker used to treat angina pectoris, congestive heart failure, and hypertension; used to treat hypertensive crisis; used to treat Raynaud's disease. For dosage, see *nifedipine*. [EH-deh-laht]. 154, 157, 163

Adam and Eve. 366

adapalene (Differin) (Derm). Topical vitamin A-type drug used to treat acne vulgaris. Gel: 0.1%. 84

AdatoSil 5000 (Oph). Injected into the posterior chamber of the eye to stop retinal detachment. Silicone oil.

Adderall, Adderall XR (Neuro, Psych) (generic *amphetamine, dextroamphetamine*). Combination central nervous system stimulant drug used to treat narcolepsy; used to treat attention-deficit/hyperactivity disorder. (Schedule II drug). Tablet: 5 mg, 7.5 mg, 10 mg, 12.5 mg, 15 mg, 20 mg, 30 mg. [EH-deh-rawl]. 274, 292

addiction. 60

addiction, drugs used to treat. 307

addictive drugs. See *schedule drugs.*

Addison's disease, drugs used to treat. 232

adefovir dipivoxil (Antivir). Nucleotide reverse transcriptase inhibitor used to treat AIDS. Orphan drug. 324

Adenocard (Cardio). Used to treat ventricular arrhythmias. For dosage, see *adenosine.* [ah-DEE-noh-kawrd]. 159

adenosine (Adenocard) (Cardio). Used to treat ventricular arrhythmias. Intravenous: 3 mg/mL. [ah-DEE-noh-seen]. 159

adenosine (Chemo). Chemotherapy drug used to treat brain tumors. Orphan drug. 347

adenosine (Derm). Used to treat stasis dermatitis. Intramuscular: 25 mg/mL. [ah-DEE-noh-seen].

ADH (abbreviation for *antidiuretic hormone*).

ADHD (abbreviation for *attention-deficit/hyperactivity disorder*).

(Adipost) (GI). No longer on the market. (Generic name *phendimetrazine*; appetite suppressant used to treat obesity).

adjuvant therapy. 339

ad lib. (abbreviation meaning *as needed*). 72

administration, drug. See *route of administration.*

Adprin-B (Analges) (generic *aspirin, calcium, magnesium*). Combination analgesic and antacid drug. Tablet: 325 mg/antacid. [EHD-prihn-B]. 301

adrenal gland dysfunction, drugs used to treat. 231

Adrenalin (Anes). Vasoconstrictor drug added to local anesthetic drug lidocaine. For dosage, see *epinephrine.* [ah-DREH-neh-lihn]. 368

Adrenalin (Emerg). Used to increase the blood pressure and initiate or increase the heart rate during emergency resuscitation. For dosage, see *epinephrine.* [ah-DREH-neh-lihn]. 180, 181, 183

adrenergic receptor. See *receptor.*

Adriamycin PFS, Adriamycin RDF (Chemo). Chemotherapy antibiotic used to treat lung cancer, gastric cancer, thyroid cancer, breast cancer, ovarian cancer, bone cancer, bladder cancer, leukemia, Hodgkin's disease, non-Hodgkin's lymphoma, and Wilm's tumor. For dosage, see *doxorubicin.* [aa-dree-ah-MY-sihn]. 342

Adrucil (Chemo). Pyrimidine antagonist chemotherapy drug used to treat breast cancer, stomach cancer, pancreatic cancer, colon cancer, and rectal cancer. For dosage, see *fluorouracil.* [EH-droo-sihl]. 340

Adsorbonac (Oph). Topical drug to reduce corneal edema after eye surgery. Ophthalmic solution: 2%, 5%. [ehd-SOHR-boh-nack].

Advair Diskus (Resp) (generic *salmeterol, fluticasone*). Combination bronchodilator and corticosteroid

drug. Diskus (inhaled powder): 100 mcg/50 mcg, 250 mcg/50 mcg, 500 mcg/50 mcg. [EHD-vehr]. 195

Advanced Formula Centrum (Misc). Multivitamin with iron nutritional supplement. Tablet.

Advanced Formula Di-Gel (GI) (generic *calcium, magnesium, simethicone*). Combination antacid and anti-gas drug. Tablet: 280 mg/128 mg/20 mg. 117

Advera (GI). Liquid nutritional supplement formulated for AIDS patients. Liquid.

Advicor (Cardio) (generic *lovastatin, niacin*). Combination of two drugs to treat hyperlipidemia. Tablet: 20 mg/500 mg, 20 mg/750 mg, 20 mg/1000 mg. [EHD-vih-kohr]. 171

Advil, Advil Liqui-Gels, Advil Migraine, Children's Advil, Junior Strength Advil, Pediatric Advil Drops (Analges, OB/GYN, Ortho). Nonsteroidal anti-inflammatory drug used to treat fever and pain in children and adults; used to treat migraine headaches; used to treat dysmenorrhea; used to treat osteoarthritis and rheumatoid arthritis. For dosage, see *ibuprofen.* 139, 304, 307

Advil Cold & Sinus (ENT) (generic *pseudoephedrine, ibuprofen*). Combination decongestant and analgesic drug. Caplet: 30 mg/200 mg.

AeroBid, AeroBid-M (Resp). Inhaled corticosteriod used to prevent acute asthma attacks. For dosage, see *flunisolide.* [EH-roh-bihd]. 196

affective disorders, drugs used to treat. See *depression* and *manic-depressive disorder.*

Afrin, Afrin Children's Nose Drops, Afrin Sinus (ENT). Decongestant. For dosage, see *oxymetazoline.* [EH-frihn]. 206

Afrin Moisturizing Saline Mist (ENT). Topical saline nasal moisturizing drug. Mist.

Afrin Tablets (ENT). Decongestant. For dosage, see *pseudoephedrine.*

Aftate for Athlete's Foot, Aftate for Jock Itch (Derm) (generic *tolnaftate*). Topical antifungal drug. Gel: 1%. Powder: 1%. Spray: 1%. [EHF-tayt]. 89

afterload (Cardio). 155

agalsidase alfa (Replagal) (Neuro). Used to replace a missing enzyme and improve cerebral blood flow in patients with Fabry's disease. Orphan drug. 275

Agenerase (Antivir). Protease inhibitor drug used to treat AIDS. For dosage, see *amprenavir.* [aa-JEH-neh-rays]. 325

Aggrastat (Cardio, Hem). Platelet aggregation inhibitor used to prevent blood clots in patients with unstable angina or myocardial infarction, or who are undergoing angioplasty or atherectomy. For dosage, see *tirofiban.* [EH-greh-staht]. 174, 187

Aggrenox (Hem, Neuro) (generic *aspirin, dipyridamole*). Combination anticoagulation drug with two platelet aggregation inhibitors used to reduce the risk of stroke in patients with transient ischemic attacks. Capsule: 25 mg/200 mg. [EH-greh-nawks]. 187, 275

AgNO₃ (chemical symbol for *silver nitrate*). See *silver nitrate*.

agonist (Misc). Category of drugs that stimulate receptors and mimic the action of a chemical on that receptor. 55

Agrylin (Hem). Used to decrease an elevated platelet count in patients with thrombocythemia. For dosage, see *anagrelide*. [EH-greh-lihn]. 188

A-Hydrocort (Endo). Injected corticosteroid anti-inflammatory drug used to treat severe inflammation in various body systems. For dosage, see *hydrocortisone*. [AA-HIGH-droh-kohrt]. 232

AIDS drugs history. Historical Notes feature. 326

AIDS, drugs used to treat. 323

AIDS-related diarrhea, drugs used to treat. 328

AIDS wasting syndrome, drugs used to treat. 327

AIDSVAX (Antivir). AIDS vaccine. Investigational drug. 327

Akarpine (Oph). Topical miotic drug used to treat glaucoma. For dosage, see *pilocarpine*. [aa-KAWR-peen]. 221

Akineton (Neuro). Anticholinergic drug used to treat Parkinson's disease. For dosage, see *biperiden*. [aa-KIHN-eh-tawn]. 269

Akwa Tears (Oph). Artificial tears. Drops. [AWK-wah].

Alamast (Oph). Topical mast cell stabilizer used to treat allergy symptoms in the eyes. For dosage, see *pemirolast*. [EHL-eh-mehst]. 220

Albalon (Oph). Topical decongestant/vasoconstrictor used to treat irritation and allergy symptoms in the eyes. For dosage, see *naphazoline*. [EHL-bah-lawn]. 220

(Albamycin) (Antibio). No longer on the market. (Generic name *novobiocin*; antibiotic).

albendazole (Albenza) (Misc). Used to treat neurocysticercosis from pork tapeworm. Tablet: 200 mg. [ehl-BEHN-dah-zohl].

Albenza (Misc). Used to treat neurocysticercosis from pork tapeworm. For dosage, see *albendazole*. [ehl-BEHN-zah].

albumin (I.V.). Intravenous blood product that contains no cellular components and is used to replace plasma protein. 381

albumin (plasma protein). 46

Albuminar-5, Albuminar-25 (I.V.). Intravenous blood product that contains no cellular components and is used to replace plasma protein. [ehl-BYOO-mih-nawr]. 381

Albunex (I.V.). Intravenous blood product that contains no cellular components and is used to replace plasma protein. 381

Albutein 5%, Albutein 25% (I.V.). Intravenous blood product that contains no cellular components and is used to replace plasma protein. [EHL-byoo-teen]. 381

albuterol (Proventil, Proventil HFA, Proventil Repetabs, Ventolin HFA, Ventolin Nebules, Ventolin Rotacaps) (Resp). Bronchodilator. Aerosol inhaler: 90 mcg/puff. Oral liquid: 2 mg/5 mL. Liquid for nebulizer: 0.083%, 0.5%. Rotahaler: 200 mcg/inhalation. Tablet: 2 mg, 4 mg, 8 mg. [ehl-BYOO-teh-rawl]. 193

Alcaine (Oph). Topical anesthetic for eyes. For dosage, see *proparacaine*. [EHL-kayn]. 222

alclometasone (Aclovate) (Derm). Topical corticosteroid anti-inflammatory drug. Cream: 0.05%. Ointment: 0.05%. [ehl-kloh-MEH-teh-zohn]. 92

alcoholism, drugs used to treat.

Aldactazide (Uro) (generic *hydrochlorothiazide, spironolactone*). Combination diuretic. Tablet: 25 mg/25 mg, 50 mg/50 mg. [ehl-DEHK-teh-zide]. 104

Aldactone (Uro). Potassium-sparing diuretic. For dosage, see *spironolactone*. [ehl-DEHK-tohn]. 104

Aldara (OB/GYN) (generic *imiquimod*). Topical drug used to treat genital/venereal warts or condyloma acuminatum. Cream: 5%. [awl-DEH-rah]. 259

aldesleukin (Proleukin) (Antivir, Chemo). Interleukin-2 chemotherapy drug used to treat colon and rectal cancer, non-Hodgkin's lymphoma, and Kaposi's sarcoma; orphan drug used to treat malignant melanoma and renal cancer; investigational drug used to treat Hodgkin's lymphoma and AIDS. Intravenous (powder to be reconstituted): (18 million IU), 1.1 mg/mL. [awl-dehs-LOO-kihn]. 325, 347

Aldochlor-150, Aldochlor-250 (Cardio) (generic *methyldopa, chlorothiazide*). Combination alpha-receptor blocker antihypertensive and diuretic drug. Tablet: 250 mg/150 mg, 250 mg/250 mg. [AHL-doh-klohr]. 166

Aldomet (Cardio). Alpha-receptor blocker used to treat hypertension. For dosage, see *methyldopa*. [AHL-doh-meht]. 165

Aldoril-15, Aldoril-25, Aldoril D30, Aldoril D50 (Cardio) (generic *methyldopa, hydrochlorothiazide*). Combination alpha-receptor blocker antihypertensive and diuretic drug. Tablet: 250 mg/15 mg, 250 mg/25 mg, 500 mg/30 mg, 500 mg/50 mg. [AHL-doh-rihl]. 167

Aldurazyme (Misc). Used to treat mucopolysaccharidosis. For dosage, see *alronidase*.

alefacept (Amevive) (Derm). Immunosuppressant drug used to treat severe, disabling psoriasis. Intravenous: 0.025 mg/kg, 0.075 mg/kg, 0.150 mg/kg. Investigational drug. 87

alemtuzumab (Campath) (Chemo). Human monoclonal antibody used to treat leukemia. Intravenous: 30 mg/3 mL. 346

alendronate (Fosamax) (OB/GYN, Ortho). Inhibits bone breakdown; used to prevent and treat postmenopausal osteoporosis; used to treat Paget's disease. Tablet: 5 mg, 10 mg, 40 mg. [ah-LEHN-droh-nayt]. 144

Alesse (OB/GYN) (generic *levonorgestrel, ethinyl estradiol*). Monophasic combination progestins and estrogen oral contraceptive. Tablet: 0.1 mg/20 mcg. 249

Aleve (Analges, OB/GYN, Ortho). Nonsteroidal anti-inflammatory drug used to treat pain; used to treat migraine headaches; used to treat dysmenorrhea; used to treat bursitis, gout, osteoarthritis, rheumatoid arthritis, and tendinitis. For dosage, see *naproxen*. [ah-LEEV]. 139, 255, 304, 307

Alfenta (Anes). Narcotic used to induce and maintain general anesthesia. (Schedule II drug). For dosage, see *alfentanil*. [ehl-FEHN-tah]. 369

alfentanil (Alfenta) (Anes). Narcotic used to induce and maintain general anesthesia. (Schedule II drug). Intravenous: 500 mcg/mL. [ehl-FEHN-tah-nihl]. 369

Alferon LDO, Alferon N (Antivir, Derm, OB/GYN). Antiviral drug used to treat genital/venereal warts or condyloma acuminatum; investigational drug used to treat AIDS. For dosage, see *interferon alfa-n3*. [EHL-feh-rawn]. 259, 326

alfuzosin (UroXatral) (Uro). Alpha$_1$-receptor blocker used to treat benign prostatic hypertrophy. 109

alglucerase (Ceredase) (GI). Used to treat Gaucher's disease. Orphan drug.

Alimentum (GI). Infant formula for infants with severe allergies or protein malabsorption. Liquid.

aliskiren (Cardio). Renin inhibitor drug used to treat hypertension. Investigational drug. 166

alitretinoin (Panretin) (Chemo, Derm). Topical vitamin A-type drug used to treat the cancerous skin lesions of Kaposi's sarcoma. Gel: 0.1%. [eh-lee-tree-tih-NOH-ihn]. 98

Alka-Mints (GI). Calcium-containing antacid. Chewable tablet: 850 mg. 116

Alka-Seltzer. See *Extra Strength Alka-Seltzer*.

Alka-Seltzer Plus Allergy Liqui-Gels, Alka-Seltzer Plus Cold Liqui-Gels (ENT) (generic *pseudoephedrine, chlorpheniramine, acetaminophen*). Combination decongestant, antihistamine, and analgesic drug. Capsule: 30 mg/2 mg/250 mg.

(Alka-Seltzer Plus Children's Cold) (ENT). No longer on the market. (Combination drug with *phenylpropanolamine*; decongestant, antihistamine, antitussive).

Alka-Seltzer Plus Cold & Cough Liqui-Gels (ENT) (generic *pseudoephedrine, chlorpheniramine, dextromethorphan, acetaminophen*). Combination decongestant, antihistamine, nonnarcotic antitussive, and analgesic drug. Liqui-Gels: 30 mg/2 mg/10 mg/250 mg.

(Alka-Seltzer Plus Cold & Cough Tablets) (ENT). No longer on the market. (Combination drug with *phenylpropanolamine*; decongestant, antihistamine, antitussive, analgesic).

Alka-Seltzer Plus Cold & Sinus Capsules (ENT) (generic *pseudoephedrine, acetaminophen*). Combination decongestant and analgesic drug. Capsule: 30 mg/325 mg.

(Alka-Seltzer Plus Cold & Sinus Tablets) (ENT). No longer on the market. (Combination drug with *phenylpropanolamine*; decongestant and aspirin).

(Alka-Seltzer Plus Cold Medicine) (ENT). No longer on the market. (Combination drug with *phenylpropanolamine*; decongestant, antihistamine, and analgesic).

Alka-Seltzer Plus Flu & Body Aches Non-Drowsy (ENT) (generic *pseudoephedrine, dextromethorphan, acetaminophen*). Combination decongestant, nonnarcotic antitussive, and analgesic drug. Liqui-Gels: 30 mg/10 mg/250 mg.

Alka-Seltzer Plus NightTime Cold Liqui-Gels (ENT) (generic *pseudoephedrine, doxylamine, dextromethorphan, acetaminophen*). Combination decongestant, antihistamine, nonnarcotic antitussive, and analgesic drug. Liqui-Gels: 30 mg/6.25 mg/10 mg/250 mg.

(Alka-Seltzer Plus NightTime Cold Tablets) (ENT). No longer on the market. (Combination drug with *phenylpropanolamine*; decongestant, antitussive, and analgesic).

Alka-Seltzer with Aspirin, Alka-Seltzer Extra Strength with Aspirin (GI) (generic *aspirin, sodium bicarbonate*). Combination aspirin and antacid drug. Effervescent tablet: 325 mg/antacid.

Alkeran (Chemo). Alkylating chemotherapy drug used to treat ovarian cancer, malignant melanoma, and multiple myeloma. For dosage, see *melphalan*. [EHL-keh-rehn]. 341

alkylating drugs (Chemo). Class of chemotherapy drugs. 341

Allegra (Derm, ENT). Antihistamine used to treat allergic rhinitis and allergic reactions with hives and itching. For dosage, see *fexofenadine*. [ah-LEH-grah]. 207

Allegra-D (ENT) (generic *pseudoephedrine, fexofenadine*). Combination decongestant and antihistamine. Tablet: 120 mg/60 mg. 211

Allerest Eye Drops (Oph). Topical decongestant/vasoconstrictor used to treat irritation and allergy symptoms in the eyes. For dosage, see *naphazo-line*. [EHL-eh-rehst]. 220

Allerest Headache Strength Advanced Formula (ENT) (generic *pseudoephedrine, chlorpheniramine, acetaminophen*). Combination decongestant, antihistamine, and analgesic drug. Tablet: 30 mg/2 mg/325 mg.

Allerest Maximum Strength (ENT) (generic *pseudoephedrine, chlorpheniramine*). Combination decongestant and antihistamine drug. Tablet: 30 mg/2 mg.

(Allerest Maximum Strength 12 Hour) (ENT). No longer on the market. (Combination drug with *phenylpropanolamine;* decongestant, antihistamine).

Allerest No Drowsiness (ENT) (generic *pseudoephedrine, acetaminophen*). Combination decongestant and analgesic drug. Caplet: 30 mg/325 mg.

Allerest Sinus Pain Formula (ENT) (generic *pseudoephedrine, chlorpheniramine, acetaminophen*). Combination decongestant, antihistamine, and analgesic drug. Tablet: 30 mg/2 mg/500 mg.

Allerest 12 Hour Nasal (ENT). Decongestant. For dosage, see *oxymetazoline*. 206

allergic reaction to a drug. 53

AllerMax Caplets (Derm, ENT). Antihistamine used to treat allergic rhinitis and allergic reactions with hives and itching. For dosage, see *diphenhydramine*. 207

allopurinol (Zyloprim) (Chemo, Ortho). Used to treat cancer patients with elevated uric acid; used to treat gout. Tablet: 100 mg, 300 mg. Intravenous (powder to be reconstituted): 500 mg. [ehl-loh-PYOUR-eh-nawl]. 146, 361

Allovectin-7 (Chemo). Chemotherapy drug used to treat malignant melanoma. Orphan drug. 347

almotriptan (Axert) (Analges). Serotonin receptor agonist drug used to treat migraine headaches. Tablet: 6.25 mg, 12.5 mg. [ehl-moh-TRIP-tehn]. 306

Alocril (Oph). Topical mast cell stabilizer used to treat allergy symptoms in the eyes. For dosage, see nedocromil. [EHL-oh-krihl]. 220

Alomide (Oph). Topical mast cell stabilizer used to treat allergy symptoms in the eyes. For dosage, see *lodoxamide*. [EHL-oh-mide]. 220

Alora (OB/GYN, Ortho). Hormone replacement therapy used to treat the symptoms of menopause; used to prevent and treat osteoporosis. For dosage, see *estradiol*. [ah-LOHR-ah]. 252

alosetron (Lotronex) (GI). Used to treat severe diarrhea in women with irritable bowel syndrome. Investigational drug.

alpha-chymotrypsin (Oph). See *chymotrypsin*.

Alphagan, Alphagan P (Oph). Topical alpha agonist drug used to treat glaucoma; orphan drug used to treat optic neuropathy. For dosage, see *brimonidine*. [EHL-fah-gehn]. 222

alpha₁-proteinase inhibitor (Prolastin) (Resp). Enzyme replacement therapy for emphysema patients with alpha₁-antitrypsin deficiency. Intravenous: 20 mg/mL.

alpha₁-receptor blockers (Cardio, Uro). Category of drugs used to treat hypertension; used to treat benign prostatic hypertrophy. 108, 165

alpha receptor. See *receptor*.

Alphatrex (Derm) (generic *betamethasone*). Topical corticosteroid anti-inflammatory drug. Cream: 0.05%. Lotion: 0.05%. Ointment: 0.05%. [EHL-fah-trehks]. 92

Alphatrex (Uro) (generic *betamethasone*). Topical corticosteroid anti-inflammatory drug used to treat phimosis (nonretractable foreskin). Cream: 0.05%. [EHL-fah-trehks]. 111

alprazolam (Xanax) (OB/GYN, Psych). Benzodiazepine drug used to treat anxiety and neurosis; used to treat panic disorder; used to treat premenstrual dysphoric disorder. (Schedule IV drug). Liquid: 0.5 mg/5 mL. Tablet: 0.25 mg, 0.5 mg, 1 mg, 2 mg. [ehl-PREH-zoh-lehm]. 254, 281, 289

alprostadil (Caverject, Edex, Muse) (Uro). Used to treat impotence due to erectile dysfunction. Injection into penis: 5 mcg/mL, 10 mcg/mL, 20 mg/mL, 40 mcg/mL. Pellet inserted into urethra: 125 mcg, 250 mcg, 500 mcg, 1000 mcg. [ehl-PRAW-stah-dihl]. 109

alprostadil (Prostin VR Pediatric) (Cardio). Used to keep the ductus arteriosus open until surgery can be performed in newborns with congenital heart defects. Intravenous: 500 mcg/mL. [ehl-PRAW-stah-dihl]. 172

Alredase (Diab). Used to treat diabetic neuropathy and retinopathy. For dosage, see *tolrestat*. [EHL-reh-days]. 241

Alrex (Oph). Topical corticosteroid used to treat inflammation of the eyes. For dosage, see *loteprednol*. 219

alronidase (Aldurazyme). Used to treat mucopolysaccharidosis. Orphan drug.

Altace (Cardio). Angiotensin-converting enzyme inhibitor used to treat hypertension and congestive heart failure; used to decrease the risk of myocardial infarction and stroke. For dosage, see *ramipril*. [AWL-tays]. 154, 164

alteplase (Activase, Cathflo Activase) (Cardio, Hem, Neuro). Tissue plasminogen activator used to dissolve blood clots from a myocardial infarction, pulmonary embolus, or stroke; used to dissolve clots in central venous catheters. Intravenous (powder to be reconstituted): 50 mg (29 million IU), 100 mg (58 million IU). [AWL-teh-plays]. 172, 188, 275

AlternaGEL (GI).   Aluminum-containing antacid. Liquid: 600 mg/5 mg. [awl-TEHR-neh-jehl]. 116

altretamine (Hexalen) (Chemo).   Alkylating chemotherapy drug used to treat ovarian cancer. Capsule: 50 mg. [awl-TREE-tah-meen]. 341

Alu-Cap (GI).   Aluminum-containing antacid. Capsule: 400 mg. [EHL-yoo-kehp]. 116

Alupent (Resp).   Bronchodilator.   For dosage, see *metaproterenol*. [EHL-yoo-pehnt]. 193

(Alurate) (Neuro).   No longer on the market. (Generic name *aprobarbital*; barbiturate used to treat insomnia).

Alu-Tab (GI).   Aluminum-containing antacid. Tablet: 500 mg. 116

Alzheimer's disease, drugs used to treat. 270

amantadine (Symmetrel) (Antivir, Neuro, Resp).   Used to treat influenza A virus respiratory tract infection; used to treat Parkinson's disease. Capsule: 100 mg. Liquid: 50 mg/5 mL. [ah-MEHN-tah-deen]. 268, 330

Amaryl (Diab).   Oral antidiabetic drug.   For dosage, see *glimepiride*. [EH-meh-rihl]. 240

ambenonium (Mytelase) (Neuro).   Anticholinesterase drug used to treat myasthenia gravis. Tablet: 10 mg. [ehm-beh-NOH-nee-uhm]. 271

Ambien (Neuro).   Nonbarbiturate drug used to treat insomnia. (Schedule IV drug).   For dosage, see *zolpidem*. [EHM-bee-ehn]. 272

AmBisome (Antifung, Antivir).   Liposomal form of amphotericin B. Used to treat severe systemic fungal and yeast infections; used to treat cryptococcal meningitis in AIDS patients.   For dosage, see *amphotericin B*. [EHM-bih-zohm]. 275, 331, 335

amcinonide (Cyclocort) (Derm).   Topical corticosteroid anti-inflammatory drug. Cream: 0.1%. Lotion: 0.1%. Ointment: 0.1%. [ehm-SIH-noh-nide]. 92

Amen (OB/GYN).   Progestins hormone drug used to treat amenorrhea; used to treat abnormal uterine bleeding.   For dosage, see *medroxyprogesterone*. 253

amenorrhea, drugs used to treat. 253

Amerge (Analges).   Serotonin receptor agonist drug used to treat migraine headaches.   For dosage, see *naratriptan*. [ah-MEHRJ]. 306

Americaine, Americaine Anesthetic (Derm, GI) (generic *benzocaine*).   Topical anesthetic for the skin and for hemorrhoids. Ointment: 20%. Spray: 20%. 94, 132

Americaine Anesthetic (ENT, GI) (generic *benzocaine*). Topical anesthetic applied to the nose and throat prior to performing laryngoscopy and esophagoscopy. Gel: 20%.

A-Methapred (Endo).   Injected corticosteroid anti-inflammatory used to treat severe inflammation in various body systems.   For dosage, see *methylprednisolone*. [AA-MEH-thah-prehd]. 232

Amevive (Derm).   Immunosuppressant drug used to treat severe, disabling psoriasis.   For dosage, see *alefacept*. 87

Amicar (Hem).   Hemostatic drug used to treat excessive bleeding in patients with certain blood clotting abnormalities.   For dosage, see *aminocaproic acid*. [EH-mih-kawr].

Amidate (Anes).   Used to induce and maintain general anesthesia.   For dosage, see *etomidate*. [EH-mih-dayt]. 369

amifostine (Ethyol) (Chemo).   Cytoprotective drug used to prevent renal toxicity in patients receiving cisplatin chemotherapy; also used to protect against xerostomia after head and neck irradiation. Intravenous (powder to be reconstituted): 500 mg. [ehmee-FAWS-teen]. 350

amikacin (Amikin) (Antibio).   Aminoglycoside antibiotic used to treat a variety of bacterial infections, including *E. coli*, *Klebsiella*, *Pseudomonas*, and *Staphylococcus*. Intramuscular or intravenous: 50 mg/mL, 250 mg/mL [eh-mih-KAY-sihn]. 316

Amikin (Antibio).   Aminoglycoside antibiotic used to treat a variety of bacterial infections, including *E. coli*, *Klebsiella*, *Pseudomonas*, and *Staphylococcus*. For dosage, see *amikacin*. [EH-mih-kihn]. 316

amiloride (Midamor) (Uro).   Potassium-sparing diuretic. Tablet: 5 mg. [eh-MIH-loh-ride]. 104

Amin-Aid (GI).   Liquid nutritional supplement formulated for patients with chronic renal disease. Powder (to be reconstituted).

Aminess 5.2% (I.V.).   Intravenous fluid for total parenteral nutrition. 376

aminocaproic acid (Amicar) (Hem).   Hemostatic drug used to treat excessive bleeding in patients with certain blood clotting abnormalities. Liquid: 250 mg/mL. Tablet: 500 mg. Intravenous: 250 mg/mL. [ah-mee-noh-keh-PROH-ihk].

aminocaproic acid (Caprogel) (Oph).   Used to treat traumatic hyphema. Orphan drug.

aminoglutethimide (Cytadren) (Chemo, Endo). Steroid drug used to suppress the adrenal cortex to treat Cushing's syndrome; also used to treat breast and prostate cancer. Tablet: 250 mg. [ah-mee-nohgloo-TEH-theh-mide]. 232, 351

aminoglycosides (Antibio).   Class of antibiotic drugs. 316

aminolevulinic acid (Levulan Kerastick) (Derm). Topical drug used to treat actinic keratoses. Liquid: 20%. [ah-mee-noh-leh-vyoo-LIH-nihk].

aminophylline (Phyllocontin) (Resp). Bronchodilator; used to prevent apnea in premature infants. Liquid: 105 mg/5 mL. Tablet: 100 mg, 200 mg, 225 mg. Suppository: 250 mg, 500 mg. Intravenous: 250 mg/10 mL. [eh-meh-NAW-feh-lihn]. 193

aminosalicylic acid (Paser Granules) (Resp). Used to treat tuberculosis. Orphan drug. 197

aminosidine (Gabbromicina) (Antivir, Resp). Used to treat *Mycobacterium avium-intracellulare* infection in AIDS patients; used to treat tuberculosis. Orphan drug. 197, 329

Aminosyn 3.5%, Aminosyn II 3.5%, Aminosyn 3.5% M, Aminosyn II 3.5% M, Aminosyn II 4.25%, Aminosyn II 4.25% M, Aminosyn 5%, Aminosyn II 5%, Aminosyn-RF 5.2%, Aminosyn 7%, Aminosyn II 7%, Aminosyn-HBC 7%, Aminosyn-PF 7%, Aminosyn 8.5%, Aminosyn II 8.5%, Aminosyn 10%, Aminosyn II 10%, Aminosyn-PF 10%, Aminosyn II 15% (I.V.). Intravenous fluid for total parenteral nutrition. 376

amiodarone (Cordarone) (Cardio). Used to treat ventricular arrhythmias. Tablet: 200 mg. Intravenous: 5 mg/mL. [eh-mee-OH-dah-rohn]. 159

amiprilose (Therafectin) (Ortho). Used to treat rheumatoid arthritis. Investigational drug. 147

amitriptyline (Elavil) (Analges, Diab, Neuro, Ortho). Tricyclic antidepressant used to treat migraines; used to treat diabetic neuropathy; used to treat postherpetic neuralgia; used to treat phantom limb pain. Tablet: 10 mg, 25 mg, 50 mg, 75 mg, 100 mg, 150 mg. Intramuscular: 10 mg/mL. [eh-mee-TRIP-teh-leen]. 147, 241, 275, 306

amitriptyline (Elavil) (Psych). Tricyclic antidepressant used to treat depression; used to treat anorexia nervosa and bulimia nervosa. Tablet: 10 mg, 25 mg, 50 mg, 75 mg, 100 mg, 150 mg. Intramuscular: 10 mg/mL. [eh-mee-TRIP-teh-leen]. 285, 291

amlexanox (Aphthasol) (ENT). Topical drug used to treat aphthous ulcers in the mouth. Paste: 5%. [ehm-LEHK-sah-nawks].

amlodipine (Norvasc) (Cardio). Calcium channel blocker used to treat angina pectoris and hypertension. Tablet: 2.5 mg, 5 mg, 10 mg. [ehm-LOH-dih-peen]. 157, 163

Ammonul (Misc) (generic *benzoate, phenylacetate*). Combination drug used to prevent and treat increased blood levels of ammonia in patients with abnormalities of the enzymes that produce urea. Orphan drug.

amobarbital (Amytal) (Anes, Neuro). Barbiturate drug used to provide preoperative sedation; used for short-term treatment of insomnia. (Schedule II drug). Intramuscular and intravenous (powder to be reconstituted): 250 mg, 500 mg. [eh-moh-BAWR-beh-tawl]. 272, 370

AMO Vitrax (Oph). Injected into the eye during eye surgery to keep the anterior chamber expanded and replace intraocular fluid. For dosage, see *sodium hyaluronate*.

amoxapine (Analges, Diab, Neuro, Ortho). Tricyclic antidepressant used to treat migraines; used to treat diabetic neuropathy; used to treat postherpetic neuralgia; used to treat phantom limb pain. Tablet: 25 mg, 50 mg, 100 mg, 150 mg. [ah-MAWK-sah-peen]. 147, 241, 275, 306

amoxapine (Psych). Tricyclic antidepressant. Tablet: 25 mg, 50 mg, 100 mg, 150 mg. [ah-MAWK-sah-peen]. 285

amoxicillin (Amoxil, Trimox, Wymox) (Antibio). Penicillin-type antibiotic used to treat various types of bacterial infections, including *Streptococcus, H. influenzae, E. coli*, gonorrhea, and *Chlamydia*; used prophylactically to prevent subacute bacterial endocarditis in at-risk patients undergoing dental or surgical procedures; used to treat *H. pylori* infection of the gastrointestinal tract. Capsule: 250 mg, 500 mg. Chewable tablet: 125 mg, 200 mg, 250 mg, 400 mg. Tablet: 500 mg, 875 mg. Liquid (powder to be reconstituted): 50 mg/mL, 125 mg/5 mL, 200 mg/5 mL, 250 mg/5 mL, 400 mg/5 mL. [ah-mawk-seh-SIH-lihn]. 120, 172, 312

Amoxil (Antibio). Penicillin-type antibiotic used to treat various types of bacterial infections, including *Streptococcus, H. influenzae, E. coli*, gonorrhea, and *Chlamydia*; used prophylactically to prevent subacute bacterial endocarditis in at-risk patients undergoing dental or surgical procedures; used to treat *H. pylori* infection of the gastrointestinal tract. For dosage, see *amoxicillin*. [ah-MAWK-sihl]. 120, 312

amphetamine (Neuro, Psych). Central nervous system stimulant used to treat narcolepsy; used to treat attention-deficit/hyperactivity disorder. (Schedule II drug). Tablet: 5 mg. [ehm-FEH-tah-meen]. 274, 291

amphetamines. Historical Notes feature. 291

amphetamines (Psych). Central nervous system stimulant class of drugs used to treat attention-deficit/hyperactivity disorder. 335

Amphocin (Antifung). Used to treat severe systemic fungal and yeast infections. For dosage, see *amphotericin B*. [EHM-foh-sihn].

Amphojel (GI). Aluminum-containing antacid. Tablet: 600 mg. Suspension: 320 mg/5 mL. [EHM-foh-jehl].

Amphotec (Antifung). Liposomal form of amphotericin B. Used to treat severe systemic fungal and yeast infections. For dosage, see *amphotericin B*. [EHM-foh-tehk]. 335

amphotericin B (Abelcet, AmBisome, Amphotec) (Antifung). Liposomal form of amphotericin B. Used to treat severe systemic fungal and yeast infections. Intravenous: 100 mg/20 mL. [ehm-foh-TEH-reh-sihn]. 331, 335

amphotericin B (Amphocin, Fungizone Intravenous) (Antifung). Used to treat severe systemic fungal and yeast infections. Intravenous (powder to be reconstituted): 50 mg. [ehm-foh-TEH-reh-sihn]. 335

amphotericin B (Fungizone) (Derm). Topical drug used to treat yeast infections. Cream: 3%. Lotion: 3%. Ointment: 3%. [ehm-foh-TEH-reh-sihn].

amphotericin B (Fungizone) (ENT). Topical drug used to treat yeast infections in the mouth. Liquid: 100 mg/mL. [ehm-foh-TEH-reh-sihn].

ampicillin (Principen, Totacillin) (Antibio). Penicillin-type antibiotic used to treat various types of bacterial infections, including *E. coli* and gonorrhea; used to prevent subacute bacterial endocarditis. Capsule: 250 mg, 500 mg. Liquid: 125 mg/5 mL, 250 mg/5 mL. Intramuscular or intravenous (powder to be reconstituted): 125 mg, 250 mg, 500 mg, 1 g, 2 g. [EHM-pih-sihl-ehn]. 313

Ampligen (Antivir, Chemo). Used to treat renal cancer and malignant melanoma; used to treat chronic fatigue syndrome; investigational drug used to treat AIDS. Orphan drug.

amprenavir (Agenerase) (Antivir). Protease inhibitor drug used to treat AIDS. Capsule: 50 mg, 150 mg. Liquid: 15 mg/mL. [ehm-PREH-nah-veer]. 325

ampule. 60

(amrinone) (Cardio). No longer on the market. (Trade name *Inocor*; used to treat congestive heart failure).

amsacrine (Amsidyl) (Chemo). Chemotherapy drug used to treat leukemia. Orphan drug. 347

Amsidyl (Chemo). Chemotherapy drug used to treat leukemia. For dosage, see *amsacrine*. 347

Amvisc, Amvisc Plus (Oph). Injected into the eye during eye surgery to keep the anterior chamber expanded and replace intraocular fluid. For dosage, see *sodium hyaluronate*. [EHM-visk].

amyl nitrite (Amyl Nitrite Aspirols) (Cardio). Nitrate drug used to prevent and treat angina pectoris. Inhalation (capsule crushed and inhaled): 0.3 mL. 156

Amyl Nitrite Aspirols (Cardio). Nitrate drug used to prevent and treat angina pectoris. For dosage, see *amyl nitrite*. 156

amyotrophic lateral sclerosis, drugs used to treat.

Amytal (Anes, Neuro). Barbiturate drug used to provide preoperative sedation; used for short-term treatment of insomnia. (Schedule II drug). For dosage, see *amobarbital*. [EH-meh-tawl]. 272, 370

anabolic steroid abuse. Focus on Healthcare Issues feature.

anabolic steroids (Antivir, Chemo, Endo, Hem). Class of drugs used to treat loss of muscle mass in AIDS wasting syndrome; also used to increase the red blood cell count in anemia; also used to treat metastatic breast cancer. Also used illegally by athletes to increase muscle mass and performance. [eh-neh-BAW-lihk STEH-roydz]. 233

Anacin, Anacin Maximum Strength (Analges) (generic *aspirin, caffeine*). Combination nonnarcotic analgesic drug and caffeine. Caplet, Tablet: 400 mg/32 mg, 500 mg/32 mg.

(Anacin-3) (Analges). No longer on the market. (Generic name *acetaminophen*; analgesic drug).

Anadrol-50 (Chemo, Endo, Hem). Anabolic steroid used to treat anemia caused by chemotherapy drugs; also used to increase red blood cell production to treat anemia; also used illegally by athletes to enhance performance. For dosage, see *oxymetholone*. [EHN-ah-drawl 50]. 234

Anafranil (OB/GYN, Psych). Tricyclic antidepressant used to treat obsessive-compulsive disorder; used to treat panic disorder; used to treat premenstrual dysphoric disorder. For dosage, see *clomipramine*. [eh-NEH-freh-nihl]. 254, 289

anagrelide (Agrylin) (Hem). Used to decrease an elevated platelet count in patients with thrombocythemia. Capsule: 0.5 mg, 1 mg. [eh-NEH-greh-lide].

Ana-Guard (Resp). Bronchodilator. For dosage, see *epinephrine*. 193

Ana-Guard Epinephrine, EpiPen Auto-Injector, EpiPen Jr. Auto-Injector (Emerg). Self-administered epinephrine to prevent anaphylactic reaction after an insect bite. For dosage, see *epinephrine*.

anakinra (Kineret) (Ortho). Interleukin-1 drug used to treat rheumatoid arthritis. Subcutaneous: 100 mg/mL. 142

Ana-Kit (Emerg). Kit containing self-administered injectable epinephrine and Chlor-Trimeton allergy tablets used to prevent anaphylactic reaction after an insect bite.

analgesic drugs (Analges). Class of drugs to relieve pain. [eh-nehl-JEE-sihk]. 61, 296

analgesics, urinary tract. 107

analog. 61

anaphylactic shock, drugs used to prevent. 54, 183

anaphylaxis. 54

Anaprox, Anaprox DS (Analges, OB/GYN, Ortho). Nonsteroidal anti-inflammatory drug used to treat pain; used to treat migraine headaches; used to treat dysmenorrhea; used to treat bursitis, gout, osteoarthritis, rheumatoid arthritis, and tendinitis. For dosage, see *naproxen*. [EH-neh-prawks]. 139, 146, 255, 304, 307

Anaspaz (GI, Uro).   Antispasmodic drug used to treat spasm of the smooth muscle of the bowel and bladder.   For dosage, see *L-hyoscyamine*. 107, 122

anastrozole (Arimidex) (Chemo).   Hormonal chemo-therapy drug used to treat breast cancer. Tablet: 1 mg. [eh-NEH-stroh-zohl]. 343

Anbesol, Baby Anbesol, Maximum Strength Anbesol (ENT) (generic *benzocaine*).   Topical anesthetic for mouth. Gel: 7.5%. Liquid: 6.3%, 20%. [EHN-beh-sawl].

Ancef (Antibio).   Cephalosporin antibiotic used to treat a variety of bacterial infections, including *Streptococcus, Staphylococcus, E. coli,* and *H. influenzae.* For dosage, see *cefazolin.* [EHN-sehf]. 315

ancestim (Stemgen) (Chemo).   Used to increase the number of blood progenitor cells collected during pheresis prior to chemotherapy or bone marrow transplant. Orphan drug.

Ancobon (Antifung).   Used to treat severe systemic fungal and yeast infections.   For dosage, see *flucytosine.* [EHN-koh-bawn]. 335

Androcur (Endo).   Used to treat severe hirsutism. For dosage, see *cyproterone.*

Androderm (Endo).   Male sex hormone used to treat the lack of production of testosterone due to absence, injury, or malfunction of the testes or malfunction of the pituitary gland; used to treat delayed puberty in boys.   For dosage, see *testosterone.* [EHN-droh-dehrm].

AndroGel (Antivir).   Used to treat AIDS wasting syndrome.   For dosage, see *testosterone.* 327

AndroGel (Endo).   Topical male sex hormone used to treat lack of production of testosterone due to absence, injury, or malfunction of the testes or malfunction of the pituitary gland. Gel: 1%. [EHN-droh- jehl].

Androgel-DHT (Antivir).   Used to treat AIDS wasting syndrome.   For dosage, see *dihydrotestosterone.* 327

Android (Chemo, Endo).   Male sex hormone used to treat breast cancer in women; used to treat the lack of production of testosterone due to absence, injury, or malfunction of the testes or malfunction of the pituitary gland; used to treat delayed puberty in boys. For dosage, see *methyltestosterone.* [EHN-droyd].

Anectine, Anectine Flo-Pack (Anes, Resp).   Muscle-relaxing drug used during surgery; used to treat patients who are intubated and on the ventilator. For dosage, see *succinylcholine.* 199, 370

Anestacon (Uro) (generic *lidocaine*).   Topical anesthetic applied to the urethra prior to cystoscopic procedures. Jelly: 2%. 111

anesthesia, drugs for. 365
   dermatologic. 94
   epidural. 368
   general. 61, 369

   inhalation. 370
   intravenous. 369
   local. 61, 368
   nerve block. 368
   regional. 368
   spinal. 368
   topical. 94, 222

anesthesia, history of. Historical Notes feature. 366

anesthetics (Anes).   Class of drugs used to completely block the sensation of pain. See also *anesthesia.* 365

Anexsia 5/500, Anexsia 7.5/650, Anexsia 10/660 (Analges) (generic *hydrocodone, acetaminophen*). Combination narcotic and nonnarcotic analgesic drug. (Schedule III drug). Tablet: 5 mg/500 mg, 7.5 mg/650 mg, 10 mg/660 mg. [ah-NECK-see-ah]. 302

angina pectoris, drugs used to treat. 155

Angiomax (Hem).   Direct thrombin inhibitor anticoagulant drug used to treat patients with unstable angina who are undergoing percutaneous transluminal coronary angioplasty.   For dosage, see *bivalirudin.*

angiotensin-converting enzyme (ACE) inhibitors (Cardio).   See *ACE inhibitors.*

angiotensin II receptor blockers (ARBs) (Cardio). Class of drugs that block angiotensin II. 164

anisindione (Miradon) (Hem).   Anticoagulant. Tablet: 50 mg. 186

(anisotropine) (GI).   No longer on the market. (Trade name *Valpin*; gastrointestinal antispasmodic drug).

anistreplase (Eminase) (Cardio, Hem).   Thrombolytic enzyme used to dissolve blood clots that cause a myocardial infarction. Intravenous (powder to be reconstituted): 30 units. [eh-nih-STREH-plays]. 172, 188

anorexia nervosa, drugs used to treat. 290

anorexients (GI).   Class of drugs also known as *appetite suppressants.* [eh-noh-REHK-see-ehnts]. 129

Ansaid (Analges, OB/GYN, Ortho).   Nonsteroidal anti-inflammatory drug used to treat migraine headaches; used to treat dysmenorrhea; used to treat gout, osteoarthritis, and rheumatoid arthritis.   For dosage, see *flurbiprofen.* [EHN-sayd]. 139, 304, 307

Antabuse. Historical Notes feature. 293

Antabuse (Psych).   Used to deter alcoholic consumption in recovering alcoholics.   For dosage, see *disulfiram.* [EHN-tah-byoos]. 293

antacids (GI).   Class of drugs used to neutralize excess acid in the gastrointestinal tract. 116

Antagon (OB/GYN).   Used to inhibit excessive gonadotropin-releasing hormone from the pituitary gland of patients taking ovulation-stimulating drugs for infertility.   For dosage, see *ganirelix.* 245

antagonism, drug. 57

antagonist (Misc).   Class of drugs used to block receptors and prevent chemicals from affecting cells. 55

Anthra-Derm (Derm) (generic *anthralin*). Topical drug used to treat psoriasis. Ointment: 0.1%, 0.25%, 0.5%, 1%. 87

anthralin (Anthra-Derm, Drithocreme, Micanol) (Derm). Topical drug used to treat psoriasis. Cream: 0.25%, 1%. Ointment: 0.1%, 0.25%, 0.5%, 1%. [ehn-THRAY-lihn]. 87

antianginal drugs (Cardio). Class of drugs used to treat or prevent angina pectoris. 155

antianxiety drugs (Psych). Class of drugs for neurosis/anxiety. Also known as *minor tranquilizers* and *anxiolytic drugs*. 280

antibiotic chemotherapy drugs (Chemo). Class of chemotherapy drugs. 341

antibiotics (Antibio). Class of anti-infective drugs used to inhibit the growth of or kill bacteria, particularly pathogens. 61, 311
 broad-spectrum. 312
 chemotherapy. 341
 ENT. 209
 ophthalmic. 218
 topical. 88
 urinary tract. 105

antibiotics in soaps and development of resistant bacteria. Focus on Healthcare Issues feature. 89

antibiotic-resistant bacteria. Focus on Healthcare Issues feature. 319

antibody. 54

anticholinergic drugs (Misc). Class of drugs that opposes the action of acetylcholine. 61, 269

anticoagulant drugs (Hem). Class of drugs used to inhibit blood clotting. 185

anticonvulsant drugs (Neuro). Class of drugs used to treat epilepsy. 263

antidepressant drugs (Psych). Class of drugs used to treat depression. 61, 285

antidiabetic drugs (Endo). Class of drugs used to treat diabetes mellitus. 236, 240

antidiarrheal drugs (GI). Class of drugs used to treat diarrhea. 122

antiemetic drugs (GI). Class of drugs used to relieve nausea and vomiting. 61, 127

antiepilepsirine (Neuro). Anticonvulsant drug used to treat tonic-clonic seizures. Orphan drug.

antiepileptic drugs (Neuro). Class of drugs used to prevent and treat seizures. 263

antiflatulance drugs (GI). Class of drugs used to treat intestinal gas and bloating. 117

antifungal drugs (Antifung, Derm). Class of drugs used to treat fungal infections. 61
 topical. 89
 systemic. 334

anti-gas drugs (GI). Class of drugs used to treat intestinal gas and bloating. 117

antigen. 54

antihistamines (Derm, ENT, Oph). Class of drugs used to block the effect of histamine (itching, redness, swelling) in allergic reactions. 61
 topical. 93
 systemic. 206

antihypertensive drugs (Cardio). Class of drugs used to treat high blood pressure. 61, 161

anti-infective drugs (Antibio). Class of drugs that includes both sulfonamides and antibiotics. 311

anti-inflammatory drugs (Derm, Ortho). Class of drugs used to decrease inflammation. 61

Antilirium (Emerg, Neuro, Psych). Tricylic antidepressant antagonist used as an antidote to reverse an overdose of a tricyclic antidepressant; used to treat ataxia as an orphan drug. For dosage, see *physostigmine*. [ehn-ty-LEER-ee-uhm]. 183, 277, 294

antimetabolite drugs (Chemo). Class of chemotherapy drugs. 339

Antiminth (Misc). Used to treat pinworms and roundworms. For dosage, see *pyrantel*.

antineoplastic drugs. See also *chemotherapy drugs*. 61

antipruritic drugs (Derm). Class of drugs used to relieve itching. 62

antipsychotic drugs (Psych). Class of drugs used to treat psychosis. Also known as *major tranquilizers* and *neuroleptics*. 283

antipyretics (Analges). Class of drugs used to treat fever. 299, 300

antiseptics (Misc). Class of topical drugs that inhibit the growth of bacteria without destroying them. 62

antispasmodic drugs (GI, Uro). Class of drugs used to stop spasm and excessive peristalsis of the smooth muscle of the bowel and bladder. 62, 107, 122

antithrombin III (Thrombate III) (Hem). Used to treat patients with antithrombin III deficiency. Intravenous: 500 IU, 1000 IU. 188

antithyroid drugs (Endo). Class of drugs used to treat hyperthyroidism. 230

antitussive drugs (ENT). Class of drugs used to suppress dry nonproductive cough. 62, 210

Antivert, Antivert/25, Antivert/50 (GI). Antiemetic drug used to treat motion sickness. For dosage, see *meclizine*. 128

antiviral drugs (Antivir). Class of drugs used to treat viral infections. 62, 323
 topical. 90
 systemic. 323

antiyeast drugs (Antifung, Derm). Class of drugs used to treat yeast infections.
 topical. 90
 systemic. 335

Antizol (Emerg). Used to reverse an overdose of ethylene glycol (antifreeze) or methanol (wood alcohol). For dosage, see *fomepizole*. 183

Antril (Chemo, Ortho). Used to prevent or treat graft-versus-host disease following bone marrow transplantation; used to treat juvenile rheumatoid arthritis. For dosage, see *interleukin-1*. 148, 361

Anturane (Ortho). Used to treat gout. For dosage, see *sulfinpyrazone*. [EHN-tyour-rayn]. 146

Anusol (GI) (generic *pramoxine*). Topical anesthetic drug used to treat hemorrhoids. Ointment: 1%. [EHN-yoo-sawl].

Anusol-HC, Anusol-HC-1 (GI) (generic *hydrocortisone*). Topical corticosteroid anti-inflammatory drug used to treat hemorrhoids. Cream: 2.5%. Ointment: 1%. Suppository: 25 mg.

anxiety, drugs used to treat. See *antianxiety drugs.*

anxiolytic drugs. See *antianxiety drugs.*

Anzemet (GI). Antiemetic drug; used to treat nausea and vomiting caused by chemotherapy. For dosage, see *dolasetron*. [EHN-zeh-meht]. 127

Aphthaid (Antivir). Used to treat aphthous stomatitis in AIDS patients. Orphan drug. For dosage, see *lactic acid*. [EHP-thayd]. 331

Aphthasol (ENT). Topical drug used to treat aphthous ulcers in the mouth. For dosage, see *amlexanox*. [EHP-theh-sawl].

A.P.L. (Endo, OB/GYN). Ovulation-stimulating drug used to treat infertility; used to treat undescended testicles and hypogonadism in men. For dosage, see *human chorionic gonadotropin*. 244

Aplisol (Resp). Diagnostic test for tuberculosis that uses purified protein derivative (PPD) from *Mycobacterium tuberculosis* injected under the skin. For dosage, see *Mantoux test*. [EH-plih-sawl].

Aplitest (Resp). Screening test device with multiple tines coated with purified protein derivative (PPD) from *Mycobacterium tuberculosis* to test for tuberculosis. For dosage, see *tine test.*

apomorphine (Neuro). Used to treat Parkinson's disease. Orphan drug. 270

apothecary system of measurement. 69

appetite suppressants (GI). Class of drugs used to treat obesity. 129

apraclonidine (Iopidine) (Oph). Topical alpha-agonist drug used to treat glaucoma. Ophthalmic solution: 0.5%, 1%. [eh-prah-CLAW-neh-deen]. 222

Apresazide 25/25, Apresazide 50/50, Apresazide 100/50 (Cardio) (generic *hydralazine, hydrochlorothiazide*). Combination antihypertensive and diuretic drug. Capsule: 25 mg/25 mg, 50 mg/50 mg, 100 mg/50 mg. [ah-PREH-sah-zide]. 167

Apresoline (Cardio). Peripheral vasodilator used to treat congestive heart failure, hypertension, and hypertensive crisis. For dosage, see *hydralazine*. [ah-PREH-soh-leen]. 166

Apri (OB/GYN) (generic *desogestrel, ethinyl estradiol*). Monophasic combination progestins and estrogen oral contraceptive. Tablet: 0.15 mg/30 mcg. [ah-PREE]. 249

(aprobarbital) (Neuro). No longer on the market. (Trade name *Alurate*; barbiturate used to treat insomnia).

aprotinin (Trasylol) (Hem). Hemostatic drug used to decrease perioperative blood loss in patients undergoing coronary artery bypass grafting. Intravenous: 10,000 KIU/mL. [eh-PROH-tih-nihn].

Aptosyn (Chemo). Chemotherapy drug used to treat prostate cancer, breast cancer, and lung cancer. Investigational drug. 347

Aquachloral Supprettes (Neuro). Nonbarbiturate drug used to treat insomnia. (Schedule IV drug). For dosage, see *chloral hydrate*. [ah-kwah-KLOHR-awl soo-PREHTZ]. 272

AquaMEPHYTON (Hem). Used to treat patients with clotting factor deficiency; used to restore normal blood clotting times after an overdose of anticoagulants other than heparin; given prophylactically to newborns to prevent hemorrhagic disease of the newborn. For dosage, see *vitamin K*. [ah-kwah-meh-FY-tohn]. 189

AquaSite (Oph). Artificial tears. Drops.

AquaTar (Derm) (generic *coal tar*). Topical drug used to treat psoriasis. Gel: 2.5%. 86

Aquatensen (Uro). Thiazide diuretic. For dosage, see *methyclothiazide*. [ah-kwah-TEHN-sihn]. 103

(Aquest) (Chemo). No longer on the market. (Generic name *estrone*; hormonal chemotherapy drug).

Ara-A (Derm, OB/GYN). See *vidarabine.*

Ara-C (Chemo). See *cytarabine.*

Aralen (Antibio, GI). Antiprotozoal drug used to treat intestinal amebiasis. For dosage, see *chloroquine*. [EH-rah-lehn]. 321

Aramine (Anes). Vasopressor used to treat hypotension that occurs with spinal anesthesia. For dosage, see *metaraminol*. [EH-rah-meen]. 371

Aranesp (Hem, Uro). Erythropoietin-type drug used to treat anemia caused by chronic renal failure. For dosage, see *darbepoetin alfa*. [EH-rah-nehsp].

Arava (Ortho). Used to treat rheumatoid arthritis. For dosage, see *leflunomide*. 142

ARB (abbreviation for *angiotensin II receptor blocker*). See *angiotensin II receptor blockers.*

(ardeparin) (Hem). No longer on the market. (Trade name *Normiflo*; anticoagulant).

Arduan (Anes). Muscle-relaxing drug used during surgery. For dosage, see *pipecuronium*. 370

Aredia (Chemo, OB/GYN, Ortho). Inhibits the breakdown of bone; used to treat hypercalcemia of malignancy; used to treat the metastatic bone lesions of breast cancer and multiple myeloma; used to prevent and treat postmenopausal osteoporosis; used to treat Paget's disease.   For dosage, see *pamidronate*. [ah-REE-dee-ah]. 144, 148, 362

Arestin (ENT).   Topical drug used to treat periodontal disease. Placed in the pockets between the gums and teeth.   For dosage, see *minocycline*.

Arfonad (Cardio).   Peripheral vasodilator used to treat hypertensive crisis.   For dosage, see *trimethaphan*. 168

argatroban (Acova) (Hem).   Direct thrombin inhibitor used to prevent or treat heparin-induced thrombocytopenia. Intravenous: 100 mg/mL.

Aricept (Neuro).   Cholinesterase inhibitor used to treat Alzheimer's disease.   For dosage, see *donepezil*. [EHR-eh-sehpt]. 271

Arimidex (Chemo).   Hormonal chemotherapy drug used to treat prostate cancer.   For dosage, see *anastrozole*. [ah-RIH-meh-dehks]. 343

Aristocort, Aristocort A (Derm) (generic *triamcinolone*).   Topical corticosteroid anti-inflammatory drug.   Cream: 0.025%, 0.1%, 0.5%. Ointment: 0.1%, 0.5%. [ah-RIHS-toh-kohrt]. 92

Aristocort (Chemo, Endo).   Oral corticosteroid anti-inflammatory drug used to treat leukemia and lymphoma; used to treat severe inflammation in various body systems; used to treat Addison's disease.   For dosage, see *triamcinolone*. [ah-RIHS-toh-kohrt]. 93, 232, 233, 351

Aristocort Forte (Ortho).   Injected corticosteroid anti-inflammatory drug used to treat severe inflammation in various body systems; also injected into a joint to treat osteoarthritis and rheumatoid arthritis.   For dosage, see *triamcinolone*. [ah-RIHS-toh-kohrt FOHR-tay]. 141, 233

Aristocort Intralesional (Derm).   Corticosteroid anti-inflammatory drug injected into skin lesions.   For dosage, see *triamcinolone*. [ah-RIHS-toh-kohrt inh-trah-LEE-shun-awl]. 92

Aristospan Intra-articular (Ortho).   Corticosteroid anti-inflammatory drug injected into a joint to treat osteoarthritis and rheumatoid arthritis.   For dosage, see *triamcinolone*. [ah-RIHS-toh-spehn inh-trah-ahr-TIHK-kyoo-lahr]. 141

Aristospan Intralesional (Derm).   Corticosteroid anti-inflammatory drug injected into skin lesions.   For dosage, see *triamcinolone*. [ah-RIHS-toh-spehn inh-trah-LEE-shun-awl]. 92

Arixtra (Hem).   Used to prevent venous thromboembolus after orthopedic surgery. For dosage, see *fondaparinux*. [ah-RIH-streh].

Arkin-Z (Cardio)   Used to treat congestive heart failure.   For dosage, see *vesnarinone*. 174

Armour Thyroid (Endo).   Thyroid hormone replacement used to treat hypothyroidism.   For dosage, see *desiccated thyroid*. [AHR-mehr THY-royd]. 229

Aromasin (Chemo).   Hormonal chemotherapy drug used to treat breast cancer.   For dosage, see *exemestane*. [ah-ROH-mah-sihn]. 343

arrhythmias, drugs used to treat. 158

arsenic trioxide (Atrivex, Trisenox) (Chemo).   Chemotherapy drug used to treat leukemia; used as an orphan drug to treat multiple myeloma. Intravenous: 1 mg/1 mL. 347

Artane, Artane Sequels (Neuro).   Anticholinergic drug used to treat Parkinson's disease.   For dosage, see *trihexyphenidyl*. [AWR-tayn]. 269

arthritis, see *osteoarthritis* or *rheumatoid arthritis*.

Arthritis Foundation Pain Reliever (Analges, Ortho).   Salicylate drug used to relieve fever and pain in children and adults; used to treat the pain and inflammation of osteoarthritis and rheumatoid arthritis in adults.   For dosage, see *aspirin*. 138, 299

Arthritis Pain Formula (Analges, Ortho) (generic *aspirin, aluminum, magnesium*).   Combination drug with aspirin and two antacids used to treat osteoarthritis and rheumatoid arthritis. Tablet: 500 mg/antacid. 138, 301

Arthropan (Analges, Ortho).   Salicylate nonaspirin analgesic drug used to treat mild-to-moderate pain and fever; used to treat inflammation; used to treat osteoarthritis and rheumatoid arthritis.   For dosage, see *choline salicylate*. [AWR-throh-pehn]. 138, 300

Arthrotec (Analges, Ortho) (generic *diclofenac, misoprostol*).   Combination nonsteroidal anti-inflammatory drug and synthetic prostaglandin; used to treat the pain of osteoarthritis and rheumatoid arthritis while protecting the stomach lining. Tablet: 50 mg/200 mcg, 75 mg/200 mcg. [AWR-throh-tehk]. 140, 305

artificial tears (Akwa Tears, AquaSite, Bion Tears, Celluvisc, Comfort Tears, Dry Eyes, GenTeal, HypoTears, HypoTears PF, Isopto Plain, Isopto Tears, Liquifilm Tears, Moisture Drops, Moisture Eyes, Murine, Murocel, Nu-Tears, Nu-Tears II, Ocucoat, Ocucoat PF, Refresh, Refresh Plus, Refresh Tears, Tears Naturale, Tears Naturale Free, Tears Naturale II, Tears Plus, Tears Renewed, Ultra Tears) (Oph).   Used to treat dry eyes. Drops.

A.S. or **AS** (abbreviation meaning *left ear*).

ASA (abbreviation for *acetylsalicylic acid*).   See *aspirin*.

ASA (abbreviation for *aminosalicylic acid*).   See *ulcerative colitis, drugs for*.

Asacol (GI).   Anti-inflammatory-type drug used to treat ulcerative colitis.   For dosage, see *mesalamine*. [AA-sah-kawl]. 126

ascorbic acid (vitamin C) (Uro). Over-the-counter (vitamin C) dietary supplement used to acidify the urine.

Ascriptin, Ascriptin A/D, Ascriptin Extra Strength (Analges, Ortho) (generic *aspirin, aluminum, calcium, magnesium*). Combination drug with aspirin and antacids used to treat fever and pain; used to treat the pain of osteoarthritis and rheumatoid arthritis. Tablet: 325 mg/50 mg/50 mg/50 mg, 325 mg/75 mg/75 mg/75 mg, 500 mg/80 mg/80 mg/80 mg. [ah-SKRIP-tihn]. 138, 301

(Asendin) (Psych). No longer on the market. (Generic name *amoxapine*; tricyclic antidepressant).

asparaginase (Elspar) (Chemo). Chemotherapy enzyme drug used to treat leukemia. Intramuscular or intravenous (powder to be reconstituted): 10,000 IU. [eh-SPEH-reh-geh-nays]. 345

Aspergum (Analges). Salicylate drug used to relieve fever and pain. For dosage, see *aspirin*. [EH-spehr-guhm].

aspirin. Historical Notes feature. 300

aspirin (Bayer Low Adult Strength, Ecotrin Adult Low Strength, Genuine Bayer Aspirin, ½ Halfprin, Halfprin 81, Heartline, St. Joseph Adult Chewable Aspirin) (Cardio, Hem, Neuro). Salicylate drug used to treat a current myocardial infarction and prevent a repeat myocardial infarction; anticoagulant; used to prevent transient ischemic attacks and strokes. Chewable tablet: 81 mg. Tablet: 81 mg, 165 mg, 325 mg. [EH-spih-rihn]. 158, 187

aspirin (Arthritis Foundation Pain Reliever, Aspergum, Bayer Children's Aspirin, Ecotrin, Ecotrin Maximum Strength, Empirin, Extended Release Bayer 8-Hour, Extra Strength Bayer Enteric 500, Genuine Bayer Aspirin, Maximum Bayer Aspirin, Norwich Extra-Strength, ZORprin) (Analges, Ortho). Salicylate drug used to relieve fever and pain in children and adults; used to treat the pain and inflammation of osteoarthritis and rheumatoid arthritis in adults. Gum: 227.5 mg. Caplet/tablet/enteric-coated tablet: 325 mg, 500 mg, 650 mg, 800 mg. Suppository: 120 mg, 200 mg, 300 mg, 600 mg. [EH-spih-rihn]. 138, 299, 300

Aspirin Free Anacin Maximum Strength (Analges, Ortho). Nonnarcotic nonaspirin analgesic drug used to treat fever and pain in children and adults; used to treat the pain of osteoarthritis. For dosage, see *acetaminophen*. 139, 301

Aspirin-Free Bayer Select Allergy Sinus (ENT) (generic *pseudoephedrine, chlorpheniramine, acetaminophen*). Combination decongestant, antihistamine, and analgesic drug. Caplet: 30 mg/2 mg/500 mg.

Aspirin-Free Bayer Select Head & Chest Cold (ENT) (generic *pseudoephedrine, dextromethorphan, guaifen-esin*). Combination decongestant, nonnarcotic antitussive, and expectorant drug. Caplet: 30 mg/10 mg/100 mg.

Asprimox, Asprimox Extra Protection for Arthritis Pain (Analges, Ortho). Combination aspirin and antacid drug. Caplet: 325 mg/antacid. Tablet: 325 mg/ antacid. [EH-sprih-mawks]. 301

Astelin (ENT). Antihistamine spray used to treat allergic rhinitis. For dosage, see *azelastine*. [EHS-teh-lihn]. 207

(astemizole) (ENT). No longer on the market. (Trade name *Hismanal*; antihistamine).

AsthmaHaler Mist (Resp). Bronchodilator. For dosage, see *epinephrine*. 193

AsthmaNefrin (Resp). Bronchodilator. For dosage, see *epinephrine*. 193

Astramorph PF (Analges, Anes, Cardio, OB/GYN). Narcotic analgesic drug used to treat moderate-to-severe pain; used as a preoperative drug to sedate and supplement anesthesia; used to treat dyspnea from congestive heart failure; used to treat the pain of childbirth. (Schedule II drug). For dosage, see *morphine*. [EH-strah-mohrf]. 173, 297

asystole, drugs used to treat. 180

Atacand (Cardio). Angiotensin II receptor blocker used to treat hypertension. For dosage, see *candesartan*. 164

Atacand HCT (Cardio) (generic *candesartan, hydrochlorothiazide*). Combination angiotensin II receptor blocker and diuretic drug used to treat hypertension. Tablet: 16/12.5 mg, 32/12.5 mg. 167

Atarax, Atarax 100 (Derm). Drug used to treat severe itching. For dosage, see *hydroxyzine*. [EH-teh-rehks].

Atarax, Atarax 100 (Psych). Drug used to treat anxiety and neurosis; used to treat hysteria; used to treat alcohol withdrawal. For dosage, see *hydroxyzine*. [EH-teh-rehks]. 282

atenolol (Tenormin) (Analges, GI, Psych). Cardioselective beta-blocker drug used to treat migraine headaches; used to prevent rebleeding from esophageal varices in patients with cirrhosis; used to treat alcohol withdrawal syndrome and performance anxiety. Tablet: 25 mg, 50 mg, 100 mg. Intravenous: 5 mg/10 mL. [ah-TEH-noh-lawl]. 132, 290, 306

atenolol (Tenormin) (Cardio). Cardioselective beta-blocker drug used to treat angina pectoris, hypertension, and ventricular arrhythmias; used to prevent repeat myocardial infarction. Tablet: 25 mg, 50 mg, 100 mg. Intravenous: 5 mg/10 mL. [ah-TEH-noh-lawl]. 157, 158, 160, 162

atevirdine mesylate (Antivir). Antiviral drug used to treat AIDS. Investigational drug. 325

athlete's foot, drugs used to treat. 89

Ativan (Anes, Neuro, Psych).   Benzodiazepine drug used as a preoperative medication to decrease anxiety and produce sedation; used to treat status epilepticus; used to treat chronic insomnia; used to treat anxiety and neurosis; used to treat alcohol withdrawal. (Schedule IV drug).   For dosage, see *lorazepam*. [EH-teh-vehn]. 267, 272, 281, 371

atorvastatin (Lipitor) (Cardio).   HMG-CoA reductase inhibitor drug used to treat hypercholesterolemia. Tablet: 10 mg, 20 mg, 40 mg. [eh-tohr-vah-STEH-tihn]. 170

atovaquone (Mepron) (Antivir).   Used to treat *Pneumocystis carinii* pneumonia in AIDS patients. Liquid: 750 mg/5 mL. 328

atracurium (Tracrium) (Anes, Resp).   Muscle-relaxing drug used during surgery; used to treat patients who are intubated and on the ventilator. Intravenous: 10 mg/mL. [eh-trah-KYOUR-ee-uhm]. 199, 370

Atragen (Chemo).   Vitamin A-type chemotherapy drug used to treat leukemia; investigational drug used to treat non-Hodgkin's lymphoma and Kaposi's sarcoma.   For dosage, see *tretinoin*. [EH-trah-jehn]. 348

Atretol (Neuro, Psych).   Anticonvulsant drug used to treat tonic-clonic and partial seizures; used to treat trigeminal neuralgia; used to treat schizophrenia; used to treat manic-depressive disorder.   For dosage, see *carbamazepine*. [EH-treh-tawl]. 265, 283, 289

Atrivex (Chemo).   Chemotherapy drug used as an orphan drug to treat multiple myeloma.   For dosage, see *arsenic trioxide*. [EH-trih-vehks]. 347

Atromid-S (Cardio).   Used to treat hypertriglyceridemia by decreasing serum triglycerides and very low-density lipoprotein levels.   For dosage, see *clofibrate*. [EH-troh-mihd S]. 171

atropine (Anes, Cardio, Emerg).   Anticholinergic drug used to facilitate endotracheal intubation by decreasing oral secretions; used as an antiarrhythmic drug to treat bradycardia; used as an emergency drug during resuscitation. Endotracheal, intracardiac, intramuscular, or intravenous: 0.05 mg/mL, 0.1 mg/mL, 0.3 mg/mL, 0.4 mg/mL, 0.5 mg/mL, 0.8 mg/mL, 1 mg/mL. [EH-troh-peen]. 159, 180, 370

atropine (Atropine Care, Atropisol, Isopto Atropine) (Oph).   Topical mydriatic drug. Ophthalmic ointment: 1%. Ophthalmic solution: 0.5%, 1%, 2%. [EH-troh-peen]. 223

Atropine Care (Oph).   Topical mydriatic drug.   For dosage, see *atropine*. [EH-troh-peen]. 223

Atropisol (Oph).   Topical mydriatic drug.   For dosage, see *atropine*. [eh-TROH-peh-sawl]. 223

Atrovent (ENT, Resp).   Used to treat allergic rhinitis; bronchodilator.   For dosage, see *ipratropium*. [EH-troh-vehnt]. 193, 214

A/T/S (Derm) (generic *erythromycin*).   Topical antibiotic used to treat acne vulgaris. Gel: 2%. Liquid: 1.5%, 2%. 84

attapulgite (Children's Kaopectate, Donnagel, Kaolin with Pectin, Kaopectate Advanced Formula, Kaopectate Maximum Strength, Parepectolin, Rheaban Maximum Strength) (GI).   Antidiarrheal drug. Caplet: 750 mg. Liquid: 750 mg/15 mL, 600 mg/15 mL. Chewable tablet: 600 mg. Suspension. 124

attention-deficit/hyperactivity disorder (ADHD), drugs used to treat. 291

A.U. or **AU** (abbreviation meaning *both ears*).

Augmentin, Augmentin ES-600 (Antibio) (generic *amoxicillin, clavulanic acid*).   Combination penicillin-type antibiotic and beta-lactimase inhibitor drug. Tablet: 250 mg/125 mg, 500 mg/125 mg, 875 mg/125 mg. Chewable tablet: 125 mg/31.25 mg, 200 mg/28.5 mg, 250 mg/62.5 mg, 400 mg/57 mg. Liquid: 124 mg/31.25 mg per 5 mL, 200 mg/28.5 mg per 5 mL, 250 mg/62.5 mg per 5 mL, 400 mg/57 mg per 5 mL. [AWG-mehn-tihn]. 320

Auralgan Otic (ENT) (generic *benzocaine*).   Topical anesthetic for the ear. Drops. [aw-RAWL-gehn].

auranofin (Ridaura) (Ortho).   Gold compound used to treat rheumatoid arthritis. Capsule: 3 mg. [aw-REH-noh-fihn]. 142

Aureomycin (Derm) (generic *chlortetracycline*).   Topical antibiotic used to treat acne vulgaris. Ointment: 3%. [aw-ree-oh-MY-sihn]. 84

Aurolate (Ortho).   Gold compound used to treat rheumatoid arthritis.   For dosage, see *gold sodium thiomalate*. 142

aurothioglucose (Solganal) (Ortho).   Gold compound used to treat rheumatoid arthritis. Intramuscular: 50 mg/mL. [aw-roh-thy-oh-GLOO-kohs]. 142

Autoplex T (Hem).   Used to treat hemophiliac patients whose bodies produce abnormal inhibitors against clotting Factor VIII.

Avalide (Cardio) (generic *irbesartan, hydrochlorothiazide*).   Combination angiotensin II receptor blocker antihypertensive and diuretic drug. Tablet: 150 mg/12.5 mg, 300 mg/12.5 mg. [EH-vah-lide]. 167

Avandia (Endo, OB/GYN).   Oral antidiabetic drug; used to treat the elevated insulin levels caused by polycystic ovary syndrome.   For dosage, see *rosiglitazone*. [ah-VEHN-dee-ah]. 240

Avapro (Cardio).   Angiotensin II receptor blocker used to treat hypertension.   For dosage, see *irbesartan*. [EH-vah-proh]. 164

(AVC) (OB/GYN). No longer on the market. (Generic name *sulfanilamide*; topical sulfa drug used to treat vaginal yeast infections).

Aveeno (Derm). Topical oatmeal used to treat itching and soothe the skin. Lotion: 1%. Powder for bath water. [ah-VEE-noh].

Aveeno Anti-Itch (Derm). Topical antipruritic drug with calamine. Cream: 3%. Lotion: 3%. [ah-VEE-noh].

Avelox (Antibio). Fluoroquinolone antibiotic used to treat a variety of infections, including *S. aureus* and *H. influenzae*. For dosage, see *moxifloxacin*. [EH-veh-lawks]. 318

Aventyl, Aventyl Pulvules (Analges, Derm, Diab, Neuro, Ortho). Tricyclic antidepressant used to treat migraines; used to treat urticaria; used to treat diabetic neuropathy; used to treat postherpetic neuralgia; used to treat phantom limb pain. For dosage, see *nortriptyline*. [ah-VEHN-tuhl]. 99, 147, 241, 276, 307

Aventyl, Aventyl Pulvules (OB/GYN, Psych). Tricyclic antidepressant used to treat depression; used to treat panic disorder; used to treat premenstrual dysphoric disorder. For dosage, see *nortriptyline*. [ah-VEHN-tuhl]. 255, 286, 289

Avita (Derm) (generic *tretinoin*). Topical vitamin A-type drug used to treat acne vulgaris. Cream: 0.025%. [ah-VEE-tah]. 84

Avitene (Hem). Topical hemostatic aide used to control bleeding during surgery. Dressing. [EH-veh-teen].

Avonex (Antivir, Chemo, GI, Neuro, OB/GYN). Used to treat AIDS; used to treat brain cancer, malignant melanoma, cutaneous T-cell lymphoma; used to treat Kaposi's sarcoma; used to treat non-A, non-B hepatitis; used to treat multiple sclerosis; used to treat genital herpes simplex type 2 infection. For dosage, see *interferon beta-1a*. [EH-voh-nehks]. 133, 148, 276, 326, 330, 346

Axert (Analges). Serotonin receptor agonist drug used to treat migraine headaches. For dosage, see *almotriptan*. [ACK-sehrt]. 306

Axid AR, Axid Pulvules (GI). H_2 blocker used to treat peptic ulcers and *H. pylori* infection. For dosage, see *nizatidine*. [EHK-sihd]. 118

Aygestin (OB/GYN). Progestins hormone drug used to treat amenorrhea; used to treat abnormal uterine bleeding; used to treat endometriosis. For dosage, see *norethindrone*. [ii-JEHS-tihn]. 248, 254

Ayr Saline (ENT). Topical saline nasal moisturizing drug. Drops. Mist.

Azactam (Antibio). Monobactam antibiotic used to treat a variety of bacterial infections, including *E. coli*, *H. influenzae*, *Klebsiella*, and *Pseudomonas*. For dosage, see *aztreonam*. [ah-ZEHK-tehm]. 317

azatadine (Optimine) (Derm, ENT). Antihistamine used to treat allergic rhinitis and allergic reactions with hives and itching. Tablet: 1 mg. [ah-ZEH-teh-deen]. 207

azathioprine (Imuran) (Ortho). Used to treat rheumatoid arthritis. Tablet: 50 mg. Intravenous: 100 mg/20 mL. [aa-zah-THY-oh-preen].

azathioprine (Imuran) (Uro). Immunosuppressant drug given after kidney transplantation to prevent rejection of the donor kidney. Tablet: 50 mg. Intravenous: 100 mg/20 mL. [aa-zah-THY-oh-preen]. 110

AZDU (Antivir). Used to treat AIDS. Orphan drug. 325

azelaic acid (Azelex, Finevin) (Derm). Topical drug used to treat acne vulgaris. Cream: 20%. [aa-zeh-LAY-ihk EH-sihd]. 84

azelastine (Astelin) (ENT). Antihistamine used to treat allergic rhinitis. Spray: 137 mcg/spray. [aa-zeh-LEH-steen]. 207

azelastine (Optivar) (Oph). Topical antihistamine used to treat allergy symptoms in the eyes. Ophthalmic solution: 0.5 mg/mL. [aa-zeh-LEH-steen]. 220

Azelex (Derm) (generic *azelaic acid*). Topical drug used to treat acne vulgaris. Cream: 20%. [AA-zeh-lehks]. 84

azidothymidine (AZT) (Antivir). See *zidovudine*.

azithromycin (Zithromax) (Antibio). Macrolide antibiotic used to treat a variety of infections, including community-acquired pneumonia, *H. influenzae*, gonorrhea, *Chlamydia*, and Legionnaire's disease. Tablet: 250 mg, 600 mg. Liquid (powder to be reconstituted): 100 mg/5 mL, 200 mg/5 mL, 1 g packet. Intramuscular or intravenous (powder to be reconstituted): 500 mg. [aa-zih-throh-MY-sihn]. 198, 319

Azmacort (Resp). Inhaled corticosteroid used to prevent acute asthma attacks. For dosage, see *triamcinolone*. [EHZ-mah-kohrt]. 196

(Azo Gantranol) (Uro). No longer on the market. (Combination sulfonamide and urinary antispasmodic drug).

(Azo Gantrisin) (Uro). No longer on the market. (Combination sulfonamide and urinary tract analgesic drug).

Azopt (Oph). Topical carbonic anhydrase inhibitor drug used to treat glaucoma. For dosage, see *brinzolamide*. [AA-zawpt]. 221

AZT (abbreviation for *azidothymidine*). See *zidovudine*.

Aztec (Antivir). Nucleoside reverse transcriptase inhibitor drug used to treat AIDS. For dosage, see *zidovudine*. 324

aztreonam (Azactam) (Antibio). Monobactam antibiotic used to treat a variety of bacterial infections, including *E. coli*, *H. influenzae*, *Klebsiella*, and *Pseudomonas*. Intramuscular or intravenous (powder to be reconstituted): 500 mg, 1 g, 2 g. [ehz-TREE-oh-nawm]. 317

Azulfidine, Azulfidine EN-tabs (GI, Ortho).   Anti-inflammatory-type drug used to treat ulcerative colitis and Crohn's disease; also used to treat rheumatoid arthritis.   For dosage, see *sulfasalazine*. [aa-ZUHL-feh-deen]. 126, 142

(bacampicillin) (Antibio).   No longer on the market. (Trade name *Spectrobid*; penicillin-type antibiotic).

Baciguent (Derm) (generic *bacitracin*).   Topical antibiotic used to treat superficial bacterial infections. Ointment. 88

Bacillus subtilis. 88

bacitracin (Antibio).   Antibiotic used only to treat staphylococcal pneumonia in infants. Intramuscular (powder to be reconstituted): 500,000 units. [beh-seh-TRAY-sehn]. 319

bacitracin (Baciguent) (Derm, Oph).   Topical antibiotic used to treat bacterial infections of the skin and eyes. Ointment: 500 units/g. Ophthalmic ointment: 500 units/g. [beh-seh-TRAY-sehn]. 88

bacitracin. Historical Notes feature. 88

Backache Maximum Strength Relief (Analges).   Salicylate nonaspirin drug used to treat pain and inflammation.   For dosage, see *magnesium salicylate*.

baclofen (Lioresal) (GI, Neuro, Ortho, Psych).   Skeletal muscle relaxant used to treat intractable hiccoughs; used to treat trigeminal neuralgia/tic douloureux; used to treat severe muscle spasticity associated with multiple sclerosis, cerebral palsy, stroke, or spinal cord injury; used to treat tardive dyskinesia caused by antipsychotic drugs. Tablet: 10 mg, 20 mg. Intrathecal: 10 mg/5 mL, 10 mg/20 mL. See also *L-baclofen*. [BEH-kloh-fehn]. 132, 145, 275, 284

bacterial infections, drugs used to treat. 311
bacterial infections of the skin, drugs used to treat. 88
bactericidal.   Acts to kill bacteria. 62
bacteriostatic.   Inhibits bacterial growth. 62
Bactine Antiseptic Anesthetic (Derm) (generic *benzalkonium, lidocaine*).   Topical combination antiseptic and anesthetic. Liquid, spray. [behk-TEEN].

(Bactocill) (Antibio).   No longer on the market. (Generic name *oxacillin*; penicillin-type antibiotic).

Bactrim, Bactrim DS, Bactrim IV, Bactrim Pediatric (Antibio) (generic *sulfamethoxazole, trimethoprim*).   Combination antibiotic and sulfonamide anti-infective drug used to treat a variety of bacterial infections, including traveler's diarrhea; also used to treat *Pneumocystis carinii* pneumonia in AIDS patients. Liquid:

200 mg/40 mg per 5 mL. Tablet: 400 mg/80 mg, 800 mg/160 mg. Intravenous: 80 mg/16 mg per 5 mL; 400 mg/80 mg per 5 mL. [BEHK-trihm]. 106, 320, 329

Bactroban, Bactroban Nasal (Derm, ENT) (generic *mupirocin*).   Topical antibiotic used to treat bacterial infections of the skin and methicillin-resistant *Staphylococcus aureus* (MRSA) infections of the nose. Cream: 2%. Ointment: 2%. [BEHK-troh-behn]. 88

baking soda (GI).   Antacid home remedy. 117

balanced salt solution (B-Salt Forte, BSS, BSS Plus, Iocare Balanced Salt) (Oph).   Irrigating solution used during eye surgery. Ophthalmic solution.

baldness, drugs used to treat.

baldness.   Historical Notes feature. 99

Balnetar (Derm) (generic *coal tar*).   Topical drug used to treat psoriasis. Liquid: 2.5%. [BAHL-neh-tahr]. 86

balsalazide (Colazal) (GI).   Anti-inflammatory-type drug used to treat ulcerative colitis. Capsule: 750 mg. 126

B&O Supprettes No. 15A, B&O Supprettes No. 16A (Analges) (generic *opium, belladonna*).   Combination narcotic analgesic and antispasmodic drug. (Schedule II drug). Suppository: 30 mg/16.2 mg, 60 mg/16.2 mg. 303

Banthine (GI).   Antispasmodic drug used to treat spasm of the smooth muscle of the bowel.   For dosage, see *methantheline*. [BEHN-theen]. 122

barbiturates (Anes, Neuro).   Class of drugs used to treat insomnia; also used to treat epilepsy; ultra-short-acting barbiturates are used to induce general anesthesia. 263

Basaljel (GI).   Aluminum-containing antacid. Capsule: 500 mg. Tablet: 500 mg. [BAY-sehl-jehl]. 116

basiliximab (Simulect) (Uro).   Immunosuppressant monoclonal antibody given after kidney transplantation to prevent rejection of the donor kidney. Intravenous: 20 mg. [bay-sih-LIHK-sih-mehb]. 110

(Baycol) (Cardio).   No longer on the market. (Generic name *cerivastatin*; used to treat hypercholesterolemia).

Bayer Aspirin, see *Genuine Bayer Aspirin*.

Bayer Buffered Aspirin, Bayer Plus Extra Strength (Analges, Ortho) (generic *aspirin, calcium, magnesium*).   Combination aspirin and antacids. Tablet: 325 mg/antacid, 500 mg/antacid. 139, 301

Bayer Children's Aspirin (Analges).   Salicylate drug used to relieve fever and pain.   For dosage, see *aspirin*. 299

Bayer Low Adult Strength (Cardio, Hem, Neuro).   Salicylate drug used to treat a current myocardial infarction and prevent a repeat myocardial infarction; anticoagulant; used to prevent transient ischemic attacks and strokes.   For dosage, see *aspirin*. 158

Bayer PM Extra Strength Aspirin Plus Sleep Aid (Analges, Neuro) (generic *aspirin, diphenhydramine*). Combination nonnarcotic analgesic and antihistamine sedative. Caplet: 500 mg/25 mg. 302

Bayer Select Chest Cold (ENT) (generic *dextromethorphan, acetaminophen*). Combination nonnarcotic antitussive and analgesic drug. Caplet: 15 mg/500 mg.

Bayer Select Flu Relief (ENT) (generic *pseudoephedrine, chlorpheniramine, dextromethorphan, acetaminophen*). Combination decongestant, antihistamine, nonnarcotic antitussive, and analgesic drug. Caplet: 30 mg/2 mg/15 mg/500 mg.

Bayer Select Head Cold Caplets (ENT) (generic *pseudoephedrine, acetaminophen*). Combination decongestant and analgesic drug. Caplet: 30 mg/500 mg.

Bayer Select Maximum Strength Backache Formula (Analges). Salicylate nonaspirin drug used to treat pain and inflammation. For dosage, see *magnesium salicylate*. 300

Bayer Select Maximum Strength Night Time Pain Relief (Neuro) (generic *acetaminophen, diphenhydramine*). Combination analgesic and antihistamine drug sleep aid. Tablet: 500 mg/25 mg. 273

Bayer Select Maximum Strength Sinus Pain Relief (ENT) (generic *pseudoephedrine, acetaminophen*). Combination decongestant and analgesic drug. Caplet: 30 mg/500 mg.

Bayer Select Night Time Cold (ENT) (generic *pseudoephedrine, triprolidine, dextromethorphan, acetaminophen*). Combination decongestant, antihistamine, nonnarcotic antitussive, and analgesic drug. Caplet: 30 mg/1.25 mg/15 mg/500 mg.

Baypress (Cardio) (generic *nitrendipine*). Calcium channel blocker used to treat hypertension. Investigational drug. 174

BayRab (Antivir). Immunoglobulin used to treat patients exposed to rabies. Intramuscular: 150 IU/mL.

BayRho-D Full Dose (OB/GYN). Immunoglobulin given after delivery to treat Rh-negative mother with an Rh-positive baby to prevent hemorrhagic disease of the newborn in a subsequent pregnancy. Intramuscular: 15–18%.

BayRho-D Mini Dose (OB/GYN). Immunoglobulin given after abortion, amniocentesis, or chorionic villus sampling to treat Rh-negative mother with an Rh-positive baby to prevent hemorrhagic disease of the newborn in a subsequent pregnancy. Intramuscular: 15–18%.

BayTet (Misc). Immunoglobulin used to treat patients exposed to tetanus because of an injury. Intramuscular: 15-18%.

BCG (Pacis, TheraCys, TICE BCG) (Chemo). Chemotherapy drug used to treat bladder cancer. Intravesical by catheter (powder to be reconstituted): 50 mg, 81 mg, 120 mg. 347

BCNU. See *carmustine*.

B-D Glucose (Diab). Used to treat hypoglycemia. For dosage, see *glucose*.

bead (drug form). 38

becaplermin (Regranex) (Derm). Topical drug used to stimulate the growth of granulation tissue in skin ulcers. Gel. 97

beclomethasone (Beclovent, QVAR, Vanceril, Vanceril Double Strength) (Resp). Corticosteroid used to prevent acute asthma attacks. Aerosol inhaler: 42 mcg/puff, 84 mcg/puff. [beh-kloh-MEH-thah-sohn]. 196

beclomethasone (Beconase, Beconase AQ, Vancenase, Vancenase AQ 84, Vancenase Pockethaler) (ENT). Topical intranasal corticosteroid used to treat allergic rhinitis. Metered-dose aerosol: 42 mcg/spray. Spray: 0.042%, 0.084%. [beh-kloh-MEH-thah-sohn]. 208

beclomethasone (orBec) (Chemo). Used to prevent graft-versus-host disease. Orphan drug. 361

Beclovent (Resp). Inhaled corticosteroid used to prevent acute asthma attacks. For dosage, see *beclomethasone*. [BEH-kloh-vehnt]. 196

Beconase, Beconase AQ (ENT). Topical intranasal corticosteroid used to treat allergic rhinitis. For dosage, see *beclomethasone*. [BEH-koh-nays]. 208

bedwetting. 111, 231

Beecham, Thomas. 13

Beepen-VK (Antibio). Penicillin antibiotic used to treat various types of bacterial infections, including *Streptococcus, Staphylococcus, Pneumococcus,* and Lyme disease. For dosage, see *penicillin V*. 313

belladonna. Historical Notes feature. 6

Bellergal-S (GI) (generic *belladona, phenobarbital*). Combination antispasmodic and sedative drug. Tablet: 0.2/40 mg. [BEH-luhr-gehl]. 122

Benadryl (GI, Neuro). Antihistamine with antiemetic effect; used to treat vertigo and motion sickness; anticholinergic effect used to treat Parkinson's disease. For dosage, see *diphenhydramine*. [BEH-nah-drihl]. 128, 269

Benadryl Allergy/Cold, Benadryl Allergy/Sinus Headache (ENT) (generic *pseudoephedrine, diphenhydramine, acetaminophen*). Combination decongestant, antihistamine, and analgesic drug. Caplet: 30 mg/12.5 mg/500 mg. Tablet: 30 mg/12.5 mg/500 mg. [BEH-nah-drihl].

Benadryl Allergy Decongestant (ENT) (generic *pseudoephedrine, diphenhydramine*). Combination decongestant and antihistamine drug. Liquid: 30 mg/12.5 mg. Tablet: 60 mg/25 mg. [BEH-nah-drihl].

Benadryl, Benadryl Allergy, Benadryl Allergy Kapseals, Benadryl Allergy Ultratabs, Benadryl Dye-Free Allergy Liqui Gels (Derm, ENT). Antihistamine used to treat allergic rhinitis and allergic reactions with hives and itching. For dosage, see *diphenhydramine*. [BEH-nah-drihl]. 207

Benadryl, Benadryl Itch Relief, Benadryl Itch Relief Children's Formula, Benadryl Itch Stopping Children's Formula, Benadryl Itch Stopping Maximum Strength, Benadryl Itch Stopping Original Strength, Maximum Strength Benadryl 2%, Maximum Strength Benadryl Itch Relief (Derm) (generic *diphenhydramine*). Topical antihistamine/antipruritic drug. Cream: 1%, 2%. Gel: 1%, 2%. Spray: 1%, 2%. [BEH-nah-drihl]. 93

benazepril (Lotensin) (Cardio). ACE inhibitor used to treat hypertension. Tablet: 5 mg, 10 mg, 20 mg, 40 mg. [beh-NEH-zeh-prihl]. 163

bendroflumethiazide (Naturetin) (Uro). Thiazide diuretic. Tablet: 5 mg, 10 mg. [behn-droh-floo-meh-THY-eh-zide]. 103

(Benemid) (Ortho). No longer on the market. (Generic name *probenecid*; used to treat gout).

Ben-Gay Original Ointment, Ben-Gay Regular Strength, Ben-Gay SPA, Ben-Gay Ultra Strength, Arthritis Formula Ben-Gay, Vanishing Scent Ben-Gay (Ortho). Topical irritant drug used to mask the pain of arthritis and muscular aches. Cream. Gel. Ointment.

benign prostatic hypertrophy (BPH), drugs used to treat. 108

benzphetamine (Didrex) (GI). Appetite suppresant used to treat obesity. Tablet: 25 mg, 50 mg.

Bentyl (GI). Antispasmodic drug. For dosage, see *dicyclomine*. [BEHN-tihl]. 122

Benylin Adult, Benylin DM, Benylin Pediatric (ENT). Nonnarcotic antitussive drug. For dosage, see *dextromethorphan*. [BEH-nih-lihn]. 210

Benylin Expectorant (ENT) (generic *dextromethorphan, guaifenesin*). Combination nonnarcotic antitussive and expectorant drug. Liquid: 5 mg/100 mg. [BEH-nih-lihn].

Benylin Multi-Symptom (ENT) (generic *pseudoephedrine, dextromethorphan, guaifenesin*). Combination decongestant, nonnarcotic antitussive, and expectorant drug. Liquid: 15 mg/5 mg/100 mg. [BEH-nih-lihn].

Benzac 5, Benzac 10, Benzac AC 2½, Benzac AC 5, Benzac AC 10, Benzac AC Wash 2½, Benzac AC Wash 5, Benzac AC Wash 10, Benzac W 5, Benzac W 10, Benzac W Wash 5, Benzac W Wash 10 (Derm) (generic *benzoyl peroxide*). Topical antibiotic used to treat acne vulgaris. Gel: 2.5%, 5%, 10%. Liquid: 2.5%, 5%, 10%. [BEHN-zehk]. 83

BenzaClin (Derm) (generic *benzoyl peroxide, clindamycin*). Topical combination antibiotic drug used to treat acne vulgaris. Gel: 5%/1%. 84

Benzamycin (Derm) (generic *benzoyl peroxide, erythromycin*). Topical combination antibiotic drug used to treat acne vulgaris. Gel. [behn-zah-MY-sihn]. 84

benzimidavir (Antivir). Used to treat cytomegalovirus infection. Investigational drug. 329

benzocaine (Americaine Anesthetic, Bicozene, Dermoplast, Lanacane, Solarcaine, Solarcaine Medicated First Aid) (Derm). Topical anesthetic. Cream: 5%, 6%. Lotion: 8%. Spray: 20%. [BEHN-zoh-kayn]. 94

benzocaine (Americaine Anesthetic) (ENT, GI). Topical anesthetic applied to instruments prior to performing nasogastric intubation, esophagoscopy, laryngoscopy, and sigmoidoscopy. Gel: 20%. [BEHN-zoh-kayn].

benzocaine (Anbesol, Baby Anbesol, Maximum Strength Anbesol, Hurricane, Numzit Teething, Orabase-B, Orabase Baby, Orabase Gel, Orabase Lip, Zilactin-B Medicated) (ENT). Topical anesthetic for the mouth. Cream: 5%. Gel: 6.3%, 7.5%, 10%, 15%, 20%. Liquid: 6.3%, 20%. Lotion: 0.2%. Paste: 20%. Spray: 20%. [BEHN-zoh-kayn].

benzocaine (Auralgan Otic, Tympagesic) (ENT). Topical anesthetic for the ear. Drops. [BEHN-zoh-kayn].

benzocaine (Cepacol Anesthetic, Cepacol Maximum Strength, Mycinettes, Spec-T, Vicks Children's Chlor- aseptic, Vicks Chloraseptic Sore Throat) (ENT). Topical anesthetic used to treat sore throats. Lozenge: 5 mg, 6 mg, 10 mg, 15 mg. Troche: 10 mg. [BEHN-zoh-kayn].

benzocaine (Vagisil) (OB/GYN). Topical anesthetic used to treat the perineum. Cream. [BEHN-zoh-kayn].

benzodiazepine drugs (Neuro, Psych). Class of drugs used to treat epilepsy; used to treat anxiety and neurosis. [behn-zoh-dy-EH-zeh-peen]. 264, 281

benzonatate (Tessalon, Tessalon Perles) (ENT). Nonnarcotic antitussive drug. Capsule: 100 mg, 200 mg. [behn-ZOH-neh-tayt]. 210

benzoyl peroxide (Benzac 5, Benzac 10, Benzac AC 2½, Benzac AC 5, Benzac AC 10, Benzac AC Wash 2½, Benzac AC Wash 5, Benzac AC Wash 10, Benzac W 5, Benzac W 10, Benzac W Wash 5, Benzac W Wash 10, Clearasil Maximum Strength, Desquam-E, Desquam-E 5, Desquam-E 10, Desquam-X 5, Desquam-X 5 Wash, Desquam-X 10, Desquam-X 10 Wash, Fostex 10% BPO, Fostex 10% Wash, Neutrogena Acne Mask, Oxy 10 Maximum Strength Advanced Formula, Oxy

10 Wash, Triaz) (Derm). Topical antibiotic drug used to treat acne vulgaris. Cream: 10%. Gel: 2.5%, 5%, 6%, 10%. Liquid: 2.5%, 5%, 10%. Lotion: 5%, 10%. Mask: 5%. [behn-zoyl peh-RAWK-side]. 83

benzphetamine (Didrex) (GI). Appetite suppressant. (Schedule III drug). Tablet: 25 mg, 50 mg. [behnz-FEH-tah-meen]. 129

(benzquinamide) (GI). No longer on the market. (Trade name *Emete-Con*; antiemetic drug).

benzthiazide (Exna) (Uro). Thiazide diuretic. Tablet: 50 mg. [behn-THY-ah-zide]. 103

benztropine (Cogentin) (Neuro). Anticholinergic drug used to treat Parkinson's disease. Tablet: 0.5 mg. Intramuscular or intravenous: 1 mg/mL. [behnz-TROH-peen]. 269

benzydamine (Tantum) (Chemo). Used to prevent oral mucositis in patients receiving radiation therapy for head and neck cancer. Orphan drug. 350

bepridil (Vascor) (Cardio). Calcium channel blocker used to treat angina pectoris. Tablet: 200 mg, 300 mg, 400 mg. [BEH-prih-dihl]. 157

beractant (Survanta) (Resp). Natural lung surfactant used to prevent and treat respiratory distress syndrome in premature newborns. Endotracheal tube: 25 mg/mL. [beh-REHK-tehnt]. 201

beraprost (Resp). Vasodilator used to treat pulmonary arterial hypertension. Orphan drug.

Berinert P (Misc). Used to treat hereditary angioedema. Orphan drug.

Berocca Parenteral Nutrition (I.V.). Intravenous combination drug of nine water-soluble and three fat-soluble vitamins. 378

Berocca Plus (Misc). Multivitamin with iron nutritional supplement. Tablet.

Berotec (Resp) (generic *fenoterol*). Bronchodilator. Investigational drug. 193

beta 1 and 2 receptors. See *receptor*.

beta-blockers (Analges, Cardio, Oph, Ortho, Psych). Class of drugs used to treat many different cardiac conditions; some beta-blockers are used to treat migraine headaches, glaucoma, essential familial tremors, situational anxiety, and other conditions. 146, 156, 160, 306

Betadine (Derm, ENT, OB/GYN) (generic *povidone iodine*). Topical iodine-containing anti-infective drug used as a hand wash and preoperative surgical skin scrub; used at the site of insertion of an I.V. or catheter; also used as a mouthwash/gargle; also used as a vaginal gel or perineal wash. Cream: 5%. Liquid: 10%. Ointment: 10%. Perineal wash: 10%. Shampoo: 7.5%. Spray: 5%. Surgical scrub: 7.5%. Swabstick: 10%. Vaginal gel: 10%. [BAY-tah-dine]. 98

Betadine Medicated Douche (OB/GYN). Antibacterial povidone iodine vaginal douche. Douche: 10%. [BAY-teh-dine].

Betagan Liquifilm (Oph). Topical beta-receptor blocker used to treat glaucoma. For dosage, see *levobunolol*. [BAY-tah-gehn]. 221

betaine (Cystadane) (Uro). Used to treat homocystinuria. Orphan drug.

beta-lactam ring. 313

beta-lactamase. 313

betamethasone (Alphatrex, Betatrex, Diprolene, Diprolene AF, Diprosone, Luxiq, Maxivate, Psorian, Teladar) (Derm). Topical corticosteroid anti-inflammatory drug used to treat various skin conditions. Cream: 0.05%, 0.1%. Foam: 1.2 mg/g. Gel: 0.05%. Lotion: 0.05%, 0.1%. Ointment: 0.05%, 0.1%. Spray: 0.1%. [bay-tah-MEH-theh-sohn]. 92

betamethasone (Alphatrex, Diprosone, Maxivate) (Uro). Topical corticosteroid anti-inflammatory drug used to treat phimosis (nonretractable foreskin). Cream: 0.05%. [bay-tah-MEH-theh-sohn]. 111

betamethasone (Celestone) (Endo). Oral and intravenous corticosteroid anti-inflammatory drug used to treat severe inflammation in various body systems. Tablet: 0.6 mg. Syrup: 0.6 mg/5 mL. Intravenous: 4 mg/mL. [bay-tah-MEH-theh-sohn]. 232

betamethasone (Celestone Soluspan) (Derm, Ortho). Corticosteroid anti-inflammatory drug injected into skin lesions; also injected into a joint to treat osteoarthritis, rheumatoid arthritis, and gouty arthritis; also injected near a joint to treat bursitis and tenosynovitis. Intra-articular, periarticular, or intradermal: 3 mg/mL. [bay-tah-MEH-theh-sohn]. 92, 141

Betapace, Betapace AF (Cardio). Nonselective beta-blocker used to treat ventricular arrhythmias. For dosage, see *sotalol*. [BAY-tah-pays]. 160

beta receptors. In Depth feature.

BetaRx (Diab). Encapsulated pig islet cells used to treat patients with diabetes mellitus. Orphan drug. 241

Betasept (Derm) (generic *chlorhexidine*). Topical anti-infective hand wash and preoperative surgical skin scrub. Liquid: 4%. [BAH-tah-sehpt]. 98

Betaseron (Antivir, Chemo, GI, Neuro, OB/GYN). Used to treat AIDS; used to treat brain cancer, malignant melanoma, cutaneous T-cell lymphoma; used to treat Kaposi's sarcoma; used to treat hepatitis; used to treat multiple sclerosis; used to treat genital herpes simplex type 2 infection. For dosage, see *interferon beta-1b*. [bay-tah-SEH-rawn]. 276, 326, 330

Betathine (Chemo). Chemotherapy drug used to treat multiple myeloma. Orphan drug. 347

Betatrex (Derm) (generic *betamethasone*). Topical corticosteroid anti-inflammatory drug. Cream: 0.1%. Lotion: 0.1%. Ointment: 0.1%. [BAY-tah-trehks]. 92

betaxolol (Betoptic, Betoptic S) (Oph). Topical beta-receptor blocker used to treat glaucoma. Ophthalmic solution: 0.25%, 0.5%. [beh-TEHK-soh-lawl]. 221

betaxolol (Kerlone) (Cardio). Cardioselective beta-blocker used to treat hypertension. Tablet: 10 mg, 20 mg. [beh-TEHK-soh-lawl]. 162

Betaxon (Oph). Topical beta-receptor blocker drug used to treat glaucoma. For dosage, see *levobetaxolol*. [beh-TEHK-sawn]. 221

bethanechol (Myotonachol) (Uro). Antispasmodic drug used to treat urinary frequency and urgency. Tablet: 5 mg, 10 mg, 25 mg, 50 mg. [beh-THEH-neh-kawl]. 107

Betimol (Oph). Topical beta-receptor blocker used to treat glaucoma. For dosage, see *timolol*. [BEH-tih-mawl]. 221

Betoptic, Betoptic S (Oph). Topical beta-receptor blocker used to treat glaucoma. For dosage, see *betaxolol*. [beh-TAWP-tihk]. 221

bexarotene (Targretin) (Chemo, Derm). Used to treat the cancerous skin lesions of cutaneous T-cell lymphoma. Capsule: 75 mg. Gel: 1%. [behk-SEH-roh-teen]. 98, 347

Bextra (Analges, OB/GYN, Ortho). Nonsteroidal anti-inflammatory and COX-2 inhibitor drug used to treat dysmenorrhea; used to treat osteoarthritis and rheumatoid arthritis. For dosage, see *valdecoxib*. [BEHK-strah]. 140, 255, 305

Bexxar (Chemo) (generic *iodine 131, tositumomab*). Combination radioactive isotope iodine 131 and monoclonal antibody used to treat non-Hodgkin's lymphoma. Orphan drug. 349

Biaxin, Biaxin XL (Antibio, GI). Macrolide antibiotic used to treat a variety of infections, including *Streptococcus*, *H. influenzae*, and *S. pneumoniae*; used to treat *Mycobacterium avium-intracellulare* in AIDS patients; used to treat *H. pylori* infection of the gastrointestinal tract. For dosage, see *clarithromycin*. [by-EHK-sihn]. 120, 319, 329

bicalutamide (Casodex) (Chemo). Hormonal chemotherapy drug used to treat prostatic cancer. Tablet: 50 mg. [by-kah-LOO-tah-mide]. 343

Bicillin L-A (Antibio). Penicillin antibiotic used to treat various types of bacterial infections, including *Streptococcus* and syphilis; used prophylactically to prevent subacute bacterial endocarditis in at-risk patients undergoing dental or surgical procedures. For dosage, see *penicillin G benzathine*. [BY-sill-ehn]. 313

BiCNU (Chemo). Alkylating chemotherapy drug used to treat multiple myeloma, Hodgkin's disease, and cutaneous T-cell lymphoma. For dosage, see *carmustine*. 341

Bicozene (Derm) (generic *benzocaine*). Topical anesthetic. Cream: 6%. 94

bicyclic antidepressants (Psych). Class of antidepressant drugs that is currently investigational.

b.i.d. (abbreviation for *twice a day*).

bile acid sequestrants (Cardio). Class of drugs used to treat hypercholesterolemia. 169

bimatoprost (Lumigan) (Oph). Topical drug used to treat glaucoma. Ophthalmic solution: 0.03%. [bih-MEH-toh-prawst]. 222

bindarit (Uro). Used to treat lupus nephritis. Orphan drug.

bioavailability. 30, 62

Biocef (Antibio). Cephalosporin antibiotic used to treat a variety of bacterial infections, including *Streptococcus*, *Staphylococcus*, *E. coli*, and *H. influenzae*. For dosage, see *cephalexin*. [BY-oh-sehf]. 315

Bion Tears (Oph). Artificial tears. Drops.

Bio-Rescue (Emerg) (generic *deferoxamine, dextran*). Combination drug used to treat iron poisoning. Orphan drug.

biotransformation. 47

BioTropin (Antivir). Human growth hormone; also used to treat AIDS wasting syndrome. For dosage, see *somatropin*. [by-oh-TROH-pihn]. 327

biperiden (Akineton) (Neuro). Anticholinergic drug used to treat Parkinson's disease. Tablet: 2 mg. [by-PEHR-eh-dehn]. 269

biphasic oral contraceptives. 250

bipolar disorder. See *manic-depressive disorder*.

birth control pills. See *contraceptives*.

bisacodyl (Correctol, Dulcolax, Feen-a-mint, Fleet Laxative, Modane) (GI). Irritant/stimulant laxative. Tablet: 5 mg. Suppository: 10 mg. 124

bismuth (Pepto-Bismol, Pepto-Bismol Maximum Strength) (GI). Antidiarrheal drug; bismuth is an ingredient in other drugs used to treat *H. pylori* infection. Caplet: 262 mg. Liquid: 130 mg/15 mL, 262 mg/15 mL, 524 mg/15 mL. Chewable tablet: 262 mg. 119, 124

Bisolvon (Oph). Used to treat Sjogren's syndrome. For dosage, see *bromhexine*.

bisoprolol (Zebeta) (Cardio). Cardioselective beta-blocker used to treat angina pectoris, hypertension, and ventricular arrhythmias. Tablet: 5 mg, 10 mg. [bih-SOH-proh-lawl]. 157, 160, 162

bitolterol (Tornalate) (Resp). Bronchodilator. Aerosol inhaler: 0.8% (0.35 mg /puff). Liquid for nebulizer: 0.2%. [by-TOHL-teh-rawl]. 193

bivalirudin (Angiomax) (Hem). Direct thrombin inhibitor anticoagulant drug used to treat patients with unstable angina who are undergoing percutaneous transluminal coronary angioplasty. Intravenous (powder to be reconstituted): 250 mg. 187

Blenoxane (Chemo, Resp). Chemotherapy antibiotic used to treat head and neck cancer, cervical cancer, testicular and penile cancer, Hodgkin's disease, and non-Hodgkin's lymphoma; an orphan drug used to treat pancreatic cancer; sclerosing drug administered via chest tube into the lung to treat malignant pleural effusion. For dosage, see *bleomycin*. [bleh-NAWK-sayn]. 342

bleomycin (Blenoxane) (Chemo, Resp). Chemotherapy antibiotic used to treat head and neck cancer, cervical cancer, testicular and penile cancer, Hodgkin's disease, and non-Hodgkin's lymphoma; an orphan drug used to treat pancreatic cancer; sclerosing drug administered via chest tube into the lung to treat malignant pleural effusion. Subcutaneous, intramuscular, or intravenous (powder for reconstitution): 15 units, 30 units. Chest tube (powder to be reconstituted): 15 units, 30 units. [blee-oh-MY-sehn]. 342

Bleph-10 (Oph). Topical sulfonamide anti-infective drug used to treat bacterial eye infections. For dosage, see *sulfacetamide*. 218

Blephamide, Blephemide Suspension (Oph) (generic *prednisolone*, *sulfacetamide*). Topical combination corticosteroid and anti-infective sulfa drug. Ophthalmic ointment: 0.2%/10%. Ophthalmic suspension: 0.2%/10%. [BLEH-fah-mide].

blindness, newborn, drugs used to prevent.

Blocadren (Analges, Ortho, Psych). Nonselective beta-blocker used to treat migraine headaches; used to treat essential familial tremors; used to treat performance anxiety. For dosage, see *timolol*. [BLAW-kah-drehn]. 146, 290, 306

Blocadren (Cardio). Nonselective beta-blocker drug used to treat hypertension and ventricular arrhythmias; used to prevent a repeat myocardial infarction. For dosage, see *timolol*. [BLAW-kah-drehn]. 158, 160, 162

blood. 378

  citrated whole. 378
  packed red blood cells (PRBCs). 379
  platelets. 380
  umbilical cord. 380
  unit of. 379
  whole. 378

blood–brain barrier. 47

blood types. Historical Notes feature. 378

BLU-U (Derm). Blue light used in conjunction with aminolevulinic acid to treat actinic keratoses.

bolus. 374

Bonamil Infant Formula with Iron (GI). Infant formula. Liquid, powder (to be reconstituted).

Bonefos (Chemo). Used to treat increased bone resorption in patients with cancer. Orphan drug.

Bonine (GI). Antiemetic drug used to treat motion sickness. For dosage, see *meclizine*. [BAW-neen]. 128

Boost (GI). Nutritional supplement. Pudding.

bore of needle. 62

Borocell (Chemo). Used to treat brain cancer. Orphan drug. 347

bosentan (Tracleer) (Resp). Endothelin receptor blocker used to dilate the pulmonary blood vessels in patients with pulmonary arterial hypertension. Tablet: 125 mg, 250 mg. 198

Botox (Oph, Neuro, Ortho). Used to treat blepharospasm, nystagmus, and strabismus caused by cervical dystonia (torticollis); used to treat muscle contractures in patients with cerebral palsy. For dosage, see *botulinum toxin type A*. [BOH-tawks]. 147, 275

botulinum toxin type A (Botox, Dysport) (Oph, Neuro, Ortho). Used to treat blepharospasm, nystagmus, and strabismus; used to treat cervical dystonia (torticollis); used to treat muscle contractures in patients with cerebral palsy. Injection (into the eye muscle or affected muscle) (powder to be reconstituted): 100 units. 147, 275

botulinum toxin type B (Myobloc) (Ortho). Used to treat the muscle contractions and abnormal head position of cervical dystonia (torticollis). Intramuscular: 2500 units/0.5 mL, 5000 units/1 mL, 10,000 units/2 mL. 147

bovine colostrum (Antivir). Used to treat diarrhea in AIDS patients. Orphan drug. 328

bovine immunoglobulin (Immuno-C, Sporidin-G) (Antivir). Cow immunoglobulin used to treat *Cryptosporidium parvum* gastrointestinal tract infection in patients with AIDS. Orphan drug. 331

bowel evacuant (GI). Class of drugs used to evacuate the colon prior to surgery or endoscopic procedures. 125

bowel prep (GI). 125

BPH (abbreviation for *benign prostatic hypertrophy*). See *benign prostatic hypertrophy*.

BranchAmin 4% (I.V.). Intravenous fluid for total parenteral nutrition. 376

brand name of drug. 22

Bravavir (Antivir). Used to treat herpes zoster infection (shingles). For dosage, see *sorivudine*. 330

breast milk, drug excretion in.

(Brethaire) (Resp). No longer on the market. (Generic name *terbutaline*; bronchodilator).

Brethine (Resp). Bronchodilator. For dosage, see *terbutaline*. 193

bretylium (Cardio). Used to treat ventricular arrhythmias. Intramuscular or intravenous: 2 mg/mL, 4 mg/mL, 50 mg/mL. [breh-TIH-lee-uhm]. 159

(Bretylol) (Cardio). No longer on the market. (Generic name *bretylium*; used to treat ventricular arrhythmias).

Brevibloc (Cardio). Cardioselective beta-blocker used to treat angina pectoris and ventricular arrhythmias. For dosage, see *esmolol*. [BREH-vih-blawk]. 157, 160, 162

Brevicon (OB/GYN) (generic *norethindrone, ethinyl estradiol*). Monophasic combination progestins and estrogen oral contraceptive. Tablet: 0.5 mg/35 mcg. [BREH-vih-kawn]. 249

Brevital (Anes). Barbiturate used to induce and maintain general anesthesia. For dosage, see *methohexital*. [BREH-vih-tawl]. 369

(Bricanyl) (OB/GYN). No longer used to stop premature labor contractions. (Generic name *terbutaline*).

Bricanyl (Resp). Bronchodilator. For dosage, see *terbutaline*. [BRIH-kah-nihl]. 193

brimonidine (Alphagan, Alphagan P) (Oph). Topical alpha-agonist drug used to treat glaucoma; orphan drug used to treat optic neuropathy. Ophthalmic solution: 0.15%, 0.2%. [brih-MOH-nih-deen]. 222

brinzolamide (Azopt) (Oph). Topical carbonic anhydrase inhibitor drug used to treat glaucoma. Ophthalmic suspension: 1%. [brihn-ZOH-lah-mide]. 221

broad-spectrum antibiotic (Antibio). Class of drugs effective against both gram-negative and gram-positive bacteria.

(bromfenac) (Analges). No longer on the market. (Trade name *Duract*; nonsteroidal anti-inflammatory drug).

bromhexine (Bisolvon) (Oph). Used to treat Sjogren's syndrome. Orphan drug.

bromocriptine (Parlodel, Parlodel Snap Tabs) (Neuro). Used to treat Parkinson's disease. Capsule: 5 mg. Tablet: 2.5 mg. [broh-moh-KRIP-teen]. 268

Bromo Seltzer (GI) (generic *acetaminophen, sodium bicarbonate*). Combination analgesic and antacid. Effervescent granules: 325 mg/2781 mg. 117

brompheniramine (Dimetapp Allergy) (Derm, ENT). Antihistamine used to treat allergic rhinitis and allergic reactions with hives and itching. Liqui-gels: 4 mg. Subcutaneous, intramuscular, or intravenous: 10 mg/mL. [brohm-feh-NEER-ah-meen]. 207

bronchodilators (Resp). Class of drugs used to dilate the pulmonary airways. 62, 193

Bronkaid Dual Action (ENT) (generic *ephedrine, guaifenesin*). Combination decongestant and expectorant drug. Caplet: 25 mg/400 mg.

(Bronkaid Mist) (Resp). No longer on the market. (Generic name *epinephrine*; bronchodilator).

Bronkodyl (Resp). Bronchodilator. For dosage, see *theophylline*. [BRAWN-koh-dihl]. 193

(Bronkometer) (Resp). No longer on the market. (Generic name *isoetharine*; bronchodilator).

(Bronkosol) (Resp). No longer on the market. (Generic name *isoetharine*; bronchodilator).

Brontex (ENT) (generic *codeine, guaifenesin*). Combination narcotic antitussive and expectorant drug. Tablet: 10 mg/300 mg.

Broxine (Chemo). Radiation sensitizer drug used to treat brain tumors. For dosage, see *broxuridine*. [BRAWK-seen]. 361

broxuridine (Broxine, Neomark) (Chemo). Radiation sensitizer drug used to treat brain tumors. Orphan drug. 361

B-Salt Forte (Oph). Irrigating solution used during eye surgery. For dosage, see *balanced salt solution*.

BSS, BSS Plus (Oph). Irrigating solution used during eye surgery. For dosage, see *balanced salt solution*.

Bucladin-S Softabs (GI). Antiemetic drug; also used to treat motion sickness. For dosage, see *buclizine*. [BYOO-kleh-dihn S]. 127, 128

buclizine (Bucladin-S Softabs) (GI). Antiemetic drug; also used to treat motion sickness. Tablet: 50 mg. [BYOO-klih-zeen]. 127, 128

budesonide (Entocort EC) (GI). Corticosteroid anti-inflammatory drug used to treat Crohn's disease. Capsule: 3 mg. [byoo-DEH-soh-nide]. 132

budesonide (Pulmicort Turbuhaler) (Resp). Inhaled corticosteroid used to prevent acute asthma attacks. Turbuhaler (inhaled powder): 200 mcg/puff. [byoo-DEH-soh-nide]. 196

budesonide (Rhinocort, Rhinocort Aqua) (ENT). Topical intranasal corticosteroid used to treat allergic rhinitis. Aerosol nasal inhaler: 32 mcg/spray. Nasal spray: 32 mcg/spray. [byoo-DEH-soh-nide]. 208

Bufferin, Tri-Buffered Bufferin (Analges, Ortho) (generic *aspirin, calcium, magnesium*). Combination aspirin and antacids. Tablet: 325 mg/antacid. 139, 301

Bufferin AF Nite Time (Neuro) (generic *diphenhydramine, magnesium*). Combination antihistamine and magnesium sleep aid. Tablet: 25 mg/500 mg. 273

bulimia nervosa, drugs used to treat. 290

bumetanide (Bumex) (Uro). Loop diuretic. Tablet: 0.5 mg, 1 mg, 2 mg. Intramuscular or intravenous: 0.25 mg/mL. [byoo-MEH-tah-nide]. 104

Bumex (Uro). Loop diuretic. For dosage, see *bumetanide*. [BYOO-mehks]. 104

Buminate 5%, Buminate 25% (I.V.). Intravenous blood product that contains no cellular components and is used to replace plasma protein. 381

bupivacaine (Marcaine, Sensorcaine, Sensorcaine MPF, Sensorcaine MPF Spinal) (Anes). Local, regional nerve block, epidural, and spinal anesthetic. Injection: 0.25%; 0.25% with 1:200,000 epinephrine; 0.5%; 0.5% with 1:200,000 epinephrine; 0.75%; 0.75% with 1:200,000 epinephrine. [byoo-PIH-vah-kayn]. 368

bupivacaine (Marcaine, Sensorcaine) (Dental, Oph, Ortho). Local anesthetic used before dental procedures; used in eye surgery; used to treat osteoarthritis or rheumatoid arthritis. Intraoral: 0.5% with 1:200,000 epinephrine. Intra-articular: 0.5% with 1:200,000 epinephrine. Retrobulbar: 0.75% with 1:200,000 epinephrine. [byoo-PIH-vah-kayn]. 147

Buprenex (Analges). Narcotic analgesic drug used to treat moderate-to-severe pain. (Schedule V drug). For dosage, see *buprenorphine*. [BYOO-preh-nehks]. 297

buprenorphine (Buprenex) (Analges). Narcotic analgesic drug used to treat moderate-to-severe pain. (Schedule V drug). Intramuscular or intravenous: 0.324 mg/mL. [byoo-preh-NOHR-feen]. 297

buprenorphine (Subutex) (Analges, Psych). Used to treat narcotic addiction. Orphan drug. 293, 308

bupropion (Wellbutrin, Wellbutrin SR, Zyban) (GI, Psych, Resp). Antidepressant used to treat depression; used to treat obesity; non-nicotine aid used to help patients stop smoking. Tablet: 75 mg, 100 mg, 150 mg. [byoo-PROH-pee-ahn]. 129, 200, 288

burns, drugs used to treat. 96

Burow's solution (Domeboro) (Derm). Topical astringent drug used to dry oozing areas of the skin. Powder or tablet to be reconstituted into a solution. 95

BuSpar (OB/GYN, Psych). Drug used to treat anxiety and neurosis; used to treat premenstrual dysphoric disorder. For dosage, see *buspirone*. [BYOO-spawr]. 254, 282

buspirone (BuSpar) (OB/GYN, Psych). Drug used to treat anxiety and neurosis; used to treat premenstrual dysphoric disorder. Tablet: 5 mg, 10 mg, 15 mg, 30 mg. [BYOO-speh-rohn]. 254, 282

busulfan (Busulfex, Myleran, Spartaject) (Chemo). Alkylating chemotherapy drug used to treat leukemia; an orphan drug used to treat brain cancer. Tablet: 2 mg. Intravenous: 6 mg/mL. [byoo-SUHL-fehn]. 341

Busulfex (Chemo). Alkylating chemotherapy drug used to treat leukemia. For dosage, see *busulfan*. [byoo-SUHL-fehks]. 341

butabarbital (Butisol) (Anes, Neuro). Barbiturate drug used to provide preoperative sedation; used for short-term treatment of insomnia. (Schedule III drug). Tablet: 15 mg, 30 mg, 50 mg, 100 mg. Liquid: 30 mg/5 mL. [byoo-tah-BAWR-beh-tawl]. 272, 370

butamben (Butesin) (Derm). Topical anesthetic. Ointment: 1%. [byoo-TEHM-behn]. 94

(Butazolidin) (Ortho). No longer on the market. (Generic name *phenylbutazone*; anti-inflammatory drug).

butenafine (Mentax) (Derm). Topical antifungal drug. Cream: 1%. [byoo-TEH-nah-feen]. 89

Butesin (Derm) (generic *butamben*). Topical anesthetic. Ointment: 1%. [BYOO-teh-sihn]. 94

Butisol (Anes, Neuro). Barbiturate drug used to provide preoperative sedation; used for short-term treatment of insomnia. (Schedule III drug). For dosage, see *butabarbital*. [BYOO-tih-sawl]. 272, 370

butoconazole (Femstat 3, Gynazole-1, Mycelex-3) (OB/GYN). Topical drug used to treat vaginal yeast infections. Vaginal cream: 2%. [byoo-toh-KAW-nah-zohl]. 256

butorphanol (Stadol, Stadol NS) (Analges, OB/GYN). Narcotic analgesic drug used to treat moderate-to-severe pain; used to treat pain during labor and delivery. (Schedule IV drug). Intramuscular or intravenous: 1 mg/mL, 2 mg/mL. Nasal spray: 10 mg/mL. [byoo-TOHR-feh-nawl]. 297

butterfly needle. 64, 65

$\bar{c}$ (symbol for *with*).

Cachexon (Antivir). Used to treat AIDS wasting syndrome. Orphan drug. 327

Cafcit (Resp). Used to prevent apnea in premature infants. For dosage, see *caffeine*.

Cafergot (Analges) (generic *ergotamine*, *caffeine*). Combination of two vasoconstrictor drugs used to treat migraine headaches. Tablet: 2 mg/100 mg. [KEH-fehr-gawt]. 307

caffeine (Cafcit) (Resp). Used to prevent apnea in premature infants. Liquid: 10 mg/mL. Intravenous: 20 mg/mL.

Caladryl (Derm) (generic *calamine*, *diphenhydramine*). Topical combination astringent and antihistamine/antipruritic drug. Cream, lotion: 8%/1%. [KEH-leh-drihl].

Caladryl Clear (Derm) (generic *diphenhydramine*, *zinc oxide*). Topical combination antihistamine/antipruritic and astringent drug. Lotion: 1%/2%. [KEH-leh-drihl].

calamine (Derm). Topical astringent drug to dry oozing skin areas. Lotion: 8%. [KEH-leh-mine].

Calamycin (Derm) (generic *benzocaine*, *calamine*, *pyrilamine*, *zinc oxide*). Topical combination anesthetic, astringent, and antihistamine/antipruritic drug. Lotion. [keh-leh-MY-sihn].

Calan (Analges). Calcium channel blocker used to treat migraine headaches. For dosage, see *verapamil*. [KAY-lehn]. 306

Calan, Calan SR (Cardio). Calcium channel blocker used to treat angina pectoris, congestive heart failure, hypertension, and atrial and ventricular arrhythmias. For dosage, see *verapamil*. [KAY-lehn]. 154, 157, 160, 163

calanolide A (Antivir). Used to treat AIDS. Investigational drug. 325

Calcibind (Uro). Used to prevent formation of kidney stones. Powder to be taken with each meal: 5 g. 111

calcifediol (Calderol) (Uro). Used to treat patients on dialysis who have hypocalcemia. Capsule: 20 mcg, 50 mcg. [kehl-sih-feh-DY-awl].

Calcijex (Uro). Used to treat patients on dialysis who have hypocalcemia. For dosage, see *calcitriol*. [KEHL-sih-jehks].

(Calcimar) (Ortho). No longer on the market. (Generic name *calcitonin-salmon*; used to treat osteoporosis).

calcipotriene (Dovonex) (Derm). Topical vitamin D-type drug used to treat psoriasis. Cream: 0.005%. Ointment: 0.005%. [kehl-sih-poh-TRY-een]. 86

calcitonin-human (Cibacalcin) (Ortho). Calcium-regulating hormone used to treat Paget's disease. Orphan drug.

calcitonin-salmon (Miacalcin) (Ortho). Calcium-regulating hormone used to prevent and treat osteoporosis; used to treat Paget's disease. Nasal spray: 200 IU/spray. Subcutaneous or intramuscular: 200 IU/mL. 143

calcitriol (Calcijex, Rocaltrol) (Uro). Used to treat patients on dialysis who have hypocalcemia. Capsule: 0.25 mcg, 0.5 mcg. Liquid: 1 mcg/mL. Intravenous: 1 mcg/mL, 2 mcg/mL. [kehl-sih-TRY-awl].

calcium channel blockers. In Depth feature.

calcium channel blockers (Analges, Cardio). Class of drugs used to treat angina pectoris, arrhythmias, hypertension; used to treat migraine headaches. 154, 157, 160, 163, 306

calcium chloride (Emerg). Used to stimulate a heart contraction during emergency resuscitation. Intracardiac or intravenous: 10%. 180, 181

Calcium Disodium Versenate (Emerg, Neuro). Used to treat lead poisoning and lead encephalopathy. For dosage, see *edetate calcium disodium*. 275

calcium EDTA. See *edetate calcium disodium*.

Caldecort. See *Maximum Strength Caldecort*.

Calderol (Uro). Used to treat patients on dialysis who have hypocalcemia. For dosage, see *calcifediol*. [KAWL-deh-rawl]. 111

calfactant (Infasurf) (Resp). Natural lung surfactant used to prevent and treat respiratory distress syndrome in newborn infants. Endotracheal tube: 35 mg/mL. [kehl-FEHK-tehnt].

Cama Arthritis Pain Reliever (Analges, Ortho) (generic *aspirin, aluminum, magnesium*). Combination aspirin and antacids. Tablet: 500 mg/antacids. [KEH-mah]. 139, 301

Campath (Chemo). Human monoclonal antibody used to treat leukemia. For dosage, see *alemtuzumab*. 346

Camptosar (Chemo). Mitosis inhibitor chemotherapy drug used to treat colon or rectal cancer. For dosage, see *irinotecan*. [KEHMP-toh-sawr]. 344

Canasa (GI). Anti-inflammatory-type drug used to treat ulcerative colitis. For dosage, see *mesalamine*. [keh-NEH-sah]. 126

cancer, drugs used to treat. 337, 351

cancer vaccines (Chemo). Class of chemotherapy drugs. 349

CancerVax (Chemo). Cancer vaccine. Investigational drug. 349

Cancidas (Antifung). Used to treat severe systemic fungal infections. For dosage, see *caspofungin*. [KEHN-keh-dahs]. 335

candesartan (Atacand) (Cardio). Angiotensin II receptor blocker used to treat hypertension. Tablet: 4 mg, 8 mg, 16 mg, 32 mg. [kehn-deh-SAWR-tehn]. 164

Candida albicans, drugs used to treat. 210, 331

candidiasis, drugs used to treat. 210

cannabinoid (GI). Active ingredient in marijuana. See *dronabinol*.

Cannabis sativa (marijuana plant).

Cantil (GI). Antispasmodic drug used to treat spasm of the smooth muscle of the bowel. For dosage, see *mepenzolate*. 122

Capastat (Resp). Antibiotic used only to treat tuberculosis. For dosage, see *capreomycin*. 197

capecitabine (Xeloda) (Chemo). Pyrimidine antagonist chemotherapy drug used to treat breast cancer and colon cancer. Tablet: 150 mg, 500 mg. [keh-peh-SIH-tah-been]. 339

Capitrol (Derm) (generic *chloroxine*). Topical anti-infective drug for seborrheic dermatitis. Shampoo: 2%. [KEH-peh-trawl]. 98

caplet. 34

Capoten (Cardio, Ortho, Uro). Angiotensin-converting enzyme inhibitor drug used to treat congestive heart failure, hypertension, and hypertensive crisis; used to improve survival rate after myocardial infarction; used to treat Raynaud's disease; used to treat rheumatoid arthritis; used to treat nephropathy in patients with diabetes. For dosage, see *captopril*. [KEH-poh-tehn]. 111, 147, 154, 158, 163

Capozide 25/15, Capozide 25/25, Capozide 50/15, Capozide 50/25 (Cardio) (generic *captopril, hydrochlorothiazide*). Combination angiotensin-converting enzyme inhibitor antihypertensive and diuretic drug. Tablet: 25 mg/15 mg, 25 mg/25 mg, 50 mg/15 mg, 50 mg/25 mg. [KEH-poh-zide]. 167

capreomycin (Capastat) (Resp). Antibiotic only used to treat tuberculosis. Intramuscular (powder to be reconstituted): 1 g. [keh-pree-oh-MY-sihn]. 197

Caprogel (Oph). Used to treat traumatic hyphema. For dosage, see *aminocaproic acid*. [KEH-proh-jehl].

capsaicin (hot pepper plant).

capsaicin (Capsin, Zostrix, Zostrix-HP) (Derm, Ortho). Topical irritant drug used to mask the pain of herpes zoster virus lesions (shingles); used to mask the pain of arthritis. Cream: 0.025%, 0.075%. Lotion: 0.025%, 0.075%. [kehp-SAY-sihn].

Capsin (Derm, Ortho). Topical irritant drug used to mask the pain of herpes zoster virus lesions (shingles); used to mask the pain of arthritis. Lotion: 0.025%, 0.075%. [KEHP-sihn].

capsule. 35

captopril (Capoten) (Cardio, Ortho, Uro). Angiotensin-converting enzyme inhibitor drug used to treat congestive heart failure, hypertension, and hypertensive crisis; used to improve survival rate after myocardial infarction; used to treat Raynaud's disease; used to treat rheumatoid arthritis; used to treat nephropathy in patients with diabetes. Tablet: 12.5 mg, 25 mg, 50 mg, 100 mg. [KEHP-toh-prihl]. 111, 147, 154, 158, 163

Carafate (GI). Used to treat peptic ulcers by binding directly to the ulcer site. For dosage, see *sucralfate*. [KEH-rah-fayt]. 119

Carafate (Chemo). Used to treat oral mucositis in patients receiving radiation therapy for head and neck cancer. For dosage, see *sucralfate*. [KEH-rah-fayt]. 350

carbachol (Carbastat, Miostat) (Oph). Miotic drug used only during eye surgery. Intraocular injection: 0.01%. [KAWR-bah-kawl].

carbachol (Carboptic, Isopto Carbachol) (Oph). Topical miotic drug used to treat glaucoma. Ophthalmic solution: 0.75%, 1.5%, 2.25%, 3%. [KAWR-bah-kawl]. 221

carbamazepine (Atretol, Carbatrol, Epitol, Tegretol, Tegretol-XR) (Neuro, Psych). Anticonvulsant drug used to treat tonic-clonic and partial seizures; used to treat trigeminal neuralgia; used to treat schizophrenia; used to treat manic-depressive disorder. Capsule: 200 mg, 300 mg. Chewable tablet: 100

mg. Tablet: 100 mg, 200 mg, 400 mg. Liquid: 100 mg/5 mL. [kawr-bah-MEH-zeh-peen]. 265, 283, 289

carbapenem antibiotics (Antibio). Antibiotic class of drugs. 317

Carbastat (Oph). Miotic drug used only during eye surgery. For dosage, see *carbachol*. [KAHR-bah-steht].

Carbatrol (Neuro, Psych). Anticonvulsant drug used to treat tonic-clonic and partial seizures; used to treat trigeminal neuralgia; used to treat schizophrenia; used to treat manic-depressive disorder. For dosage, see *carbamazepine*. [KAWR-bah-trawl]. 265, 283, 289

carbenicillin (Geocillin) (Antibio). Penicillin-type antibiotic used to treat a variety of bacterial infections, including *E. coli* and *Pseudomonas*. Tablet: 382 mg. [kawr-beh-nih-SIH-lihn]. 313

Carbex (Neuro, Psych). Used to treat Parkinson's disease. Pending use to treat depression. For dosage, see *selegiline*. 269

carbidopa (Lodosyn) (Neuro). Used to treat Parkinson's disease. Tablet: 25 mg. [kawr-beh-DOH-pah]. 268

carbinoxamine (ENT). Antihistamine used to treat allergic rhinitis. Liquid: 2 mg/5 mL. 207

Carbocaine (Anes). Local, regional nerve block, and epidural anesthetic drug. For dosage, see *mepivacaine*. [KAWR-boh-kayn]. 368

carbonic anhydrase inhibitors (Oph). Class of drugs used to treat glaucoma.

carboplatin (Paraplatin) (Chemo). Chemotherapy platinum drug used to treat ovarian cancer. Intravenous (powder to be reconstituted): 50 mg, 150 mg, 450 mg. [kawr-boh-PLEH-tihn]. 345

carboprost (Hemabate) (OB/GYN). Prostaglandin used to produce abortion; used to treat postpartum uterine bleeding. Intramuscular: 250 mcg/ml. [KAWR-boh-prawst]. 248, 255

Carboptic (Oph). Topical miotic drug used to treat glaucoma. For dosage, see *carbachol*. [kawr-BAWP-tihk]. 221

carbovir (Antivir). Antiviral drug used to treat AIDS. Orphan drug. 326

Cardene, Cardene I.V., Cardene SR (Cardio). Calcium channel blocker used to treat angina pectoris, congestive heart failure, and hypertension; used to treat hypertensive crisis. For dosage, see *nicardipine*. 154, 157, 163, 168

cardiac glycosides. In Depth feature. 152

cardiac glycosides (Cardio). Class of digitalis drugs used to treat congestive heart failure. 151

Cardio-Green (Oph). Dye used during angiography of the eye. For dosage, see *indocyanine green*.

cardioplegic solution (Plegisol) (Cardio). Electrolyte solution injected at the beginning of open heart surgery to induce cardiac arrest. Intra-arterial (into the aortic root).

(Cardioquin) (Cardio). No longer on the market. (Generic name *quinidine*; used to treat atrial and ventricular arrhythmias).

cardioselective beta-blockers. 162

cardiovascular drugs. 150

Cardizem, Cardizem CD, Cardizem SR (Cardio). Calcium channel blocker used to treat angina pectoris, hypertension, and atrial and ventricular arrhythmias; used to treat Raynaud's disease. For dosage, see *diltiazem*. [KAWR-dih-zehm]. 157, 160, 163

Cardura (Cardio, Uro). Alpha₁-receptor blocker used to treat hypertension; used to treat benign prostatic hypertrophy. For dosage, see *doxazosin*. [kawr-DYOUR-ah]. 109, 165

carisoprodol (Soma) (Ortho). Skeletal muscle relaxant used to treat minor muscle spasms associated with injuries. Tablet: 350 mg. [kawr-ih-SOH-proh-dawl]. 144

carmustine (BiCNU, Gliadel) (Chemo). Alkylating chemotherapy drug used to treat brain cancer, multiple myeloma, Hodgkin's disease, and cutaneous T-cell lymphoma. Intracranial wafer: 7.7 mg. Intravenous (powder to be reconstituted): 100 mg. [kawr-MUHS-teen]. 341

Carnation Follow-up, Carnation Good Start (GI). Infant formula. Liquid, powder (to be reconstituted).

Carnitor (Antivir). Used to protect against toxicity in patients receiving zidovudine. For dosage, see *levocarnitine*. 331

carprofen (Rimadyl) (Analges, Ortho). Nonsteroidal anti-inflammatory drug for rheumatoid arthritis and osteoarthritis. Already approved for use by veterinarians in cats and dogs. Investigational drug for humans. 147, 304

carteolol (Cartrol) (Cardio). Nonselective beta-blocker used to treat angina pectoris and hypertension. Tablet: 2.5 mg, 5 mg. [kawr-TEE-oh-lawl]. 157, 162

carteolol (Ocupress) (Oph). Topical beta receptor blocker used to treat glaucoma. Ophthalmic solution: 1%. [kawr-TEE-oh-lawl]. 221

Cartrol (Cardio). Nonselective beta-blocker drug used to treat angina pectoris and hypertension. For dosage, see *carteolol*. [KAWR-trawl]. 157, 162

carvedilol (Coreg) (Cardio). Alpha₁ and nonselective beta-receptor blocker used to treat angina pectoris, congestive heart failure, and hypertension. Tablet: 3.125 mg, 6.25 mg, 12.5 mg, 25 mg. [kawr-VEE-dih-lawl]. 155, 157, 165

cascara (GI). Irritant/stimulant laxative. Liquid. Tablet: 325 mg. 124

Casodex (Chemo). Hormonal chemotherapy drug used to treat prostatic cancer. For dosage, see *bicalutamide*. [KEH-soh-dehks]. 343

caspofungin (Cancidas) (Antifung). Used to treat severe systemic fungal infections. Intravenous (powder for reconstitution): 50 mg, 70 mg. [kehs-poh-FUHN-jehn]. 335

castor oil (GI). Laxative. Liquid. 125

Cataflam (Analges, OB/GYN, Ortho). Nonsteroidal anti-inflammatory drug used to treat pain; used to treat dysmenorrhea; used to treat osteoarthritis and rheumatoid arthritis. For dosage, see *diclofenac*. [KEH-teh-flehm]. 139, 255, 304

Catapres (Endo). Alpha-receptor blocker used to diagnose pheochromocytoma of the adrenal cortex. For dosage, see *clonidine*. [KEH-teh-prehs].

Catapres, Catapres-TTS-1, Catapres-TTS-2, Catapres-TTS-3 (Cardio, Resp). Alpha-receptor blocker used to treat hypertension and atrial arrhythmias; used to help patients stop smoking. For dosage, see *clonidine*. [KEH-teh-prehs]. 159, 165, 199

Catapres, Catapres-TTS-1, Catapres-TTS-2, Catapres-TTS-3 (Chemo). Alpha-receptor blocker used to treat severe pain in cancer patients; used to treat cyclosporine-induced nephrotoxicity. For dosage, see *clonidine*. [KEH-teh-prehs]. 361

Catapres, Catapres-TTS-1, Catapres-TTS-2, Catapres-TTS-3 (Derm, Neuro). Alpha-receptor blocker used to treat postherpetic neuralgia/shingles; used to treat hyperhidrosis (excessive sweating). For dosage, see *clonidine*. [KEH-teh-prehs]. 275

Catapres, Catapres-TTS-1, Catapres-TTS-2, Catapres-TTS-3 (Analges, GI, Ortho, Psych). Alpha-receptor blocker used to treat narcotic withdrawal; used to treat ulcerative colitis; used to treat restless legs syndrome; used to treat psychosis and schizophrenia; used to treat the mania of manic-depressive syndrome; used to treat Tourette's syndrome; used to treat attention-deficit/hyperactivity disorder; used to treat alcohol withdrawal. For dosage, see *clonidine*. [KEH-teh-prehs]. 132, 147, 284, 288, 292, 308

(Catarase) (Oph). No longer on the market. (Generic name *chymotrypsin*; used to free the lens during cataract surgery).

Catatrol (Neuro, Psych). Bicyclic antidepressant; used to treat narcolepsy. For dosage, see *viloxazine*. 274

Cathflo Activase (Cardio, Hem). Used to dissolve clots in central venous catheters. For dosage, see *alteplase*. 188, 275

Caverject (Uro). Used to treat impotence due to erectile dysfunction. Injection into penis: 5 mcg/mL, 10 mcg/mL, 20 mg/mL, 40 mcg/mL. 109

cc (abbreviation for *cubic centimeter*).

CCNU. See *lomustine*.

CD (abbreviation for *controlled dose*).

CDDP. See *cisplatin*.

CD4 human immunoglobulin (Antivir). Antiviral drug used to treat AIDS. Orphan drug. 326

CEA-Cide Y-90 (Chemo) (generic *monoclonal antibody, yttrium 90*). Combination monoclonal antibody and radioactive isotope yttrium 90 used to treat ovarian cancer. Orphan drug. 349

Ceclor, Ceclor CD, Ceclor Pulvules (Antibio). Cephalosporin antibiotic used to treat various bacterial infections, including *Streptococcus, Staphylococcus, E. coli,* and *H. influenzae*. For dosage, see *cefaclor*. [SEE-klohr]. 315

Cedax (Antibio). Cephalosporin antibiotic used to treat a variety of bacterial infections, including *Streptococcus* and *H. influenzae*. For dosage, see *ceftibuten*. [SEE-dehks]. 316

CeeNu (Chemo). Alkylating chemotherapy drug used to treat brain cancer and Hodgkin's disease. For dosage, see *lomustine*. 341

cefaclor (Ceclor, Ceclor CD, Ceclor Pulvules) (Antibio). Cephalosporin antibiotic used to treat various bacterial infections, including *Streptococcus, Staphylococcus, E. coli,* and *H. influenzae*. Capsule: 250 mg, 500 mg. Tablet: 375 mg, 500 mg. Liquid: 125 mg/5 mL, 187 mg/5 mL, 250 mg/5 mL, 375 mg/5 mL. [SEH-fah-klohr]. 315

cefadroxil (Duricef) (Antibio). Cephalosporin antibiotic used to treat a variety of bacterial infections, including *Streptococcus, Staphylococcus,* and *E. coli*. Capsule: 500 mg. Tablet: 1 g. Liquid: 125 mg/5 mL, 250 mg/5 mL, 500 mg/5 mL. [seh-fah-DRAWK-sihl]. 315

Cefadyl (Antibio). Cephalosporin antibiotic used to treat a variety of bacterial infections, including *Streptococcus, Staphylococcus, E. coli,* and *H. influenzae*. For dosage, see *cephapirin*. [SEH-fah-dill]. 315

cefamandole (Mandol) (Antibio). Cephalosporin antibiotic used to treat a variety of bacterial infections, including *Streptococcus, Staphylococcus, E. coli,* and *H. influenzae*. Intramuscular or intravenous (powder to be reconstituted): 1 g, 2 g. [seh-fah-MEHN-dawl]. 315

cefazolin (Ancef, Kefzol, Zolicef) (Antibio). Cephalosporin antibiotic used to treat a variety of bacterial infections, including *Streptococcus, Staphylococcus, E. coli,* and *H. influenzae*. Intramuscular or intravenous: 500 mg, 1 g. [seh-fah-ZOH-lihn]. 315

cefdinir (Omnicef) (Antibio). Cephalosporin antibiotic used to treat a variety of bacterial infections, including *Streptococcus, Staphylococcus,* community-acquired pneumonia, and *H. influenzae*. Capsule: 300 mg. Liquid: 125 mg/5 mL. [SEHF-dih-neer]. 316

cefditoren (Spectracef) (Antibio). Cephalosporin antibiotic used to treat bronchitis, pharyngitis, tonsillitis, and skin infections. Tablet: 200 mg. [sehf-dih-TOH-rehn]. 315

cefepime (Maxipime) (Antibio). Cephalosporin antibiotic used to treat a variety of bacterial infections, including *Streptococcus, Staphylococcus,* and *E. coli*. Intramuscular and intravenous (powder to be reconstituted): 500 mg, 1 g, 2 g. [SEH-feh-peem]. 316

cefixime (Suprax) (Antibio). Cephalosporin antibiotic used to treat various types of bacterial infections, including *Streptococcus, E. coli, H. influenzae,* and gonorrhea. Tablet: 200 mg, 400 mg. Liquid (powder to be reconstituted): 100 mg/5 mL. 316

Cefizox (Antibio). Cephalosporin antibiotic used to treat various types of bacterial infections, including *Streptococcus, Staphylococcus, E. coli, H. influenzae,* and gonorrhea. For dosage, see *ceftizoxime*. [SEH-fih-zawks]. 316

cefmetazole (Zefazone) (Antibio). Cephalosporin antibiotic used to treat a variety of bacterial infections, including *Staphylococcus, E. coli,* and *H. influenzae*. Intravenous: 1 g/50 mL, 2 g/50 mL. [sehf-MEH-tah-zohl]. 316

Cefobid (Antibio). Cephalosporin antibiotic used to treat various types of bacterial infections, including *Streptococcus, Staphylococcus, E. coli,* and gonorrhea. For dosage, see *cefoperazone*. [SEH-foh-bihd]. 316

cefonicid (Monocid) (Antibio). Cephalosporin antibiotic used to treat a variety of bacterial infections, including *Streptococcus, Staphylococcus, E. coli,* and *H. influenzae*. Intramuscular or intravenous (powder to be reconstituted): 1 g. [seh-foh-NY-sihd]. 316

cefoperazone (Cefobid) (Antibio). Cephalosporin antibiotic used to treat various types of bacterial infections, including *Streptococcus, Staphylococcus, E. coli,* and gonorrhea. Intramuscular or intravenous (powder to be reconstituted): 1 g, 2 g. [sehf-foh-PEH-rah-zohn]. 316

Cefotan (Antibio). Cephalosporin antibiotic used to treat various types of bacterial infections, including *Streptococcus, Staphylococcus, E. coli, H. influenzae,* and gonorrhea. For dosage, see *cefotetan*. [SEH-foh-tehn]. 316

cefotaxime (Claforan) (Antibio). Cephalosporin antibiotic used to treat a variety of bacterial infections, including *Streptococcus, Staphylococcus, E. coli,* and *H. influenzae*. Intramuscular or intravenous (powder to be reconstituted): 500 mg, 1 g, 2 g. [seh-foh-TEHK-seem]. 316

cefotetan (Cefotan) (Antibio). Cephalosporin antibiotic used to treat various types of bacterial infections, including *Streptococcus, Staphylococcus, E. coli,*

H. influenzae, and gonorrhea. Intramuscular or intravenous (powder to be reconstituted): 1 g, 2 g. [seh-foh-TEE-tehn]. 316

cefoxitin (Mefoxin) (Antibio). Cephalosporin antibiotic used to treat various types of bacterial infections, including *Streptococcus, Staphylococcus, E. coli, H. influenzae*, and gonorrhea. Intramuscular or intravenous (powder to be reconstituted): 1 g, 2 g. [seh-FAWK-sih-tihn]. 316

cefpodoxime (Vantin) (Antibio). Cephalosporin antibiotic used to treat various types of bacterial infections, including *H. influenzae*, staphylococci, *E. coli*, and gonorrhea. Tablet: 100 mg, 200 mg. Granules (to be reconstituted): 50 mg/5 mL, 100 mg/5 mL. [sehf-poh-DAWK-zeem]. 316

cefprozil (Cefzil) (Antibio). Cephalosporin antibiotic used to treat a variety of bacterial infections, including *Streptococcus* and *H. influenzae*. Tablet: 250 mg, 500 mg. Liquid: 125 mg/5 mL, 250 mg/5 mL. [sehf-PROH-zill]. 316

ceftazidime (Ceptaz, Fortaz, Tazicef, Tazidime) (Antibio). Cephalosporin antibiotic used to treat a variety of bacterial infections, including *Streptococcus, Staphylococcus, E. coli*, and *H. influenzae*. Intramuscular or intravenous (powder to be reconstituted): 500 mg, 1 g, 2 g. [sehf-TEH-zeh-deem]. 316

ceftibuten (Cedax) (Antibio). Cephalosporin antibiotic used to treat a variety of bacterial infections, including *Streptococcus* and *H. influenzae*. Capsule: 400 mg. Liquid: 90 mg/5 mL, 180 mg/5 mL. [sehf-tih-BYOO-tehn]. 316

Ceftin (Antibio). Cephalosporin antibiotic used to treat various types of infections, including *Streptococcus, Staphylococcus, H. influenzae, E. coli*, and gonorrhea. For dosage, see *cefuroxime*. [SEHF-tihn]. 316

ceftizoxime (Cefizox) (Antibio). Cephalosporin antibiotic used to treat various types of bacterial infections, including *Streptococcus, Staphylococcus, E. coli, H. influenzae*, and gonorrhea. Intramuscular or intravenous (powder to be reconstituted): 500 mg, 1 g, 2 g. [sehf-tih-ZAWK-seem]. 316

ceftriaxone (Rocephin) (Antibio). Cephalosporin antibiotic used to treat various types of bacterial infections, including *Streptococcus, Staphylococcus, H. influenzae, E. coli*, gonorrhea, and Lyme disease. Intramuscular or intravenous (powder to be reconstituted): 250 mg, 500 mg, 1 g, 2 g. [sehf-try-ECK-zohn]. 316

cefuroxime (Ceftin, Kefurox, Zinacef) (Antibio). Cephalosporin antibiotic used to treat various types of infections, including *Streptococcus, Staphylococcus, H. influenzae, E. coli*, and gonorrhea. Tablet: 125 mg, 250 mg, 500 mg. Liquid: 125 mg/5 mL, 250 mg/5

mL. Intramuscular or intravenous (powder to be reconstituted): 1.5 g. [seh-fyoor-AWK-zeem]. 316

Cefzil (Antibio). Cephalosporin antibiotic used to treat a variety of bacterial infections, including *Streptococcus* and *H. influenzae*. For dosage, see *cefprozil*. [SEHF-zill]. 316

Celebrex (Analges, GI, OB/GYN, Ortho). Nonsteroidal anti-inflammatory and cyclooxygenase-2 inhibitor drug used to treat pain; used to decrease the number of colonic polyps in patients with familial adenomatous polyposis; used to treat dysmenorrhea; used to treat the pain of osteoarthritis and rheumatoid arthritis. For dosage, see *celecoxib*. [SEH-leh-brehks]. 132, 140, 305

celecoxib (Celebrex) (Analges, GI, OB/GYN, Ortho). Nonsteroidal anti-inflammatory and cyclooxygenase-2 inhibitor drug used to treat pain; used to decrease the number of colonic polyps in patients with familial adenomatous polyposis; used to treat dysmenorrhea; used to treat the pain of osteoarthritis and rheumatoid arthritis. Capsule: 100 mg, 200 mg. [sehl-ah-KAWK-sihb]. 132, 140, 305

Celestone (Endo). Corticosteroid anti-inflammatory drug used to treat severe inflammation in various body systems. For dosage, see *betamethasone*. [seh-LEHS-tohn]. 232

Celestone Soluspan (Derm, Ortho). Corticosteroid anti-inflammatory drug injected into skin lesions; also injected into a joint to treat osteoarthritis, rheumatoid arthritis, and gouty arthritis; also injected near a joint to treat bursitis and tenosynovitis. For dosage, see *betamethasone*. [seh-LEHS-tohn SAWL-yoo-spehn]. 92, 141

Celexa (OB/GYN, Psych). Selective serotonin reuptake inhibitor antidepressant used to treat depression; used to treat panic disorder; used to treat social anxiety disorder/social phobias; used to treat premenstrual dysphoric disorder. For dosage, see *citalopram*. [seh-LEHK-zah]. 254, 287, 289, 290

celiprolol (Selecor) (Cardio). Selective beta$_2$-blocker for hypertension and angina pectoris. Investigational drug. 172

CellCept (Cardio, GI, Uro). Immunosuppressant drug given after organ transplantation to prevent rejection of the donor heart, liver, or kidney. For dosage, see *mycophenolate*. 110, 133, 174

Celluvisc (Oph). Artificial tears. Drops.

Celontin (Neuro). Anticonvulsant drug used to treat absence seizures. For dosage, see *methsuximide*. [seh-LAWN-tihn]. 264

Cenestin (OB/GYN). Hormone replacement therapy used to treat the symptoms of menopause. For dosage, see *conjugated estrogens*. [seh-NEHS-tihn]. 252

Centovir (Antivir). Used to treat cytomegalovirus in patients wiith bone marrow transplant. Orphan drug. 329

Centoxin (Antibio). Used to treat gram-negative bacteremia and shock. For dosage, see *nebacumab*. 321

(Centrax) (Psych). No longer on the market. (Generic name *prazepam*; benzodiazepine antianxiety drug).

Ceo-Two (GI). Mechanical laxative that releases CO_2 gas. Suppository. 125

Cepacol Anesthetic, Cepacol Maximum Strength (ENT) (generic *benzocaine*). Topical anesthetic used to treat sore throats. Lozenge: 10 mg. Troche: 10 mg.

cephalexin (Biocef, Keflex, Keftab) (Antibio). Cephalosporin antibiotic used to treat a variety of bacterial infections, including *Streptococcus*, *Staphylococcus*, *E. coli*, and *H. influenzae*. Capsule: 250 mg, 500 mg. Tablet: 250 mg, 500 mg, 1 g. Liquid: 125 mg/5 mL, 250 mg/5 mL. 315

cephalosporins (Antibio). Class of antibacterial drugs. 314

(cephalothin) (Antibio). No longer on the market. (Trade name *Keflin*; cephalosporin antibiotic).

cephapirin (Cefadyl) (Antibio). Cephalosporin antibiotic used to treat a variety of bacterial infections, including *Streptococcus*, *Staphylococcus*, *E. coli*, and *H. influenzae*. Intramuscular or intravenous: 1 g. [seh-fah-PEER-ehn]. 315

cephradine (Velosef) (Antibio). Cephalosporin antibiotic used to treat a variety of bacterial infections, including *Streptococcus*, *Staphylococcus*, *E. coli*, and *H. influenzae*. Capsule: 250 mg, 500 mg. Liquid: 125 mg/5 mL, 250 mg/5 mL. Intramuscular or intravenous: 250 mg, 500 mg, 1 g. [SEH-frah-deen]. 315

Cephulac (GI). Used to decrease blood ammonia in patients with liver disease and encephalopathy. For dosage, see *lactulose*. [SEH-fyoo-lehk]. 133

Ceptaz (Antibio). Cephalosporin antibiotic used to treat a variety of bacterial infections, including *Streptococcus*, *Staphylococcus*, *E. coli*, and *H. influenzae*. For dosage, see *ceftazidime*. [SEHP-tehz]. 316

Cerebyx (Neuro). Anticonvulsant drug used to treat status epilepticus. For dosage, see *fosphenytoin*. [SEHR-eh-bihks]. 265, 267

Ceredase (GI). Used to treat Gaucher's disease. For dosage, see *alglucerase*.

Ceresine (Neuro). Used to treat severe head injury. Orphan drug. 275

Cerezyme (GI). An enzyme drug used to treat Gaucher's disease. For dosage, see *imiglucerase*. [SEH-reh-zime].

(cerivastatin) (Cardio). No longer on the market. (Trade name *Baycol*; used to treat hypercholesterolemia).

Cernevit-12 (I.V.). Intravenous combination drug of nine water-soluble and three fat-soluble vitamins. 378

Cerose DM (ENT) (generic *phenylephrine, chlorpheniramine, dextromethorphan*). Combination decongestant, antihistamine, and nonnarcotic antitussive drug. Liquid: 10 mg/4 mg/15 mg.

Cerubidine (Chemo). Chemotherapy antibiotic used to treat leukemia. For dosage, see *daunorubicin*. [seh-ROO-beh-deen]. 342

Cerumenex (ENT). Topical drug used to soften hardened cerumen in the ear. Drops. [seh-ROO-meh-nehks].

cervical ripening, drugs used to produce. 247

cervical ripening. In Depth feature. 247

Cervidil (OB/GYN). Prostaglandin drug used to ripen the cervix for delivery. For dosage, see *dinoprostone*. [SEHR-veh-dill].

Cetacaine (Derm, ENT) (generic *benzocaine, butamben, tetracaine*). Combination topical anesthetic drug. Gel. Liquid. Ointment. Spray. [SEE-tah-kayn]. 94

Cetamide (Oph). Topical sulfonamide anti-infective drug used to treat bacterial eye infections. For dosage, see *sulfacetamide*. [SEE-tah-mide]. 218

Cetapred (Oph) (generic *prenisolone, sulfacetamide*). Topical combination corticosteroid and anti-infective sulfa drug. Ophthalmic ointment: 0.25%/10%. [SEE-tah-prehd].

cetirizine (Zyrtec) (Derm, ENT). Antihistamine used to treat allergic rhinitis and allergic reactions with hives and itching. Liquid: 5 mg/5 mL. Tablet: 5 mg, 10 mg. [seh-TEER-eh-zeen]. 207

cetrorelix (Cetrotide) (OB/GYN). Used to inhibit excessive gonadotropin-releasing hormone from the pituitary gland of patients taking ovulation-stimulating drugs for infertility. Subcutaneous: 0.25 mg, 3 mg. 245

Cetrotide (OB/GYN). Used to inhibit excessive gonadotropin-releasing hormone released from the pituitary gland of patients taking ovulation-stimulating drugs for infertility. For dosage, see *cetrorelix*. [SEE-troh-tide]. 245

cetuximab (Chemo). Monoclonal antibody used to treat head and neck cancer. Orphan drug. 346

cevimeline (Evoxac) (ENT). Used to treat dry mouth due to Sjogren's syndrome. Capsule: 30 mg.

charcoal, see *activated charcoal*.

Chemet (Emerg, Neuro, Uro). Chelating drug used to treat arsenic, lead, and mercury poisoning and lead encephalopathy; used to treat cystine kidney stones. For dosage, see *succimer*. 112, 277

chemical name of drug. 22

chemoreceptor trigger zone. 127

chemotherapy drugs. 337

chemotherapy enzyme drugs (Chemo). Class of chemotherapy drugs. 345

chemotherapy protocols. 349

chemotherapy toxicity, drugs used to treat. 350

Chenix (GI). Used to dissolve gallstones in patients who cannot have surgery. For dosage, see *chenodiol*. [CHEE-nihks]. 129

chenodiol (Chenix) (GI). Used to dissolve gallstones in patients who cannot have surgery. Tablet: 250 mg. [chee-noh-DY-awl]. 129

Cheracol Cough (ENT) (generic *codeine, guaifenesin*). Combination narcotic antitussive and expectorant drug. Syrup: 10 mg/100 mg. [CHEH-rah-kawl].

Cheracol Nasal (ENT). Decongestant. For dosage, see *oxymetazoline*. [CHEH-rah-kawl]. 206

(Cheracol Plus) (ENT). No longer on the market. (Combination drug with *phenylpropanolamine;* decongestant, antihistamine, and nonnarcotic antitussive drug).

CHF (abbreviation for *congestive heart failure*). See *congestive heart failure*.

Chibroxin (Oph). Topical antibiotic used to treat bacterial eye infections. For dosage, see *norfloxacin*. [cheh-BRAWK-sehn]. 218

Children's Advil, see *Advil*.

(Children's Allerest) (ENT). No longer on the market. (Combination drug with *phenylpropanolamine;* decongestant and antihistamine).

Children's Cepacol (ENT) (generic *pseudoephedrine, acetaminophen*). Combination decongestant and analgesic drug. Liquid: 15 mg/160 mg.

Children's Dramamine (GI). Antihistamine used to treat vertigo and motion sickness. For dosage, see *dimenhydrinate*. 128

Childrens' Feverall (Analges). Nonnarcotic non-aspirin analgesic drug used to treat fever and pain in children. For dosage, see *acetaminophen*. 301

Children's Kaopectate (GI). Antidiarrheal drug. For dosage, see *attapulgite*. 124

Children's Motrin, see *Motrin*.

Children's Nostril, see *Nostril*.

Children's Panadol, see *Panadol*.

Children's Tylenol, Children's Tylenol Soft Chews, see *Tylenol*.

Children's Tylenol Cold (ENT) (generic *pseudoephedrine, chlorpheniramine, acetaminophen*). Combination decongestant, antihistamine, and analgesic drug. Liquid: 15 mg/1 mg/160 mg. Tablet: 7.5 mg/0.5 mg/80 mg.

Children's Tylenol Cold Plus Cough (ENT) (generic *pseudoephedrine, chlorpheniramine, dextromethorphan, acetaminophen*). Combination decongestant, antihistamine, nonnarcotic antitussive, and analgesic drug. Chewable tablet: 7.5 mg/0.5 mg/2.5 mg/80 mg.

Chlamydia, drugs used to treat. 258

chloral hydrate (Aquachloral Supprettes) (Neuro). Nonbarbiturate drug used to treat insomnia. (Schedule IV drug). Capsule: 500 mg. Liquid: 250 mg/5 mL. Suppository: 324 mg, 648 mg. [klohr-awl HY-drayt]. 272

(chlorambucil) (Chemo). No longer on the market. (Trade name *Leukeran*; alkylating chemotherapy drug).

chloramphenicol (Chloromycetin) (ENT). Topical antibiotic for external auditory canal ear infections. Drops: 0.5%. [klohr-ehm-FEH-neh-kawl].

chloramphenicol (Chloromycetin, Chloroptic, Chloroptic S. O. P.) (Oph). Topical antibiotic used to treat bacterial eye infections. Ophthalmic solution: 5 mg/mL. Ophthalmic ointment: 10 mg/g. Powder to be reconstituted: 25 mg. [klohr-ehm-FEH-neh-kawl]. 218

chloramphenicol (Chloromycetin) (Antibio). Antibiotic used to treat a variety of bacterial infections, including *H. influenzae* and rickettsiae. Capsule: 250 mg. Intravenous (powder to be reconstituted): 100 mg/mL. [klohr-ehm-FEH-neh-kawl]. 319

(Chloraseptic) (ENT). No longer on the market. (Topical anesthetic for the mouth).

chlordiazepoxide (Librium). Historical Notes feature.

chlordiazepoxide (Librium, Mitran, Reposans-10) (Anes, Neuro, Psych). Benzodiazepine drug used as a preoperative medication to relieve anxiety and provide sedation; used to treat anxiety and neurosis; used to treat alcohol withdrawal amd prevent seizures. (Schedule IV drug). Capsule: 5 mg, 10 mg, 25 mg. Intramuscular or intravenous (powder to be reconstituted): 100 mg. [klohr-dy-eh-zeh-PAWK-zide]. 267, 281

Chloresium (Derm) (generic *chlorophyll derivative*). Topical drug that promotes healing of skin ulcers and wounds and controls odors. Liquid: 0.2%. Ointment: 0.5%. [klohr-EE-see-uhm].

chlorhexidine (Betasept, Hibiclens, Hibistat) (Derm). Topical anti-infective hand wash and preoperative surgical skin scrub. Hand rinse: 0.5%. Liquid: 4%. Sponge brush, towelettes. 98

chlorhexidine (Peridex, PerioGard) (Chemo, ENT). Topical mouthwash drug used to treat oral mucositis in chemotherapy patients; used to treat gingivitis. Liquid oral rinse: 0.12%.

(chlormezanone) (Psych). No longer on the market. (Trade name *Trancopal*; antianxiety drug).

(chloroform) (Anes). No longer on the market. (Inhaled gas for general anesthesia). 366

Chloromycetin (ENT) (generic *chloramphenicol*). Topical antibiotic used to treat external auditory canal ear infections. Drops: 0.5%. [klohr-oh-my-SEE-tihn].

Chloromycetin (Antibio). Antibiotic used to treat a variety of bacterial infections, including *H. influenzae* and rickettsiae. For dosage, see *chloramphenicol*. [klohr-oh-my-SEE-tihn]. 319

Chloromycetin (Antibio, Oph). Topical antibiotic used to treat bacterial eye infections. For dosage, see *chloramphenicol*. [klohr-oh-my-SEE-tihn].

chlorophyll derivative (Chloresium) (Derm). Topical drug used to promote healing of skin ulcers and wounds and control odors. Liquid: 0.2%. Ointment: 0.5%.

chloroprocaine (Nesacaine, Nesacaine MPF) (Anes). Local, regional nerve block, and epidural anesthetic. Injection: 1%, 2%, 3%. 368

Chloroptic, Chloroptic S.O.P. (Oph). Topical antibiotic used to treat bacterial eye infections. For dosage, see *chloramphenicol*. [klohr-AWP-tihk].

chloroquine (Aralen) (Antibio, GI). Antiprotozoal drug used to treat intestinal amebiasis. Tablet: 250 mg, 500 mg. Intramuscular: 50 mg/mL. [KLOR-oh-kwihn]. 321

chlorothiazide (Diuril) (Uro). Thiazide diuretic. Liquid: 250 mg/5 mL. Tablet: 250 mg, 500 mg. Intravenous: 500 mg/20 mL. [klohr-oh-THY-eh-zide]. 103

(chlorotrianisene) (Chemo, OB/GYN). No longer on the market. (Trade name *Tace*; estrogen replacement for menopause, hormonal chemotherapy drug).

chloroxine (Capitrol) (Derm). Topical anti-infective drug for seborrheic dermatitis. Shampoo: 2%. 98

chlorphenesin (Maolate) (Ortho). Skeletal muscle relaxant used to treat minor muscle spasms associated with injuries. Tablet: 400 mg. 144

chlorpheniramine (Chlor-Trimeton Allergy 4 Hour, Chlor-Trimeton Allergy 8 Hour, Chlor-Trimeton Allergy 12 Hour) (ENT). Antihistamine used to treat allergic rhinitis. Chewable tablet: 2 mg. Liquid: 2 mg/5 mL. Tablet: 4 mg, 8 mg, 12 mg. Subcutaneous or intramuscular: 10 mg/mL. [klohr-feh-NEER-eh-meen]. 207

chlorpromazine (Thorazine, Thorazine Spansules) (GI). Antiemetic drug; used to treat nausea and vomiting caused by chemotherapy; also used to treat intractable hiccoughs. Capsule: 30 mg, 75 mg, 150 mg. Liquid: 30 mg/mL, 100 mg/mL. Syrup: 10 mg/5 mL. Tablet: 10 mg, 25 mg, 50 mg, 100 mg, 200 mg. Suppository: 25 mg, 100 mg. Intramuscular or intravenous: 25 mg/mL. [klohr-PROH-mah-zeen]. 127

chlorpromazine (Thorazine, Thorazine Spansules) (Psych). Phenothiazine drug used to treat psychosis; used to treat manic-depressive disorder; used

as short-term treatment for explosive, impulsive behavior and mood lability in children; used to treat attention-deficit/hyperactivity disorder. Capsule: 30 mg, 75 mg, 150 mg. Liquid: 30 mg/mL, 100 mg/mL. Syrup: 10 mg/5 mL. Tablet: 10 mg, 25 mg, 50 mg, 100 mg, 200 mg. Suppository: 25 mg, 100 mg. Intramuscular or intravenous: 25 mg/mL. [klohr-PROH-mah-zeen]. 283, 289, 292

chlorpropamide (Diabinese) (Diab). Oral antidiabetic drug. Tablet: 100 mg, 250 mg. [klohr-PROH-pah-mide]. 240

(chlorprothixene) (Psych). No longer on the market. (Trade name *Taractan*; antipsychotic drug).

chlortetracycline (Aureomycin) (Derm). Topical antibiotic used to treat acne vulgaris. Ointment: 3%. [klohr-teh-trah-SY-kleen]. 84

chlorthalidone (Hygroton) (Uro). Thiazide-like diuretic. Tablet: 15 mg, 25 mg, 50 mg, 100 mg. [klohr-THEHL-ih-dohn]. 103

(Chlor-Trimeton Allergy-Sinus) (ENT). No longer on the market. (Combination drug with *phenylpropanolamine*; decongestant, antihistamine, and analgesic).

Chlor-Trimeton Allergy 4 Hour, Chlor-Trimeton Allergy 8 Hour, Chlor-Trimeton Allergy 12 Hour (ENT). Antihistamine used to treat allergic rhinitis. For dosage, see *chlorpheniramine*. [klohr-TRIH-meh-tawn]. 207

Chlor-Trimeton 4 Hour Relief (ENT) (generic *pseudoephedrine, chlorpheniramine*). Combination decongestant and antihistamine drug. Tablet: 60 mg/4 mg. [klohr-TRIH-meh-tawn].

Chlor-Trimeton 12 Hour Relief (ENT) (generic *pseudoephedrine, chlorpheniramine*). Combination decongestant and antihistamine drug. Tablet: 120 mg/8 mg. [klohr-TRIH-meh-tawn].

chlorzoxazone (Paraflex, Parafon Forte DSC) (Ortho). Skeletal muscle relaxant used to treat minor muscle spasms associated with injuries. Caplet: 250 mg, 500 mg. Tablet: 250 mg, 500 mg. [klohr-ZAWK-sah-zohn]. 144

Choice dm (Diab, GI). Liquid nutritional supplement formulated for patients with diabetes mellitus. Liquid.

Choledyl SA (Resp). Bronchodilator. For dosage, see *oxtriphylline*. [koh-LEE-dihl]. 193

Cholestin (Cardio). Food supplement used to lower cholesterol levels. [koh-LEH-stihn]. 171

cholestyramine (LoCHOLEST, LoCHOLEST Light, Prevalite, Questran, Questran Light) (Cardio, Emerg). Bile acid sequestrant drug used to treat hypercholesterolemia; used to treat digitalis toxicity; used to treat thyroid hormone overdose or pesticide poisoning. Powder (to be reconstituted): 4 g. Tablet: 1 g. [koh-leh-STY-rah-meen]. 153, 169

cholinergic receptors. See *receptor*. 62

choline salicylate (Arthropan) (Analges, Ortho). Salicylate nonaspirin analgesic drug used to treat mild-to-moderate pain and fever; used to treat inflammation; used to treat osteoarthritis and rheumatoid arthritis. Liquid: 870 mg/5 mL. [KOH-leen sah-LIH-seh-layt]. 138, 300

(Choloxin) (Cardio). No longer on the market. (Generic name *dextrothyroxine*; used to treat hypercholesterolemia).

Chooz (GI). Calcium-containing antacid. Chewable tablet: 500 mg. 116

choriogonadotropin alfa (Ovidrel) (OB/GYN). Ovulation-stimulating drug used to treat infertility. Subcutaneous (powder to be reconstituted): 250 mcg. [koh-ree-oh-goh-neh-doh-TROH-pihn ehl-fah]. 244

Chromagen (Cardio). Combination iron, intrinsic factor, vitamin B_{12}, and vitamin C drug used to treat iron deficiency anemia and pernicious anemia. Capsule: 66 mg/100 mg/10 mcg/250 mg. 172

Chromagen FA (Misc). Combination iron, vitamin B_{12}, vitamin C, and folic acid nutritional supplement. Capsule.

Chromagen Forte (Misc). Combination iron, vitamin B_{12}, vitamin C, and folic acid nutritional supplement. Capsule.

Chromelin Complexion Blender (Derm) (generic *dihydroxyacetone*). Topical drug used to darken areas of hypopigmented skin in patients with vitiligo. Liquid: 5%. 98

chronotherapy. 48

Chronulac (GI). Laxative. For dosage, see *lactulose*. 125

(Chymodiactin) (Ortho, Neuro). No longer on the market. (Generic name *chymopapain*; used to dissolve a herniated disk).

(chymopapain) (Ortho, Neuro). No longer on the market. (Trade name *Chymodiactin*; used to dissolve a herniated disk).

(chymotrypsin) (Oph). No longer on the market. (Trade name *Catarase*; used to free lens during cataract surgery).

Cibacalcin (Ortho). Calcium-regulating hormone used to treat Paget's disease. For dosage, see *calcitonin-human*. 147

(Cibalith-S) (Antivir, Chemo, Psych). No longer on the market. (Generic name *lithium*; used to treat manic-depressive disorder; used to treat neutropenia in AIDS and chemotherapy patients).

ciclopirox (Loprox, Penlac Nail Lacquer) (Derm). Topical antifungal drug. Cream: 0.77%. Liquid nail solution: 8%. Lotion: 0.77%. [sih-kloh-PEER-awks]. 89

cidofovir (Forvade) (Antivir). Antiviral drug used to treat genital herpes. Investigational drug. 330

cidofovir (Vistide) (Antivir, Oph). Antiviral drug used to treat cytomegalovirus retinitis in AIDS patients; investigational drug used to treat Kaposi's sarcoma. Intravenous: 75 mg/mL. [sy-doh-FOH-veer]. 329

cifenline (Cipralan) (Cardio). Used to treat arrhythmias. Investigational drug. 172

cilazapril (Inhibace) (Cardio). Angiotensin-converting enzyme inhibitor used to treat hypertension and congestive heart failure. Investigational drug. 172

ciliary neurotrophic factor (Neuro). Used to treat amyotrophic lateral sclerosis. Orphan drug. 275

cilostazol (Pletal) (Cardio). Vasodilator used to treat peripheral vascular disease. Tablet: 50 mg, 100 mg. [sih-LAW-steh-zohl]. 172

Ciloxan (Oph). Topical antibiotic used to treat bacterial eye infections. For dosage, see *ciprofloxacin*. [sih-LAWK-sehn]. 218

cimetidine (Tagamet, Tagamet HB 200) (Derm, GI). H_2 blocker used in conjunction with standard antihistamines to treat chronic itching and hives; used to treat peptic ulcers and *H. pylori* infection. Liquid: 200 mg/5 mL, 300 mg/5 mL. Tablet: 200 mg, 300 mg, 400 mg, 800 mg. Intramuscular or intravenous: 150 mg/mL, 300 mg/2 mL. [sy-MEH-tih-deen]. 94, 118

Cinobac (Antibio). Quinolone antibiotic used only to treat urinary tract infections. For dosage, see *cinoxacin*. [SIH-noh-behk]. 105, 318

cinoxacin (Cinobac) (Antibio). Quinolone antibiotic used only to treat urinary tract infections. Capsule: 250 mg, 500 mg. [seh-NAWK-sah-sihn]. 105, 318

Cipralan (Cardio) (generic *cifenline*). Used to treat arrhythmias. Investigational drug. 172

Cipro, Cipro I.V. (Antibio). Fluoroquinolone antibiotic used to treat many types of infections, including *Streptococcus*, *Staphylococcus*, *H. influenzae*, *E. coli*, *Klebsiella pneumonia*, *Pseudomonas aeruginosa*, and gonorrhea; used to treat traveler's diarrhea; used to treat cutaneous or inhaled anthrax from bioterrorism. For dosage, see *ciprofloxacin*. [SIH-proh]. 98, 105, 123, 318

ciprofloxacin (Cipro, Cipro I.V.) (Antibio). Fluoroquinolone antibiotic used to treat many types of infections, including *Streptococcus*, *Staphylococcus*, *H. influenzae*, *E. coli*, *Klebsiella pneumonia*, *Pseudomonas aeruginosa*, and gonorrhea; used to treat traveler's diarrhea; used to treat cutaneous or inhaled anthrax from bioterrorism. Liquid: 5 g/100 mL. Tablet: 100 mg, 250 mg, 500 mg, 750 mg. Intravenous: 200

mg/20 mL, 400 mg/40 mL. [sih-proh-FLAWK-sah-sihn]. 318

ciprofloxacin (Ciloxan) (Oph).   Topical antibiotic used to treat bacterial eye infections. Ophthalmic solution: 3.5 mg/mL. Ophthalmic ointment: 3.33 mg/g. [sih-proh-FLAWK-sah-sehn]. 218

Cipro HC Otic (ENT) (generic *hydrocortisone, ciprofloxacin*).   Combination topical corticosteroid and antibiotic for the ears. Drops: 10 mg/2 mg per mL.

(cisapride) (GI).   No longer on the market. (Trade name *Propulsid*; gastric stimulant used to treat heartburn and gastroesophageal reflux disease).

cisatracurium (Nimbex) (Anes, Resp).   Muscle-relaxing drug used during surgery; used to treat patients who are intubated and on the ventilator. Intravenous: 2 mg/mL, 10 mg/mL. [sihs-eh-trah-KYOUR-ee-uhm]. 199, 370

cisplatin (Platinol-AQ) (Chemo).   Chemotherapy platinum drug used to treat ovarian cancer, testicular cancer, and bladder cancer. Intravenous: 1 mg/mL. [sihs-PLEH-tehn]. 345

cis-platinum (Chemo).   See *cisplatin*.

citalopram (Celexa) (OB/GYN, Psych).   Selective serotonin reuptake inhibitor antidepressant used to treat depression; used to treat panic disorder; used to treat social anxiety disorder/social phobias; used to treat premenstrual dysphoric disorder. Tablet: 20 mg, 40 mg. Liquid: 10 mg/5 mL. [seh-TEH-loh-prehm]. 254, 287, 289, 290

Citanest (ENT).   Local and regional nerve block anesthetic for dental procedures.   For dosage, see *prilocaine*.

Citrolith (Ortho) (generic *potassium citrate, sodium citrate*).   Used to treat gout. Tablet: 50 mg/950 mg.

Citrotein (GI).   Liquid nutritional supplement. Liquid. Powder (to be reconstituted).

citrovorum factor.   See *leucovorin*.

Citrucel (GI).   Bulk-producing laxative.   For dosage, see *methylcellulose*. [SIH-treh-sehl]. 125

cladribine (Leustatin, Mylinax) (Chemo, Neuro).   Purine antagonist chemotherapy drug used to treat leukemia, non-Hodgkin's lymphoma, and cutaneous T-cell lymphoma; orphan drug used to treat multiple sclerosis. Intravenous: 1 mg/mL. [KLEH-dreh-been]. 275, 339

Claforan (Antibio).   Cephalosporin antibiotic used to treat a variety of bacterial infections, including *Streptococcus, Staphylococcus, E. coli*, and *H. influenzae*. For dosage, see *cefotaxime*. [KLEH-foh-rehn]. 316

Clarinex (Derm, ENT).   Antihistamine used to treat idiopathic urticaria; used to treat allergic rhinitis. For dosage, see *desloratadine*. [KLEH-reh-nehks]. 207

clarithromycin (Biaxin, Biaxin XL) (Antibio, GI).   Macrolide antibiotic used to treat a variety of infections, including *Streptococcus, H. influenzae*, and *S. pneumoniae*; used to treat *Mycobacterium avium-intracellulare* in AIDS patients; used to treat *H. pylori* infection of the gastrointestinal tract. Tablet: 250 mg, 500 mg. Liquid (granules to be reconstituted): 125 mg/5 mL, 250 mg/5 mL. [kleh-rih-throh-MY-sihn]. 120, 319, 329

Claritin, Claritin Reditabs (Derm, ENT).   Antihistamine used to treat allergic rhinitis and allergic reactions with hives and itching.   For dosage, see *loratadine*. 207

Claritin-D (ENT) (generic *pseudoephedrine, loratadine*).   Combination decongestant and antihistamine drug. Capsule: 120 mg/5 mg. [KLEH-reh-tihn].

Claritin-D 24-Hour (ENT) (generic *pseudoephedrine, loratadine*).   Combination decongestant and antihistamine drug. Tablet: 240 mg/10 mg.

Clearasil Maximum Strength (Derm) (generic *benzoyl peroxide*).   Topical antibiotic used to treat acne vulgaris. Cream: 10%. 83

Clearasil Medicated Deep Cleanser (Derm) (generic *salicylic acid*).   Topical keratolytic used to treat acne vulgaris. Liquid: 0.5%. 83

clemastine (Tavist) (Derm, ENT).   Antihistamine used to treat allergic rhinitis and allergic reactions with hives and itching. Liquid: 0.67 mg/5 mL. Tablet: 1.34 mg, 2.68 mg. [kleh-MEH-steen]. 207

Cleocin, Cleocin Pediatric (Antibio, OB/GYN).   Antibiotic used to treat a variety of serious bacterial infections, including *Staphylococcus, Streptococcus, Pneumococcus*; used to treat central nervous system toxoplasmosis in AIDS patients; used to treat *Pneumocystis carinii* pneumonia in AIDS patients; used to treat bacterial vaginal infections; used to treat *Chlamydia* vaginal infections.   For dosage, see *clindamycin*. [KLEE-oh-sihn]. 319, 328, 331

Cleocin T (Derm) (generic *clindamycin*).   Topical antibiotic used to treat acne vulgaris. Gel: 10 mg/mL. Liquid: 10 mg/mL. Lotion: 10 mg/mL. [KLEE-oh-sihn]. 84

Cleocin, Cleocin Vaginal Ovules (OB/GYN) (generic *clindamycin*).   Topical antibiotic used to treat bacterial vaginal infections. Cream: 2%. Suppositories: 100 mg/2.5 g. [KLEE-oh-sihn]. 256

clidinium (Quarzan) (GI).   Antispasmodic drug. Capsule: 2.5 mg, 5 mg. [klih-DIH-nee-uhm]. 122

climacteric.   Historical Notes feature. 252

Climara (OB/GYN, Ortho).   Hormone replacement therapy used to treat the symptoms of menopause; used to prevent and treat osteoporosis.   For dosage, see *estradiol*. [kly-MEH-rah]. 252

clindamycin (Cleocin, Cleocin Pediatric) (Antibio, OB/GYN). Antibiotic used to treat a variety of serious bacterial infections, including *Staphylococcus, Streptococcus, Pneumococcus*; used to treat central nervous system toxoplasmosis in AIDS patients; used to treat *Pneumocystis carinii* pneumonia in AIDS patients; used to treat bacterial vaginal infections; used to treat *Chlamydia* vaginal infections. Capsule: 75 mg, 150 mg, 300 mg. Liquid: 75 mg/5 mL. Intramuscular or intravenous: 150 mg/mL. [klihn-dah-MY-sihn]. 319, 328, 331

clindamycin (Cleocin T, C/T/S) (Derm). Topical antibiotic for acne vulgaris. Gel: 10 mg/mL. Liquid: 10 mg/mL. Lotion: 10 mg/mL. [klihn-dah-MY-sihn]. 84

clindamycin (Cleocin, Cleocin Vaginal Ovules) (OB/GYN). Topical antibiotic used to treat bacterial vaginal infections. Cream: 2%. Suppositories: 100 mg/2.5 g. [klihn-dah-MY-sihn]. 256

Clinoril (Analges, Ortho). Nonsteroidal anti-inflammatory drug used to treat bursitis, gout, osteoarthritis, rheumatoid arthritis, and tendinitis. For dosage, see *sulindac*. [KLIH-noh-rihl]. 139, 146, 304

clioquinol (Derm). Topical antifungal drug. Cream: 3%. [klee-OH-kwih-nawl]. 89

(Clistin) (ENT). No longer on the market. (Generic name *carbinoxamine*; antihistamine).

clobazam (Frisium) (Neuro, Psych). Used to treat epilepsy; used to treat anxiety. Investigational drug. 265, 282

clobetasol (Cormax, Olux, Temovate) (Derm). Topical corticosteroid anti-inflammatory drug. Cream: 0.05%. Foam: 0.05%. Gel: 0.05%. Liquid: 0.05%. Ointment: 0.05%. [kloh-BEH-teh-sawl]. 92

clocortolone (Cloderm) (Derm). Topical corticosteroid anti-inflammatory drug. Cream: 0.1%. [kloh-KOHR-toh-lohn]. 92

Cloderm (Derm) (generic *clocortolone*). Topical corticosteroid anti-inflammatory drug. Cream: 0.1%. [KLOH-dehrm]. 92

clofibrate (Atromid-S) (Cardio). Used to treat hypertriglyceridemia by decreasing serum triglycerides and very low-density lipoprotein levels. Capsule: 500 mg. [kloh-FY-brayt]. 171

Clomid (OB/GYN). Ovulation-stimulating hormone drug used to treat infertility. For dosage, see *clomiphene*. [KLOH-mihd]. 244

clomiphene (Clomid, Serophene) (OB/GYN). Ovulation-stimulating hormone drug used to treat infertility. Tablet 50 mg. [KLOH-meh-feen]. 244

clomipramine (Anafranil) (OB/GYN, Psych). Antidepressant used to treat obsessive-compulsive disorder; used to treat panic disorder; used to treat premenstrual dysphoric disorder. Capsule: 25 mg, 50 mg, 75 mg. [kloh-MIH-prah-meen]. 254, 289

clonazepam (Klonopin) (Neuro, Psych). Benzodiazepine drug used to treat absence seizures; used to treat Lennox–Gastaut syndrome; used to treat the muscular symptoms of Parkinson's disease; used to treat neuralgia; used to treat schizophrenia; used to treat the manic phase of manic-depressive disorder. (Schedule IV drug). Tablet: 0.5 mg, 1 mg, 2 mg. [klawn-EH-zeh-pehm]. 264, 270, 283, 288

clonidine (Catapres, Catapres-TTS-1, Catapres-TTS-2, Catapres-TTS-3) (Cardio, Resp). Alpha-receptor blocker used to treat hypertension and atrial arrhythmias; used to help patients stop smoking. Tablet: 0.1 mg, 0.2 mg, 0.3 mg. Transdermal patch: 0.1 mg/24 hr, 0.2 mg/24 hr, 0.3 mg/24 hr. [KLAW-neh-deen]. 159, 165, 199

clonidine (Catapres, Catapres-TTS-1, Catapres-TTS-2, Catapres-TTS-3) (Chemo). Alpha-receptor blocker used to treat severe pain in cancer patients; used to treat cyclosporine-induced nephrotoxicity. Tablet: 0.1 mg, 0.2 mg, 0.3 mg. Transdermal patch: 0.1 mg/24 hr, 0.2 mg/24 hr, 0.3 mg/24 hr. [KLAW-neh-deen]. 361

clonidine (Catapres, Catapres-TTS-1, Catapres-TTS-2, Catapres-TTS-3) (Derm, Neuro). Alpha-receptor blocker used to treat postherpetic neuralgia/shingles; used to treat hyperhidrosis (excessive sweating). Tablet: 0.1 mg, 0.2 mg, 0.3 mg. Transdermal patch: 0.1 mg/24 hr, 0.2 mg/24 hr, 0.3 mg/24 hr. [KLAW-neh-deen]. 275

clonidine (Catapres) (Endo). Alpha-receptor blocker used to diagnose pheochromocytoma of the adrenal cortex. Tablet: 0.1 mg, 0.2 mg, 0.3 mg. [KLAW-neh-deen].

clonidine (Catapres, Catapres-TTS-1, Catapres-TTS-2, Catapres-TTS-3) (Analges, GI, Ortho, Psych). Alpha-receptor blocker used to treat narcotic withdrawal; used to treat ulcerative colitis; used to treat restless legs syndrome; used to treat psychosis and schizophrenia; used to treat the mania of manic-depressive syndrome; used to treat Tourette's syndrome; used to treat attention-deficit/hyperactivity disorder; used to treat alcohol withdrawal. Tablet: 0.1 mg, 0.2 mg, 0.3 mg. Transdermal patch: 0.1 mg/24 hr, 0.2 mg/24 hr, 0.3 mg/24 hr. [KLAW-neh-deen]. 132, 147, 284, 288, 292, 308

clonidine (Duraclon) (Analges). Nonnarcotic analgesic drug used to treat severe pain. Epidural: 100 mcg/mL, 500 mcg/mL. [KLAW-neh-deen]. 299

clopidogrel (Plavix) (Cardio, Hem, Neuro). Platelet aggregation inhibitor used to prevent blood clots and reduce the risk of myocardial infarction or stroke in patients with atherosclerosis and previous history of myocardial infarction or stroke. Tablet: 75 mg. 172, 187, 275

clorazepate (Tranxene, Tranxene-SD, Tranxene-SD Half Strength, Tranxene-T) (Neuro, Psych). Benzodiazepine drug used to treat anxiety and neurosis; used to treat alcohol withdrawal; used to treat partial seizures. (Schedule IV drug). Capsule: 3.75 mg, 7.5 mg, 11.25 mg, 15 mg, 22.5 mg. [klohr-EH-zeh-payt]. 264, 281

Clorpactin WSC-90 (Derm) (generic *oxychlorosene*). Topical antibacterial, antifungal, and antiviral drug used to irrigate wounds. Powder to be reconstituted into a solution. 99

clotrimazole (Gyne-Lotrimin 3, Gyne-Lotrimin 7, Mycelex-7) (OB/GYN). Topical drug used to treat vaginal yeast infections. Vaginal cream: 1%, 2%, Vaginal suppository: 100 mg, 200 mg. [kloh-TRIH-meh-zohl]. 256

clotrimazole (Cruex, Desenex, Lotrimin, Lotrimin AF 1%) (Derm). Topical antifungal and antiyeast drug. Cream: 1%. Liquid: 1%. Lotion: 1%. [kloh-TRIH-meh-zohl]. 89

clotrimazole (Mycelex) (ENT). Topical drug used to treat yeast infections in the mouth. Troche: 10 mg. [kloh-TRIH-meh-zohl]. 211

cloxacillin (Cloxapen) (Antibio). Penicillin-type antibiotic used to treat a variety of bacterial infections, including staphylococci. Capsule: 250 mg, 500 mg. Liquid: 125 mg/5 mL. {KLAWK-seh-sih-lihn}. 313

Cloxapen (Antibio). Penicillin-type antibiotic used to treat a variety of bacterial infections, including staphylococci. For dosage, see *cloxacillin*. [KLAWK-seh-pehn]. 313

clozapine (Clozaril) (Psych). Drug used to treat psychosis and schizophrenia. Tablet: 25 mg, 100 mg. [KLOH-zah-peen]. 284

Clozaril (Psych). Drug used to treat psychosis and schizophrenia. For dosage, see *clozapine*. [KLOH-zah-rihl]. 284

CMV (abbreviation for *cytomegalovirus*). See *cytomegalovirus*.

Coagulin-B (Hem) (generic *gene for coagulation Factor IX*). This drug, carried on a virus vector, is used to treat hemophilia B. Intramuscular. Orphan drug.

coal tar. Historical Notes feature. 86

coal tar drugs used to treat psoriasis. 86

cocaine (coca bush leaves). 13, 367

cocaine (Cocaine Viscous) (ENT). Topical ear, nose, and throat vasoconstrictor and anesthetic. Liquid: 4%, 10%. Powder. [koh-KAYN]. 214

codeine (Analges). Narcotic analgesic used to treat mild-to-moderate pain. (Schedule II drug). Tablet: 15 mg, 30 mg, 60 mg. Liquid: 15 mg/5 mL. Subcutaneous or intramuscular: 30 mg/mL, 60 mg/mL. [KOH-deen]. 297

codeine (ENT). Narcotic antitussive used to treat nonproductive cough. (Schedule II drug). Tablet: 15 mg, 30 mg, 60 mg. [KOH-deen]. 210

Code of Hammurabi. 12

Cogentin (Neuro). Anticholinergic drug used to treat Parkinson's disease. For dosage, see *benztropine*. [koh-JEHN-tihn]. 269

Cognex (Neuro). Cholinesterase inhibitor used to treat Alzheimer's disease. For dosage, see *tacrine*. [KAWG-nehks]. 271

Colace (GI). Stool softener laxative. For dosage, see *docusate*. [KOH-lays]. 125

Colazal (GI). Anti-inflammatory-type drug used to treat ulcerative colitis. For dosage, see *balsalazide*. 126

colchicine (Neuro, Ortho). Orphan drug used to treat multiple sclerosis; also used to treat gout. Tablet: 0.5 mg, 0.6 mg. [KOHL-cheh-seen]. 146, 275

Colchicum autumnale (meadow saffron flower).

cold sores. See *herpes simplex virus*.

colesevelam (Welchol) (Cardio). Bile acid sequestrant used to treat hypercholesterolemia. Tablet: 625 mg. 169

Colestid (Cardio). Bile acid sequestrant used to treat hypercholesterolemia and digitalis toxicity. For dosage, see *colestipol*. [koh-LEHS-tihd]. 153, 169

colestipol (Colestid) (Cardio). Bile acid sequestrant used to treat hypercholesterolemia and digitalis toxicity. Granules: 5 g. Tablet: 1 g. [koh-LEHS-tih-pohl]. 153, 169

colfosceril (Exosurf Neonate) (Resp). Synthetic lung surfactant used to prevent and treat respiratory distress syndrome in premature newborns. Endotracheal tube (powder to be reconstituted): 108 mg. [kohl-foh-SKEHR-ihl].

colistimethate (Coly-Mycin M) (Antibio). Antibiotic used to treat infections, including *E. coli*, *Pseudomonas aeruginosa*, and *Klebsiella pneumoniae*. Intramuscular or intravenous (powder to be reconstituted): 150 mg. [koh-lihs-tih-MEH-thayt]. 319

collagenase (Santyl) (Derm). Topical enzyme drug used to debride burns and wounds. Ointment. [koh-LEH-jeh-nays]. 96

Collyrium Fresh (Oph). Topical decongestant/vasoconstrictor used to treat irritation and allergy symptoms in the eyes. For dosage, see *tetrahydrozoline*.

Colomed (Chemo). Used to treat radiation proctitis. Orphan drug. 361

Coly-Mycin M (Antibio).   Antibiotic used to treat infections, including *E. coli, Pseudomonas aeruginosa,* and *Klebsiella pneumoniae.*   For dosage, see *colistimethate.* [koh-lee-MY-sihn M]. 319

Coly-Mycin S Otic (ENT) (generic *hydrocortisone, colistin, neomycin*).   Combination topical drug with a corticosteroid and two antibiotics for the ears. Drops: 1%/3 mg/4.71 mg. [koh-lee-MY-sihn S OH-tihk]. 212

CoLyte (GI) (generic *polyethylene glycol, electrolyte solution*).   Bowel evacuant/bowel prep. Oral liquid (powder to be reconstituted). 125

Combipatch (OB/GYN) (generic *norethindrone, estradiol*).   Combination progestins and estrogen drug used to treat symptoms of menopause. Transdermal patch (twice weekly): 0.014 mg/0.05 mg (9 cm^2), 0.25 mg/0.05 mg (16 cm^2). [KAWM-bee-patch]. 253

Combipres 0.1, Combipres 0.2, Combipres 0.3 (Cardio) (generic *clonidine, chlorthalidone*).   Combination alpha-receptor blocker antihypertensive and diuretic drug. Tablet: 0.1 mg/15 mg, 0.2 mg/15 mg, 0.3 mg/15 mg. [KAWM-bih-prehs]. 167

Combivent (Resp) (generic *albuterol, ipratropium*). Combination bronchodilator drug. Aerosol inhaler: 103 mcg/18 mcg per puff. [KAWM-bih-vehnt]. 195

Combivir (Antivir) (generic *lamivudine, zidovudine*). Combination of two nucleoside reverse transcriptase inhibitor drugs used to treat AIDS. Tablet: 150 mg/300 mg. [KAWM-bih-veer]. 325

Comfort Tears (Oph).   Artificial tears. Drops.

Compassionate Use Investigational New Drug application. 16

Compazine (GI).   Phenothiazine drug used to treat nausea and vomiting.   For dosage, see *prochlorperazine.* [KAWM-pah-zeen]. 127

Compazine (Psych).   Phenothiazine drug used to treat psychosis; used to treat anxiety.   For dosage, see *prochlorperazine.* [KAWM-pah-zeen]. 282, 283

Compleat Modified Formula (GI).   Liquid nutritional supplement. Liquid.

Compound W (Derm) (generic *salicylic acid*).   Topical keratolytic drug used to treat warts. Gel: 17%. Liquid: 17%. 91

Comprehensive Drug Abuse Prevention and Control Act, The. 16

computer, drugs designed by. 25

COMP (abbreviation for *catechol-O-methyltransferase*).

Compoz Gel Caps, Compoz Nighttime Sleep Aid (Neuro).   Antihistamine drug sleep aid.   For dosage, see *diphenhydramine.* 273

COMT inhibitors (Neuro).   Class of drugs used to treat Parkinson's disease. 269

Comtan (Neuro).   COMT inhibitor used to treat Parkinson's disease.   For dosage, see *entacapone.* [KAWM-tehn]. 269

Comtrex Allergy-Sinus (ENT) (generic *pseudoephedrine, chlorpheniramine, acetaminophen*).   Combination decongestant, antihistamine, and analgesic drug. Caplet: 30 mg/2 mg/500 mg. Tablet: 30 mg/2 mg/500 mg.

Comtrex Liquid (ENT) (generic *pseudoephedrine, chlorpheniramine,   dextromethorphan,   acetaminophen*). Combination decongestant, antihistamine, nonnarcotic antitussive, and analgesic drug. Liquid: 10 mg/0.67 mg/3.3 mg/108.3 mg.

(Comtrex Liqui-Gels) (ENT).   No longer on the market. (Combination drug with *phenylpropanolamine;* decongestant, antihistamine, nonnarcotic antitussive, and analgesic drug).

Comtrex Maximum Strength Multi-Symptom Cold & Flu Relief Caplet/Tablet (ENT) (generic *pseudoephedrine, chlorpheniramine, dextromethorphan, acetaminophen*).   Combination decongestant, antihistamine, nonnarcotic antitussive, and analgesic drug. Caplet: 30 mg/2 mg/15 mg/500 mg. Tablet: 30 mg/2 mg/15 mg/500 mg.

(Comtrex Maximum Strength Multi-Symptom Cold & Flu Relief Liqui-Gels) (ENT).   No longer on the market. (Combination drug with *phenylpropanolamine;* decongestant, antihistamine, nonnarcotic antitussive, and analgesic drug).

Comtrex Maximum Strength Non-Drowsy (ENT) (generic *pseudoephedrine, dextromethorphan, acetaminophen*).   Combination decongestant, nonnarcotic antitussive, and analgesic drug. Caplet: 30 mg/15 mg/500 mg.

Concerta (Neuro, Psych).   Central nervous system stimulant used to treat narcolepsy; used to treat attention-deficit/hyperactivity disorder. (Schedule II drug).   For dosage, see *methylphenidate.* [kawn-SEHR-tah]. 274, 292

condyloma acuminatum (genital warts), drugs used to treat. 259, 330

Condylox (OB/GYN) (generic *podofilox*).   Topical drug used to treat genital/venereal warts or condyloma acuminatum. Gel: 0.5%. Liquid: 0.5%. [KAWN-dih-lawks]. 259

congestive heart failure, drugs used to treat. 151

conjugated estrogens (Cenestin) (OB/GYN).   Hormone replacement therapy used to treat the symptoms of menopause. Tablet: 0.625 mg, 0.9 mg, 1.25 mg. [kawn-joo-GAY-tehd EHS-troh-jehns]. 252

conjugated estrogens (Premarin Vaginal Cream) (OB/GYN).   Topical hormone replacement therapy used to treat atrophic vaginitis of menopause.

Cream: 0.625 mg. [kawn-joo-GAY-tehd EHS-troh-jehns]. 252

conjugated estrogens (Premarin, Premarin Intravenous) (Chemo, OB/GYN, Ortho). Hormonal chemotherapy drug used to treat breast and prostate carcinoma; hormone replacement therapy used to treat the symptoms of menopause; used to treat abnormal uterine bleeding; used to prevent and treat osteoporosis. Tablet: 0.3 mg, 0.625 mg, 0.9 mg, 1.25 mg, 2.5 mg. Intramuscular or intravenous: 25 mg/5 mL. [kawn-joo-GAY-tehd EHS-troh-jehns]. 252, 254, 343

(Constant-T) (Resp). No longer on the market. (Generic name *theophylline*; bronchodilator).

constipation, drugs used to treat. See *laxatives*.

Contac Cough & Chest Cold (ENT) (generic *pseudoephedrine, dextromethorphan, guaifenesin*). Combination decongestant, nonnarcotic antitussive, and expectorant drug. Liquid: 15 mg/5 mg/50 mg.

Contac Cough & Sore Throat (ENT) (generic *dextromethorphan, acetaminophen*). Combination nonnarcotic antitussive and analgesic drug. Liquid: 5 mg/125 mg.

Contac Day & Night Allergy/Sinus (ENT) (generic *pseudoephedrine, diphenhydramine, acetaminophen*). Combination decongestant, antihistamine, and analgesic drug. Caplets: 60 mg/50 mg/650 mg.

Contac Day & Night Cold & Flu (ENT) (generic *pseudoephedrine, diphenhydramine, dextromethorphan, acetaminophen*). Combination decongestant, antihistamine, nonnarcotic antitussive, and analgesic drug. Caplet: 60 mg/50 mg/30 mg/650 mg.

(Contac Maximum Strength 12 Hour) (ENT). No longer on the market. (Combination drug with *phenylpropanolamine*; decongestant and antihistamine drug).

Contac Severe Cold & Flu, Contac Severe Cold & Flu Nighttime (ENT) (generic *pseudoephedrine, chlorpheniramine, dextromethorphan, acetaminophen*). Combination decongestant, antihistamine, nonnarcotic antitussive, and analgesic drug. Caplet: 30 mg/2 mg/15 mg/500 mg. Liquid: 10 mg/0.67 mg/5 mg/167 mg.

(Contac 12 Hour) (ENT). No longer on the market. (Combination drug with *phenylpropanolamine*; decongestant and antihistamine drug).

contraceptives (OB/GYN). Class of drugs used to prevent pregnancy. 248

controlled substances. 16, 18, 60

Controlled Substances Act of 1970, The. 16

Copaxone (Neuro). Immunosuppressant drug used to treat multiple sclerosis. For dosage, see *glatiramer*. [koh-PEHK-zohn]. 276

Cordarone (Cardio). Used to treat ventricular arrhythmias. For dosage, see *amiodarone*. [KOHR-deh-rohn]. 159

Cordran, Cordran SP (Derm) (generic *flurandrenolide*). Topical corticosteroid anti-inflammatory drug. Cream: 0.025%, 0.05%. Lotion: 0.05%. Ointment: 0.025%, 0.05%. Tape: 4 mcg/cm². [KOHR-drehn]. 92

Coreg (Cardio). Alpha₁ and nonselective beta-receptor blocker used to treat angina pectoris, congestive heart failure, and hypertension. For dosage, see *carvedilol*. [KOH-rehg]. 155, 157, 165

Corgard (Analges, GI, Ortho, Neuro, Psych). Cardioselective beta-blocker used to treat migraine headaches; used to prevent rebleeding from esophageal varices in patients with cirrhosis; used to treat essential familial tremor; used to treat the tremors of Parkinson's disease; used to treat aggressive behavior; used to treat the side effects of muscle tremor and restlessness from antipsychotic drugs; used to treat performance anxiety. For dosage, see *nadolol*. [KOHR-gawrd]. 134, 146, 269, 306

Corgard (Cardio). Nonselective beta-blocker used to treat angina pectoris, hypertension, and ventricular arrhythmias. For dosage, see *nadolol*. [KOHR-gawrd]. 157, 160, 162

Coricidin, Coricidin HB (ENT) (generic *chlorpheniramine, acetaminophen*). Combination antihistamine and analgesic drug. Tablet: 2 mg/325 mg. [koh-rih-SEE-dihn].

(Coricidin D, Coricidin Maximum Strength Sinus Headache) (ENT). No longer on the market. (Combination drug with *phenylpropanolamine*; decongestant, antihistamine, and analgesic drug).

Corlopam (Cardio). Peripheral vasodilator used to treat hypertensive crisis. For dosage, see *fenoldopam*. [KOHR-loh-pehm]. 168

Cormax (Derm) (generic *clobetasol*). Topical corticosteroid anti-inflammatory drug. Ointment: 0.05%.

Correctol (GI). Irritant/stimulant laxative. For dosage, see *bisacodyl*. 124

Cortaid Intensive Therapy, Cortaid with Aloe, Maximum Strength Cortaid (Derm) (generic *hydrocortisone*). Topical corticosteroid anti-inflammatory drug. Cream: 0.5%, 1%. Ointment: 0.5%, 1%. Spray: 1%. 92

Cort-Dome (Derm) (generic *hydrocortisone*). Topical corticosteroid anti-inflammatory drug. Cream: 0.5%, 1%. 92

Cort-Dome High Potency (GI) (generic *hydrocortisone*). Topical corticosteroid anti-inflammatory drug used to treat hemorrhoids. Suppository: 25 mg. 133

Cortef (Endo). Corticosteroid anti-inflammatory drug used to treat severe inflammation in various body systems. For dosage, see *hydrocortisone*. [KOHR-tehf]. 232

Cortenema (GI). Topical corticosteroid anti-inflammatory drug used to treat ulcerative colitis. For dosage, see *hydrocortisone*. [KORT-eh-ne-mah]. 126

corticosteroids. In Depth feature. 93

corticosteroids (Derm). Topical class of drugs used to decrease inflammation and itching. [kohr-teh-koh-STEH-roydz]. 92

corticosteroids (Chemo, Derm, ENT, Oph, Ortho, Resp). Class of drugs used as part of chemotherapy protocols; used to treat severe inflammation in various body systems. [kohr-teh-koh-STEH-roydz]. 62, 92, 141, 196, 232, 350

corticotropin (ACTH, Acthar) (Endo). Adrenocorticotropic hormone replacement therapy used to treat Addison's disease; used during diagnostic testing to determine adrenal cortex function. Intramuscular, intravenous, or subcutaneous (powder to be reconstituted): 25 units, 40 units. [kohr-teh-koh-TROH-pihn]. 232

corticotropin-releasing factor (Xerecept) (Neuro). Used to decrease edema around a brain tumor. Orphan drug. 275

Cortifoam (GI). Topical corticosteroid anti-inflammatory drug used to treat ulcerative colitis. For dosage, see *hydrocortisone*. [KOHR-teh-fohm]. 126

cortisone (Cortone) (Endo). Corticosteroid anti-inflammatory drug used to treat severe inflammation in various body systems. Tablet: 5 mg, 10 mg, 25 mg. [KOHR-teh-zohn]. 232

cortisone, discovery of. Historical Notes feature. 233

Cortisporin (Derm) (generic *hydrocortisone, neomycin, polymyxin B*). Topical combination corticosteroid and antibiotic drug. Cream, ointment. [kohr-teh-SPOHR-ehn]. 88

Cortisporin (Oph) (generic *bacitracin, hydrocortisone, neomycin, polymyxin B*). Topical combination corticosteroid and antibiotic drug. Ophthalmic ointment: 400 units/1%/0.35%/10,000 units. [kohr-teh-SPOHR-ehn].

Cortisporin Ophthalmic Suspension (Oph) (generic *hydrocortisone, neomycin, polymyxin B*). Topical combination corticosteroid and antibiotic drug. Ophthalmic suspension: 1%/0.35%/10,000 units. [kohr-teh-SPOHR-ehn].

Cortisporin Otic (ENT) (generic *hydrocortisone, neomycin, polymyxin B*). Combination topical corticosteroid and antibiotic drug for the ears. Drops: 1%/5 mg/10,000 units. [kohr-teh-SPOHR-ehn].

Cortisporin-TC Otic (ENT) (generic *hydrocortisone, colistin, neomycin*). Combination topical corticosteroid and antibiotic drug for the ears. Drops: 1%/3 mg/3.3 mg. [kohr-teh-SPOHR-ehn].

Cortizone-5, Cortizone-10 (Derm) (generic *hydrocortisone*). Topical corticosteroid anti-inflammatory drug. Cream: 0.5%. Ointment: 0.5%, 1%. 92

Cortone (Endo). Corticosteroid anti-inflammatory drug used to treat severe inflammation in various body systems. For dosage, see *cortisone*. [KOHR-tohn]. 232

(Cortril) (Derm). No longer on the market. (Generic name *hydrocortisone*; topical corticosteroid anti-inflammatory drug).

Cortrosyn (Endo). Used during diagnostic testing to determine adrenal cortex function. For dosage, see *cosyntropin*. [KOHR-troh-sihn].

Corvert (Cardio). Used to treat atrial arrhythmias. For dosage, see *ibutilide*. [KOHR-vehrt].

Corzide 40/5, Corzide 80/5 (Cardio) (generic *nadolol, bendroflumethiazide*). Combination beta-blocker antihypertensive and diuretic drug. Tablet: 40 mg/5 mg, 80 mg/5 mg. 167

Cosmegen (Chemo). Chemotherapy antibiotic used to treat uterine cancer, bone cancer, testicular cancer, rhabdomyosarcoma, and Wilm's tumor. For dosage, see *dactinomycin*. [KAWS-meh-jehn]. 342

Cosopt (Oph) (generic *dorzolamide, timolol*). Topical combination carbonic anhydrase inhibitor and beta-receptor blocker drug used to treat glaucoma. Ophthalmic solution: 2%. [KOH-sawpt]. 222

cosyntropin (Cortrosyn) (Endo). Used during diagnostic testing to determine adrenal cortex function. Intramuscular or intravenous (powder to be reconstituted): 0.25 mg. [koh-sihn-TROH-pihn].

Cotazym, Cotazym-S (GI) (generic *amylase, lipase, protease*). Combination drug replacement therapy for digestive enzymes. Capsule, tablet: 30,000 units/8000 units/30,000 units; 20,000 units/5000 units/20,000 units. [KOH-tah-zime]. 132

Cough Formula Comtrex (ENT) (generic *pseudoephedrine, dextromethorphan, guaifenesin*). Combination decongestant, nonnarcotic antitussive, and expectorant drug. Liquid: 15 mg/7.5 mg/50 mg.

Coumadin (Hem). Anticoagulant. For dosage, see *warfarin*. 186

coumarin (Onkolox) (Chemo). Chemotherapy drug used to treat renal cancer. Orphan drug. 347

Covera-HS (Cardio). Calcium channel blocker used to treat angina pectoris, congestive heart failure, hypertension, and atrial and ventricular arrhythmias. For dosage, see *verapamil*. [koh-VEH-rah]. 154, 157, 160, 163

Coviracil (Antivir). Nucleoside reverse transcriptase inhibitor drug used to treat AIDS. For dosage, see *emtricitabine*. [koh-VEER-ah-sihl]. 324

COX (abbreviation for *cyclooxygenase*). See *COX-2 inhibitors*.

COX-1 and COX-2 enzymes. In Depth feature. 140

COX-2 inhibitors (Ortho). Class of drugs used to treat the pain and inflammation of osteoarthritis and rheumatoid arthritis. 140, 304

Cozaar (Cardio). Angiotensin II receptor blocker used to treat hypertension. For dosage, see *losartan*. [KOH-zahr]. 164

CR (controlled-release) tablet. See also *tablet*. 62

crash cart (Emerg). Portable cart holding all emergency resuscitation drugs/devices.

creams, topical. 35

Crinone (OB/GYN). Progestins hormone used to treat infertility; used to treat amenorrhea; used to treat functional uterine bleeding. For dosage, see *progesterone*. [KRY-nohn]. 245, 254

Criticare HN (GI). Liquid nutritional supplement. Liquid.

Crixivan (Antivir). Protease inhibitor drug used to treat AIDS. For dosage, see *indinavir*. [KRIHK-sih-vehn]. 325

Crolom (Oph). Topical mast cell stabilizer used to treat allergic symptoms in the eyes. For dosage, see *cromolyn*. [KROH-lawm]. 220

cromolyn (Children's NasalCrom, Crolom, NasalCrom, Opticrom) (ENT, Oph). Topical mast cell stabilizer used to treat allergic symptoms in the nose and eyes; orphan drug used to treat vernal keratoconjunctivitis. Nasal spray: 40 mg/mL, 5.2 mg/spray. Ophthalmic solution: 4%. [KROH-moh-lihn]. 208, 220

cromolyn (Gastrocrom) (GI). Mast cell stabilizer taken orally for food allergies. Liquid concentrate: 100 mg/5 mL. [KROH-moh-lihn]. 132

cromolyn (Intal) (Resp). Mast cell stabilizer used to prevent acute asthma attacks. Aerosol inhaler: 800 mcg/puff. Liquid for nebulizer: 20 mg/2 mL. [KROH-moh-lihn]. 197

Cronassial (Oph). Used to treat retinitis pigmentosa. For dosage, see *gangliosides*.

crotamiton (Eurax) (Derm). Topical drug used to treat scabies (mites). Cream: 10%. Lotion: 10%. [kroh-TEH-mih-tawn]. 95

Cruex (Derm) (generic *clotrimazole*). Topical antifungal drug. Cream: 1%. [KROO-ehks]. 89

cryoprecipitate (I.V.). General term for any intravenous blood product with no cellular components; used to replace plasma proteins and clotting factors. [kry-oh-pree-SIH-pih-tayt]. 188, 381

Cryptaz (Antivir, GI). Used to treat protozoal diarrhea; used to treat *Cryptosporidium parvum* parasitic diarrhea in AIDS patients. For dosage, see *nitazoxanide*. [KRIHP-tehz]. 134, 331

crystalloid (I.V.). General term for normal saline and lactated Ringer's intravenous fluids. [KRIH-stah-loyd]. 376

(Crystodigin) (Cardio). No longer on the market. (Generic name *digitoxin*; cardiac glycoside used to treat congestive heart failure and atrial flutter/fibrillation).

C/T/S (Derm) (generic *clindamycin*). Topical antibiotic used to treat acne vulgaris. Liquid: 10 mg/mL. 84

cubic centimeter (cc). 70

(curare) (Anes). No longer on the market. (Neuromuscular blocker used during general anesthesia). 367

Curosurf (Resp). Natural lung surfactant used to prevent and treat respiratory distress syndrome in newborn infants; used to treat respiratory distress syndrome in adults. For dosage, see *poractant alfa*. [KYOUR-oh-sehrf].

Cushing's syndrome, drugs used to treat. 231

Cutivate (Derm) (generic *fluticasone*). Topical corticosteroid anti-inflammatory drug. Cream: 0.05%. Ointment: 0.005%. [KYOO-tih-vayt]. 92

cyanocobalamin (Nascobal) (Cardio). Vitamin B_{12}. Given orally, this drug is considered to be a nutritional supplement. Given nasally or intramuscularly, it is used to treat pernicious anemia. Intranasal gel (Nascobal): 500 mcg/0.1 mL. Lozenge: 100 mcg, 250 mcg, 500 mcg. Tablet: 100 mcg, 500 mcg, 1000 mcg, 5000 mcg. Intramuscular: 100 mcg/mL, 1000 mcg/mL. [sy-eh-no-koh-BAWL-ah-meen]. 172

(Cyclan) (Cardio). No longer on the market. (Generic name *cyclandelate*; vasodilator used to treat peripheral vascular disease).

(cyclandelate) (Cardio). No longer on the market. (Trade name *Cyclan*; vasodilator used to treat peripheral vascular disease).

Cyclessa (OB/GYN, Ortho) (generic *desogestrel, ethinyl estradiol*). Triphasic combination progestins and estrogen oral contraceptive. Tablet: 0.1 mg/25 mcg then 0.125 mg/25 mcg then 0.15 mg/25 mcg. [sy-KLEH-sah]. 251

cyclizine (Marezine) (GI). Antiemetic; also used to treat motion sickness. Tablet: 50 mg. 127, 128

cyclobenzaprine (Ortho). Skeletal muscle relaxant used to treat minor muscle spasms associated with injuries. Tablet: 10 mg. [sy-kloh-BEHN-zah-preen]. 144

Cyclocort (Derm) (generic *amcinonide*). Topical corticosteroid anti-inflammatory drug. Cream: 0.1%. Lotion: 0.1%. Ointment: 0.1%. [SY-kloh-kohrt]. 92

Cyclogyl (Oph). Topical mydriatic drug. For dosage, see *cyclopentolate*. [SY-kloh-jihl]. 223

Cyclomydril (Oph). Topical combination mydriatic and ophthalmic decongestant drug. Ophthalmic solution: 0.2%/1%. [sy-kloh-MY-drihl]. 223

cyclopentolate (Cyclogyl, Pentolair) (Oph). Topical mydriatic drug. Ophthalmic solution: 0.5%, 1%, 2%. [sy-kloh-PEHN-toh-layt]. 223

cyclophosphamide (Cytoxan, Cytoxan Lyophilized, Neosar) (Chemo, Uro). Alkylating chemotherapy drug used to treat Hodgkin's disease, non-Hodgkin's lymphoma, multiple myeloma, leukemia, brain cancer, eye cancer, cutaneous T-cell lymphoma, and cancer of the breast and ovary; used to treat pediatric nephrotic syndrome. Tablet: 25 mg, 50 mg. Intravenous: 100 mg. [sy-kloh-FAWS-fah-mide]. 111, 341

(cyclopropane) (Anes). No longer on the market. (Inhaled gas for general anesthesia). 367

cycloserine (Seromycin Pulvules) (Resp). Used to treat tuberculosis. Capsule: 250 mg. [sy-kloh-SEH-reen]. 197

cyclosporine (Gengraf, Neoral, Sandimmune, SangCya) (Cardio, GI, Uro). Immunosuppressant drug given after organ transplantation to prevent rejection of the donor heart, liver, or kidney. Capsule: 25 mg, 50 mg, 100 mg. Liquid: 100 mg/mL. Intravenous: 50 mg/mL. [sy-kloh-SPOHR-een]. 110, 132, 173

cyclosporine (Neoral) (Derm, Ortho). Immunosuppressant drug used to treat severe, disabling psoriasis and rheumatoid arthritis. Capsule: 25 mg, 100 mg. Liquid: 100 mg/mL. [sy-kloh-SPOHR-een]. 87

cyclosporine (Optimmune) (Oph). Used to treat Sjogren's syndrome. Orphan drug. [sy-kloh-SPOHR-een].

Cycrin (OB/GYN). Progestins hormone drug used to treat amenorrhea; used to treat abnormal uterine bleeding. For dosage, see *medroxyprogesterone*. [SY-krihn]. 253

Cyklokapron (Hem). Hemostatic drug used to prevent or treat hemorrhage in hemophiliac patients; used during tooth extractions in these patients. For dosage, see *tranexamic acid*.

Cylert (Neuro, Psych). Central nervous system stimulant used to treat narcolepsy; used to treat attention-deficit/hyperactivity disorder. (Schedule IV drug). For dosage, see *pemoline*. [SY-lehrt]. 274, 292

Cymeval (Antivir). Antiviral drug used to treat cytomegalovirus retinitis. For dosage, see *valganciclovir*. [SIH-meh-vehl]. 330

cyproheptadine (Periactin) (Antivir, Derm, ENT). Antihistamine used to treat AIDS wasting syndrome; used to treat allergic rhinitis and allergic reactions with hives and itching. Liquid: 2 mg/5 mL. Tablet: 4 mg. [sih-proh-HEHP-tah-deen]. 207, 327

cyproterone (Androcur) (Endo). Used to treat severe hirsutism. Orphan drug.

Cystadane (Uro). Used to treat homocystinuria. For dosage, see *betaine*.

Cystagon (Uro). Used to treat nephropathic cystinosis. For dosage, see *cysteamine*.

cysteamine (Cystagon) (Uro). Used to treat nephropathic cystinosis. Orphan drug.

Cystex (Uro) (generic *methenamine, sodium salicylate*). Combination drug used to treat urinary tract infections. Tablet: 162 mg/162.5 mg. [SIHS-tehks].

cystic fibrosis, drugs used to treat.

Cystospaz, Cystospaz-M (GI, Uro). Antispasmodic drug used to treat spasm of the smooth muscle of the bowel and bladder. For dosage, see *L-hyoscyamine*. 107

Cytadren (Chemo, Endo). Steroid drug used to suppress the adrenal cortex to treat Cushing's syndrome; used to treat breast and prostate cancer. For dosage, see *aminoglutethimide*. [SY-tah-drehn]. 232, 351

cytarabine (Cytosar-U, Tarabine PFS) (Chemo). Pyrimidine antagonist chemotherapy drug used to treat leukemia. Subcutaneous, intravenous, or intrathecal: 20 mg/mL, (powder to be reconstituted): 100 mg, 500 mg, 1 g, 2 g. [sy-TEH-rah-been]. 340

cytarabine (DepoCyt) (Chemo). Liposomal form of pyrimidine antagonist chemotherapy drug used to treat malignant meningitis. Injection into lumbar sac or into an intraventricular reservoir: 10 mg/mL. [sy-TEH-rah-been]. 361

CytoGam (Antivir). Antiviral immunoglobulin used to prevent cytomegalovirus infection in patients with an organ transplant. For dosage, see *cytomegalovirus immunoglobulin*. [SY-toh-gehm].

Cytoimplant (Chemo). Chemotherapy drug used to treat pancreatic cancer. Orphan drug. 347

cytolin (Antivir). Monoclonal antibody used to treat AIDS. Investigational drug. 326

cytomegalovirus (CMV) infection/retinitis, drugs used to treat. 329

cytomegalovirus immunoglobulin (CytoGam) (Antivir). Used to prevent cytomegalovirus infection in patients with an organ transplant. Orphan drug.

Cytomel (Endo). Thyroid hormone replacement. For dosage, see *liothyronine*. [SY-toh-mehl]. 229

Cytosar-U (Chemo). Pyrimidine antagonist chemotherapy drug. For dosage, see *cytarabine*. [SY-toh-sahr]. 340

Cytotec (GI, OB/GYN). Used to prevent ulcers in patients taking aspirin or nonsteroidal anti-inflammatory drugs; used to induce labor; used to assist in abortion. For dosage, see *misoprostol*. [SY-toh-tehk]. 119, 148, 255, 309

Cytovene (Antivir, Oph). Antiviral drug used to treat cytomegalovirus retinitis; used to treat cytomegalovirus in organ transplant recipients. For dosage, see *ganciclovir*. [SY-toh-veen]. 330

Cytoxan, Cytoxan Lyophilized (Chemo, Uro). Alkylating chemotherapy drug used to treat Hodgkin's disease, non-Hodgkin's lymphoma, multiple myeloma, leukemia, brain cancer, eye cancer, cutaneous T-cell lymphoma, and cancer of the breast and ovary; used to treat pediatric nephrotic syndrome. For dosage, see *cyclophosphamide*. [sy-TAWK-sihn]. 111, 341

dacarbazine (DTIC-Dome) (Chemo, Endo). Alkylating chemotherapy drug used to treat malignant melanoma and Hodgkin's disease; used to treat pheochromocytoma of the adrenal cortex. Intravenous: 10 mg/mL. [dah-KAWR-bah-zeen]. 341

daclizumab (Zenapax) (Uro). Immunosuppressant monoclonal antibody given after kidney transplantation to prevent rejection of the donor kidney. Intravenous: 25 mg/5 mL. [dah-KLIH-zoo-mehb]. 110

dactinomycin (Cosmegen) (Chemo). Chemotherapy antibiotic used to treat uterine cancer, bone cancer, testicular cancer, rhabdomyosarcoma, and Wilm's tumor. Intravenous (powder to be reconstituted): 0.5 mg. [dehk-tihn-oh-MY-sihn]. 342

Dalalone, Dalalone D.P., Dalalone L.A. (Derm, Ortho, Neuro). Corticosteroid anti-inflammatory drug injected into a joint to treat osteoarthritis and rheumatoid arthritis; also injected near a joint to treat bursitis and tenosynovitis; also given intravenously to treat cerebral edema; also injected into skin lesions. For dosage, see *dexamethasone*. [DEH-lah-lohn]. 92, 141, 275

(Dalgan) (Analges). No longer on the market. (Generic name *dezocine*; nonnarcotic analgesic drug).

Dalmane (Neuro). Nonbarbiturate benzodiazepine drug used to treat insomnia. (Schedule IV drug). For dosage, see *flurazepam*. [dehl-MAYN]. 272

dalteparin (Fragmin) (Hem). Low molecular weight heparin anticoagulant. Subcutaneous: 2500 IU (16 mg/0.2 mL), 5000 IU (32 mg/0.2 mL), 10,000 IU (64 mg/mL). [dawl-teh-PEH-rihn]. 186

danaparoid (Orgaran) (Hem). Low molecular weight heparin-like anticoagulant. Subcutaneous: 750 anti-Xa units/0.6 mL. 186

danazol (Danocrine) (Endo, OB/GYN). Male sex hormone used to treat precocious puberty; used to treat gynecomastia; used to treat endometriosis; used to treat fibrocystic breast disease; used to treat hereditary angioedema. Capsule: 50 mg, 100 mg, 200 mg. [DEH-nah-zawl]. 248

Danocrine (Endo, OB/GYN). Male sex hormone used to treat precocious puberty; used to treat gynecomastia; used to treat endometriosis; used to treat fibrocystic breast disease; used to treat heredi-

tary angioedema. For dosage, see *danazol*. [DEH-noh-krihn]. 248

Dantrium (Anes, Ortho, Psych). Skeletal muscle relaxant; used to treat intraoperative malignant hyperthermia; used to treat severe muscle spasticity associated with multiple sclerosis, cerebral palsy, stroke, or spinal cord injury; used to treat neuroleptic malignant syndrome caused by an adverse reaction to antipsychotic drugs. For dosage, see *dantrolene*. [DEHN-tree-uhm]. 145, 293, 371

dantrolene (Dantrium) (Anes, Ortho, Psych). Skeletal muscle relaxant; used to treat intraoperative malignant hyperthermia; used to treat severe muscle spasticity associated with multiple sclerosis, cerebral palsy, stroke, or spinal cord injury; used to treat neuroleptic malignant syndrome caused by an adverse reaction to antipsychotic drugs. Capsule: 25 mg, 50 mg, 100 mg. Intravenous (powder to be reconstituted): 20 mg. [DEHN-troh-leen]. 145, 293, 371

dapiprazole (Rev-Eyes) (Oph). Topical alpha-receptor blocker used to treat glaucoma. Ophthalmic solution (powder to be reconstituted): 25 mg/5 mL (0.5%). [deh-PIH-preh-zohl]. 221

dapsone (Antivir, Ortho). Drug used to treat leprosy; used to treat *Pneumocystis carinii* pneumonia in AIDS patients; used to treat leishmaniasis; used to treat rheumatoid arthritis. Tablet: 25 mg, 100 mg. [DEHP-zohn]. 147, 328

Daranide (Oph). Carbonic anhydrase inhibitor used to treat glaucoma. For dosage, see *dichlorphenamide*. 221

darbepoetin alfa (Aranesp) (Uro). Erythropoietin-type drug used to treat anemia in patients with chronic renal failure. Subcutaneous or intravenous: 25 mcg, 40 mcg, 60 mcg, 100 mcg, 200 mcg. [dahr-bee-poy-EE-tihn]. 111

(Darbid) (GI). No longer on the market. (Generic name *isopropamide*; GI antispasmodic drug).

(Daricon) (GI). No longer on the market. (Generic name *oxyphencyclimine*; GI antispasmodic drug).

Darvocet-N 50, Darvocet-N 100 (Analges) (generic *propoxyphene, acetaminophen*). Combination narcotic and nonnarcotic drug. (Schedule IV drug). Tablet: 50 mg/326 mg, 100 mg/650 mg. [DAWR-voh-seht]. 302

Darvon Compound-65 (Analges) (generic *propoxyphene, aspirin*). Combination narcotic and nonnarcotic drug. (Schedule IV drug). Pulvules: 65 mg/389 mg. [DAWR-vawn]. 302

Darvon-N, Darvon Pulvules (Analges). Narcotic analgesic drug used to treat mild-to-moderate pain. (Schedule IV drug). For dosage, see *propoxyphene*. [DAWR-vawn]. 298

(Datril) (Analges). No longer on the market. (Generic name *acetaminophen*; analgesic drug).

daunorubicin (Cerubidine) (Chemo). Chemotherapy antibiotic used to treat leukemia. Intravenous: 5 mg/mL, (powder to be reconstituted) 20 mg, 50 mg. [daw-noh-ROO-beh-sihn]. 342

daunorubicin (DaunoXome) (Chemo). Liposomal form of chemotherapy antibiotic used to treat Kaposi's sarcoma. Intravenous: 2 mg/mL. [daw-noh-ROO-beh-sihn]. 342

DaunoXome (Antivir). Liposomal form of chemotherapy antibiotic used to treat Kaposi's sarcoma. For dosage, see *daunorubicin*. [DAW-noh-zohm]. 342

Daypro (Analges, Ortho). Nonsteroidal anti-inflammatory drug used to treat osteoarthritis and rheumatoid arthritis. For dosage, see *oxaprozin*. [DAY-proh]. 139, 304

DCF. See *pentostatin*.

DDAVP. See *desmopressin*.

ddC (abbreviation for *dideoxycytidine*). See *zalcitabine*.

ddI (abbreviation for *dideoxyinosine*). See *didanosine*.

DEA (abbreviation for *Drug Enforcement Administration*). See *Drug Enforcement Administration*.

de Angelcy, Marquis. 366

DEA number. 17, 79

Debacterol (ENT). Topical chemical cautery drug that debrides necrotic tissue and kills bacteria. Used to treat canker sores and ulcerating mouth lesions. Liquid.

debridement, drugs used for tissue. 96

Debrisan (Derm) (generic *dextranomer*). Topical drug used to absorb drainage from burns, skin ulcers, and wounds. Beads, paste. [deh-BREE-sehn]. 96

Debrox (ENT). Topical drug used to soften hardened cerumen in the ear. Drops.

Decabid (Cardio) (generic *indecainide*). Antiarrhythmic drug. Investigational drug. 173

Decadron (Chemo, Derm, Endo). Oral corticosteroid anti-inflammatory drug used to treat severe inflammation in various body systems; used to diagnose Cushing's syndrome; used as part of chemotherapy treatment. For dosage, see *dexamethasone*. [DEH-kah-drawn]. 93, 232, 351

Decadron (Derm) (generic *dexamethasone*). Topical corticosteroid anti-inflammatory drug. Cream: 0.1%. [DEH-kah-drawn]. 92

Decadron (Oph). Topical corticosteroid used to treat inflammation of the eyes. For dosage, see *dexamethasone*. [DEH-kah-drawn].

Decadron, Decadron-LA (Ortho, Neuro). Corticosteroid anti-inflammatory drug injected into a joint to treat osteoarthritis and rheumatoid arthritis; also injected near a joint to treat bursitis and tenosynovi-

tis; also given intravenously to treat cerebral edema. For dosage, see *dexamethasone*. [DEH-kah-drawn]. 141, 275

(Decadron Respihaler) (Resp). No longer on the market. (Generic name *dexamethasone*; corticosteroid for asthma).

(Decadron Turbinaire) (ENT). No longer on the market. (Generic name *dexamethasone*; topical intranasal corticosteroid).

Decadron with Xylocaine (Ortho) (generic *dexamethasone, lidocaine*). Combination corticosteroid anti-inflammatory and anesthetic drug used to treat bursitis and tenosynovitis. Periarticular injection: 4 mg/10mg per mL. 148

Deca-Durabolin (Chemo, Endo, Hem). Anabolic steroid used to treat metastatic breast cancer; also used to increase red blood cell production to treat anemia; also used illegally by athletes. For dosage, see *nandrolone*. [DEH-kah-dyoor-EH-boh-lihn]. 234

Decapeptyl (Chemo). Chemotherapy drug used to treat ovarian cancer. For dosage, see *triptorelin*. [deh-kah-PEHP-tuhl]. 343

Decaspray (Derm) (generic *dexamethasone*). Topical corticosteroid anti-inflammatory drug. Spray: 0.04%. 92

Decholin (GI). Used to thin bile secretions in patients prone to bile duct obstruction. For dosage, see *dehydrocholic acid*. [DEH-koh-lihn]. 132

decitabine (Chemo). Chemotherapy drug used to treat leukemia; used to treat myelodysplastic syndrome. Orphan drug. 347

Declomycin (Antibio, Endo). Tetracycline-type antibiotic; also used to treat SIADH. For dosage, see *demeclocycline*. [deh-kloh-MY-sihn]. 231, 317

Deconamine (ENT) (generic *pseudoephedrine, chlorpheniramine*). Combination decongestant and antihistamine drug. Syrup: 30 mg/2 mg. Tablet: 60 mg/4 mg. [dee-KAW-nah-meen].

Deconamine CX (ENT) (generic *pseudoephedrine, hydrocodone, guaifenesin*). Combination decongestant, narcotic antitussive, and expectorant drug. Liquid: 60 mg/5 mg/200 mg. Tablet: 30 mg/5 mg/300 mg. [dee-KAW-nah-meen].

Deconamine SR (ENT) (generic *pseudoephedrine, chlorpheniramine*). Combination decongestant and antihistamine drug. Capsule: 120 mg/8 mg. [dee-KAW-nah-meen].

decongestants (ENT). Class of drugs used to decrease congestion of mucous membranes of sinuses and nose. 62, 206

Defy (Oph). Topical antibiotic used to treat bacterial eye infections. For dosage, see *tobramycin*. [dee-FY]. 218

Dehydrex (Oph). Used to treat corneal erosions. For dosage, see *dextran 70*.

dehydrocholic acid (Decholin) (GI). Used to thin bile secretions in patients prone to bile duct obstruction. Tablet: 250 mg. [dee-hy-droh-KOH-lihk]. 132

Delaprem (OB/GYN). Ovulation-stimulating drug used to treat infertility. For dosage, see *hexoprenaline*. [DEH-lah-prehm]. 246

Delatestryl (Chemo, Endo). Male sex hormone used to treat breast cancer in women; used to treat the lack of production of testosterone due to absence, injury, malfunction of the testes or malfunction of the pituitary gland; used to treat delayed puberty in boys. For dosage, see *testosterone*. [deh-lah-TEHS-trihl]. 343

delavirdine (Rescriptor) (Antivir). Nonnucleoside reverse transcriptase inhibitor drug used to treat AIDS. Tablet: 100 mg, 200 mg. [deh-lah-VEER-deen]. 325

Delestrogen (Chemo, OB/GYN). Hormone chemotherapy drug used to treat prostate carcinoma; hormone replacement therapy used to treat the symptoms of menopause. For dosage, see *estradiol valerate*. [deh-LEHS-troh-jehn]. 252, 343

(Delta-Cortef) (Endo, Ortho). No longer on the market. (Generic name *prednisolone*; corticosteroid anti-inflammatory drug).

Deltasone (Chemo, Endo). Oral corticosteroid anti-inflammatory drug used to treat severe inflammation in various body systems; used as part of chemotherapy treatment. For dosage, see *prednisone*. [DEHL-teh-sohn]. 232, 351

Demadex (Uro). Loop diuretic. For dosage, see *torsemide*. [DEH-mah-dehks]. 104

(Demazin) (ENT). No longer on the market. (Combination drug with *phenylpropanolamine*; decongestant and antihistamine drug).

demecarium (Humorsol) (Oph). Topical cholinesterase inhibitor drug used to treat glaucoma. Ophthalmic solution: 0.125%, 0.25%. [deh-meh-KEH-ree-uhm]. 221

demeclocycline (Declomycin) (Antibio, Endo). Tetracycline-type antibiotic; also used to treat SIADH. Capsule: 150 mg. Tablet: 150 mg, 300 mg. [deh-meh-kloh-SY-kleen]. 231, 317

Demerol (Analges, Anes, OB/GYN). Narcotic analgesic used to treat moderate-to-severe pain; given preoperatively to produce sedation and relieve pain; used for pain relief during childbirth. (Schedule II drug). For dosage, see *meperidine*. [DEH-meh-rawl]. 297, 371

Demser (Endo). Inhibits the enzyme that helps to produce epinephrine and norepinephrine. Used to treat hypertension caused by excessive epinephrine and norepinephrine from a pheochromocytoma of the adrenal medulla. For dosage, see *metyrosine*. [DEHM-zehr].

Demulen 1/35, Demulen 1/50 (OB/GYN) (generic *ethynodiol, ethinyl estradiol*). Monophasic combination progestins and estrogen oral contraceptive. Tablet: 35 mcg/1 mg, 50 mcg/1 mg. [DEH-myoo-lehn]. 249

Denavir (Derm, ENT) (generic *penciclovir*). Topical antiviral drug used to treat herpes simplex virus, type 1 (cold sores) infections. Cream: 10 mg/g. [DEH-nah-veer]. 91

denileukin (Ontak) (Chemo). Chemotherapy recombinant DNA drug that combines interleukin-2 and diphtheria toxin protein that is kept frozen until thawed for use; used to treat cutaneous T-cell lymphoma. Intravenous: 140 mcg/mL. [deh-nee-LOO-kihn]. 347

Denorex, Extra Strength Denorex (Derm) (generic *coal tar*). Topical drug used to treat psoriasis. Shampoo: 9%, 12.5%. [DEH-noh-rehks]. 86

Dentipatch (Anes) (generic *lidocaine*). Topical dental anesthetic. Patch: 23/2 cm^2, 46.1/2 cm^2.

deoxycoformycin. See *pentostatin*.

Depacon (Analges, Neuro, Psych). Used to treat migraine headaches, used to treat absence and complex partial seizures; used to treat the mania of manic-depressive disorder. For dosage, see *valproic acid*. [DEH-pah-kawn]. 265, 288, 307

Depakene (Analges, Neuro, Psych). Used to treat migraine headaches, used to treat absence and complex partial seizures; used to treat the mania of manic-depressive disorder. For dosage, see *valproic acid*. [DEH-pah-keen]. 265, 288, 307

Depakote, Depakote ER (Analges, Neuro, Psych). Used to treat migraine headaches, used to treat absence and complex partial seizures; used to treat the mania of manic-depressive disorder. For dosage, see *valproic acid*. [DEH-pah-koht]. 265, 288, 307

dependence, physical/psychological.

depGynogen (OB/GYN). Hormone replacement therapy used to treat the symptoms of menopause. For dosage, see *estradiol cypionate*. [dehp-GY-noh-jehn]. 252

DepoCyt (Chemo). Liposomal form of pyrimidine antagonist chemotherapy drug used to treat malignant meningitis. For dosage, see *cytarabine*. [DEH-poh-siht]. 361

Depo-Estradiol Cypionate (OB/GYN). Hormone replacement therapy used to treat the symptoms of menopause. For dosage, see *estradiol cypionate*. [deh-poh-ehs-trah-DY-awl SIH-pee-oh-nayt]. 252

DepoGen (OB/GYN).   Hormone replacement therapy used to treat the symptoms of menopause.   For dosage, see *estradiol cypionate*. [DEH-poh-jehn]. 252

Depo-Medrol (Derm, Endo, Ortho).   Corticosteroid anti-inflammatory drug used to treat Addison's disease; also injected into a joint to treat osteoarthritis and rheumatoid arthritis; also injected near a joint to treat bursitis and tenosynovitis; also injected into skin lesions.   For dosage, see *methylprednisolone*. [deh-poh-MEH-drawl]. 92, 141, 232

Deponit (Cardio).   Nitrate drug used to prevent and treat angina pectoris.   For dosage, see *nitroglycerin*. [DEH-poh-niht]. 156

Depopred-40, Depopred-80 (Derm, Endo, Ortho).   Corticosteroid anti-inflammatory drug used to treat Addison's disease; also injected into a joint to treat osteoarthritis and rheumatoid arthritis; also injected near a joint to treat bursitis and tenosynovitis; also injected into skin lesions.   For dosage, see *methylprednisolone*. [DEH-poh-prehd]. 92, 141, 232

Depo-Provera (Chemo, OB/GYN).   Hormonal chemotherapy drug used to treat breast cancer, uterine cancer, and kidney cancer; progestins-only 3-month contraceptive.   For dosage, see *medroxyprogesterone*. [deh-poh-proh-VEH-rah]. 251, 343

Depo-Testadiol (OB/GYN) (generic *testosterone, estradiol cypionate*).   Combination androgen and estrogen drug used to treat symptoms of menopause. Intramuscular: 50 mg/2 mg. [deh-poh-TEHS-teh-dy-awl]. 253

Depo-Testosterone (Endo).   Male sex hormone used to treat the lack of production of testosterone due to absence, injury, malfunction of the testes or malfunction of the pituitary gland; used to treat delayed puberty in boys.   For dosage, see *testosterone*. [deh-poh-tehs-TAW- steh-rohn].

depression caused by Accutane. 85

depression, drugs used to treat. 285

(Deprol) (Psych).   No longer on the market. (Generic names *benactyzine, meprobamate*; combination antidepressant drug).

Dermacort (Derm) (generic *hydrocortisone*).   Topical corticosteroid anti-inflammatory drug. Cream: 1%. Lotion: 1%. 92

Dermamycin (Derm) (generic *diphenhydramine*).   Topical antihistamine/antipruritic drug. Cream: 2%. Spray: 2%. 93

Derma-Smoothe/FS (Derm) (generic *fluocinolone*). Topical corticosteroid anti-inflammatory drug. Oil: 0.01%. 92

dermatology drugs. 82

Dermatop (Derm) (generic *prednicarbate*).   Topical corticosteroid anti-inflammatory drug. Cream: 0.1%. 92

Dermolate (Derm) (generic *hydrocortisone*).   Topical corticosteroid anti-inflammatory drug. Cream: 0.5%. [DEHR-moh-layt]. 92

Dermoplast (Derm) (generic *benzocaine*).   Topical anesthetic. Lotion: 8%. Spray: 20%. [DEHR-moh-PLEHST]. 94

Dermuspray (Derm) (generic *trypsin*).   Topical enzyme drug used to debride burns and wounds. Spray. [DEHR-moo-sprah]. 96

Desenex (Derm) (generic *clotrimazole*).   Topical antifungal drug. Cream: 1%. [DEH-seh-nehks]. 89

desflurane (Suprane) (Anes).   Used to induce and maintain general anesthesia. Inhaled gas. [dehs-FLOH-rayn]. 370

desiccated thyroid (Armour Thyroid) (Endo).   Thyroid hormone replacement used to treat hypothyroidism. Capsule: 60 mg (1 grain), 120 mg (2 grains), 180 mg (3 grains), 300 mg (5 grains). Tablet: 15 mg (¼ grain), 30 mg (½ grain), 60 mg (1 grain), 90 mg (1½ grains), 120 mg (2 grains), 180 mg (3 grains), 240 mg (4 grains), 300 mg (5 grains). [DEH-seh-kay-tehd THY-royd]. 229

desipramine (Norpramin) (Analges, Derm, Diab, Neuro, Ortho).   Tricyclic antidepressant used to treat migraines; used to treat urticaria; used to treat diabetic neuropathy; used to treat postherpetic neuralgia; used to treat phantom limb pain. Tablet: 10 mg, 25 mg, 50 mg, 75 mg, 100 mg, 150 mg. [deh-SIP-rah-meen]. 98, 147, 241, 275, 307

desipramine (Norpramin) (OB/GYN, Psych).   Tricyclic antidepressant used to treat depression; used to treat panic disorder; used to treat anorexia nervosa and bulimia nervosa; used to treat the symptoms of cocaine withdrawal; used to treat premenstrual dysphoric disorder. Tablet: 10 mg, 25 mg, 50 mg, 75 mg, 100 mg, 150 mg. [deh-SIP-rah-meen]. 254, 285, 289, 291

Desitin (Derm) (generic *vitamin A, zinc oxide*).   Topical combination drug with vitamin A plus an astringent to dry oozing skin. Ointment. [DEH-sih-tihn]. 95

desloratadine (Clarinex) (Derm, ENT).   Antihistamine used to treat idiopathic urticaria; used to treat allergic rhinitis. Tablet: 5 mg. [dehs-loh-REH-tah-deen]. 207

deslorelin (Somagard) (Endo).   Used to treat precocious puberty. Orphan drug.

desmopressin (DDAVP, Stimate) (Endo, Hem).   Antidiuretic hormone replacement used to treat diabetes insipidus and bleeding in hemophiliacs. Tablet: 0.1 mg, 0.2 mg. Nasal spray: 0.1 mg/mL (10 mcg/spray) (400 IU), 1.5 mg/mL. Intravenous or subcutaneous: 4 mcg/mL. [dehz-moh-PREH-sihn]. 188, 231 desmopressin (DDAVP, Stimate) (Uro). Antidiuretic hormone replacement used to treat enuresis. Nasal spray: 0.1 mg/mL (10 mcg/spray) (400 IU), 1.5 mg/mL. [dehz-moh-PREH-sihn]. 111

Desogen (OB/GYN) (generic *desogestrel, ethinyl estradiol*). Monophasic combination progestins and estrogen oral contraceptive. Tablet: 0.15 mg/30 mcg. [DEH-soh-jehn]. 249

desonide (DesOwen, Tridesilon) (Derm). Topical corticosteroid anti-inflammatory drug. Cream: 0.05%. Lotion: 0.05%. Ointment: 0.05%. [DEH-soh-nide]. 92

DesOwen (Derm) (generic *desonide*). Topical corticosteroid anti-inflammatory drug. Cream: 0.05%. Lotion: 0.05%. Ointment: 0.05%. 92

desoximetasone (Topicort, Topicort LP) (Derm). Topical corticosteroid anti-inflammatory drug. Cream: 0.05%, 0.25%. Gel: 0.05%. Ointment: 0.25%. [deh-sawk-see-MEH-tah-sohn]. 92

desoxyephedrine (Vicks Inhaler) (ENT). Decongestant. Nasal inhaler: 50 mg/puff. [deh-sawk-see-eh-FEH-drihn]. 206

Desoxyn, Desoxyn Gradumet (Neuro, Psych). Central nervous system stimulant used to treat narcolepsy; used to treat attention-deficit/hyperactivity disorder. (Schedule II drug). For dosage, see *methamphetamine*. [deh-SAWK-sehn]. 274, 291

Desquam-E, Desquam-E 5, Desquam-E 10, Desquam-X 5, Desquam-X 5 Wash, Desquam-X 10, Desquam-X 10 Wash (Derm) (generic *benzoyl peroxide*). Topical antibiotic used to treat acne vulgaris. Gel: 2.5%, 5%, 10%. Liquid: 5%, 10%. [DEHS-kwahm]. 83

Desyrel, Desyrel Dividose (Psych). Tetracyclic antidepressant used to treat depression; used to treat panic disorder. For dosage, see *trazodone*. [DEH-seh-rehl]. 288, 289

Detrol, Detrol LA (Uro). Used to treat overactive bladder. For dosage, see *tolterodine*. [DEH-trawl].

Dexacidin, Dexacidin Ophthalmic Suspension (Oph) (generic *dexamethasone, neomycin, polymyxin B*). Topical combination corticosteroid and antibiotic drug. Ophthalmic ointment: 0.1%/0.25%/10,000 units. Ophthalmic suspension: 0.1%/0.25%/10,000 units. [DEHK-sah-sy-dihn].

Dexameth (Chemo, Endo). Corticosteroid anti-inflammatory drug used to treat severe inflammation in various body systems; used to diagnose Cushing's syndrome; used as part of chemotherapy treatment. For dosage, see *dexamethasone*. [DEHK-sah-meth]. 232, 351

dexamethasone (Dalalone, Dalalone D.P., Dalalone L.A., Decadron, Decadron-LA, Hexadrol) (Derm, Ortho, Neuro). Corticosteroid anti-inflammatory drug injected into a joint to treat osteoarthritis and rheumatoid arthritis; also injected near a joint to treat bursitis and tenosynovitis; also injected into skin lesions; also given intravenously to treat cerebral edema. Intra-articular, periarticular, intradermal, or intravenous: 4 mg/mL, 8 mg/mL, 10 mg/mL, 16 mg/mL, 20 mg/mL, 24 mg/mL. [dehk-sah-MEH-theh-zohn]. 92, 141, 275

dexamethasone (Decadron, Decaspray) (Derm). Topical corticosteroid anti-inflammatory drug. Cream: 0.1%. Spray: 0.04%. [dehk-sah-MEH-theh-zohn]. 92

dexamethasone (Decadron, Dexameth, Dexamethasone Intensol, Dexone, Hexadrol) (Chemo, Derm, Endo). Corticosteroid anti-inflammatory drug used to treat severe inflammation in various body systems; used to diagnose Cushing's syndrome; used as part of chemotherapy treatment. Elixir: 0.5 mg/5 mL. Liquid: 0.5 mg/0.5 mL, 0.5 mg/5 mL. Tablet: 0.25 mg, 0.5 mg, 0.75 mg, 1 mg, 1.5 mg, 2 mg, 4 mg, 6 mg. Tablets pack: Six 1.5 mg and eight 0.75 mg. [dehk-sah-MEH-theh-zohn]. 93, 232, 351

dexamethasone (Decadron, Maxidex) (Oph). Topical corticosteroid used to treat inflammation of the eyes. Ophthalmic solution: 0.1%. Ophthalmic suspension: 0.1%. Ophthalmic ointment: 0.05%. [dehk-sah-MEH-theh-zohn].

Dexamethasone Intensol (Chemo, Endo). Corticosteroid anti-inflammatory drug used to treat severe inflammation in various body systems; used to diagnose Cushing's syndrome; used as part of chemotherapy treatment. For dosage, see *dexamethasone*. [dehk-sah-MEH-theh-zohn ehn-TEHN-sawl]. 232, 351

(Dexasporin) (Oph). No longer on the market. (Combination corticosteroid and antibiotic drug for the eye).

(Dexatrim) (GI). No longer on the market. (Generic name *phenylpropanolamine*; appetite suppressant).

dexchlorpheniramine (Polaramine, Polaramine Repetabs) (Derm, ENT). Antihistamine used to treat allergic rhinitis and allergic reactions with hives and itching. Liquid: 2 mg/5 mL. Tablet: 2 mg, 4 mg, 6 mg. [dehks-klohr-feh-NEER-ah-meen]. 207

Dexedrine, Dexedrine Spansules (Neuro, Psych). Central nervous system stimulant used to treat narcolepsy; used to treat attention-deficit/hyperactivity disorder. (Schedule II drug). For dosage, see *dextroamphetamine*. [DEHK-seh-dreen]. 274, 291

(dexfenfluramine) (GI). No longer on the market. (Trade name *Redux*; appetite suppressant used to treat obesity).

dexloxiglumide (GI). Cholecystokinin receptor blocker used to treat irritable bowel syndrome. Investigational drug. 133

dexmedetomidine (Precedex) (Anes, Resp). Nonbarbiturate drug used as a preoperative sedative; used to sedate patients who are intubated and on the ventilator. Intravenous: 100 mcg/mL. [decks-meh-deh-TOH-meh-deen]. 371

dexmethylphenidate (Focalin) (Psych). Central nervous system stimulant used to treat attention-deficit/hyperactivity disorder. Tablet: 2 mg, 5 mg, 10 mg. [dehks-meh-thuhl-FEH-neh-dayt]. 292

Dexone (Chemo, Endo). Oral corticosteroid anti-inflammatory drug used to treat severe inflammation in various body systems; used to diagnose Cushing's syndrome; used as part of chemotherapy treatment. For dosage, see *dexamethasone*. [DEHK-zohn]. 232, 350

dexpanthenol (Ilopan) (GI). Gastric stimulant used to treat paralytic ileus. Intramuscular or intravenous: 250 mg/mL. [dehks-PEHN-theh-nawl]. 126

dexpanthenol (Panthoderm) (Derm). Topical antipruritic drug. Cream: 2%. [dehks-PEHN-theh-nawl]. 95

dexrazoxane (Zinecard) (Cardio). Cytoprotective drug used to prevent cardiomyopathy in patients receiving doxorubicin chemotherapy. Intravenous (powder to be reconstituted): 10 mg/mL; 250 mg, 500 mg. [dehks-rah-ZAWK-zayn]. 173, 350

dextran 40 (Gentran 40, Rheomacrodex) (I.V.). Intravenous nonblood plasma volume expander. 382

dextran 1 (Promit) (I.V.). Given intravenously before a dextran infusion to prevent an anaphylactic reaction. Intravenous: 150 mg/mL. 383

dextran 70 (Dehydrex) (Oph). Used to treat corneal erosions. Orphan drug.

dextran 70 (Gentran 70, Macrodex) (I.V.). Intravenous nonblood plasma volume expander. 382

dextran 75 (Gentran 75) (I.V.). Intravenous nonblood plasma volume expander. 382

dextranomer (Debrisan) (Derm). Topical drug used to absorb drainage from burns, skin ulcers, and wounds. Beads, paste. 96

dextran sulfate (Antivir). Used to treat AIDS. Orphan drug. 326

dextran sulfate (Uendex) (Resp). Used to treat cystic fibrosis. Aerosol inhaler. Orphan drug.

dextroamphetamine (Dexedrine, Dexedrine Spansules, Dextrostat) (Neuro, Psych). Central nervous system stimulant used to treat narcolepsy; used to treat attention-deficit/hyperactivity disorder. (Schedule II drug). Capsule: 5 mg, 10 mg, 15 mg. Tablet: 5 mg, 10 mg. [dehks-troh-ehm-FEH-tah-meen]. 274, 291

dextromethorphan (Benylin Adult, Benylin DM, Benylin Pediatric, Drixoral Cough Liquid Caps, Pediatric Vicks 44d Dry Hacking Cough and Head Congestion, Pertussin CS, Pertussin ES, Robitussin Cough Calmers, Robitussin Pediatric, St. Joseph Cough Suppressant, Sucrets Cough Control, Sucrets 4-Hour Cough, Vicks Dry Hacking Cough) (ENT). Nonnarcotic antitussive drug. Capsule: 30 mg. Liquid/syrup: 3.5 mg/5 mL, 7.5 mg/5 mL, 10 mg/5 mL, 15 mg/5 mL, 10 mg/15 mL, 15 mg/15 mL. Lozenge: 5 mg, 7.5 mg, 15 mg. [dehks-troh-meh-THOHR-fehn].210

dextrorotary. 62

dextrose 50% in water, dextrose 5% in water (D-5-W), dextrose 40% in water, dextrose 70% in water, dextrose 60% in water, dextrose 10% in water (D-10-W), dextrose 20% in water, dextrose 25% in water, dextrose 2.5% in water (D-2.5-W) (I.V.). Intravenous fluid of dextrose and water. 375

dextrose 5% with lactated Ringer's (D5/LR) (I.V.). Intravenous fluid of dextrose with sodium, potassium, calcium, chloride, and lactate. 376

dextrose 5% with normal saline (D5/NS), dextrose 5% with half normal saline (D5/0.45% NaCl), dextrose 10% with normal saline (D10/NS), dextrose 10% with half normal saline (D10/0.45% NaCl) (I.V.). Intravenous fluid of dextrose with saline. 376

Dextrostat (Neuro, Psych). Central nervous system stimulant used to treat narcolepsy; used to treat attention-deficit/hyperactivity disorder. (Schedule II drug). For dosage, see *dextroamphetamine*. 274, 291

(dextrothyroxine) (Cardio). No longer on the market. (Trade name *Choloxin*; used to treat hypercholesterolemia).

(dezocine) (Analges). No longer on the market. (Trade name *Dalgan*; nonnarcotic analgesic drug).

d4T. See *stavudine*.

D.H.E. 45 (Analges). Used to treat migraine headaches. For dosage, see *dihydroergotamine*. 307

DiaBeta (Diab). Oral antidiabetic drug. For dosage, see *glyburide*. [dy-ah-BAY-teh]. 240

diabetes insipidus, drugs used to treat. 231

diabetes mellitus, drugs used to treat. 236

diabetic neuropathy, drugs used to treat. 241

Diabinese (Diab). Oral antidiabetic drug. For dosage, see *chlorpropamide*. [dy-EH-beh-neez]. 240

(Dialose) (GI). No longer on the market. (Generic name *docusate*; laxative).

Diamox, Diamox Sequels (Cardio, Neuro, Oph). Carbonic anhydrase inhibitor used to treat edema in congestive heart failure; used to treat absence seizures; used to treat glaucoma. For dosage, see *acetazolamide*. [DY-ah-mawks]. 172, 221, 265

(Diapid) (Endo). No longer on the market. (Generic name *lypressin*; used to treat diabetes insipidus).

diarrhea, drugs used to treat. See *antidiarrheal drugs*.

Diastat (Neuro). Benzodiazepine drug used to treat status epilepticus. (Schedule IV drug). For dosage, see *diazepam*. 267

diazepam (Diastat, Valium) (Emerg, Neuro, Psych). Benzodiazepine drug used to treat status epilepticus and acute alcohol withdrawal. (Schedule IV drug). Endotracheal, intramuscular, or intravenous: 5 mg/mL. [dy-EH-zeh-pehm]. 267

diazepam (Diazepam Intensol, Valium) (Neuro, Ortho). Benzodiazepine drug used as a skeletal muscle relaxant to treat minor muscle spasms associated with injuries; used to treat severe muscle spasticity associated with multiple sclerosis, cerebral palsy, stroke, or spinal cord injury; used to treat epilepsy. (Schedule IV drug). Liquid: 1 mg/mL, 5 mg/mL, 5 mg/5 mL. Tablet: 2 mg, 5 mg, 10 mg. Rectal gel: 2.5 mg, 10 mg, 15 mg, 20 mg. Intramuscular or intravenous: 5 mg/mL. [dy-EH-zeh-pehm]. 144, 264

diazepam (Diazepam Intensol, Valium) (Psych). Benzodiazepine drug used to treat anxiety and neurosis; used to treat panic disorder; used to treat alcohol withdrawal. (Schedule IV drug). Liquid: 5 mg/5 mL, 5 mg/mL. Tablet: 2 mg, 5 mg, 10 mg. [dy-EH-zeh-pehm]. 281

diazepam (Valium). Historical Notes feature. 281

diazepam (Valium) (Anes). Benzodiazepine drug used preoperatively to decrease anxiety and provide sedation. (Schedule IV drug). Intramuscular or intravenous: 5 mg/mL. [dy-EH-zeh-pehm]. 371

Diazepam Intensol (Neuro, Ortho). Benzodiazepine drug used as a skeletal muscle relaxant to treat minor muscle spasms associated with injuries; used to treat severe muscle spasticity associated with multiple sclerosis, cerebral palsy, stroke, or spinal cord injury. (Schedule IV drug). Liquid: 5 mg/mL, 5 mg/5 mL. Tablet: 2 mg, 5 mg, 10 mg. Intramuscular or intravenous: 5 mg/mL. [dy-EH-zeh-pehm]. 144, 264

Diazepam Intensol (Psych). Benzodiazepine drug used to treat anxiety and neurosis; used to treat panic disorder; used to treat alcohol withdrawal. (Schedule IV drug). Liquid: 5 mg/5 mL, 5 mg/mL. Tablet: 2 mg, 5 mg, 10 mg. [dy-EH-zeh-pehm]. 281

diaziquone (Chemo). Chemotherapy drug used to treat brain cancer. Orphan drug. 347

diazoxide (Hyperstat) (Cardio). Peripheral vasodilator used to treat hypertensive crisis. Intravenous: 15 mg/mL. [dy-ah-ZAWK-side]. 167

diazoxide (Proglycem) (Diab). Used to treat hypoglycemia. Capsule: 50 mg. Liquid: 50 mg/mL. [dy-ah-ZAWK-side].

dibucaine (Nupercainal) (Derm). Topical anesthetic. Cream: 0.5%. Ointment: 1%. [DIH-byoo-kayn]. 94

dichlorphenamide (Daranide) (Oph). Carbonic anhydrase inhibitor used to treat glaucoma. Tablet: 50 mg. [dy-klohr-FEH-nah-mide]. 221

diclofenac (Cataflam, Voltaren, Voltaren-XR) (Analges, OB/GYN, Ortho). Nonsteroidal anti-inflammatory drug used to treat pain; used to treat dysmenorrhea; used to treat osteoarthritis and rheumatoid arthritis. Tablet: 25 mg, 50 mg, 75 mg, 100 mg. [dy-KLOH-feh-nack]. 139, 255, 304

diclofenac (Solaraze) (Derm). Nonsteroidal anti-inflammatory drug used to treat actinic keratoses. Gel: 3%. [dy-KLOH-feh-nack]. 98

diclofenac (Voltaren) (Oph). Topical nonsteroidal anti-inflammatory drug used to treat inflammation in the eyes. Ophthalmic solution: 1%. [dy-KLOH-feh-nack]. 219

dicloxacillin (Dycill, Dynapen, Pathocil) (Antibio). Penicillin-type antibiotic used to treat a variety of bacterial infections, including staphylococci. Capsule: 250 mg, 500 mg. Liquid: 62.5 mg/5 mL. [dy-klawk-sah-SIH-lihn]. 313

(dicumarol) (Hem). No longer on the market. (Anticoagulant).

dicyclomine (Bentyl, Di-Spaz) (GI). Antispasmodic drug. Capsule: 10 mg, 20 mg. Tablet: 20 mg. Syrup: 10 mg/5 mL. Intramuscular: 10 mg/mL. [dy-SY-kloh-meen]. 122

didanosine (ddI) (Videx, Videx EC) (Antivir). Nucleoside reverse transcriptase inhibitor drug used to treat AIDS. Capsule: 125 mg, 200 mg, 250 mg, 400 mg. Tablet: 25 mg, 50 mg, 100 mg, 150 mg, 200 mg. Liquid (powder to be reconstituted): 100 mg, 167 mg; 250 mg, 2 g, 4 g. [dy-DEH-noh-seen]. 324

dideoxycytidine (ddC). See *zalcitabine*.

dideoxyinosine (ddI). See *didanosine*.

Didrex (GI). Appetite suppressant used to treat obesity. (Schedule III drug). For dosage, see *benzphetamine*. 129

Didronel, Didronel IV (Chemo, OB/GYN, Ortho). Inhibits the breakdown of bone; used to treat hypercalcemia of malignancy; used to prevent and treat postmenopausal osteoporosis; used to treat Paget's disease. For dosage, see *etidronate*. [DIH-droh-nell]. 141, 361

dienestrol (Ortho Dienestrol Vaginal Cream) (OB/GYN). Topical hormone replacement therapy used to treat atrophic vaginitis of menopause. Cream: 0.01%. [dy-eh-NEHS-trawl]. 252

diethyldithiocarbamate (Imuthiol) (Antivir). Used to treat AIDS. Orphan drug. 326

diethylpropion (Tenuate, Tenuate Dospan) (GI). Appetite suppressant used to treat obesity. (Schedule IV drug). Tablet: 25 mg, 75 mg. [dy-eh-thul-PROH-pee-awn]. 129

(diethylstilbestrol) (Chemo). No longer on the market. (Trade name *Stilphostrol*; hormonal chemotherapy drug).

difenoxin (Motofen) (GI). Narcotic antidiarrheal drug. Tablet: 1 mg. [dy-feh-NAWK-sihn]. 123

Differin (Derm) (generic *adapalene*). Topical vitamin A-type drug used to treat acne vulgaris. Gel: 0.1%. [DIH-feh-rihn]. 84

diflorasone (Florone, Florone E, Maxiflor, Psorcon E) (Derm). Topical corticosteroid anti-inflammatory drug. Cream: 0.05%. Ointment: 0.05%. [dy-FLOHR-ah-zohn]. 92

Diflucan (Antifung). Used to treat severe topical and systemic fungal and yeast infections; used to treat cryptococcal meningitis in AIDS patients. For dosage, see *fluconazole*. [dy-FLOO-kehn]. 331, 335

diflunisal (Dolobid) (Analges, Ortho). Salicylate nonaspirin drug used to treat mild-to-moderate pain; used to treat pain and inflammation of osteoarthritis and rheumatoid arthritis. Tablet: 250 mg, 500 mg. [dy-FLOO-neh-sawl]. 138, 300

"dig" (Cardio). Slang term for *digitalis* or *digoxin*. Pronounced "dij." 152

Di-Gel (GI) (generic *aluminum, magnesium, simethicone*). Combination antacid and anti-gas drug. Liquid: 200 mg/20 mg. See also *Advanced Formula Di-Gel*. 117

Digibind (Cardio). Antidote used to treat the effects of digitalis overdose or toxicity. For dosage, see *digoxin immune Fab*. [DIH-jah-bind]. 153

(Digidote) (Cardio). No longer on the market. (Generic name *digoxin immune Fab*; antidote for digitalis toxicity).

Digitalis lanata (plant). 151

digitalis toxicity. 152, 153

(digitoxin) (Cardio). No longer on the market. (Trade name *Crystodigin*; cardiac glycoside used to treat congestive heart failure and atrial flutter/fibrillation).

digoxin (Lanoxicaps, Lanoxin) (Cardio). Cardiac glycoside drug used to treat atrial flutter/fibrillation and congestive heart failure. Capsule: 0.05 mg, 0.1 mg, 0.2 mg. Liquid: 0.05 mg/mL. Tablet: 0.125 mg, 0.25 mg, 0.5 mg. Intravenous: 0.1 mg/mL, 0.25 mg/mL. [dih-JAWK-sihn] 152, 160

digoxin immune Fab (Digibind) (Cardio). Antidote used to treat the effects of digitalis overdose or toxicity. Intravenous (powder to be reconstituted): 38 mg. [dih-JAWK-sihn]. 153

dihydroergotamine (D.H.E. 45, Migranal) (Analges). Used to treat migraine headaches. Nasal spray: 4 mg/mL. Intramuscular or intravenous: 1 mg/mL. [dy-hy-droh-ehr-GAW-tah-meen]. 307

dihydrotestosterone (Androgel-DHT) (Antivir). Used to treat AIDS wasting syndrome. Orphan drug. 327

dihydroxyacetone (Chromelin Complexion Blender) (Derm). Topical drug used to darken hypopigmented areas of skin in patients with vitiligo. Liquid: 5%. 98

Dilacor XR (Cardio). Calcium channel blocker used to treat angina pectoris, hypertension, and atrial and ventricular arrhythmias; used to treat Raynaud's disease. For dosage, see *diltiazem*. [DIH-lah-kohr]. 157, 160, 163

Dilantin Infatabs, Dilantin Kapseals, Dilantin-125 (Neuro). Anticonvulsant drug used to treat tonic-clonic and complex partial seizures; used to treat status epilepticus. For dosage, see *phenytoin*. [dy-LEHN-tehn]. 264, 267

Dilaudid, Dilaudid-5, Dilaudid HP (Analges). Narcotic analgesic used to treat moderate-to-severe pain. (Schedule II drug). For dosage, see *hydromorphone*. [dy-LAW-dihd]. 297

Dilaudid Cough (ENT) (generic *hydromorphone, guaifenesin*). Combination narcotic antitussive and expectorant drug. Syrup: 1 mg/100 mg. [dy-LAW-dihd]. 211

dilevalol (Unicard) (Cardio). Beta-blocker used to treat hypertension. Investigational drug. 173

diltiazem (Cardizem, Cardizem CD, Cardizem SR, Dilacor XR, Tiamate) (Cardio). Calcium channel blocker used to treat angina pectoris, hypertension, and atrial and ventricular arrhythmias; used to treat Raynaud's disease. Capsule: 60 mg, 90 mg, 120 mg, 180 mg, 240 mg, 300 mg, 360 mg, 420 mg. Tablet: 30 mg, 60 mg, 90 mg, 120 mg, 180 mg. 240 mg. Injection: 5 mg/mL. [dihl-TY-ah-zehm]. 157, 160, 163

diluent. 62

dimenhydrinate (Children's Dramamine, Dramamine) (ENT, GI). Antihistamine used to treat vertigo and motion sickness. Liquid: 12.5 mg/5 mL. Chewable tablet: 50 mg. Tablet: 50 mg. Intramuscular or intravenous: 50 mg/mL. [dy-mehn-HY-drih-nayt]. 128

Dimetane Decongestant (ENT) (generic *phenylephrine, brompheniramine*). Combination decongestant and antihistamine drug. Caplet: 10 mg/4 mg. Elixir: 5 mg/2 mg. [DY-meh-tayn].

Dimetapp Allergy (Derm, ENT). Antihistamine used to treat allergic rhinitis and allergic reactions with hives and itching. For dosage, see *brompheniramine*. [DY-meh-tehp]. 207

(Dimetapp Cold & Allergy, Dimetapp Elixir, Dimetapp Extentabs, Dimetapp 4-Hour Liqui-Gels, Dimetapp Tablets) (ENT). No longer on the market. (Combination drug with *phenylpropanolamine*; decongestant and antihistamine drug).

(Dimetapp Cold & Flu) (ENT). No longer on the market. (Combination drug with *phenylpropanolamine*; decongestant, antihistamine, and analgesic).

(Dimetapp DM) (ENT). No longer on the market. (Combination drug with *phenylpropanolamine*; decongestant, antihistamine, and nonnarcotic antitussive drug).

Dimetapp-DX Cough (ENT) (generic *pseudoephedrine, brompheniramine, dextromethorphan*). Combination decongestant, antihistamine, and nonnarcotic antitussive drug. Syrup: 30 mg/2 mg/10 mg. [DY-meh-tehp].

Dimetapp Sinus (ENT) (generic *pseudoephedrine, ibuprofen*). Combination decongestant and analgesic drug. Caplet: 30 mg/200 mg. [DY-meh-tehp].

dimethyl sulfoxide (DMSO) (Rimso-50) (Uro). Urinary tract analgesic. Solution (instilled into bladder): 50%. 107

dinoprostone (Cervidil, Prepidil) (OB/GYN). Prostaglandin drug used to ripen the cervix for delivery. Vaginal gel: 0.5 mg. Vaginal insert: 10 mg. [dy-noh-PRAW-stohn].

dinoprostone (Prostin E2) (OB/GYN). Prostaglandin drug used to produce abortion. Vaginal suppository: 20 mg. [dy-noh-PRAW-stohn]. 255

Diovan (Cardio). Angiotensin II receptor blocker used to treat congesteive heart failure and hypertension. For dosage, see *valsartan*. [DY-oh-vehn]. 155, 164

Diovan HCT (Cardio) (generic *valsartan, hydrochlorothiazide*). Combination angiotensin II receptor blocker antihypertensive and diuretic drug. Tablet: 80 mg/12.5 mg, 160 mg/12.5 mg, 160 mg/25 mg. [DY-oh-vehn]. 167

Dipentum (GI). Anti-inflammatory-type drug used to treat ulcerative colitis. For dosage, see *olsalazine*. [dy-PEHN-tuhm]. 126

diphenhydramine (AllerMax Caplets, Benadryl, Benadryl Allergy Kapseals, Benadryl Allergy Ultratabs, Benadryl Dye-Free Allergy Liqui Gels) (Derm, ENT). Antihistamine used to treat allergic rhinitis and allergic reactions with hives and itching; used to control coughing. Capsule: 25 mg, 50 mg. Chewable tablet: 12.5 mg. Liquid: 12.5 mg/5 mL. Tablet: 25 mg, 50 mg. Intramuscular or intravenous: 50 mg/mL. [dy-phen-HY-drah-meen]. 207

diphenhydramine (Benadryl, Benadryl Itch Relief, Benadryl Itch Relief Children's Formula, Benadryl Itch Stopping Maximum Strength, Benadryl Itch Stopping Children's Formula, Benadryl Itch Stopping Original Strength, Dermamycin, Maximum Strength Benadryl 2%, Maximum Strength Benadryl Itch Relief) (Derm). Topical antihistamine and antipruritic drug. Cream: 1%, 2%. Gel: 1%, 2%. Lotion: 1%. Spray:1%, 2%. [dy-phen-HY-drah-meen]. 93

diphenhydramine (Benadryl) (GI, Neuro). Antihistamine with antiemetic effect; used to treat vertigo and motion sickness; anticholinergic effect used to treat Parkinson's disease. Capsule: 25 mg, 50 mg. Chewable tablet: 12.5 mg. Liquid: 12.5 mg/5 mL. Tablet: 25 mg, 50 mg. Intramuscular or intravenous: 50 mg/mL. [dy-phen-HY-drah-meen]. 128, 269

diphenhydramine (Compoz Gel Caps, Compoz Nighttime Sleep Aid, Maximum Strength Nytol, Maximum Strength Unisom Sleep Gels, Midol PM, Miles Nervine, Nytol, Sleep-eze 3, Sominex) (Neuro). Antihistamine drug sleep aid. Capsule: 25 mg, 50 mg. Tablet: 25 mg, 50 mg. [dy-phen-HY-drah-meen].

(diphenidol) (GI). No longer on the market. (Trade name *Vontrol*; antiemetic drug used to treat motion sickness).

diphenoxylate (Lomotil) (GI). Narcotic antidiarrheal drug. Liquid: 2.5 mg/5 mL. Tablet: 2.5 mg. [dy-feh-NAWK-seh-layt]. 123

dipivefrin (Propine) (Oph). Topical alpha/beta-agonist drug used to treat glaucoma. Ophthalmic solution: 0.1%. [dih-PIH-veh-frihn]. 222

Diprivan (Anes). Used to induce and maintain general anesthesia; used to sedate patients who are intubated and on the ventilator. For dosage, see *propofol*. [DIH-proh-vehn]. 199, 369

Diprolene, Diprolene AF (Derm) (generic *betamethasone*). Topical corticosteroid anti-inflammatory drug. Cream: 0.05%. Gel: 0.05%. Lotion: 0.05%. Ointment: 0.05%. [DIH-proh-leen]. 92

Diprosone (Derm) (generic *betamethasone*). Topical corticosteroid anti-inflammatory drug. Cream: 0.05%. Lotion: 0.05%. Ointment: 0.05%. Spray: 0.1%. [DIH-proh-sohn]. 92

Diprosone (Uro) (generic *betamethasone*). Topical corticosteroid anti-inflammatory drug used to treat phimosis (nonretractable foreskin). Cream: 0.05%. [DIH-proh-sohn]. 111

dipyridamole (Persantine) (Cardio). Coronary artery vasodilator used diagnostically to provoke angina in patients with coronary artery disease who cannot tolerate exercise stress testing; a platelet aggregation inhibitor used to prevent blood clot after cardiac valve replacement surgery. Tablet: 25 mg, 50 mg, 75 mg. [dy-py-RIH-dah-mohl]. 173, 187

dirithromycin (Dynabac) (Antibio). Macrolide antibiotic used to treat a variety of infections, including community-acquired pneumonia, *H. influenzae*, and Legionnaire's disease. Tablet: 250 mg. [deh-rih-throh-MY-sihn]. 198, 319

Disalcid (Analges, Ortho). Salicylate nonaspirin drug used to treat pain; used to treat the pain and inflammation of osteoarthritis and rheumatoid arthritis. For dosage, see *salsalate*. [dy-SEHL-sihd]. 138, 300

disinfectants. Chemical agents used to kill bacteria on instruments and surfaces. 62

Disophrol (ENT) (generic *pseudoephedrine, dexbrompheniramine*). Combination decongestant and antihistamine drug. Tablet: 60 mg/2 mg.

disopyramide (Norpace, Norpace CR) (Cardio). Used to treat ventricular arrhythmias. Capsule: 100 mg, 150 mg. 159

Di-Spaz (GI). Antispasmodic drug. For dosage, see *dicyclomine*. 122

distribution, drug. 46

disulfiram (Antabuse) (Psych). Used to deter alcohol consumption in recovering alcoholics. Tablet: 250 mg, 500 mg. [dy-SUHL-fih-rehm]. 293

Ditropan, Ditropan XL (Uro). Antispasmodic drug used to treat urinary urgency and frequency. For dosage, see *oxybutynin*. [DIH-troh-pehn]. 107

Diucardin (Uro). Thiazide diuretic. For dosage, see *hydroflumethiazide*. [dy-yoo-KAWR-dihn]. 103

(Diupres) (Cardio). No longer on the market. (Generic names *reserpine, chlorothiazide*; combination antihypertensive and diuretic drug).

Diurese (Uro). Thiazide diuretic. For dosage, see *trichlormethiazide*. [DY-yoo-rees]. 103

diuretic drugs, diuretics (Uro). Class of drugs that excrete excess water and sodium; used to treat hypertension, congestive heart failure, and renal failure. 62
    loop. 104
    potassium-sparing. 104
    potassium-wasting. 104
    thiazide. 103

Diuril (Uro). Thiazide diuretic. For dosage, see *chlorothiazide*. 103

(Dizac) (Neuro, Ortho, Psych). No longer on the market. (Generic name *diazepam*; anticonvulsant, skeletal muscle relaxant, antianxiety drug).

DMSO (abbreviation for *dimethyl sulfoxide*). See *dimethyl sulfoxide*.

DNA, recombinant. See *recombinant DNA technology*.

dobutamine (Dobutrex) (Cardio, Emerg). Nonselective beta-blocker used to treat decompensated congestive heart failure; vasopressor used to treat hypotension during emergency resuscitation. Intravenous: 12.5 mg/mL. [doh-BYOO-tah-meen]. 173, 181

Dobutrex (Cardio, Emerg). Nonselective beta-blocker used to treat decompensated congestive heart failure; vasopressor used to treat hypotension during emergency resuscitation. For dosage, see *dobutamine*. [doh-BYOO-trehks]. 173, 181

docetaxel (Taxotere) (Chemo). Mitosis inhibitor chemotherapy drug used to treat breast cancer, lung cancer, head and neck cancer, gastric cancer, pancreatic cancer, ovarian cancer, prostatic cancer, bladder cancer, malignant melanoma, and non-Hodgkin's lymphoma. Intravenous: 20 mg, 80 mg. [dawk-seh-TACK-sehl]. 344

Dr. Scholl's Wart Removal (Derm) (generic *salicylic acid*). Topical keratolytic drug used to treat warts. Liquid, disk.

docosanol (Abreva) (Antivir, Derm, ENT). Topical drug used to treat herpes simplex type 1 infections (cold sores). Cream: 10%. [doh-KOH-sah-nawl]. 91

docusate (Colace, ex-lax stool softener, Modane Soft, Phillips' Liqui-Gels, Surfak Liquigels) (GI). Stool softener laxative. Capsule: 50 mg, 100 mg, 250 mg. Liquid: 150 mg/5 mL. Syrup: 60 mg/15 mL. Tablet: 100 mg. Caplet: 100 mg. [DAW-kyoo-sayt]. 125

dofetilide (Tikosyn) (Cardio). Used to treat atrial arrhythmias. Capsule: 125 mcg, 250 mcg, 500 mcg. [doh-FEH-tih-lide].

dolasetron (Anzemet) (GI). Antiemetic drug; used to treat nausea and vomiting caused by chemotherapy. Tablet: 50 mg, 100 mg. Intravenous: 20 mg/mL. 127

Dole, Bob.

(Dolene) (Analges). No longer on the market. (Generic name *propoxyphene*; narcotic analgesic drug).

Dolobid (Analges, Ortho). Salicylate nonaspirin drug used to treat mild-to-moderate pain; used to treat pain and inflammation of osteoarthritis and rheumatoid arthritis. For dosage, see *diflunisal*. [DOH-loh-bihd]. 138, 300

Dolophine (Analges). Narcotic analgesic used to treat severe pain; used to manage dependence and withdrawal from narcotics. (Schedule II drug). For dosage, see *methadone*. [DOH-loh-feen]. 297, 308

Dolsed (Uro) (generic *L-hyoscyamine, methenamine, methylene blue*). Combination urinary tract antispasmodic and anti-infective drug. Tablet. 107

Domeboro (Derm) (generic *Burow's solution*). Topical astringent solution used to dry oozing areas on the skin. Powder or tablet to be reconstituted into a solution. [DOHM-bohr-oh].

domperidone (Motilium) (GI). Antiemetic drug; used to treat nausea and vomiting caused by chemotherapy. Investigational drug. 128

donepezil (Aricept) (Neuro). Cholinesterase inhibitor used to treat Alzheimer's disease. Tablet: 5 mg 10 mg. [daw-NEH-peh-zill]. 271

Donnagel (GI). Antidiarrheal drug. For dosage, see *attapulgite*. [DAW-nah-jehl]. 124

Donnatal, Donnatal Extentabs (GI) (generic *L-hyoscyamine, scopolamine, phenobarbital*). Combination antispasmodic and sedative drug. Capsule: 0.1037 mg/0.0065 mg/16.2 mg. Tablet: 0.1037 mg/0.0065 mg/16.2 mg. Elixir: 0.1037 mg/0.0065 mg/16.2 mg. [DAW-nah-tawl]. 122

Donnazyme (GI) (generic *amylase, lipase, pancreatin, protease*). Combination replacement drug for digestive enzymes. Capsule, tablet: 12,500 units/1000 units/500 mg/12,500 units. [DAW-nah-zime]. 133

dopamine. In Depth feature. 268

dopamine (Intropin) (Cardio, Emerg, Resp). Vasopressor used to treat decompensated congestive heart failure; used to treat hypotension during emergency resuscitation; used to treat chronic obstructive pulmonary disease; used to treat respiratory distress syndrome in infants. Intravenous: 40 mg/mL, 80 mg/mL, 160 mg/mL. [DOH-pah-meen]. 173, 181

dopamine (neurotransmitter).

(Dopar) (Neuro). No longer on the market. (Generic name *levodopa*; used to treat Parkinson's disease).

Doral (Neuro). Nonbarbiturate benzodiazepine drug used to treat insomnia. (Schedule IV drug). For dosage, see *quazepam*. 272

Dorcol Children's Cough (ENT) (generic *pseudoephedrine, dextromethorphan, guaifenesin*). Combination decongestant, nonnarcotic antitussive, and expectorant drug. Syrup: 15 mg/5 mg/50 mg.

(Doriden) (Neuro). No longer on the market. (Generic name *glutethimide*; nonbarbiturate used to treat insomnia).

dornase alfa (Pulmozyme) (Resp). Enzyme that breaks apart the DNA in mucus and thins it in patients with cystic fibrosis. Liquid for nebulizer: 1 mg/mL.

Doryx (Antibio). Tetracycline-type antibiotic used to treat a variety of infections, including traveler's diarrhea, gonorrhea, syphilis, and *Chlamydia*; used to treat cutaneous or inhaled anthrax from bioterrorism. For dosage, see *doxycycline*. [DOH-rihks]. 98, 123, 317

dorzolamide (Trusopt) (Oph). Topical carbonic anhydrase inhibitor drug used to treat glaucoma. Ophthalmic solution: 2%. [dohr-ZOH-lah-mide]. 221

dose.
loading. 64
maintenance. 64
toxic. 53

dothiepin (Prothiaden) (Psych). Tricyclic antidepressant used to treat depression. Investigational drug. 285

double-blind clinical trial. 65

Double Strength Gaviscon-2 (GI) (generic *aluminum, magnesium, sodium bicarbonate*). Combination antacid. Tablet: 160 mg. See also *Gaviscon*. 117

Dovonex (Derm) (generic *calcipotriene*). Topical vitamin D-type drug used to treat psoriasis. Cream: 0.005%. Ointment: 0.005%. [DOH-voh-nehks]. 86

doxacurium (Nuromax) (Anes, Resp). Muscle relaxant used during surgery; used to treat patients who are intubated and on the ventilator. Intravenous: 1 mg/mL. [dawk-sah-KYOUR-ee-uhm]. 199, 370

doxazosin (Cardura) (Cardio, Uro). Alpha₁-receptor blocker used to treat hypertension; used to treat benign prostatic hypertrophy. Tablet: 1 mg, 2 mg, 4 mg, 8 mg. [dawk-sah-ZOH-sihn]. 109, 165

doxepin (Sinequan, Sinequan Concentrate) (Analges, Derm, Diab, Neuro, Ortho). Tricyclic antidepressant used to treat migraines; used to treat urticaria; used to treat diabetic neuropathy; used to treat postherpetic neuralgia; used to treat phantom limb pain. Capsule: 10 mg, 25 mg, 50 mg, 75 mg, 100 mg, 150 mg. Liquid: 10 mg/mL. [DAWK-seh-pihn]. 98, 147, 241, 275, 282, 307

doxepin (Sinequan, Sinequan Concentrate) (Psych). Tricyclic antidepressant used to treat depression; also used to treat anxiety and neurosis. Capsule: 10 mg, 25 mg, 50 mg, 75 mg, 100 mg, 150 mg. Liquid: 10 mg/mL. [DAWK-seh-pihn]. 285

doxepin (Zonalon) (Derm). Topical antihistamine/antipruritic drug. Cream: 5%. [DAWK-seh-pihn]. 93

Doxidan (GI) (generic *docusate, casanthranol*). Combination stool softener and irritant/stimulant laxative. Capsule. [DAWK-sih-dehn]. 125

Doxil (Chemo). Liposomal form of chemotherapy antibiotic used to treat Kaposi's sarcoma; orphan drug used to treat ovarian cancer. For dosage, see *doxorubicin*. [DAWK-sill]. 342

doxorubicin (Adriamycin PFS, Adriamycin RDF, Rubex) (Chemo). Chemotherapy antibiotic used to treat lung cancer, gastric cancer, liver cancer, thyroid cancer, breast cancer, ovarian cancer, bone cancer, bladder cancer, leukemia, Hodgkin's disease, non-Hodgkin's lymphoma, and Wilm's tumor. Intravenous: 2 mg/mL, (powder to be reconstituted): 10 mg, 20 mg, 50 mg, 100 mg, 150 mg. [dawk-soh-ROO-beh-sihn]. 342

doxorubicin (Doxil) (Chemo). Liposomal form of chemotherapy antibiotic used to treat Kaposi's sarcoma; orphan drug used to treat ovarian cancer. Intravenous: 20 mg/10 mL. [dawk-soh-ROO-beh- sihn]. 342

doxorubicin MTC-DOX. See *MTC-DOX*.

doxycycline (Doryx, Vibramycin, Vibramycin IV, Vibra-Tabs) (Antibio). Tetracycline-type antibiotic used to treat a variety of infections, including traveler's diarrhea, gonorrhea, syphilis, and *Chlamydia*; used to treat cutaneous or inhaled anthrax from bioterrorism. Capsule: 50 mg, 100 mg. Tablet: 50 mg, 100 mg. Liquid (powder to be reconstituted): 25 ml/5 mL. Syrup: 50 mg/5 mL. Intravenous (powder to be reconstituted): 100 mg, 200 mg. [dawk-see-SY-kleen]. 98, 123, 317

doxycycline (Periostat) (Antibio, ENT). Used to treat periodontal disease. Capsule: 20 mg. [dawk-see-SY-kleen].

doxylamine (Unisom Nighttime Sleep-Aid) (Neuro). Sleep aid. Tablet: 25 mg.

Dracula. 6

dram. 69

Dramamine (GI). Antihistamine used to treat vertigo and motion sickness. For dosage, see *dimenhydrinate*. [DREH-mah-meen]. 128

Dristan Cold (ENT) (generic *pseudoephedrine, acetaminophen*). Combination decongestant and analgesic drug. Caplet: 30 mg/500 mg.

Dristan Cold Multi-Symptom Formula (ENT) (generic *phenylephrine, chlorpheniramine, acetaminophen*). Combination decongestant, antihistamine, and analgesic drug. Tablet: 5 mg/2 mg/325 mg.

Dristan Nasal (ENT) (generic *phenylephrine, pheniramine*). Combination decongestant and antihistamine drug. Spray: 0.5%/0.2%.

Dristan Saline Spray (ENT). Topical saline nasal moisturizing drug. Mist.

Dristan Sinus (ENT) (generic *pseudoephedrine, ibuprofen*). Combination decongestant and analgesic drug. Caplet: 30 mg/200 mg.

Dristan 12 Hr Nasal (ENT). Decongestant. For dosage, see *oxymetazoline*. 206

Drithocreme (Derm) (generic *anthralin*). Topical drug used to treat psoriasis. Cream: 0.25%. [DRIH-oh-kreem]. 87

Drixoral (ENT) (generic *pseudoephedrine, brompheniramine*). Combination decongestant and antihistamine drug. Syrup: 30 mg/2 mg. [drihk-SOHR-awl].

Drixoral Cold & Allergy (ENT) (generic *pseudoephedrine, dexbrompheniramine*). Combination decongestant and antihistamine drug. Tablet: 120 mg/6 mg. [drihk-SOHR-awl].

Drixoral Cold & Flu, Drixoral Plus (ENT) (generic *pseudoephedrine, dexbrompheniramine, acetaminophen*). Combination decongestant, antihistamine, and analgesic. Tablet: 60 mg/3 mg/500 mg. [drihk-SOHR-awl].

Drixoral Cough & Congestion (ENT) (generic *pseudoephedrine, dextromethorphan*). Combination decongestant and nonnarcotic antitussive drug. Liquid Caps: 60 mg/30 mg. [drihk-SOHR-awl].

Drixoral Cough and Sore Throat Liquid Caps (ENT) (generic *dextromethorphan, acetaminophen*). Combination nonnarcotic antitussive and analgesic drug. Gelcap: 15 mg/325 mg. [drihk-SOHR-awl].

Drixoral Cough Liquid Caps (ENT). Nonnarcotic antitussive drug. For dosage, see *dextromethorphan*. [drihk-SOHR-awl]. 210

Drixoral Non-Drowsy Formula (ENT). Decongestant. For dosage, see *pseudoephedrine*. [drihk-SOHR-awl]. 206

dronabinol (Marinol) (Antivir, GI). Appetite stimulant used to treat AIDS patients; antiemetic drug used to treat nausea and vomiting caused by chemotherapy. Capsule: 2.5 mg, 5 mg, 10 mg. [droh-NEH-bih-nawl]. 128, 327

droperidol (Inapsine) (Anes). Preoperative drug used to produce sedation; used to induce and maintain general anesthesia. Intramuscular or intravenous: 2.5 mg/mL. [droh-PEH-rih-dawl]. 369

drops (drug measurement). 70

dropsy. 152

Dr Scholl's Clear Away Plantar, Dr Scholl's Wart Remover (Derm) (generic *salicylic acid*). Topical keratolytic drug used to treat warts. Disk: 40%. Liquid: 17%. 91

drotrecogin alfa (Xigris) (Antibio). Used to treat severe sepsis. Intravenous (powder to be reconstituted): 5 mg, 20 mg. [droh-treh-KAW-gehn EHL-fah]. 321

drug absorption. 46

drug advertisements. 13

drug cycle, steps in the. 45

drug design. 21, 25

drug distribution in the body. 46

drug–drug reaction. 56, 57

drug effect. 50

drug excretion. 48

drug–food reaction. 57

Drug Enforcement Administration (DEA), The. 16

Drug Enforcement Administration (DEA) number. 17

drug forms. 33

drug idiosyncrasy. 55

drug label. 29

drug legislation. 12

drug marketing. 21, 31

drug metabolism. 47

drug names, spelling of. See also *brand, chemical, generic,* and *trade name.* 22

drug of choice. 62

drug patent. 29

drug recalls. 30

drugs.
ancient. 5
computer design of. 25
cost of prescription. Focus on Healthcare Issues feature. 31
definition of. 2
derived from animals. 7, 24
derived from minerals. 7, 24
derived from plants. 6, 24
fat-soluble. 48
1800s and 1900s. 7
linguistic origin of. 2
medicinal uses of. 2

origins of new. 24

recombinant DNA. 26

testing of new. 27

water-soluble. 48

drug tolerance. 63

Dry Eyes (Oph).   Artificial tears. Drops.

DS (abbreviation for *double strength*); part of the trade name of a drug. 63

DTIC-Dome (Chemo, Endo).   Alkylating chemotherapy drug used to treat malignant melanoma and Hodgkin's disease; used to treat pheochromocytoma of the adrenal cortex.   For dosage, see *dacarbazine.* 341

Dulcolax (GI).   Irritant/stimulant laxative.   For dosage, see *bisacodyl.* [DUHL-koh-lehks]. 124

duloxetine (Uro).   Used to treat stress urinary incontinence. Investigational drug. 111

DuoDerm (Derm).   Topical drug used to absorb drainage from burns, skin ulcers, and wounds. Granules, paste. 96

Duodopa (Neuro) (generic names *carbidopa, levodopa*). Combination drug used to treat Parkinson's disease. Orphan drug. 270

DuoFilm (Derm) (generic *salicylic acid*).   Topical keratolytic drug used to treat warts. Liquid: 17%. Patch: 40%. 91

DuoNeb (Resp) (generic *albuterol, ipratropium*).   Combination bronchodilator used to treat asthma. Nebulizer unit: 3 mg/0.5 mg. 195

DuoPlant (Derm) (generic *salicylic acid*).   Topical keratolytic drug used to treat warts. Gel: 17%. 91

(Duo-Medihaler) (Resp).   No longer on the market. (Generic name *isoproterenol, phenylephrine*; combination bronchodilator and decongestant).

Duracap.   Part of the trade name of a drug indicating a time-release capsule. 63

Duraclon (Analges).   Nonnarcotic analgesic drug used to treat severe pain via epidural administration. For dosage, see *clonidine.* [DUHR-eh-klawn]. 299

(Duract) (Analges).   No longer on the market. (Generic name *bromfenac*; nonsteroidal anti-inflammatory drug).

Duradrin (Analges) (generic *isometheptene, dichloralphenazone, acetaminophen*).   Combination vasoconstrictor, sedative, and analgesic used to treat migraine headaches. Capsule: 65 mg/100 mg/325 mg. [DUHR-ah-drihn]. 307

Duragesic-25, Duragesic-50, Duragesic-75, Duragesic-100 (Analges).   Narcotic analgesic drug used to treat chronic severe pain. (Schedule II drug).   For dosage, see *fentanyl.* [duhr-ah-GEE-sihk]. 297

Duramist Plus (ENT).   Decongestant.   For dosage, see *oxymetazoline.* 206

Duramorph, Duramorph PF (Analges, Anes, Cardio, OB/GYN).   Narcotic analgesic drug used to treat moderate-to-severe pain; used as a preoperative drug to sedate and supplement anesthesia; used to treat dyspnea from congestive heart failure; used to treat the pain of childbirth. (Schedule II drug).   For dosage, see *morphine.* [DUHR-ah-mohrf]. 173, 297

Duranest, Duranest MPF (Anes, OB/GYN, Oph). Regional nerve block anesthetic; used for regional anesthesia for cesarean section; used for retrobulbar anesthesia during eye surgery.   For dosage, see *etidocaine.* 368

Duratears Naturale (Oph).   Artificial tears for the eyes. Ophthalmic ointment.

Duration (ENT).   Decongestant.   For dosage, see *oxymetazoline.* 206

Durham-Humphrey Amendment. 14

Duricef (Antibio).   Cephalosporin antibiotic used to treat a variety of bacterial infections, including *Streptococcus, Staphylococcus*, and *E. coli.*   For dosage, see *cefadroxil.* [DUHR-ah-sehf]. 315

dutasteride (Derm, Uro).   First drug in the class of 5-alpha-reductase inhibitors used to treat benign prostatic hypertrophy; in clinical trials for treating male pattern baldness. [doo-TEH-steh-ride]. 98, 109

(Duvoid) (Uro).   No longer on the market. (Generic name *bethanechol*; urinary antispasmodic).

Dyazide (Uro) (generic *hydrochlorothiazide, triamterene*). Combination diuretic. Capsule: 50 mg/37.5 mg. [DY-ah-zide]. 104

Dycill (Antibio).   Penicillin-type antibiotic used to treat a variety of bacterial infections, including staphylococci.   For dosage, see *dicloxacillin.* [DY-sill]. 313

Dyclone (Anes, GI, Resp, Uro).   Topical anesthetic applied to the throat prior to esophagoscopy or bronchoscopy or to the urethra prior to cystoscopy. Solution: 0.5%, 1%.

dyclonine (Dyclone) (Anes, GI, Resp, Uro).   Topical anesthetic applied to the throat prior to esophagoscopy or bronchoscopy or to the urethra prior to cystoscopy. Solution: 0.5%, 1%. [dy-KLOH-neen].

dyclonine (Sucrets, Sucrets Children's Sore Throat, Sucrets Maximum Strength) (ENT).   Topical anesthetic used to treat a sore throat. Lozenge: 1.2 mg, 3 mg. Throat spray: 0.1%. [dy-KLOH-neen].

(Dymelor) (Diab).   No longer on the market. (Generic name *acetohexamide*; oral antidiabetic drug).

Dynabac (Antibio).   Macrolide antibiotic used to treat a variety of infections, including community-acquired pneumonia, *H. influenzae*, and Legionnaire's disease.   For dosage, see *dirithromycin.* [DY-nah-back]. 198, 319

Dynacin (Antibio).   Tetracycline-type antibiotic used to treat a variety of infections, including acne vulgaris, gonorrhea, syphilis, and *Chlamydia*; used to treat malignant pleural effusion.   For dosage, see *minocycline*. [DY-nah-sihn]. 84, 317

DynaCirc, DynaCirc CR (Cardio).   Calcium channel blocker used to treat hypertension.   For dosage, see *isradipine*. [DY-nah-sirk]. 163

Dynapen (Antibio).   Penicillin-type antibiotic used to treat a variety of bacterial infections, including staphylococci.   For dosage, see *dicloxacillin*. [DY-nah-pehn]. 313

dyphylline (Lufyllin, Lufyllin-400) (Resp).   Bronchodilator. Liquid: 100 mg/15 mL, 160 mg/15 mL. Tablet: 200 mg, 400 mg. Intramuscular: 250 mg/mL. [DY-feh-lihn]. 193

Dyrenium (Uro).   Potassium-sparing diuretic.   For dosage, see *triamterene*. 104

dysmenorrhea, drugs used to treat. 255

Dysport (Oph, Neuro, Ortho).   Used to treat blepharospasm; used to treat cervical dystonia (torticollis); used to treat muscle contractures in patients with cerebral palsy. Orphan drug. 147, 275

ear, nose, and throat drugs. 206

(Easprin) (Analges, Ortho).   No longer on the market. (Generic name *aspirin*; nonnarcotic analgesic drug).

ECCO11 (Chemo).   Chemotherapy drug of the class of membrane metalloprotease inhibitors; used to treat lung cancer. Investigational drug. 347

echothiophate iodide (Phospholine Iodide) (Oph).   Topical cholinesterase inhibitor drug used to treat glaucoma. Ophthalmic solution (powder to be reconstituted): 1.5 mg/5 mL (0.03%), 6.25 mg/5 mL (0.125%). [ehk-oh-THY-oh-fayt].

E. coli (abbreviation for *Escherichia coli*).   Common cause of urinary tract infections.

EC-Naprosyn, see *Naprosyn*.

econazole (Spectazole) (Derm).   Topical antifungal and antiyeast drug. Cream: 1%. [ee-KAW-nah-zohl]. 89

Econopred, Econopred Plus (Oph).   Topical corticosteroid used to treat inflammation of the eyes.   For dosage, see *prednisolone*. [ee-KAW-noh-prehd]. 219

Ecotrin Adult Low Strength (Cardio, Hem, Neuro).   Salicylate drug used to treat current myocardial infarction and prevent repeat myocardial infarction; anticoagulant; used to prevent transient ischemic attacks and strokes.   For dosage, see *aspirin*. [EH-koh-trihn]. 158

Ecotrin, Ecotrin Maximum Strength (Analges, Ortho).   Salicylate drug used to relieve fever and pain; used to treat the pain and inflammation of osteoarthritis and rheumatoid arthritis.   For dosage, see *aspirin*. [EH-koh-trihn]. 299

ED (abbreviation for *erectile dysfunction*).   See *erectile dysfunction*.

Edecrin (Uro).   Loop diuretic.   For dosage, see *ethacrynic acid*. 104

edetate (Endrate) (Cardio).   Used to treat ventricular arrhythmias caused by digitalis toxicity; used to treat hypercalcemia. Intravenous: 150 mg/mL. [EH-deh-tayt].

edetate calcium disodium (calcium EDTA) (Calcium Disodium Versenate) (Emerg, Neuro).   Used to treat lead poisoning and lead encephalopathy. Subcutaneous, intramuscular, or intravenous: 200 mg/mL. 275

Edex (Uro).   Used to treat impotence due to erectile dysfunction. Injection into penis: 5 mcg/mL, 10 mcg/mL, 20 mg/mL, 40 mcg/mL. 109

edrophonium (Enlon, Reversol, Tensilon) (Neuro).   Anticholinesterase drug used to diagnose (not treat) myasthenia gravis. Intramuscular or intravenous: 10 mg/mL. [eh-droh-FOH-nee-uhm]. 275

E.E.S. 200, E.E.S. 400 (Antibio).   Macrolide antibiotic used to treat a variety of infections, including *Streptococcus*, *H. influenzae*, gonorrhea, syphilis, *Chlamydia*, and Legionnaire's disease; used to prevent subacute bacterial endocarditis.   For dosage, see *erythromycin*. 319

efalizumab (Xanelim) (Derm).   Monoclonal antibody used to treat severe psoriasis. Subcutaneous: 1 mg/kg, 2 mg/kg. 87

efavirenz (Sustiva) (Antivir).   Nonnucleoside reverse transcriptase inhibitor drug used to treat AIDS. Capsule: 50 mg, 100 mg, 200 mg. [eh-FEH-vih-rehnz]. 325

effect.
   adverse. 52
   allergic. 53
   drug. 50
   first-pass. 47
   local. 50
   negative chronotropic. 152
   positive inotropic. 152
   side. 51
   systemic. 50
   therapeutic. 27, 51
   toxic. 53

Effexor, Effexor XR (Psych).   Antidepressant used to treat depression; used to treat anxiety.   For dosage, see *venlafaxine*. [ee-FEHK-sohr]. 282, 288

Efidac/24 (ENT).   Decongestant.   For dosage, see *pseudoephedrine*. [EH-fih-dack]. 206

eflornithine (Ornidyl) (Antivir). Used to treat *Pneumocystis carinii* pneumonia in AIDS patients. Intravenous: 200 mg/mL. [eh-FLOHR-nih-theen]. 328

eflornithine (Vaniqa) (Derm). Topical drug that slows the growth of unwanted facial hair in women. Cream: 13.9%. [eh-FLOHR-nih-theen]. 98

Efudex (Derm) (generic *fluorouracil*). Topical chemotherapy drug used to treat keratoses and superficial basal cell carcinoma. Cream: 1%, 5%. Liquid: 1%, 2%, 5%. [EH-fyoo-dehks]. 98

(Elase) (Derm). No longer on the market. (Topical enzyme drug used to debride burns and wounds).

Elavil (Analges, Diab, Neuro, Ortho). Tricyclic antidepressant used to treat migraines; used to treat diabetic neuropathy; used to treat postherpetic neuralgia; used to treat phantom limb pain. For dosage, see *amitriptyline*. [EHL-ah-vill]. 147, 241, 275, 306

Elavil (Psych). Tricyclic antidepressant used to treat depression; used to treat anorexia nervosa and bulimia nervosa. For dosage, see *amitriptyline*. [EHL-ah-vill]. 285, 291

elcatonin (Analges). Used to treat severe pain. Intrathecal injection. Orphan drug. 309

Eldepryl (Neuro, Psych). Used to treat Parkinson's disease. Pending use to treat depression. For dosage, see *selegiline*. [EHL-deh-prill]. 269

Eldisine (Chemo). Chemotherapy drug. Investigational drug. 344

Elidel (Derm) (generic *pimecrolimus*). Topical nonsteriodal anti-inflammatory drug used to treat infant eczema. Cream. 95

Eligard (Chemo). Hormonal chemotherapy drug used to treat prostate cancer. For dosage, see *leuprolide*. [EH-leh-gahrd]. 343

Elimite (Derm) (generic *permethrin*). Topical drug used to treat scabies (mites) and pediculosis (lice). Cream: 5%. 95

elixir. 36

Elixophyllin (Resp). Bronchodilator. For dosage, see *theophylline*. [ee-lihks-AW-fih-lihn]. 193

Elixophyllin GG, Elixophyllin-Kl (Resp) (generic *theophylline, guaifenesin* or *potassium iodide*). Combination bronchodilator and expectorant drug. Liquid: 80 mg/130 mg, 100 mg/100 mg. [ee-lihks-AW-fih-lihn]. 195

Ellence (Chemo). Chemotherapy antibiotic used to treat breast cancer. For dosage, see *epirubicin*. 342

Elliott's B Solution (Chemo). Diluent used when methotrexate or cytarabine are administered intrathecally. Orphan drug. 361

Elmiron (Uro). Urinary tract analgesic. For dosage, see *pentosan*. [ehl-MY-rawn]. 107

Elocon (Derm) (generic *mometasone*). Topical corticosteroid anti-inflammatory drug. Cream: 0.1%. Lotion: 0.1%. Ointment: 0.1%. [EHL-oh-kawn]. 92

Eloxatin (Chemo). Chemotherapy platinum drug used to treat ovarian cancer and colon cancer. For dosage, see *oxaliplatin*. 345

Elspar (Chemo). Chemotherapy enzyme drug used to treat leukemia. For dosage, see *asparaginase*. [EHL-spahr]. 345

Emadine (Oph). Topical antihistamine used to treat allergy symptoms in the eyes. For dosage, see *emedastine*. [EH-mah-deen]. 220

Emcyt (Chemo). Alkylating and hormone chemotherapy drug used to treat prostate cancer. For dosage, see *estramustine*. [EHM-siht]. 341, 343

emedastine (Emadine) (Oph). Topical antihistamine used to treat allergy symptoms in the eyes. Ophthalmic solution: 0.05%. [eh-mee-DAH-steen]. 220

emergency resuscitation, drugs used for. 178

(Emete-Con) (GI). No longer on the market. (Trade name *benzquinamide*; antiemetic drug).

emetics (Emerg). Class of drugs used to treat overdose and poisoning by inducing vomiting. 182

Emetrol (GI). Antiemetic drug. For dosage, see *phosphorated carbohydrate solution*. [EH-meh-trawl]. 127

Emgel (Derm) (generic *erythromycin*). Topical antibiotic used to treat acne vulgaris. Gel: 2%. Ointment: 2%. [EHM-jehl]. 84

Eminase (Cardio, Hem). Thrombolytic enzyme used to dissolve blood clots that cause a myocardial infarction. For dosage, see *anistreplase*. [EH-mih-nays]. 172, 188

EMLA (Derm) (generic *lidocaine, prilocaine*). Combination topical anesthetic drug. Cream: 2.5%. [EHM-lah]. 94

Empirin (Analges, Ortho). Salicylate drug used to relieve fever and pain; used to treat the pain and inflammation of osteoarthritis and rheumatoid arthritis. For dosage, see *aspirin*. [EHM-peh-rihn]. 300

Empirin with Codeine No. 3 (Analges) (generic *codeine, aspirin*). Combination narcotic and nonnarcotic analgesic drug. (Schedule III drug). Tablet: 30 mg/325 mg. [EHM-peh-rihn]. 302

Empirin with Codeine No. 4 (Analges) (generic *codeine, aspirin*). Combination narcotic and nonnarcotic analgesic drug. (Schedule III drug). Tablet: 60 mg/325 mg. [EHM-peh-rihn]. 302

emtricitabine (FTC) (Coviracil) (Antivir). Nucleoside reverse transcriptase inhibitor drug used to treat AIDS. Investigational drug. 324

emulsion (drug form). 37

E-Mycin (Antibio). Macrolide antibiotic used to treat a variety of infections, including *Streptococcus, H. in-*

fluenzae, gonorrhea, syphilis, *Chlamydia*, and Legionnaire's disease; used to prevent subacute bacterial endocarditis. For dosage, see *erythromycin*. [ee-MY-sihn]. 319

Enable (Ortho) (generic *tenidap*). Anti-inflammatory cytokine inhibitor used to treat rheumatoid arthritis. Investigational drug. 148

enalapril (Vasotec, Vasotec I.V.) (Cardio, Uro). Angiotensin-converting enzyme inhibitor drug used to treat hypertension and congestive heart failure; used to treat hypertensive crisis; used to treat diabetic nephropathy. Tablet: 2.5 mg, 5 mg, 10 mg, 20 mg. Intravenous: 1.25 mg/mL. [eh-NEH-lah-prihl]. 111, 154, 163, 167

Enbrel (Ortho). Used to treat rheumatoid arthritis. For dosage, see *etanercept*. 142

(encainide) (Cardio). No longer on the market. (Trade name *Enkaid*; ACE inhibitor used to treat arrhythmias).

Endocodone (Analges, Neuro). Narcotic analgesic used to treat moderate-to-severe pain; used to treat neuralgia from herpes zoster virus infection (shingles). (Schedule II drug). For dosage, see *oxycodone*. [ehn-doh-KOH-dohn]. 276, 297

endocrine drugs (Endo). 228

endometriosis, drugs used to treat. 248

endorphins. 297

Endostatin (Chemo). Angiogenesis inhibiting drug used to treat pancreatic cancer. Orphan drug. 347

endotracheal intubation. Historical Notes feature. 367

endotracheal tube, administration of drugs by. 42, 179

Endrate (Cardio). Used to treat ventricular arrhythmias caused by digitalis toxicity; used to treat hypercalcemia. For dosage, see *edetate*.

Enduron (Uro). Thiazide diuretic. For dosage, see *methyclothiazide*. [EHN-dyour-awn]. 103

Enduronyl, Enduronyl Forte (Cardio) (generic *deserpidine, methyclothiazide*). Combination antihypertensive and diuretic drug. Tablet: 0.25 mg/5 mg, 0.5 mg/5 mg. [ehn-dyour-AW-nihl]. 167

enema. 125

Enfamil, Enfamil LactoFree, Enfamil Next Step, Enfamil with Iron, Enfamil Premature Formula (GI). Infant formula. Liquid, concentrated liquid, powder (to be reconstituted).

enflurane (Ethrane) (Anes). Used to induce and maintain general anesthesia. Inhaled gas. [ehn-FLUH-rayn]. 370

Engerix-B (GI). Hepatitis B vaccine. For dosage, see *hepatitis B vaccine*. 133

(Enkaid) (Cardio). No longer on the market. (Generic name *encainide*; Angiotensin-converting enzyme inhibitor used to treat arrhythmias).

Enlon (Neuro). Anticholinesterase drug used to diagnose (not treat) myasthenia gravis. For dosage, see *edrophonium*. [EHN-lawn]. 275

Enlon-Plus (Anes) (generic *edrophonium, atropine*). Combination anticholinesterase and atropine drug used to reverse the effect of neuromuscular blocking drugs used during general anesthesia. Intravenous: 10 mg/0.14 mg. [EHN-lawn]. 371

(Enovid) (OB/GYN). No longer on the market. (Generic names *estrogen, progestins;* used to treat endometriosis, hypermenorrhea, irregular menstruation).

enoxacin (Penetrex) (Antibio). Fluoroquinolone antibiotic used to treat urinary tract infections and gonorrhea. Tablet: 200 mg, 400 mg. [eh-NAWK-seh-sihn]. 105, 318

enoxaparin (Lovenox) (Hem). Low molecular weight heparin anticoagulant; used to prevent deep venous thrombosis in patients with restricted mobility. Subcutaneous: 30 mg/0.3 mL, 40 mg/0.4 mL, 60 mg/0.6 mL, 80 mg/0.8 mL, 100 mg/mL. [eh-nawk-sah-PEH-rihn]. 186

Ensure, Ensure HN, Ensure High Protein, Ensure Plus, Ensure Plus HN (GI). Liquid nutritional supplement. Liquid, powder, pudding.

ENT drugs (ENT). Class of drugs used to treat ear, nose, and throat diseases. 206

entacapone (Comtan) (Neuro). COMT inhibitor used to treat Parkinson's disease. Tablet: 200 mg. 269

enteric-coated tablet. See *tablet*.

(Entex) (ENT). No longer on the market. (Combination drug with *phenylpropanolamine;* decongestant and expectorant).

(Entex LA) (ENT). No longer on the market. (Combination drug with *phenylpropanolamine;* decongestant and expectorant).

Entex PSE (ENT) (generic *pseudoephedrine, guaifenesin*). Combination decongestant and expectorant drug. Tablet: 120 mg/600 mg.

Entocort EC (GI). Corticosteroid anti-inflammatory drug used to treat Crohn's disease. For dosage, see *budesonide*. 132

Enuclene (Oph). Solution to clean and wet an artificial eye. For dosage, see *tyloxapol*.

ephedrine (ENT). Decongestant. Jelly: 1%. Spray: 0.25%. 206

ephedrine (Neuro). Central nervous system stimulant used to treat narcolepsy and myasthenia gravis. Intravenous: 50 mg/mL.

ephedrine (Resp). Bronchodilator. Capsule: 25 mg. Intravenous: 50 mg/mL. 193

"epi" (slang term for *epinephrine*). 181

Epifrin (Oph). Topical alpha/beta-agonist drug used to treat glaucoma. For dosage, see *epinephrine*. [EH-pih-frehn]. 221

epilepsy, drugs used to treat. 263

E-Pilo-1, E-Pilo-2, E-Pilo-4, E-Pilo-6 (Oph) (generic *pilocarpine, epinephrine*). Topical combination miotic and alpha/beta-receptor agonist drug used to treat glaucoma. Ophthalmic solution: 1%/1%, 2%/1%, 4%/1%, 6%/1%. 222

Epinal (Oph). Topical alpha/beta-agonist drug used to treat glaucoma. For dosage, see *epinephryl*. [EH-pih-nawl]. 222

epinephrine (Adrenalin) (Anes). Vasoconstrictor drug added to local anesthetic drug lidocaine. Injection: 1:50,000; 1:100,000; 1:200,000. [eh-pih-NEH-frihn]. 368

epinephrine (Adrenalin) (Emerg). Used to increase blood pressure and initiate or increase heart rate during emergency resuscitation. Endotracheal, intracardiac, or intravenous: 1:200 (5 mg/mL), 1:1000 (1 mg/mL), 1:2000 (0.5 mg/mL), 1:10,000 (0.1 mg/mL), 1:100,000 (0.01 mg/mL). [eh-pih-NEH-frihn]. 180, 181, 183

epinephrine (Ana-Guard Epinephrine, EpiPen Auto-Injector, EpiPen Jr. Auto-Injector) (Emerg). Self-administered epinephrine used to prevent anaphylactic reaction after an insect bite. Intramuscular: 1:1000, 1:2000. [eh-pih-NEH-frihn]. 183

epinephrine (Ana-Guard, AsthmaHaler Mist, AsthmaNefrin, microNefrin, Primatene Mist) (Resp). Bronchodilator. Aerosol inhaler: 0.16 mg/puff, 0.2 mg/puff. Liquid for nebulizer: 1:100, 1:1000, 2.25%. Subcutaneous, intramuscular, or intravenous: 1:1000 (1 mg/mL), 1:10,000 (0.1 mg/mL). [eh-pih-NEH-frihn]. 193

epinephrine (Epifrin, Glaucon) (Oph). Topical alpha/beta-agonist drug used to treat glaucoma. Ophthalmic solution: 0.1%, 0.5%, 1%, 2%. [eh-pih-NEH-frihn]. 221

epinephrine (neurotransmitter). 161

epinephryl (Epinal) (Oph). Topical alpha/beta-agonist drug used to treat glaucoma. Ophthalmic solution: 0.5%, 1%. [eh-pih-NEH-frill]. 222

EpiPen Auto-Injector, EpiPen Jr. Auto-Injector (Emerg). Self-administered injectable epinephrine used to prevent anaphylactic reaction after an insect bite. For dosage, see *epinephrine*. 183

epirubicin (Ellence) (Chemo). Chemotherapy antibiotic used to treat breast cancer. Intravenous: 2 mg/mL. [eh-pee-ROO-beh-sihn]. 342

Epitol (Neuro, Psych). Anticonvulsant drug used to treat tonic-clonic and partial seizures; used to treat trigeminal neuralgia; used to treat schizophrenia; used to treat manic-depressive disorder. For dosage, see *carbamazepine*. [EH-pih-tawl]. 265, 283, 289

Epivir, Epivir-HBV (Antivir, GI). Nucleoside reverse transcriptase inhibitor drug used to treat AIDS; used to treat hepatitis B. For dosage, see *lamivudine*. [EH-pih-veer]. 324

epoetin alfa (Epogen, Procrit) (Antivir, Chemo, Hem, Uro). Erythropoietin-type drug that stimulates red blood cell production in patients with AIDS, patients on chemotherapy, and patients with anemia or chronic renal failure. Subcutaneous or intravenous: 2000 units/mL, 3000 units/mL, 4000 units/mL, 10,000 units/mL, 20,000 units/mL. [eh-poh-EE-tihn EHL-fah]. 111, 331, 361

epoetin beta (Marogen) (Uro). Erythropoietin-type drug used to treat anemia in patients with end-stage renal disease. Orphan drug. 111

Epogen (Antivir, Chemo, Hem, Uro). Erythropoietin-type drug that stimulates red blood cell production in patients with AIDS, patients on chemotherapy, and patients with anemia or chronic renal failure. For dosage, see *epoetin alfa*. 111, 331, 361

epoprostenol (Flolan) (Resp). Vasodilator used to treat primary pulmonary hypertension. Intravenous (powder to be reconstituted): 0.5 mg, 1.5 mg. Administered continously via central venous catheter and computer-controlled drug pump. [eh-poh-PRAW-steh-nawl]. 198

eprosartan (Teveten) (Cardio). Angiotensin II receptor blocker used to treat hypertension. Tablet: 400 mg, 600 mg. [eh-proh-SAWR-tehn]. 164

Epsom salt (GI). Magnesium-containing laxative. Granules. 124

eptifibatide (Integrilin) (Cardio, Hem). Platelet aggregation inhibitor used to prevent blood clots in patients with unstable angina or myocardial infarction, or who are undergoing angioplasty or atherectomy. Intravenous: 0.75 mg/mL, 2 mg/mL. [ehp-tih-FIH-bah-tide]. 173, 187

Equagesic (Analges, Psych) (generic *meprobamate, aspirin*). Combination antianxiety and aspirin drug. Tablet: 200 mg/325 mg. [eh-kwah-GEE-sihk]. 293, 302

Equanil (Psych). Drug used to treat anxiety and neurosis. (Schedule IV drug). For dosage, see *meprobamate*. [EH-kwah-nihl]. 282

erectile dysfunction, drugs used to treat. 109

Ergamisol (Chemo). Chemotherapy drug used to treat colon cancer. For dosage, see *levamisole*. [ehr-GEH-meh-sawl]. 348

ergoloid mesylates (Gerimal, Hydergine, Hydergine LC) (Neuro). Used to treat the dementia of Alzheimer's disease. Capsule: 1 mg. Tablet: 0.5 mg, 1 mg. Sublingual tablet: 1 mg. Liquid: 1 mg/mL. [EHR-goh-loyd meh-seh-laytz]. 271

Ergomar (Analges). Used to treat migraine headaches. For dosage, see *ergotamine*. [EHR-goh-mawr]. 307

ergonovine (Ergotrate) (OB/GYN).   Used to treat postpartum or postabortion uterine bleeding. Intramuscular or intravenous: 0.2 mg/mL. [ehr-goh-NOH-veen]. 248

ergotamine (Ergomar) (Analges).   Used to treat migraine headaches. Sublingual tablet: 2 mg. [ehr-GAW-tah-meen]. 307

(Ergostat) (Analges).   No longer on the market. (Generic name *ergotamine*; used to treat migraine headaches).

Ergotrate (OB/GYN).   Used to treat postpartum or postabortion uterine bleeding.   For dosage, see *ergonovine*. [EHR-goh-trayt]. 248

ertapenem (Invanz) (Antibio).   Carbapenem antibiotic used to treat a variety of infections. Intramuscular or intravenous: 1 g. [ehr-tah-PEH-nehm]. 317

Erwinase (Chemo).   Chemotherapy enzyme drug used to treat leukemia.   For dosage, see *erwinia L-asparaginase*. [EHR-wih-nays]. 345

erwinia L-asparaginase (Erwinase) (Chemo). Chemotherapy enzyme drug used to treat leukemia. Orphan drug. [erh-WIH-nee-ah L eh-SPEH-reh-geh-nays]. 345

ERYC (Antibio).   Macrolide antibiotic used to treat a variety of infections, including *Streptococcus*, *H. influenzae*, gonorrhea, syphilis, *Chlamydia*, and Legionnaire's disease; used to prevent subacute bacterial endocarditis.   For dosage, see *erythromycin*. [eh-ree-SEE].

Eryderm (Derm) (generic *erythromycin*).   Topical antibiotic used to treat acne vulgaris. Liquid: 2%. [EH-ree-dehrm]. 84

Erygel (Derm) (generic *erythromycin*).   Topical antibiotic used to treat acne vulgaris. Gel: 2%. [EH-ree-jehl]. 84

EryPed 200, EryPed 400 (Antibio).   Macrolide antibiotic used to treat a variety of infections, including *Streptococcus*, *H. influenzae*, gonorrhea, syphilis, *Chlamydia*, and Legionnaire's disease; used to prevent subacute bacterial endocarditis.   For dosage, see *erythromycin*. [eh-ree-PEED]. 319

Ery-Tab (Antibio).   Macrolide antibiotic used to treat a variety of infections, including *Streptococcus*, *H. influenzae*, gonorrhea, syphilis, *Chlamydia*, and Legionnaire's disease; used to prevent subacute bacterial endocarditis.   For dosage, see *erythromycin*. [eh-ree-TEHB]. 319

Erythrocin (Antibio).   Macrolide antibiotic used to treat a variety of infections, including *Streptococcus*, *H. influenzae*, gonorrhea, syphilis, *Chlamydia*, and Legionnaire's disease; used to prevent subacute bacterial endocarditis.   For dosage, see *erythromycin*. [eh-REE-throh-sihn]. 319

erythromycin (E.E.S. 200, E.E.S. 400, E-Mycin, ERYC, EryPed, EryPed 200, EryPed 400, Ery-Tab, Erythrocin, Ilotycin, PCE Dispertab) (Antibio). Macrolide antibiotic used to treat a variety of infections, including *Streptococcus*, *H. influenzae*, gonorrhea, syphilis, *Chlamydia*, and Legionnaire's disease; used to prevent subacute bacterial endocarditis. Chewable tablet: 220 mg. Tablet: 250 mg, 400 mg, 500 mg. Enteric tablet: 333 mg. Liquid: 100 mg/2.5 mL, 125 mg/5 mL, 200 mg/5 mL, 250 mg/5 mL, 400 mg/5 mL. Intravenous (powder to be reconstituted): 500 mg, 1 g. [eh-reh-throh-MY-sihn]. 319

erythromycin (A/T/S, Emgel, Eryderm, Erygel, Staticin, T-Stat) (Derm).   Topical antibiotic used to treat acne vulgaris. Gel: 2%. Liquid: 1.5%, 2%. Ointment: 2%. [eh-reh-throh-MY-sihn]. 84

erythromycin (Ilotycin) (Oph).   Topical antibiotic used to treat bacterial eye infections; used to prevent gonorrhea-caused blindness and *Chlamydia* eye infections in newborns. Ophthalmic ointment: 0.5%. [eh-reh-throh-MY-sihn].

erythropoietin.   See *epoetin alfa*.

Esclim (OB/GYN, Ortho).   Hormone replacement therapy used to treat the symptoms of menopause; used to prevent and treat osteoporosis.   For dosage, see *estradiol*. [EHS-klihm]. 252

(Eserine) (Oph).   No longer on the market. (Generic name *physostigmine*; used to treat glaucoma).

Esidrix (Uro).   Thiazide diuretic.   For dosage, see *hydrochlorothiazide*. [EH-sih-drihks]. 103

Esimil (Cardio) (generic *guanethidine, hydrochlorothiazide*).   Combination antihypertensive and diuretic drug. Tablet: 10 mg/25 mg. 167

Eskalith, Eskalith CR (Psych).   Antipsychotic drug used to treat the mania of manic-depressive disorder; used to treat tardive dyskinesia, a side effect of antipsychotic drugs; used to treat bulimia nervosa. For dosage, see *lithium*. [EHS-kah-lith]. 284, 288, 291

Eskalith, Eskalith CR (Analges, Antivir, Chemo, Endo).   Antipsychotic drug used to prevent cluster headaches; used to treat neutropenia in AIDS patients receiving zidovudine; used to treat chemotherapy-induced neutropenia; used to treat syndrome of inappropriate antidiuretic hormone.   For dosage, see *lithium*. [EHS-kah-lith]. 231, 331, 362

esmolol (Brevibloc) (Cardio).   Cardioselective beta-blocker used to treat angina pectoris and ventricular arrhythmias. Intravenous: 10 mg/mL, 250 mg/mL. [EHS-moh-lawl]. 157, 160, 162

esomeprazole (Nexium) (GI).   Proton pump inhibitor drug used to treat heartburn, gastroesophageal reflux disease, and *H. pylori* infection. Capsule: 20 mg, 40 mg. [eh-soh-MEH-prah-zohl]. 121

Esoterica (Derm) (generic *hydroquinone*). Topical drug used to lighten areas of hyperpigmented skin. Cream: 1.5%. [eh-soh-TEH-rih-kah]. 99

Estar (Derm) (generic *coal tar*). Topical drug used to treat psoriasis. Gel: 5%. [EHS-tawr]. 86

estazolam (ProSom) (Neuro). Nonbarbiturate drug used to treat insomnia. (Schedule IV drug). Tablet: 1 mg, 2 mg. [eh-STEH-zoh-lehm]. 272

esterified estrogens (Estratab, Menest) (Chemo, OB/GYN, Ortho). Hormonal chemotherapy drug used to treat breast and prostate carcinoma; hormone replacement therapy used to treat the symptoms of menopause; used to prevent and treat osteoporosis. Tablet: 0.3 mg, 0.625 mg, 1.25 mg, 2.5 mg. [eh-STEH-rih-fyd EHS-troh-jehns]. 252, 343

Estinyl (Chemo, OB/GYN). Hormonal chemotherapy drug used to treat breast cancer and prostate cancer; hormone replacement therapy used to treat menopause. For dosage, see *ethinyl estradiol*. [EHS-tih-nill]. 252, 343

Estrace Vaginal Cream (OB/GYN). Topical hormone replacement therapy used to treat atrophic vaginitis of menopause. Cream: 0.1 mg. [EHS-trays]. 252

Estrace (Chemo, OB/GYN, Ortho). Estrogen used to treat breast and prostatic carcinoma; hormone replacement therapy to treat the symptoms of menopause; used to treat osteoporosis. For dosage, see *estradiol*. [EHS-trays]. 252, 343

Estraderm (OB/GYN, Ortho). Hormone replacement therapy used to treat the symptoms of menopause; used to prevent and treat osteoporosis. For dosage, see *estradiol*. [EHS-trah-dehrm]. 252

estradiol (Alora, Climara, Esclim, Estraderm, Fem-Patch, Vivelle, Vivelle-Dot) (OB/GYN, Ortho). Hormone replacement therapy used to treat the symptoms of menopause; used to prevent and treat osteoporosis. Patch: 0.025 mg/24 hr, 0.0375 mg/24 hr, 0.05 mg/24 hr, 0.075 mg/24 hr, 0.1 mg/24 hr. [ehs-trah-DY-awl]. 352

estradiol (Estrace Vaginal Cream) (OB/GYN). Topical hormone replacement therapy used to treat atrophic vaginitis of menopause. Cream: 0.1 mg. [ehs-trah-DY-awl]. 250

estradiol (Estrace) (Chemo, OB/GYN, Ortho). Hormone chemotherapy drug used to treat breast and prostate carcinoma; hormone replacement therapy used to treat the symptoms of menopause; used to prevent and treat osteoporosis. Tablet: 0.5 mg, 1 mg, 1.5 mg, 2 mg. [ehs-trah-DY-awl]. 252, 343

estradiol (Estring) (OB/GYN). Topical hormone replacement therapy used to treat atrophic vaginitis of menopause. Vaginal ring: 2 mg. [ehs-trah-DY-awl]. 252

estradiol cypionate (Depo-Estradiol Cypionate, dep-Gynogen, DepoGen). Hormone replacement therapy used to treat the symptoms of menopause. Intramuscular: 5 mg/mL. [ehs-trah-DY-awl SIH-pee-oh-nayt]. 252

estradiol hemihydrate (Vagifem) (OB/GYN). Hormone replacement therapy used to treat atrophic vaginitis of menopause. Vaginal tablet: 25 mcg. [ehs-trah-DY-awl heh-mee-HY-drayt]. 252

estradiol valerate (Delestrogen, Gynogen L.A. 20, Valergan 20, Valergan 40). (Chemo, OB/GYN). Hormone chemotherapy drug used to treat prostate carcinoma; hormone replacement therapy used to treat the symptoms of menopause. Intramuscular: 10 mg/mL, 20 mg/mL, 40 mg/mL. [ehs-trah-DY-awl VEH-leh-rayt]. 252, 343

(Estradurin) (Chemo). No longer on the market. (Generic name *polyestradiol*; hormonal chemotherapy drug).

estramustine (Emcyt) (Chemo). Alkylating and hormone chemotherapy drug used to treat prostatic cancer. Capsule: 140 mg. [ehs-trah-MUH-steen]. 341, 343

Estratab (Chemo, OB/GYN, Ortho). Estrogen used to treat breast and prostate carcinoma; hormone replacement therapy used to treat the symptoms of menopause; used to prevent and treat osteoporosis. For dosage, see *esterified estrogens*. [EHS-trah-tehb]. 252, 343

Estratest, Estratest H.S. (OB/GYN) (generic *methyltestosterone, esterified estrogens*). Combination androgen and estrogen drug used to treat symptoms of menopause. [EHS-trah-tehst]. 253

Estring (OB/GYN). Topical hormone replacement therapy used to treat atrophic vaginitis of menopause. For dosage, see *estradiol*. [EHS-tring]. 252

estrogen replacement therapy (OB/GYN, Ortho). Class of drugs used to relieve the symptoms of menopause and prevent or treat postmenopausal osteoporosis. 252

estrone (Kestrone 5) (Chemo, OB/GYN). Hormonal chemotherapy drug used to treat prostate cancer; hormone replacement therapy used to treat the symptoms of menopause. Intramuscular: 5 mg/mL. [EHS-trohn]. 252, 343

estropipiate (Ogen, Ortho-Est) (OB/GYN, Ortho). Hormone replacement therapy used to treat the symptoms of menopause; used to prevent or treat osteoporosis. Tablet: 0.625 mg, 1.25 mg, 2.5 mg, 5 mg. [ehs-troh-PIH-pee-ate]. 252

Estrostep Fe, Estrostep 21 (Derm, OB/GYN, Ortho) (generic *norethindrone, ethinyl estradiol*). Triphasic combination progestins and estrogen oral contraceptive; used to treat acne vulgaris; used to prevent post-menopausal osteoporosis. Tablet: 1 mg/20 mcg then 1 mg/30 mcg then 1 mg/35 mcg. [EHS-troh-stehp]. 251

(Estrovis) (OB/GYN).   No longer on the market. (Generic name *quinestrol*; estrogen replacement therapy for menopause).

etanercept (Enbrel) (Ortho).   Used to treat rheumatoid arthritis. Subcutaneous (powder to be reconstituted): 25 mg. [eh-TEH-nehr-sehpt]. 142

ethacrynic acid (Edecrin) (Uro).   Loop diuretic. Tablet: 25 mg, 50 mg. Intravenous: 50 mg/50 mL. [eh-thah-KRIH-nihk EH-sihd]. 104

ethambutol (Myambutol) (Resp).   Bactericidal antibiotic used only to treat tuberculosis. Tablet: 100 mg, 400 mg. [eh-THAHM-byoo-tawl]. 197

Ethamolin (Cardio, GI).   Sclerosing drug used to treat varicose veins; also used to stop bleeding from esophageal varices.   For dosage, see *ethanolamine*. [eh-THAH-moh-lihn]. 133

ethanolamine (Ethamolin) (Cardio, GI).   Sclerosing drug used to treat varicose veins; used to stop bleeding esophageal varices. Intravenous (injection into the varicose vein or esophageal varix): 5%. [eh-thah-NOH-lah-meen]. 133

ethaverine (Cardio, Neuro).   Peripheral vasodilator used to treat blood vessel spasms in peripheral vascular disease and cerebrovascular disease. Tablet: 100 mg. [eh-THAH-veh-reen]. 168, 173

(ethchlorvynol) (Neuro).   No longer on the market. (Trade name *Placidyl*; nonbarbiturate used to treat insomnia).

(ether) (Anes).   No longer on the market. (Inhaled gas for general anesthesia). 366

(ethinamate) (Neuro).   No longer on the market. (Trade name *Valmid*; nonbarbiturate used to treat insomnia).

ethinyl estradiol (Estinyl) (Chemo, OB/GYN).   Hormonal chemotherapy drug used to treat breast cancer and prostate cancer; hormone replacement therapy used to treat menopause. Tablet: 0.02 mg, 0.05, 0.5 mg. [EH-theh-nill ehs-trah-DY-awl]. 252, 343

ethiofos (Chemo).   Cytoprotective drug used to prevent toxicity in patients receiving cisplatin and cyclophosphamide chemotherapy. Orphan drug. 350

ethionamide (Trecator-SC) (Resp).   Used to treat tuberculosis. Tablet: 250 mg. 197

Ethmozine (Cardio).   Used to treat ventricular arrhythmias.   For dosage, see *moricizine*. [EHTH-moh-zeen]. 159

(ethopropazine) (Neuro).   No longer on the market. (Trade name *Parsidol*; used to treat Parkinson's disease).

ethosuximide (Zarontin) (Neuro).   Anticonvulsant drug used to treat absence seizures. Capsule: 250 mg. Liquid: 250 mg/5mL. [eh-thoh-SUHK-seh-mide]. 264

ethotoin (Peganone) (Neuro).   Anticonvulsant drug used to treat tonic-clonic and psychomotor seizures. Tablet: 250 mg. 264

Ethrane (Anes).   Used to induce and maintain general anesthesia. Inhaled gas. [EE-thrayn]. 370

Ethyol (Chemo).   Cytoprotective drug used to prevent renal toxicity in patients receiving cisplatin chemotherapy; also used to prevent xerostomia after head and neck irradiation.   For dosage, see *amifostine*. 350

etidocaine (Duranest, Duranest MPF) (Anes).   Regional nerve block anesthetic. Injection: 1%; 1% with 1:200,000 epinephrine. [eh-TEE-doh-kayn]. 368

etidocaine (Duranest, Duranest MPF) (OB/GYN).   Regional anesthesia for cesarean section. Injection: 1%, 1.5%. [eh-TEE-doh-kayn]. 368

etidocaine (Duranest, Duranest MPF) (Oph).   Retrobulbar anesthesia for eye surgery. Injection: 1%, 1.5%. [eh-TEE-doh-kayn].

etidronate (Didronel, Didronel IV) (Chemo, OB/GYN, Ortho).   Inhibits the breakdown of bone; used to treat hypercalcemia of malignancy; used to prevent and treat postmenopausal osteoporosis; used to treat Paget's disease. Tablet: 200 mg, 400 mg. Intravenous: 300 mg/6 mL. [eh-TIH-droh-nayt]. 144, 361

Ethypharm (Chemo).   Chemotherapy drug used to treat brain cancer. Biodegradable microspheres for implant. Orphan drug.

etodolac (Lodine, Lodine XL) (Analges, Ortho).   Nonsteroidal anti-inflammatory drug used to treat pain; used to treat bursitis, gout, osteoarthritis, rheumatoid arthritis, and tendinitis. Capsule: 200 mg, 300 mg. Tablet: 400 mg, 500 mg, 600 mg. [eh-TOH-doh-lack]. 139, 304

etomidate (Amidate) (Anes).   Used to induce and maintain general anesthesia. Intravenous: 2 mg/mL. [eh-TAW-mih-dayt]. 369

Etopophos (Chemo).   Mitosis inhibitor chemotherapy drug used to treat lung cancer, testicular cancer, liver cancer, ovarian cancer, uterine cancer, breast cancer, gastric cancer, leukemia, Hodgkin's disease, non-Hodgkin's lymphoma, rhabdomyosarcoma, and Kaposi's sarcoma.   For dosage, see *etoposide*. [eh-TOH-poh-faws]. 344

etoposide (Etopophos, Toposar, VePesid) (Chemo). Mitosis inhibitor chemotherapy drug used to treat lung cancer, testicular cancer, liver cancer, ovarian cancer, uterine cancer, breast cancer, gastric cancer, leukemia, Hodgkin's disease, non-Hodgkin's lymphoma, rhabdomyosarcoma, and Kaposi's sarcoma. Capsule: 50 mg. Intravenous: 20 mg/mL, (powder to be reconstituted) 100 mg. [eh-TOH-poh-side]. 344

Etrafon, Etrafon-A, Etrafon-Forte, Etrafon 2-10 (Psych) (generic *amitriptyline, perphenazine*). Combination antidepressant and antipsychotic drug. Tablet: 10 mg/2 mg, 25 mg/2 mg, 10 mg/4 mg, 25 mg/4 mg, 50 mg/4 mg. [EH-trah-fawn]. 293

(etretinate) (Derm). No longer on the market. (Trade name *Tegison*; vitamin A-type drug used to treat psoriasis).

Eucalyptamint, Eucalyptamint Maximum Strength (Ortho). Topical irritant drug used to mask the pain of arthritis and muscular aches. Gel. Ointment.

Eulexin (Chemo, Endo). Hormonal chemotherapy drug used to treat prostatic cancer; also used to treat hirsutism. For dosage, see *flutamide*. [yoo-LEHK-sihn]. 343

Eurax (Derm) (generic *crotamiton*). Topical drug used to treat scabies (mites). Cream: 10%. Lotion: 10%. [YOOR-acks]. 95

(Euthroid) (Endo). No longer on the market. (Generic name *liotrix*; thyroid hormone replacement).

Evac-Q-Kwik (GI) (generic *magnesium/potassium citrate, bisacodyl*). Bowel evacuant/bowel prep kit. Oral liquid, oral tablets, and suppository. 125

Evista (OB/GYN, Ortho). Selective estrogen receptor modulator (SERM) used to prevent and treat osteoporosis after menopause. For dosage, see *raloxifene*. [ee-VIHS-tah]. 144

Evoxac (ENT). Used to treat dry mouth due to Sjogren's syndrome. For dosage, see *cevimeline*.

Eloxatin (Chemo). Chemotherapy platinum drug used to treat ovarian cancer and colon cancer. For dosage, see *oxaliplatin*. [eh-LAWK-sah-tihn].

Excedrin Aspirin Free (Analges) (generic *acetaminophen, caffeine*). Combination analgesic and caffeine drug. Caplet, Geltab: 500 mg/65 mg. [ehk-SEH-drihn].

Excedrin Extra Strength, Excedrin Migraine (Analges) (generic *acetaminophen, aspirin, caffeine*). Combination of two nonnarcotic analgesics and caffeine drug. Caplet, Gelcap, Tablet: 250 mg/250 mg/65 mg. [ehk-SEH-drihn].

Excedrin P.M., Excedrine P.M. Liquigels (Neuro) (generic *acetaminophen, diphenhydramine*). Combination analgesic and antihistamine sleep aid. Capsule: 500 mg/25 mg. Tablet: 500 mg/25 mg. Liquid: 167 mg/8.3 mg per 5 mL, 1000 mg/50 mg per 30 mL. [ehk-SEH-drihn].

excretion, drug. 48

Exelderm (Derm) (generic *sulconazole*). Topical antifungal drug. Cream: 1%. Liquid: 1%. [EHK-sehl-dehrm]. 89

Exelon (Neuro). Cholinesterase inhibitor used to treat Alzheimer's disease. For dosage, see *rivastigmine*. [EHK-seh-lawn]. 271

exemestane (Aromasin) (Chemo). Hormonal chemotherapy drug used to treat breast cancer. Tablet: 25 mg. [ehk-seh-MEHS-tayn]. 343

exisulind (Aptosyn) (Chemo). Chemotherapy drug used to treat prostate cancer, breat cancer, and lung cancer. Investigational drug. 347

ex-lax, ex-lax chocolated, Maximum Strength ex-lax (GI). Irritant/stimulant laxative. For dosage, see *sennosides*. 124

ex-lax stool softener (GI). Stool softener laxative. For dosage, see *docusate*. 125

Exna (Uro). Thiazide diuretic. For dosage, see *benzthiazide*. 103

Exosurf Neonate (Resp). Synthetic lung surfactant used to prevent and treat respiratory distress syndrome in premature newborns. For dosage, see *colfosceril*.

expectorants (ENT). Class of drugs that thins mucus to facilitate productive coughing. 63, 210

Extencaps. Part of the trade name of a drug, indicating a time-release capsule. 63

Extended Release Bayer 8-Hour. See *Genuine Bayer Aspirin.*

Extentab. Part of the trade name of a drug, indicating a time-release tablet. 63

Extra Strength Alka-Seltzer, Original Alka-Seltzer (GI) (generic *aspirin, sodium bicarbonate*). Combination analgesic and antacid. Effervescent tablet: 325 mg/1700 mg, 500 mg/1985 mg. 117

Extra Strength Bayer Enteric 500. See *Genuine Bayer Aspirin.*

Extra Strength Denorex. See *Denorex.*

Extra Strength Doan's (Analges). Salicylate nonaspirin drug used to treat pain and inflammation. For dosage, see *magnesium salicylate*. 300

Extra Strength Doan's P.M. (Neuro) (generic *diphenhydramine, magnesium*). Combination antihistamine and magnesium sleep aid. Tablet: 25 mg/500 mg. 273

Extra Strength Maalox, Extra Strength Maalox Plus (GI) (generic *aluminum, magnesium, simethicone*). Combination antacid and anti-gas drug. Suspension: 500 mg/450 mg/40 mg. See also *Maalox*. 117

Extra Strength Tums. See *Tums.*

Extra Strength Tylenol PM, Extra Strength Tylenol PM Gelcaps (Neuro) (generic *acetaminophen, diphen-*

hydramine).   Combination analgesic and antihistamine sleep aid. Capsule: 500 mg/25 mg. Tablet: 500 mg/25 mg. 273

Eyesine (Oph).   Topical decongestant/vasoconstrictor used to treat irritation and allergy symptoms in the eyes.   For dosage, see *tetrahydrozoline*.

Fabrase (Misc).   Alpha-galactosidase-A drug used as replacement therapy to treat this missing enzyme in Fabry's disease. Orphan drug.

famciclovir (Famvir) (Antivir, Derm, OB/GYN). Drug used to treat herpes zoster virus infections; used to treat genital herpes (condyloma acuminatum). Tablet: 125 mg, 250 mg, 500 mg. [fehm-SIH-kloh-veer]. 330

famotidine (Pepcid, Pepcid AC, Pepcid AC Acid Controller, Pepcid RPD) (GI).   H$_2$ blocker used to treat peptic ulcers and *H. pylori* infection. Chewable tablet: 10 mg. Orally disintegrating tablet: 20 mg, 40 mg. Gelcap: 10 mg. Liquid (reconstituted powder): 40 mg/5 mL. Tablet: 10 mg, 20 mg, 40 mg. Intravenous: 2 mg/mL, 4 mg/mL, 10 mg/mL, 20 mg/mL. [feh-MOH-teh-deen]. 118

fampridine (Neurelan) (Neuro).   Used to treat multiple sclerosis. Orphan drug. 275

Famvir (Antivir, Derm, OB/GYN).   Used to treat herpes zoster virus infections; used to treat genital herpes (condyloma acuminatum).   For dosage, see *famciclovir*. [FEHM-veer]. 330

Fareston (Chemo).   Hormonal chemotherapy drug used to treat breast cancer.   For dosage, see *toremifene*. [FEHR-eh-stuhn]. 343

Fastin (GI).   Appetite suppressant used to treat obesity. (Schedule IV drug).   For dosage, see *phentermine*. 129

FDA (abbreviation for *Food and Drug Administration*). See *Food and Drug Administration*.

Feen-a-Mint (GI).   Irritant/stimulant laxative.   For dosage, see *bisacodyl*. 124

felbamate (Felbatol) (Neuro).   Anticonvulsant drug used to treat partial seizures; used to treat Lennox–Gestaut syndrome. Tablet: 400 mg, 600 mg. Liquid: 600 mg/5 mL. [FEHL-bah-mayt]. 265

Felbatol (Neuro).   Anticonvulsant drug used to treat partial seizures; used to treat Lennox–Gestaut syndrome.   For dosage, see *felbamate*. [FEHL-bah-tawl]. 265

Feldene (Analges, OB/GYN, Ortho).   Nonsteroidal anti-inflammatory drug used to treat dysmenorrhea; used to treat osteoarthritis and rheumatoid arthritis. For dosage, see *piroxicam*. [FEHL-deen]. 139, 255, 304

felodipine (Plendil) (Cardio).   Calcium channel blocker used to treat congestive heart failure, hypertension, and Raynaud's disease. Tablet: 2.5 mg, 5 mg, 10 mg. [feh-LOH-dih-peen]. 154, 163

Femara (Chemo).   Hormonal chemotherapy drug used to treat breast cancer.   For dosage, see *letrozole*. [fee-MEH-rah]. 343

(Femcare) (OB/GYN).   No longer on the market. (Generic drug *clotrimazole*; used to treat vaginal yeast infections).

Femhrt (Derm, OB/GYN, Ortho) (generic *norethindrone, estradiol*).   Combination progestins and estrogen drug used to treat acne vulgaris; used to treat symptoms of menopause; used to prevent or treat postmenopausal osteoporosis. Tablet: 5 mcg/1 mg. 253

FemPatch (OB/GYN, Ortho).   Hormone replacement therapy used to treat the symptoms of menopause; used to prevent and treat osteoporosis.   For dosage, see *estradiol*. 252

Femstat 3 (OB/GYN) (generic *butoconazole*).   Topical drug used to treat vaginal yeast infections. Vaginal cream: 2%. [FEHM-steht]. 256

(fenfluramine) (GI).   No longer on the market. (Trade name *Pondimin*; appetite suppressant used to treat obesity).

fenofibrate (Tricor) (Cardio).   Used to treat hypercholesterolemia by decreasing low-density lipoproteins; used to treat hypertriglyceridemia by decreasing serum triglyercides and very low-density lipoprotein levels. Capsule: 67 mg, 134 mg, 200 mg. 171

fenoldopam (Corlopam) (Cardio).   Peripheral vasodilator used to treat hypertensive crisis. Intravenous: 10 mg/mL. [feh-NOHL-doh-pehm]. 168

fenoprofen (Nalfon Pulvules) (Analges, Ortho). Nonsteroidal anti-inflammatory drug used to treat pain; used to treat migraine headaches; used to treat osteoarthritis and rheumatoid arthritis. Capsule: 200 mg, 300 mg. Tablet: 600 mg. [feh-noh-PROH-fehn]. 139, 304, 307

fenoterol (Berotec) (Resp).   Bronchodilator. Investigational drug. 193

fen-phen. 52, 130

fenretinide (Chemo).   Chemotherapy drug used to treat breast cancer, bladder cancer, and head and neck cancer. Investigational drug. 347

fentanyl (Actiq) (Analges).   Narcotic analgesic drug used to treat breakthrough pain in patients already on other narcotics. (Schedule II drug). Oral lozenge on a stick, "lollipop": 200 mcg, 400 mcg, 600 mcg, 800 mcg, 1200 mcg, 1600 mcg. [FEHN-teh-nill]. 297

fentanyl (Duragesic-25, Duragesic-50, Duragesic-75, Duragesic-100) (Analges).   Narcotic analgesic drug used to treat chronic severe pain. (Schedule II drug). Transdermal patch: 25 mcg/hr, 50 mcg/hr, 75 mcg/hr, 100 mcg/hr. [FEHN-teh-nill]. 297

fentanyl (Sublimaze) (Anes).   Preoperative narcotic drug used to provide sedation; used to induce and maintain general anesthesia. (Schedule II drug). Intramuscular and intravenous: 0.05 mg/mL. [FEHN-teh-nill]. 369

(Fentanyl Oralet) (Analges).   No longer on the market. (Generic name *fentanyl*; narcotic used to treat pain).

Fero-Folic-500 (Misc).   Combination iron, vitamin C, and folic acid nutritional supplement. Filmtab.

Ferotrinsic (Cardio).   Combination iron, intrinsic factor, vitamin B_{12}, vitamin C, and folic acid drug used to treat iron deficiency anemia and pernicious anemia. Capsule: 110 mg/240 mg/15 mcg/75 mg/0.5 mg.

Ferrlecit (Cardio).   Used to treat iron deficiency anemia in hemodialysis patients. Intravenous: 62.4 mg/5 mL.

Fertinex (Endo, OB/GYN).   Ovulation-stimulating hormone drug used to treat infertility; orphan drug used to treat low sperm count and infertility in men with pituitary gland malfunction.   For dosage, see *urofollitropin*. [FUHR-tih-nehks]. 244

fexofenadine (Allegra) (Derm, ENT).   Antihistamine used to treat allergic rhinitis and allergic reactions with hives and itching. Capsule: 60 mg. Tablet: 30 mg, 60 mg, 180 mg. [fehk-soh-FEH-nah-deen]. 207

FFP (fresh frozen plasma) (I.V.).   Intravenous blood product that contains no cellular components and is used to replace plasma proteins and clotting factors.

Fiberall (GI).   Bulk-producing laxative.   For dosage, see *psyllium*. 125

FiberCon (GI).   Bulk-producing laxative.   For dosage, see *polycarbophil*. 125

fight or flight. 161

filgrastim (Neupogen) (Antivir, Chemo, Hem).   Granulocyte colony-stimulating factor used to treat neutropenia in AIDS patients; used with chemotherapy and bone marrow transplants; used to treat aplastic anemia. Subcutaneous or intravenous: 300 mcg/mL. 331, 361

finasteride (Propecia) (Derm).   Oral drug used to treat male pattern baldness. Tablet: 1 mg. [fih-NEH-steh-ride]. 98

finasteride (Proscar) (Uro).   Used to treat benign prostatic hypertrophy. Tablet: 5 mg. [fih-NEH-steh-ride]. 108

Finevin (Derm) (generic *azelaic acid*).   Topical drug used to treat acne vulgaris. Cream: 20%. 84

Fioricet (Analges) (generic *acetaminophen, caffeine, butalbital*).   Combination nonnarcotic analgesic, stimulant, and barbiturate drug. Tablet: 325 mg/40 mg/50 mg. [fee-OHR-eh-seht]. 302

Fioricet with Codeine (Analges) (generic *codeine, acetaminophen, butalbital*).   Combination narcotic, nonnarcotic, and barbiturate analgesic/sedative drug. (Schedule III drug). Capsule: 30 mg/325 mg/50 mg. [fee-OHR-eh-seht]. 303

Fiorinal (Analges) (generic *aspirin, caffeine, butalbital*).   Combination nonnarcotic analgesic, stimulant, and barbiturate drug. Capsule: 325 mg/40 mg/50 mg. [fee-OHR-eh-nawl]. 302

Fiorinal with Codeine (Analges) (generic *codeine, aspirin, butalbital*).   Combination narcotic, nonnarcotic, and barbiturate analgesic/sedative drug. (Schedule III drug). Capsule: 30 mg/325 mg. [fee-OHR-eh-nawl]. 303

first-pass effect. 47

5-FU. See *fluorouracil*.

5-HT4 blocker (GI).   A class of drugs that blocks 5-HT4 (serotonin) receptors.

Flagyl, Flagyl 375 (GI, OB/GYN).   Antibacterial and antiprotozoal drug used to treat intestinal amebiasis; used to treat *Trichomonas vaginalis* vaginal infection, a sexually transmitted disease.   For dosage, see *metronidazole*. [FLEH-jyool].

Flagyl, Flagyl ER, Flagyl 375, Flagyl IV, Flagyl IV RTU (Antibio, GI).   Antibacterial and antiprotozoal drug used to treat a variety of infections, including *Bacteroides*, Crohn's disease, and *H. pylori* infections of the gastrointestinal tract.   For dosage, see *metronidazole*. [FLEH-jyool]. 120

Flarex (Oph).   Topical corticosteroid used to treat inflammation of the eyes.   For dosage, see *fluorometholone*. [FLEH-rehks]. 219

flavoxate (Urispas) (Uro).   Antispasmodic drug used to treat urinary frequency and urgency. Tablet: 100 mg. [flay-VAWK-sayt]. 107

flecainide (Tambocor) (Cardio).   Used to treat atrial and ventricular arrhythmias. Tablet: 50 mg, 100 mg, 150 mg. [FLEH-keh-nide]. 159

Fleet (GI) (generic *sodium phosphate*).   Enema.

Fleet Babylax (GI).   Mechanical laxative. Rectal liquid: 4 mL per applicator. 125

Fleet Bisacodyl (GI) (generic *bisacodyl*).   Enema. 126

Fleet Laxative (GI).   Irritant/stimulant laxative. For dosage, see *bisacodyl*. 124

Fleet Mineral Oil (GI) (generic *mineral oil*).   Enema. 126

Fleet Prep Kit 1 (GI) (generic *phosphosoda, bisacodyl*).   Bowel evacuant/bowel prep kit. Oral liquid, oral tablets, suppository. 125

Fleet Prep Kit 2 (GI) (generic *phosphosoda, bisacodyl*).   Bowel evacuant/bowel prep kit. Oral liquid, oral tablets, enema. 125

Fleet Prep Kit 3 (GI) (generic *phosphosoda, bisacodyl*). Bowel evacuant/bowel prep kit. Oral liquid, oral tablets, enema. 125

Fletcher's Castoria (GI).   Irritant/stimulant laxative. For dosage, see *sennosides*. 124

Flexall Ultra Plus, Maximum Strength Flexall 454 (Ortho).   Topical irritant drug used to mask the pain of arthritis and muscular aches. Gel.

(Flexeril) (Ortho).   No longer on the market. (Generic name *cyclobenzaprine;* skeletal muscle relaxant).

Flocor (Hem, Neuro).   Used to treat sickle cell crisis; used to treat subarachnoid hemorrhage and ruptured cerebral aneurysm. Orphan drug. 275

Flolan (Resp).   Vasodilator used to treat pulmonary arterial hypertension.   For dosage, see *epoprostenol*. 198

Flomax (Uro).   Alpha$_1$-receptor blocker used to treat benign prostatic hypertrophy.   For dosage, see *tamsulosin*. [FLOH-mehks]. 109

Flonase (ENT).   Topical intranasal corticosteroid used to treat allergic rhinitis.   For dosage, see *fluticasone*. [FLOH-nays]. 208

Florinef (Endo).   Used to treat Addison's disease. For dosage, see *fludrocortisone*. [FLOHR-eh-nehf]. 232

Florone, Florone E (Derm) (generic *diflorasone*).   Topical corticosteroid anti-inflammatory drug. Cream: 0.05%. 92

Flovent, Flovent Diskus, Flovent Rotadisk (Resp).   Inhaled corticosteroid used to prevent acute asthma attacks.   For dosage, see *fluticasone*. [FLOH-vehnt]. 196

Floxin (Antibio).   Fluoroquinolone antibiotic used to treat a variety of infections, including *H. influenzae, E. coli*, and gonorrhea.   For dosage, see *ofloxacin*. [FLAWK-sihn]. 105, 318

floxuridine (FUDR) (Chemo).   Pyrimidine antagonist chemotherapy drug used to treat gastrointestinal cancer. Intra-arterial (powder to be reconstituted): 500 mg. [flawks-YOUR-eh-deen]. 340

fluconazole (Diflucan) (Antifung).   Used to treat severe topical and systemic fungal and yeast infections; used to treat cryptococcal meningitis in AIDS patients. Tablet: 50 mg, 100 mg, 150 mg, 200 mg. Liquid (powder to be reconstituted): 10 mg/mL. Intravenous: 2 mg/mL. [floo-KAW-neh-zohl]. 331, 335

flucytosine (Ancobon) (Antifung).   Used to treat severe systemic fungal and yeast infections. Capsule: 250 mg, 500 mg. [floo-SY-toh-seen]. 335

Fludara (Chemo).   Purine antagonist chemotherapy drug used to treat leukemia, Hodgkin's disease, non-Hodgkin's lymphoma, and cutaneous T-cell lymphoma.   For dosage, see *fludarabine*. [floo-DEH-rah]. 339

fludarabine (Fludara) (Chemo).   Purine antagonist chemotherapy drug used to treat leukemia, Hodgkin's disease, non-Hodgkin's lymphoma, and cutaneous T-cell lymphoma. Intravenous (powder to be reconstituted): 50 mg. [floo-DEHR-ah-been]. 339

fludrocortisone (Florinef) (Endo).   Used to treat Addison's disease. Tablet: 0.1 mg. [floo-droh-KOHR-teh-sohn]. 232

Flumadine (Antivir).   Antiviral drug used to prevent and treat influenza A virus infection.   For dosage, see *rimantadine*. [FLOO-mah-deen]. 330

flumazenil (Romazicon) (Emerg, Psych).   Benzodiazepine antagonist used as an antidote to reverse the effect of an overdose of a benzodiazepine antianxiety drug. Intravenous: 0.1 mg/mL. [floo-MAH-zeh-nill]. 182, 293

flunarizine (Sibelium) (Neuro).   Used to treat alternating hemiplegia. Orphan drug. 275

flunisolide (AeroBid, AeroBid-M) (Resp).   Corticosteroid used to prevent acute asthma attacks. Aerosol inhaler: 250 mcg/puff. [floo-NIH-soh-lide]. 196

flunisolide (Nasalide) (ENT).   Topical intranasal corticosteroid used to treat allergic rhinitis. Spray: 0.025%, 25 mcg/spray. 208

flunitrazepam (Rohypnol) (Psych).   Illegal drug not approved for use in the United States. So-called "date-rape drug." 293

fluocinolone (Derma-Smoothe/FS, Flurosyn, Synalar, Synalar-HP) (Derm).   Topical corticosteroid anti-inflammatory drug. Cream: 0.01%, 0.025%, 0.2%. Liquid: 0.01%. Oil: 0.01%. Ointment: 0.025%. [floo-oh-SIH-noh-lohn]. 92

fluocinonide (Lidex, Lidex-E) (Derm).   Topical corticosteroid anti-inflammatory drug. Cream: 0.05%. Gel: 0.05%. Liquid: 0.05%. Ointment: 0.05%. [floo-oh-SIH-noh-nide]. 92

Fluoracaine (Oph) (generic *fluorescein, proparacaine*).   Topical combination ophthalmic dye and anesthetic drug. Ophthalmic solution: 0.25%/0.5%. [FLOHR-ah-kayn].

fluorescein (Fluorescite, Fluorets, Ful-Glo) (Oph).   Topical yellow-green dye that shows corneal abrasions and ulcers; used during angiography of the eye. Ophthalmic solution: 2%. Ophthalmic strips: 0.6 mg, 1 mg. Intravenous: 10%, 25%. [FLOHR-eh-seen].

Fluorescite (Oph).   Topical yellow-green dye that shows corneal abrasions and ulcers; used during angiography of the eye.   For dosage, see *fluorescein*. [FLOHR-eh-site].

Fluoresoft (Oph).   Topical dye used to assist in fitting contact lenses.   For dosage, see *fluorexon*.

Fluorets (Oph). Topical yellow-green dye that shows corneal abrasions and ulcers. For dosage, see *fluorescein*. [FLOHR-ehts].

fluorexon (Fluoresoft) (Oph). Topical dye used to assist in fitting contact lenses. Ophthalmic solution 0.35%. [flohr-EHK-sawn].

fluorometholone (Flarex, Fluor-Op, FML, FML Forte, FML S.O.P.) (Oph). Topical corticosteroid used to treat inflammation of the eyes. Ophthalmic suspension: 0.1%, 0.25%. Ophthalmic ointment: 0.1%. [flohr-oh-MEH-theh-lohn]. 219

Fluor-Op (Oph). Topical corticosteroid used to treat inflammation of the eyes. For dosage, see *fluorometholone*. 219

fluoroquinolones (Antibio, Uro). Class of antibiotics. 318

fluorouracil (5-FU, Adrucil) (Chemo). Pyrimidine antagonist chemotherapy drug used to treat breast cancer, stomach cancer, pancreatic cancer, colon cancer, and rectal cancer. Intravenous: 50 mg/mL. [flohr-oh-YOUR-ah-sill]. 340

fluorouracil (Efudex) (Derm). Topical chemotherapy drug used to treat keratoses and superficial basal cell carcinoma. Cream: 1%, 5%. Liquid: 1%, 2%, 5%. [flohr-oh-YOUR-ah-sill]. 98

fluorouracil (5-FU) (Chemo). Chemotherapy drug used to treat brain cancer. Biodegradable microspheres for implant. Orphan drug. 340

(Fluothane) (Anes). No longer on the market. (Generic name *halothane*; inhaled general anesthetic).

fluoxetine (Prozac, Prozac Weekly) (Analges, Neuro). Selective serotonin reuptake inhibitor antidepressant used to treat migraine headaches; used to treat narcolepsy; used to treat levodopa-induced dyskinesia. Tablet: 10 mg. Pulvule: 10 mg, 20 mg, 40 mg. Liquid: 20 mg/5 mL. [floo-AWK-seh-teen]. 270, 274, 307

fluoxetine (Prozac, Prozac Weekly) (Diab). Selective serotonin reuptake inhibitor used to treat diabetic peripheral neuropathy. Capsule: 90 mg. Tablet: 10 mg. Pulvule: 10 mg, 20 mg, 40 mg. Liquid: 20 mg/5 mL. [floo-AWK-seh-teen].

fluoxetine (Prozac, Prozac Weekly) (Psych). Selective serotonin reuptake inhibitor antidepressant used to treat depression; used to treat obsessive-compulsive disorder; used to treat bulimia nervosa and anorexia nervosa; used to treat attention-deficit/hyperactivity disorder; used to treat manic-depressive disorder; used to treat kleptomania; used to treat posttraumatic stress disorder; used to treat psychosis and schizophrenia; used to treat autism; used to treat social anxiety disorder/social phobias; used to treat panic disorder. Tablet: 10

mg. Pulvule: 10 mg, 20 mg, 40 mg. Liquid: 20 mg/5 mL. [floo-AWK-seh-teen]. 284, 287, 289, 290, 291, 292

fluoxetine (Sarafem) (OB/GYN). Selective serotonin reuptake inhibitor antidepressant used to treat premenstrual dysphoric disorder. Tablet: 10 mg. Pulvule: 10 mg, 20 mg, 40 mg. Liquid: 20 mg/5 mL. [floo-AWK-seh-teen]. 254

fluoxymesterone (Halotestin) (Chemo, Endo). Male sex hormone used to treat breast cancer in women; used to treat the lack of production of testosterone due to absence, injury, malfunction of the testes or malfunction of the pituitary gland; used to treat delayed puberty in boys. Tablet: 2 mg, 5 mg, 10 mg. [floo-awk-see-MEHS-teh-rohn]. 343

flupirtine (Analges). Nonnarcotic analgesic. Investigational drug. 309

fluphenazine (Permitil, Prolixin) (Psych). Phenothiazine drug used to treat psychosis and schizophrenia. Tablet: 1 mg, 2.5 mg, 5 mg, 10 mg. Liquid: 2.5 mg/mL, 5 mg/mL. Subcutaneous or intramuscular: 25 mg/mL. [floo-FEH-nah-zeen]. 283

flurandrenolide (Cordran, Cordran SP) (Derm). Topical corticosteroid anti-inflammatory drug. Cream: 0.025%, 0.05%. Lotion: 0.05%. Ointment: 0.025%, 0.05%. Tape: 4 mcg/cm². [flohr-ehn-DREH-noh-lide]. 92

Flurate (Oph) (generic *benoxinate, fluorescein*). Topical combination anesthetic and ophthalmic dye drug. Ophthalmic solution: 0.4%/0.25%.

flurazepam (Dalmane) (Neuro). Nonbarbiturate benzodiazepine drug used to treat insomnia. (Schedule IV drug). Capsule: 15 mg, 30 mg. [flohr-EH-zeh-pehm]. 272

flurbiprofen (Ansaid) (Analges, OB/GYN, Ortho). Nonsteroidal anti-inflammatory drug used to treat migraine headaches; used to treat dysmenorrhea; used to treat gout, osteoarthritis, and rheumatoid arthritis. Tablet: 50 mg, 100 mg. [flohr-bih-PROH-fehn]. 139, 304, 307

flurbiprofen (Ocufen) (Oph). Topical nonsteroidal anti-inflammatory drug used only to prevent miosis during eye surgery. Ophthalmic solution: 0.03%. [flohr-bih-PROH-fehn].

Flurosyn (Derm) (generic *fluocinolone*). Topical corticosteroid anti-inflammatory drug. Cream: 0.01%, 0.025%. Ointment: 0.025%. [FLOHR-oh-sihn]. 92

FluShield (Antivir, Resp). Vaccine to prevent influenza A virus infection. For dosage, see *influenza vaccine*.

"flu shot." See *influenza vaccine*.

flutamide (Eulexin) (Chemo, Endo). Hormonal chemotherapy drug used to treat prostatic cancer;

also used to treat hirsutism. Capsule: 125 mg. [FLOO-teh-mide]. 343

Flutex (Derm) (generic *triamcinolone*). Topical corticosteroid anti-inflammatory drug. Cream: 0.025%, 0.1%, 0.5%. Ointment: 0.025%, 0.1%, 0.5%. [FLOO-tehks]. 92

fluticasone (Cutivate) (Derm). Topical corticosteroid anti-inflammatory drug. Cream: 0.05%. Ointment: 0.005%. 92

fluticasone (Flonase) (ENT). Topical intranasal corticosteroid used to treat allergic rhinitis. Spray: 0.05%. 208

fluticasone (Flovent, Flovent Diskus, Flovent Rotadisk) (Resp). Corticosteroid used to prevent acute asthma attacks. Aerosol inhaler: 44 mcg/puff, 110 mcg/puff, 220 mcg/puff. Rotadisk (inhaled powder): 50 mcg, 100 mcg, 250 mcg. 196

fluvastatin (Lescol, Lescol XL) (Cardio). HMG-CoA reductase inhibitor drug used to treat hypercholesterolemia. Capsule: 20 mg, 40 mg. Tablet; 80 mg. [floo-vah-STEH-tihn]. 170

Fluvirin (Antivir, Resp). Vaccine to prevent influenza A virus infection. For dosage, see *influenza vaccine*. 330

fluvoxamine (Luvox) (OB/GYN). Selective serotonin reuptake inhibitor antidepressant used to treat premenstrual dysphoric disorder. Tablet: 25 mg, 50 mg, 100 mg. [floo-VAWK-seh-meen]. 255

fluvoxamine (Luvox) (Psych). Selective serotonin reuptake inhibitor antidepressant used to treat depression; used to treat anxiety; used to treat obsessive-compulsive disorder; used to treat autism; used to treat social anxiety disorder; used to treat panic disorder; used to treat posttraumatic stress disorder. Tablet: 25 mg, 50 mg, 100 mg. [floo-VAWK-seh-meen]. 282, 287, 289, 290

Fluzone (Antivir, Resp). Vaccine to prevent influenza A virus infection. For dosage, see *influenza vaccine*.

FML, FML Forte, FML S.O.P. (Oph). Topical corticosteroid used to treat inflammation of the eyes. For dosage, see *fluorometholone*. 219

foam (drug form). 37

Focalin (Psych). Central nervous system stimulant used to treat attention-deficit/hyperactivity disorder. For dosage, see *dexmethylphenidate*. [FOH-kah-lihn]. 292

FocalSeal-L (Resp). Topical drug used to seal lung tissue during surgery. Solution activated by light.

FocalSeal-S (Neuro). Topical drug used to seal the dura during neurosurgery. Solution activated by light.

Focus on Healthcare Issues features.
Accutane and suicide attempts. 53, 85
anabolic steroid abuse. 233
antibiotics in soaps and the development of resistant bacteria. 89
antibiotic-resistant bacteria. 319
beef/pork insulin off the market. 7, 240
cost of prescription drugs. 31
legalization of marijuana. 17
OxyContin as drug of abuse. 17, 298
prescription drugs changed to over-the-counter drugs. 19
Ritalin and Prozac prescriptions for preschoolers. 292
treatment of drug addicts. 308
tuberculosis treatment. 198
umbilical cord blood. 380

(Folex) (Chemo, Derm). No longer on the market. (Generic name *methotrexate*; folic acid antagonist chemotherapy drug; used to treat severe psoriasis).

folic acid (Folvite) (Hem, Neuro, OB/GYN). Water-soluble vitamin used to treat megaloblastic anemia; given to pregnant women to prevent neural tube defects in the baby. Tablet: 0.4 mg, 0.8 mg, 1 mg. Subcutaneous, intramuscular, or intravenous: 5 mg/mL. [FOH-lihk EH-sihd]. 245

folinic acid. See *leucovorin*.

Follistim (OB/GYN). Ovulation-stimulating drug used to treat infertility. For dosage, see *follitropin beta*. [FOH-leh-stihm]. 244

follitropin alfa (Gonal-F) (Endo, OB/GYN). Ovulation-stimulating hormone drug used to treat infertility; orphan drug used to treat decreased sperm count and infertility in men. Subcutaneous (powder to be reconstituted): 37.5 IU, 75 IU, 150 IU. [foh-leh-TROH-pihn EHL-fah]. 244

follitropin beta (Follistim) (OB/GYN). Ovulation-stimulating drug used to treat infertility. Subcutaneous or intramuscular (powder to be reconstituted): 75 IU. [foh-leh-TROH-pihn BAY-tah]. 244

Folvite (Hem, Neuro, OB/GYN). Used to treat megaloblastic anemia; given to pregnant women to prevent neural tube defects in the baby. For dosage, see *folic acid*. [FOHL-vite].

fomepizole (Antizol) (Emerg). Used to reverse the effects of an overdose of ethylene glycol (antifreeze) or methanol (wood alcohol). Intravenous: 1 g/mL. [foh-MEH-peh-zohl]. 183

fomivirsen (Vitravene) (Antivir, Oph). Antiviral drug used to treat cytomegalovirus retinitis in AIDS patients. Intraocular injection: 6.6 mg/mL. [foh-mih-VEHR-sehn]. 329

fondaparinux (Arixtra) (Hem).   Used to prevent venous thromboembolus after orthopedic surgery. Subcutaneous: 2.5 mg/0.5 mL.

Food and Drug Administration (FDA), The. 14

Food and Drug Administration (FDA) Modernization Act of 1997, The. 15

Food and Drugs Act of 1906, The. 14

Food, Drug, and Cosmetic Act of 1938, The. 14

Foradil Aerolizer (Resp).   Bronchodilator.   For dosage, see *formoterol.* [FOHR-ah-dihl]. 193

Forane (Anes).   Used to induce and maintain general anesthesia. Inhaled gas. [FOH-rayn]. 370

formoterol (Foradil Aerolizer) (Resp).   Bronchodilator. Aerolizer Inhaler: Powder. [fohr-MOH-teh-rawl]. 193

formula, infant (GI). 131

Forta Drink, Forta Shake (GI).   Liquid nutritional supplement. Powder (to be reconstituted).

Fortaz (Antibio).   Cephalosporin antibiotic used to treat a variety of bacterial infections, including *Streptococcus, Staphylococcus, E. coli,* and *H. influenzae.* For dosage, see *ceftazidime.* [FOHR-tehz]. 316

Fortovase (Antivir).   Protease inhibitor drug used to treat AIDS.   For dosage, see *saquinavir.* [FOHR-toh-vays]. 325

Forvade (Antivir).   Antiviral drug used to treat genital herpes.   For dosage, see *cidofovir.* 330

Fosamax (OB/GYN, Ortho).   Inhibits bone breakdown; used to prevent and treat postmenopausal osteoporosis; used to treat Paget's disease.   For dosage, see *alendronate.* [FAW-sah-mehks]. 144

Foscan (Chemo).   Chemotherapy drug used to treat head and neck cancer.   For dosage, see *temoporfin.* [FAWS-kehn]. 348

foscarnet (Foscavir) (Antivir).   Antiviral drug used to treat AIDS; used to treat cytomegalovirus retinitis; used to treat herpes simplex virus infection. Intravenous: 24 mg/mL. [FAWS-kahr-neht]. 326, 329, 330

Foscavir (Antivir).   Antiviral drug used to treat AIDS; used to treat cytomegalovirus retinitis; used to treat herpes simplex virus infection.   For dosage, see *foscarnet.* [FAWS-kah-veer]. 326, 329, 330

fosfomycin (Monurol) (Uro).   Urinary anti-infective drug. Granules administered with a meal: 3 g. 106

fosinopril (Monopril) (Cardio).   Angiotensin-converting enzyme inhibitor used to treat congestive heart failure and hypertension. Tablet: 10 mg, 20 mg, 40 mg. 154, 163

fosphenytoin (Cerebyx) (Neuro).   Anticonvulsant drug used to treat status epilepticus. Intramuscular or intravenous: 150 mg/2 mL, 750 mg/10 mL. [fahs-FEHN-toh-ehn]. 265, 267

Fostex 10% BPO, Fostex 10% Wash (Derm) (generic *benzoyl peroxide*).   Topical antibiotic used to treat acne vulgaris. Gel: 10%. Liquid: 10%. 83

4-aminosalicylic acid (Pamisyl, Rezipas) (GI).   Used to treat ulcerative colitis. Orphan drug. 126

4-ASA (abbreviation for *4-aminosalicylic acid*).   See *4-aminosalicylic acid.*

4-Way Fast Acting Original (ENT) (generic *naphazoline, phenylephrine, pyrilamine*).   Combination decongestant and antihistamine drug. Spray: 0.05%/0.5%/ 0.2%.

4-Way Long Lasting Nasal (ENT).   Decongestant. For dosage, see *oxymetazoline.* 206

foxglove (plant).   Historical Notes feature. 6, 151, 152

Fragmin (Hem).   Low molecular weight heparin anticoagulant.   For dosage, see *dalteparin.* [FREHG-mihn]. 186

FreAmine III 3%, FreAmine III 8.5%, FreAmine HBC 6.9%, FreAmine III 10% (I.V.).   Intravenous fluid for total parenteral nutrition. [free-ah-MEEN]. 376

fresh frozen plasma (FFP) (I.V.).   Intravenous blood product that contains no cellular components and is used to replace plasma proteins and clotting factors.

Frisium (Neuro, Psych) (generic *clobazam*).   Used to treat epilepsy; used to treat anxiety. Investigational drug. 265, 282

Frova (Analges).   Serotonin receptor agonist drug used to treat migraine headaches.   For dosage, see *frovatriptan.* 306

frovatriptan (Frova) (Analges).   Serotonin receptor agonist drug used to treat migraine headaches. Tablet: 2.5 mg. [froh-vah-TRIHP-tehn]. 306

FUDR (Chemo).   Pyrimidine antagonist chemotherapy drug used to treat gastrointestinal cancer.   For dosage, see *floxuridine.* 340

Ful-Glo (Oph).   Topical yellow-green dye that shows corneal abrasions and ulcers.

Fulvicin P/G, Fulvicin U/F (Antifung, Derm).   Used to treat severe topical fungal infections.   For dosage, see *griseofulvin.* [FOOL-veh-sihn]. 90, 334

(Funduscein) (Oph).   No longer on the market. (Generic name *fluorescein*; topical yellow dye that shows corneal abrasions).

fungal infections, drugs used to treat. 334, 335

fungal infections of the skin, drugs used to treat. 89

Fungizone (Derm) (generic *amphotericin B*).   Topical antiyeast drug. Cream: 3%, Lotion: 3%. Ointment: 3%. [FUHN-jeh-zohn].

Fungizone (ENT).   Topical drug used to treat yeast infections in the mouth.   For dosage, see *amphotericin B.* [FUHN-jeh-zohn].

Fungizone Intravenous (Antifung). Used to treat severe systemic fungal and yeast infections. For dosage, see *amphotericin B*. [FUHN-jeh-zohn]. 335

Fungoid, Fungoid Creme, Fungoid Tincture (Derm) (generic *triacetin*). Topical antifungal drug. Cream, liquid. [FUHN-goyd]. 89

Furacin (Derm) (generic *nitrofurazone*). Topical antibiotic used to treat severe burns. Cream: 0.2%. Liquid: 0.2%. Ointment: 0.2%. [FYOUR-eh-sihn]. 97

Furadantin (Antibio, Uro). Antibiotic used only to treat urinary tract infections. For dosage, see *nitrofurantoin*. [fyour-eh-DEHN-tihn]. 106, 319

furazolidone (Furoxone) (Antibio, GI). Antibacterial and antiprotozoal drug for traveler's diarrhea. Liquid: 50 mg/15 mL. Tablet: 100 mg. 124, 319

furosemide (Lasix) (Endo, Uro). Loop diuretic; used to treat syndrome of inappropriate antidiuretic hormone. Liquid: 10 mg/mL, 40 mg/5 mL. Tablet: 20 mg, 40 mg, 80 mg. Intramuscular or intravenous: 10 mg/mL. [fyour-OH-seh-mide]. 104, 231

Furoxone (Antibio, GI). Antibacterial and antiprotozoal drug for traveler's diarrhea. For dosage, see *furazolidone*. [fyour-AWK-zohn]. 124, 319

g (abbreviation for *gram*). 69

gabapentin (Neurontin) (Analges, Derm, Neuro, Psych). Used to treat migraine headaches; used to treat postherpetic neuralgia; used to treat the partial seizures of epilepsy; used to treat multiple sclerosis and amyotrophic lateral sclerosis; used to treat manic-depressive disorder. Capsule: 100 mg, 300 mg, 400 mg. Tablet: 600 mg, 800 mg. Liquid: 250 mg/5 mL. [gah-bah-PEHN-tihn]. 265, 276

Gabbromicina (Antivir, Resp). Used to treat *Mycobacterium avium-intracellulare* infection in AIDS patients; used to treat tuberculosis. For dosage, see *aminosidine*. 197, 329

Gabitril Filmtabs (Neuro). Anticonvulsant drug used to treat simple and complex partial seizures. For dosage, see *tiagabine*. [GAH-bih-trill]. 265

galantamine (Reminyl) (Neuro). Cholinesterase inhibitor used to treat Alzheimer's disease. Tablet: 4 mg, 8 mg, 12 mg. Liquid: 4 mg/mL. [gah-LAHN-tah-meen]. 271

Galardin (Oph). Used to treat corneal ulcers. Orphan drug.

gallium nitrate (Ganite) (Chemo). Used to treat the hypercalcemia of malignancy; investigational drug used to treat non-Hodgkin's lymphoma. Orphan drug. 359, 361

Gallo, Robert. 327

gallstones, drugs used to treat. 129

Galzin (Misc). Used to treat Wilson's disease. For dosage, see *zinc acetate*.

Gamimune N (Antivir). Immunoglobulin used to treat AIDS. Orphan drug.

gamma hydroxybutyrate (GHB) (Neuro). Used to treat narcolepsy. (Schedule I drug). Previously, this drug was illegal and abused as a sedative in sexual assaults. Orphan drug. 16, 274

ganciclovir (Cytovene, Vitrasert) (Antivir). Antiviral drug used to treat cytomegalovirus retinitis; used to treat cytomegalovirus in organ transplant recipients. Capsule: 250 mg, 500 mg. Intravenous (powder to be reconstituted): 500 mg. Ocular implant. [gehn-SIH-kloh-veer]. 329, 330

gangliosides (Cronassial) (Oph). Used to treat retinitis pigmentosa. Orphan drug.

ganirelix (Antagon) (OB/GYN). Used to inhibit excessive gonadotropin-releasing hormone from the pituitary gland of patients taking ovulation-stimulating drugs for infertility. Subcutaneous: 250 mcg/0.5 mL. [geh-nih-RAY-lihks]. 245

Ganite (Chemo). Used to treat the hypercalcemia of malignancy. For dosage, see *gallium nitrate*.

Gantanol (Antibio, Uro). Sulfonamide used to treat urinary tract and other types of infections. For dosage, see *sulfamethoxazole*. [GEHN-tah-nawl]. 106, 312

Gantrisin (Oph). Topical sulfonamide anti-infective drug used to treat bacterial eye infections. For dosage, see *sulfisoxazole*. [GEHN-trah-sihn].

Gantrisin Pediatric (Antibio, Uro). Sulfonamide used to treat urinary tract and other infections. For dosage, see *sulfisoxazole*. [GEHN-trehn-sihn]. 106, 312

Garamycin (Antibio). Aminoglycoside antibiotic used to treat a variety of bacterial infections, including *E. coli*, *Klebsiella*, *Pseudomonas*, and *Staphylococcus*. For dosage, see *gentamicin*. [geh-rah-MY-sihn]. 316

Garamycin (Derm, Oph) (generic *gentamicin*). Topical antibiotic used to treat bacterial skin and eye infections. Cream: 0.1%. Ointment: 0.1%. Ophthalmic solution: 3 mg/mL. Ophthalmic ointment: 3 mg/g. [geh-rah-MY-sihn]. 88

gastric stimulants (GI). Class of drugs used to increase peristalsis in the gastrointestinal tract. 122

Gastrocrom (GI). Mast cell stabilizer used to treat food allergies. For dosage, see *cromolyn*. 132

gastroesophageal reflux disease (GERD), drugs used to treat. 120

gastrointestinal drugs. 115

Gastrosed (GI, Uro). Antispasmodic drug used to treat spasm of the smooth muscle of the bowel and bladder. For dosage, see *L-hyoscyamine*. [GEHS-troh-sehd]. 122

gastrostomy tube, administration of drugs by. 40

Gastrozepine (GI) (generic *pirenzepine*). Used to treat peptic ulcers. Investigational drug. 134

Gas-X, Extra-Strength Gas-X (GI). Antiflatulence drug. For dosage, see *simethicone*. 118

gatifloxacin (Tequin) (Antibio). Fluoroquinolone antibiotic used to treat various types of infections, including staphylococcus, *H. influenzae*, *E. coli*, community-acquired pneumonia, and gonorrhea; used to treat Legionnaire's disease. Tablet: 200 mg, 400 mg. Intravenous: 200 mg/20 mL, 400 mg/40 mL. [geh-tih-FLAWK-sah-sihn]. 105, 198, 318

gauge of needle. 63

Gaviscon Extra Strength Relief Formula Liquid (GI) (generic *aluminum, magnesium, simethicone*). Combination antacid and anti-gas drug. Liquid. [GEH-vih-skawn]. 117

Gaviscon Liquid (GI) (generic *aluminum, magnesium*). Combination antacid. Liquid. [GEH-vih-skawn]. 117

Gaviscon Tablet, Gaviscon Extra Strength Relief Formula Tablet (GI) (generic *aluminum, calcium, magnesium, sodium bicarbonate*). Combination antacid. Tablet. [GEH-vih-skawn]. 117

G-CSF. See *filgrastim*.

gel (drug form). 35

Gelfilm, Gelfilm Ophthalmic (Hem). Topical hemostatic drug used to control bleeding during surgery. Gelatin film.

Gelfoam (Hem). Topical hemostatic drug used to control bleeding during surgical procedures. Cone. Pack. Powder. Sponge.

Gelusil (GI) (generic *aluminum, magnesium, simethicone*). Combination antacid and anti-gas drug. Tablet: 200 mg/200 mg/25 mg. [JEHL-yoo-sihl]. 117

gemcitabine (Gemzar) (Chemo). Pyrimidine antagonist chemotherapy drug used to treat lung cancer. Intravenous (powder to be reconstituted): 20 mg/mL. [jehm-SIH-tah-been]. 340

gemfibrozil (Lopid) (Cardio). Used to treat hypertriglyceridemia by decreasing serum triglyercides and very low-density liproprotein levels. Tablet: 600 mg. [jehm-FIH-broh-zihl]. 171

gemtuzumab (Mylotarg) (Chemo). Monoclonal antibody used to treat leukemia. Intravenous: 5 mg/20 mL. 346

Gemzar (Chemo). Pyrimidine antagonist chemotherapy drug. For dosage, see *gemcitabine*. [JEHM-zawr]. 340

Gendex 75 (I.V.). Intravenous nonblood plasma volume expander. 382

gene splicing. See *recombinant DNA technology*.

generic name of drug. 22

Genasense (Chemo). Chemotherapy drug used to treat leukemia and malignant melanoma. Orphan drug. 347

genetic engineering. See *recombinant DNA technology*.

Genevax-HIV (Antivir). AIDS vaccine. Investigational drug. 327

Gengraf (Cardio, GI, Uro). Immunosuppressant drug given after organ transplantation to prevent rejection of the donor heart, liver, or kidney. For dosage, see *cyclosporine*. [JEHN-grehf]. 110, 132, 173

genome, human. 26

Genoptic, Genoptic S.O.P. (Oph). Topical antibiotic used to treat bacterial eye infections. For dosage, see *gentamicin*. [jehn-AWP-tihk]. 218

(Genora) (OB/GYN). No longer on the market. (Oral contraceptive).

Genotropin, Genotropin MiniQuick (Endo). Growth hormone replacement for adults and children with growth failure; also used to treat growth failure of infants who are small for gestational age. For dosage, see *somatropin*. [jee-noh-TROH-pihn]. 230

Gentacidin (Oph). Topical antibiotic used to treat bacterial eye infections. For dosage, see *gentamicin*. [jehn-tah-SY-dihn]. 218

Gentak (Oph). Topical antibiotic used to treat bacterial eye infections. For dosage, see *gentamicin*. [JEHN-tehk]. 218

gentamicin (Garamycin) (Derm). Topical antibiotic used to treat bacterial skin infections. Cream: 0.1%. Ointment: 0.1%. [jehn-tah-MY-sihn]. 88

gentamicin (Garamycin, Genoptic, Genoptic S.O.P., Gentacidin, Gentak) (Oph). Topical antibiotic used to treat bacterial eye infections. Ophthalmic solution: 3 mg/mL. Ophthalmic ointment: 3 mg/g. [jehn-tah-MY-sihn].

gentamicin (Garamycin) (Antibio). Aminoglycoside antibiotic used to treat a variety of bacterial infections, including *E. coli*, *Klebsiella*, *Pseudomonas*, and *Staphylococcus*. Intramuscular or intravenous: 40 mg/mL, 10 mg/mL. [jehn-tah-MY-sihn]. 316

gentamicin beads (Septopal) (Ortho). Antibiotic used to treat osteomyelitis. Implanted drug beads on a wire. [jehn-tah-MY-sihn]. 148

gentamicin liposomal (Maitec) (Antivir). Antibiotic used to treat *Mycobacterium avium-intracellulare* in AIDS patients. Orphan drug. 329

Gen Teal (Oph). Artificial tears. Drops.

gentian violet (Derm). Topical purple antibacterial and antifungal dye. Liquid: 1%, 2%. [jehn-shun VY-oh-leht]. 99

Gentle Strength ex-lax (GI) (generic *docusate, sennosides*). Combination stool softener and irritant/stimulant laxative. Caplet: 65 mg/10 mg.

Gentran 40, Gentran 70 (I.V.). Intravenous nonblood plasma volume expander. 382

Genuine Bayer Aspirin (Cardio, Hem, Neuro). Salicylate drug used to treat current myocardial infarction and prevent repeat myocardial infarction; anticoagulant; used to prevent transient ischemic attacks and strokes. For dosage, see *aspirin*. 158

Genuine Bayer Aspirin, Maximum Bayer Aspirin, Extended Release Bayer 8-Hour, Extra Strength Bayer Enteric 500 (Analges, Ortho). Salicylate drug used to relieve fever and pain; used to treat the pain and inflammation of osteoarthritis and rheumatoid arthritis. For dosage, see *aspirin*. 300

Geocillin (Antibio). Penicillin-type antibiotic used to treat a variety of bacterial infections, including *E. coli* and *Pseudomonas*. For dosage, see *carbenicillin*. [GEE-oh-sill-ihn]. 313

Geodon (Psych). Drug used to treat psychosis and schizophrenia. For dosage, see *ziprasidone*. [GEE-oh-dawn]. 284

gepirone (Psych). Used to treat anxiety and depression. Investigational drug. 282

Gerber Baby Formula with Iron, Gerber Soy Formula (GI). Infant formula. Liquid, powder (to be reconstituted).

GERD (abbreviation for *gastroesophageal reflux disease*). See *gastroesophageal reflux disease.*

Geref (Antivir, Endo, OB/GYN). Used to treat AIDS wasting syndrome; used to treat growth hormone deficiency; used to treat infertility due to failure to ovulate. For dosage, see *sermorelin*. [JEH-rehf]. 230, 244, 327

Gerimal (Neuro). Used to treat the dementia of Alzheimer's disease. For dosage, see *ergoloid mesylates*. [JEH-reh-mawl]. 271

Geritol Complete, Geritol Tonic (Misc). Multivitamin with iron nutritional supplement. Liquid. Tablet.

GHB (abbreviation for *gamma hydroxybutyrate*). See *gamma hydroxybutyrate.*

glatiramer (Copaxone) (Neuro). Immunosuppressant drug used to treat multiple sclerosis. Subcutaneous: 20 mg/2 mL. 276

glaucoma, drugs used to treat. 220

Glaucon (Oph). Topical alpha/beta-agonist drug used to treat glaucoma. For dosage, see *epinephrine*. [GLAH-kawn]. 221

GlaucTabs (Oph). Carbonic anhydrase inhibitor used to treat glaucoma. For dosage, see *methazolamide*. 221

Gleevec (Chemo). Chemotherapy drug used to treat leukemia. For dosage, see *imatinib*. [GLEE-vehk]. 348

Gliadel (Chemo). Alkylating chemotherapy drug used to treat brain cancer. For dosage, see *carmustine*. [GLEE-ah-dell]. 341

glimepiride (Amaryl) (Diab). Oral antidiabetic drug. Tablet: 1 mg, 2 mg, 4 mg. [glih-MEH-pih-ride]. 240

glipizide (Glucotrol, Glucotrol XL) (Diab). Oral antidiabetic drug. Tablet: 2.5 mg, 5 mg, 10 mg. [GLIH-peh-zide]. 240

glucagon (Diab). Used to treat hypoglycemia. Intravenous (powder to be reconstituted): 1 mg. [GLOO-kah-gawn].

Glucerna (Diab, GI). Liquid nutritional supplement formulated for patients with diabetes mellitus. Liquid. [gloo-SEHR-nah].

Glucophage, Glucophage XR (Diab, OB/GYN). Oral antidiabetic drug; used to treat the elevated insulin levels caused by polycystic ovary syndrome. For dosage, see *metformin*. [GLOO-koh-fawj]. 241

glucose (B-D Glucose, Insta-Glucose) (Diab). Used to treat hypoglycemia. Gel. Tablet.

Glucotrol, Glucotrol XL (Diab). Oral antidiabetic drug. For dosage, see *glipizide*. [GLOO-koh-trawl]. 240

Glucovance (Diab) (generic *glyburide, metformin*). Combination oral antidiabetic drug. Tablet: 1.25 mg/250 mg, 2.5 mg/500 mg, 5 mg/500 mg. [GLOO-koh-vehns]. 241

glutamic acid (GI). Gastric acid replacement. Capsule: 340 mg. [gloo-TEH-mihk EH-sihd]. 133

glutethimide (Neuro). Nonbarbiturate drug used to treat insomnia. (Schedule II drug). Tablet: 250 mg. [gloo-TEH-theh-mide]. 272

glyburide (DiaBeta, Glynase PresTab, Micronase) (Diab). Oral antidiabetic drug. Tablet: 1.25 mg, 1.5 mg, 2.5 mg, 3 mg, 4.5 mg, 5 mg, 6 mg. [GLY-byour-ide]. 240

glycerin (Colace, Fleet Babylax) (GI). Mechanical laxative. Rectal liquid: 4 mL per applicator. Suppository. 125

glycerin (Ophthalgan) (Oph). Topical drug used to treat corneal edema. Ophthalmic solution.

glycopyrrolate (Robinul, Robinul Forte) (GI). Antispasmodic drug. Tablet: 1 mg, 2 mg. Intramuscular or intravenous: 0.2 mg/mL. [gly-koh-PY-roh-layt]. 122

Glynase PresTab (Diab). Oral antidiabetic drug. For dosage, see *glyburide*. [GLY-nays]. 240

Glypressin (GI). Sclerosing drug used to stop bleeding from esophageal varices. For dosage, see *terlipressin*. [gly-PREH-sihn]. 135

Glyset (Diab). Oral antidiabetic drug. For dosage, see *miglitol*. 241

GM-CSF. See *sargramostim*.

gold compounds (Ortho). Class of anti-inflammatory drugs used to treat rheumatoid arthritis. 142

gold sodium thiomalate (Aurolate) (Ortho). Gold compound used to treat rheumatoid arthritis. Intramuscular: 50 mg/mL. 142

GoLYTELY (GI) (generic *polyethylene glycol, eletrolyte solution*). Bowel evacuant/bowel prep. Oral liquid (powder to be reconstituted). 125

gonadorelin (Lutrepulse) (OB/GYN). Pituitary gland hormone drug used to treat amenorrhea. Orphan drug. 253

Gonak (Oph). Injected into the eye during surgery to keep the anterior chamber expanded and replace intraocular fluid. For dosage, see *methylcellulose*. [GOH-nack].

Gonal-F (Endo, OB/GYN). Ovulation-stimulating hormone drug used to treat infertility; orphan drug used to treat decreased sperm count and infertility in men. For dosage, see *follitropin alfa*. [GOH-nawl F]. 244

Goniosol (Oph). Injected into the eye during surgery to keep the anterior chamber expanded and replace intraocular fluid. For dosage, see *methylcellulose*. [GOH-nee-oh-sawl].

gonorrhea, drugs used to treat. 257

goserelin (Zoladex) (Chemo, OB/GYN). Hormonal chemotherapy drug used to treat breast cancer; used to treat prostate cancer; used to treat endometriosis. Subcutaneous implant: 3.6 mg, 10.8 mg. [gah-seh-RAY-lihn]. 248, 343

gout, drugs used to treat. 146

grain (gr). 69

gram (g). 69

granisetron (Kytril) (GI). Antiemetic drug; used to treat nausea and vomiting caused by chemotherapy. Tablet: 1 mg. Intravenous: 1 mg/mL. [greh-NIH-seh-trawn]. 128

Granulderm, Granulex, GranuMed (Derm) (generic *trypsin*). Topical enzyme drug used to debride burns and wounds. Spray. 96

(grepafloxacin) (Antibio). No longer on the market. (Trade name *Raxar*; fluoroquinolone antibiotic).

(Grifulvin V) (Antifung). No longer on the market. (Generic name *griseofulvin*; used to treat severe topical fungal infections).

Grisactin 250, Grisactin 500, Grisactin Ultra (Antifung, Derm). Used to treat severe topical fungal infections. For dosage, see *griseofulvin*. [grih-ZACK-tihn]. 90, 334

griseofulvin (Fulvicin P/G, Fulvicin U/F, Grisactin 250, Grisactin 500, Grisactin Ultra, Griseofulvin Ultramicrosize) (Antifung, Derm). Used to treat severe topical fungal infections. Capsule: 250 mg. Tablet: 125 mg, 165 mg, 250 mg, 330 mg, 500 mg. [grih-zee-oh-FOOL-vihn]. 90, 334

Griseofulvin Ultramicrosize (Antifung, Derm). Used to treat severe topical fungal infections. For dosage, see *griseofulvin*. [grih-zee-oh-FOOL-vihn]. 90

growth hormone replacement drugs (Endo). Class of drugs used to treat decreased growth in children. 230

gt. (abbreviation for *drop*), **gtt.** (abbreviation for *drops*).

guaifenesin (Humibid L.A., Humibid Sprinkle, Naldecon Senior EX, Organidin NR, Robitussin) (ENT, OB/GYN). Expectorant; used to thin cervical mucus to treat infertility. Capsule: 200 mg, 300 mg. Liquid/syrup: 100 mg/5 mL, 200 mg/5 mL. Tablet: 100 mg, 200 mg, 575 mg, 600 mg, 1200 mg. [gwy-eh-FEH-neh-sihn]. 210

guanabenz (Wytensin) (Cardio). Alpha$_2$-receptor blocker used to treat hypertension. Tablet: 4 mg, 8 mg. [GWAH-neh-behns]. 165

guanadrel (Hylorel) (Cardio). Blocks the release of norepinephrine from the adrenal medulla; used to treat hypertension. Tablet: 10 mg. [GWAH-neh-drehl]. 166

guanethidine (Ismelin) (Cardio, Neuro). Blocks the release of norepinephrine from the adrenal medulla; used to treat hypertension; used to treat sympathetic dystrophy and causalgia. Tablet: 10 mg, 25 mg. [gwah-NEH-theh-deen]. 166, 276

guanfacine (Tenex) (Cardio, Psych). Alpha$_2$-receptor blocker used to treat hypertension; used to treat withdrawal from heroin; an orphan drug used to treat fragile X syndrome. Tablet: 1 mg, 2 mg. [gwahn-FEH-seen]. 165, 293

guanidine (Neuro). Anticholinesterase drug used to treat the muscle weakness of Eaton–Lambert syndrome. Tablet: 125 mg. [GWAH-nih-deen]. 276

(gusperimus) (Uro). No longer on the market. (Trade name *Spanidin*; used to treat rejection of kidney transplant).

Gustase (GI) (generic *amylase, protease*). Combination replacement drug for digestive enzymes. Tablet: 30 mg/6 mg. 133

Gustase Plus (GI) (generic *amylase, protease, phenobarbital*). Combination replacement therapy for digestive enzymes and sedative drug. Tablet: 30 mg/6 mg/8 mg. 133

Gynazole-1 (OB/GYN) (generic *butoconazole*). Topical drug used to treat vaginal yeast infections. Vaginal cream: 2%. [GY-neh-zohl]. 256

Gyne-Lotrimin 3, Gyne-Lotrimin 7 (OB/GYN). Topical drug used to treat vaginal yeast infections. Vaginal cream: 1%, 2%. Vaginal suppository: 100 mg, 200 mg. [gy-nee-LOH-trih-mihn]. 256

Gynogen L.A. 20 (Chemo, OB/GYN). Hormone chemotherapy drug used to treat prostate carcinoma; hormone replacement therapy used to treat the symptoms of menopause. For dosage, see *estradiol valerate*. [GY-noh-jehn]. 252, 343

Gyrocaps. Part of the trade name of a drug; it indicates a slow-release capsule. 63

H₁ receptor. See *receptor*.

H₂ blockers (GI). Class of drugs used to treat peptic ulcers. 118

H₂ receptor. See *receptor*.

Habitrol (Resp, Psych). Nicotine drug used to stop smoking; used to treat Tourette's syndrome. Transdermal patch: 7 mg/24 hr, 14 mg/24 hr, 21 mg/24 hr. [HEH-bih-trawl]. 199, 294

(halazepam) (Psych). No longer on the market. (Trade name *Paxipam*; benzodiazepine antianxiety drug).

halcinonide (Halog, Halog-E) (Derm). Topical corticosteroid anti-inflammatory drug. Cream: 0.025%, 0.1%. Liquid: 0.1%. Ointment: 0.1%. [hehl-SIH-noh-nide]. 92

Halcion (Neuro). Nonbarbiturate benzodiazepine drug used to treat insomnia. (Schedule IV drug). For dosage, see *triazolam*. [HEHL-see-awn]. 272

Haldol, Haldol Decanoate 50, Haldol Decanoate 100 (Psych). Drug used to treat psychosis; used to treat Tourette's syndrome; used as short-term treatment for explosive, impulsive behavior and mood lability in children. For dosage, see *haloperidol*. [HEHL-dawl]. 284

Haley's M-O (GI) (generic *magnesium, mineral oil*). Combination magnesium-containing laxative and mineral oil. Liquid: 900 mg/15 mL. 125

half-life. 52, 63

half normal saline (0.45% NaCl) (I.V.). Intravenous fluid of sodium and water at half the concentration of tissue fluids. 376

Halfprin 81, ½ Halfprin (Cardio, Hem, Neuro). Salicylate drug used to treat current myocardial infarction and prevent repeat myocardial infarction; anticoagulant; used to prevent transient ischemic attacks and strokes. For dosage, see *aspirin*. 158

halobetasol (Ultravate) (Derm). Topical corticosteroid anti-inflammatory drug. Cream: 0.05%. Ointment: 0.05%. [heh-loh-BAY-teh-sawl]. 92

halofuginone (Stenorol) (Misc). Used to treat systemic sclerosis. Orphan drug.

Halog, Halog-E (Derm) (generic *halcinonide*). Topical corticosteroid anti-inflammatory drug. Cream: 0.025%, 0.1%. Liquid: 0.1%. Ointment: 0.1%. 92

haloperidol (Haldol, Haldol Decanoate 50, Haldol Decanoate 100) (Psych). Drug used to treat psychosis; used to treat Tourette's syndrome; used as short-term treatment for explosive, impulsive behavior and mood lability in children. Tablet: 0.5 mg, 1 mg, 2 mg, 5 mg, 10 mg, 20 mg. Liquid: 2 mg/mL. Intramuscular or intravenous: 5 mg/mL, 50 mg/mL, 100 mg/mL. [heh-loh-PEH-reh-dawl]. 284

haloprogin (Halotex) (Derm). Topical antifungal drug. Cream: 1%. Liquid: 1%. 89

Halotestin (Chemo, Endo). Male sex hormone used to treat breast cancer in women; used to treat the lack of production of testosterone due to absence, injury, or malfunction of the testes or malfunction of the pituitary gland; used to treat delayed puberty in boys. For dosage, see *fluoxymesterone*. [heh-loh-TEHS-tihn]. 343

Halotex (Derm) (generic *haloprogin*). Topical antifungal drug. Cream: 1%. Liquid: 1%. 89

halothane (Anes). Used to induce and maintain general anesthesia. Inhaled gas. [HEH-loh-thayn]. 367, 370

Haltran (Analges, OB/GYN, Ortho). Nonsteroidal anti-inflammatory drug used to treat fever and pain; used to treat migraine headaches; used to treat dysmenorrhea; used to treat osteoarthritis and rheumatoid arthritis. For dosage, see *ibuprofen*. [HAWL- trehn]. 139, 304

Hamlet. 6

Harrison Narcotics Act of 1914, The. 16

Havrix (GI). Hepatitis A vaccine. For dosage, see *hepatitis A vaccine*. [HEHV-rihks].

HCG or hCG (OB/GYN) (abbreviation for *human chorionic gonadotropin*).

HCTZ (abbreviation for *hydrochlorothiazide*). See *hydrochlorothiazide*.

Healon, Healon GV (Oph). Injected into the eye during surgery to keep the anterior chamber expanded and replace intraocular fluid. For dosage, see *sodium hyaluronate*. [HEE-lawn].

Healon Yellow (Oph) (generic *fluorescein dye, sodium hyaluronate*). Combination drug injected into the eye during surgery to keep the anterior chamber expanded and help visualize tissues. Ophthalmic solution: 0.005 mg/10 mg per mL. [HEE-lawn].

Heartline (Cardio, Hem, Neuro). Salicylate drug used to treat current myocardial infarction and prevent repeat myocardial infarction; anticoagulant; used to prevent transient ischemic attacks and strokes. For dosage, see *aspirin*. 158

Helicobacter pylori **infection,** drugs used to treat. 119

Helidac (GI) (generic *bismuth, metronidazole, tetracycline*). Combination antibacterial and antiprotozoal drug used to treat peptic ulcers caused by *Helicobacter pylori*. Capsule: 262.4 mg/250 mg/500 mg. Tablet: 262.4 mg/250 mg/500 mg. [HEE-lih-dack]. 120

Hemabate (OB/GYN). Prostaglandin used to produce abortion; used to treat postpartum uterine bleeding. For dosage, see *carboprost*. [HEE-mah-bayt]. 248, 255

Hematrol (Hem). Used to treat immune thrombocytopenic purpura. Orphan drug.

Hemex (Misc) (generic name *hemin, zinc mesoporphyrin*). Used to treat acute intermittent porphyria. Orphan drug.

hemin (Panhematin). Used to treat acute intermittent porphyria. Orphan drug.

Hemofil M (Hem). Clotting factor VIII used to treat hemophiliac patients. Intravenous (powder to be reconstituted): 12.5 mg/mL.

hemophiliacs and AIDS. Historical Notes feature. 382

henbane (herb). 6

Hepacid (Chemo). Chemotherapy drug used to treat liver cancer. Orphan drug. 347

heparin (Hem). Anticoagulant. Subcutaneous or intravenous: 1000 units/mL, 2000 units/mL, 2500 units/mL, 5000 units/mL, 7500 units/mL, 10,000 units/mL, 20,000 units/mL, 40,000 units/mL. [HEH-pah-rihn]. 186

heparin, low molecular weight. 186

heparin lock. 186, 374

HepatAmine (I.V.). Intravenous fluid for total parenteral nutrition, especially for patients with hepatic failure. 378

Hepatic-Aid II (GI). Liquid nutritional supplement formulated for patients with chronic liver disease. Powder (to be reconstituted).

hepatitis A vaccine (Havrix, Vaqta). Vaccine to protect against hepatitis A. Intramuscular (HAV protein): 25 U/0.5 mL, 50 U/1 mL. Intramuscular (viral antigen): 720 EL.U./0.5 mL, 1440 EL.U./1 mL.

hepatitis B vaccine (Engerix-B, Recombivax HB). Vaccine to protect against hepatitis B. Intramuscular (hepatitis B surface antigen): 5 mcg/0.5 mL, 10 mcg/0.5 mL, 10 mcg/mL, 20 mcg/mL.

Herceptin (Chemo). Human monoclonal antibody used to treat breast cancer and pancreatic cancer. For dosage, see *trastuzumab*. [hehr-SEHP-tihn]. 346

heroin. Historical Notes feature. 16, 298

herpes simplex virus type 1 infections, drugs used to treat. 91, 330

herpes simplex virus type 2 infections, drugs used to treat. 330

herpes zoster virus infections, drugs used to treat. 91, 330

(Herplex) (Oph). No longer on the market. (Generic name *idoxuridine*; topical drug for herpes infection of eye).

(Hespan) (I.V.). No longer on the market. (Generic name *hetastarch*; intravenous nonblood plasma volume expander).

hetastarch (I.V.). Intravenous nonblood plasma volume expander. 381

hexachlorophene (pHisoHex) (Derm). Topical antibacterial skin cleanser. Liquid: 3%. 99

Hexadrol (Chemo, Derm, Endo). Corticosteroid anti-inflammatory drug used to treat severe inflammation in various body systems; used to diagnose Cushing's syndrome; used as part of chemotherapy treatment. For dosage, see *dexamethasone*. [HEHK-sah-drawl]. 93, 232, 351

Hexadrol (Ortho, Neuro). Corticosteroid anti-inflammatory drug injected into a joint to treat osteoarthritis and rheumatoid arthritis; injected near a joint to treat bursitis and tenosynovitis; given intravenously to treat cerebral edema. For dosage, see *dexamethasone*. [HEHK-sah-drawl]. 141, 275

Hexalen (Chemo). Alkylating chemotherapy drug used to treat ovarian cancer. For dosage, see *altretamine*. [HECK-sah-lehn]. 341

hexamethylmelamine. See *altretamine*.

(hexocyclium) (GI). No longer on the market. (Trade name *Tral*; GI antispasmodic drug).

hexoprenaline (Delaprem) (OB/GYN). Ovulation-stimulating drug used to treat infertility. Investigational drug. 246

HFA (abbreviation for *hydrofluoroalkane*). Propellant in inhaler. 194

Hibiclens (Derm). Topical anti-infective hand wash and preoperative surgical scrub. Liquid: 4%. Sponge brush. 98

Hibistat (Derm). Topical anti-infective hand rinse. Rinse: 0.5%. Towelettes. 98

hiccups, drugs used to treat. 132

Hiprex (Antibio, Uro). Anti-infective drug only used to treat urinary tract infections. For dosage, see *methenamine*. [HIH-prehks]. 106, 319

(Hismanal) (ENT). No longer on the market. (Generic name *astemizole*; antihistamine). Historical Notes feature.

histamine. 53, 54

histamine (Maxamine) (Chemo). Used to treat leukemia and malignant melanoma. Orphan drug. 361

Historical Notes features
  AIDS drugs history. 326
  amphetamines. 291
  anesthesia, anesthetic drugs. 366

Antabuse. 293

aspirin. 300

bacitracin. 88

baldness. 99

belladonna. 6

blood types. 378

chlordiazepoxide (Librium). 281

Civil War drug addiction. 298

coal tar. 86

cortisone, discovery of. 233

endotracheal intubation. 367

foxglove. 152

hemophiliacs and AIDS. 382

heroin and morphine. 298

Hismanal and Seldane off the market. 207

H₂ blockers. 118

MAO inhibitors. 285

meprobamate. 280

neuromuscular blocking drugs. 367

nitrogen mustard. 341

patent drug advertisement. 13

penicillin discovered. 314

phenobarbital and phenytoin. 263

plasmapheresis. 382

psychiatric drugs. 280, 281, 283

sulfonamide drugs discovered. 312

thalidomide, history of. 15, 328

Thorazine. 283

tricyclic antidepressants. 285

tuberculosis drugs. 197

Tylenol cyanide murders. 301

histrelin (Supprelin) (Endo). Used to treat precocious puberty. Intramuscular: 120 mcg/0.6 mL, 300 mcg/0.6 mL, 600 mcg/0.6 mL. [hihs-TRAY-lihn].

HIV (human immunodeficiency virus). See *AIDS*.

HIV immunoglobulin (Hivig) (Antivir). Used to treat AIDS. Orphan drug. 326

Hivid (Antivir). Nucleoside reverse transcriptase inhibitor drug used to treat AIDS. For dosage, see *zalcitabine*. [HIH-vihd]. 324

HMG-CoA reductase inhibitors (Cardio). Used to treat hypercholesterolemia. 169

Hivig (Antivir) (generic *HIV immunoglobulin*). Used to treat AIDS drug. Orphan drug. 326

HMS. See *medrysone*.

homatropine (Isopto Homatropine) (Oph). Topical mydriatic drug. Ophthalmic solution: 2%, 5%. [hoh-mah-TROH-peen]. 223

hormonal chemotherapy drugs (Chemo). Class of chemotherapy drugs. 343

hormone replacement therapy (HRT) (OB/GYN, Ortho). Class of drugs used to relieve the symptoms of menopause and prevent or treat postmenopausal osteoporosis. 252

household measurement of drugs. 70

H. pylori. See *Helicobacter pylori*.

HRT (abbreviation for *hormone replacement therapy*). See *hormone replacement therapy*.

h.s. (abbreviation for *hours of sleep*).

HTN (abbreviation for *hypertension*). See *hypertension*.

H₂ blockers. Historical Notes feature. 118

H₂ blockers (GI). Class of drugs used to treat peptic ulcers. 118

Humalog (Diab). Rapid-acting human recombinant DNA lispro insulin. Subcutaneous: 100 units/mL. [HYOO-mah-lawg]. 238

Humalog Mix 75/25 (Diab) (generic *NPH insulin, human recombinant DNA lispro regular insulin*). Combination of intermediate-acting and fast-acting insulin. Subcutaneous: 75 units/25 units per mL. [HYOO-mah-lawg]. 239

human B-type natriuretic peptides (hBHP) (Cardio). Class of drugs used to treat severely decompensated congestive heart failure. 155

human chorionic gonadotropin (HCG) (A.P.L. Pregnyl, Profasi) (Endo, OB/GYN). Ovulation-stimulating drug used to treat infertility; used to treat undescended testicles and hypogonadism in men. Intramuscular: 500 units/mL, 1000 units/mL, 2000 units/mL. [hyoo-mehn koh-ree-AW-nick goh-NEH-dah-troh-pihn]. 244

Humatin (Antibio, GI). Aminoglycoside antibiotic and amebicide used to treat intestintal amebiasis and hepatic coma. For dosage, see *paromomycin*. [HYOO-mah-tihn]. 134, 317

Humatrope (Endo). Growth hormone replacement for adults and children with growth failure; also used to treat growth failure of infants who are small for gestational age. For dosage, see *somatropin*. [HYOO-mah-trohp]. 230

HuMax-CD4 (Ortho). Used to treat rheumatoid arthritis. Investigational drug. 148

Humegon (OB/GYN). Ovulation-stimulating drug used to treat infertility. For dosage, see *menotropins*. [HYOO-meh-gawn]. 244

Humibid DM, Humibid DM Sprinkle (ENT) (generic *dextromethorphan, guaifenesin*). Combination nonnarcotic antitussive and expectorant drug. Capsule: 15 mg/300 mg. Tablet: 30 mg/600 mg. [HYOO-mih-bihd].

Humibid L.A., Humibid Sprinkle (ENT, OB/GYN). Expectorant; used to thin cervical mucus to treat infertility. For dosage, see *guiafenesin*. [HYOO-mih-bihd]. 210

Humorsol (Oph). Topical cholinesterase inhibitor drug used to treat glaucoma. For dosage, see *demecarium*. [HYOO-muhr-sawl]. 221

Humulin 50/50 (Diab) (generic *human recombinant DNA NPH and regular insulins*).   Combination of intermediate-acting and fast-acting insulin. Subcutaneous: 50 units/50 units per mL. [HYOO-myoo-lihn]. 239

Humulin 70/30 (Diab) (generic *human recombinant DNA NPH and regular insulins*).   Combination of intermediate-acting and fast-acting insulin. Subcutaneous: 70 units/30 units per mL. [HYOO-myoo-lihn]. 239

Humulin R Regular U-500 Concentrated (Diab).   Concentrated DNA recombinant human insulin. Subcutaneous: 500 unit/mL. [HYOO-myoo-lihn]. 239

Humulin L (Diab).   Intermediate-acting lente insulin. Subcutaneous: 100 units/mL. [HYOO-myoo-lihn]. 238

Humulin N (Diab).   Intermediate-acting NPH insulin. Subcutaneous: 100 units/mL. [HYOO-myoo-lihn]. 238

Humulin R (Diab).   Fast-acting regular insulin. Subcutaneous: 100 units/mL. [HYOO-myoo-lihn]. 238

Humulin U Ultralente (Diab).   Long-acting ultralente insulin. Subcutaneous: 100 units/mL. [HYOO-myoo-lihn]. 238

Hurricane (ENT) (generic *benzocaine*).   Topical anesthetic for the mouth. Gel: 20%. Spray: 20%.

Hyalgan (Ortho).   Used to maintain the lubricating quality of synovial fluid in patients with osteoarthritis.   For dosage, see *hyaluronic acid derivative*. [hy-EHL-gehn]. 141

hyaluronic acid derivative (Hyalgan, Synvisc) (Ortho).   Used to maintain the lubricating quality of synovial fluid in patients with osteoarthritis. Intra-articular: 16 mg/2 mL, 20 mg/2 mL. [hy-ehl-your-AW-nihk EH-sihd]. 141

Hycamtin (Chemo).   Mitosis inhibitor chemotherapy drug used to treat lung cancer and ovarian cancer. For dosage, see *topotecan*. [hy-KEHMP-tihn]. 344

Hycodan (ENT).   Narcotic antitussive drug.   For dosage, see *hydrocodone*. [HY-koh-dehn]. 210

Hycomine Compound (ENT) (generic *phenylephrine, chlorpheniramine, hydrocodone, acetaminophen*).   Combination decongestant, antihistamine, narcotic antitussive, and analgesic drug. Tablet: 10 mg/2 mg/5 mg/250 mg. [HY-koh-mihn].

(Hycomine Pediatric Syrup, Hycomine Syrup) (ENT).   No longer on the market. (Combination drug with *phenylpropanolamine*; decongestant and narcotic antitussive drug).

Hycort (Derm) (generic *hydrocortisone*).   Topical corticosteroid anti-inflammatory drug. Cream: 1%. Ointment: 1%. 92

Hycotuss Expectorant (ENT) (generic *hydrocodone, guaifenesin*).   Combination narcotic antitussive and expectorant drug. Syrup: 5 mg/100 mg.

hydantoins (Neuro).   Class of drugs used to treat epilepsy. 264

Hydeltrasol (Derm, Endo, Neuro, Ortho).   Corticosteroid anti-inflammatory injected into skin lesions; used to treat severe inflammation in various body systems; used to treat multiple sclerosis; injected into a joint to treat osteoarthritis and rheumatoid arthritis; injected near a joint to treat bursitis and tenosynovitis.   For dosage, see *prednisolone*. [hy-DELL-trah-zawl]. 141, 232, 277

Hydergine, Hydergine LC (Neuro).   Used to treat the dementia of Alzheimer's disease.   For dosage, see *ergoloid mesylates*. [HY-dehr-jeen]. 271

hydralazine (Apresoline) (Cardio).   Peripheral vasodilator used to treat congestive heart failure, hypertension, and hypertensive crisis. Tablet: 10 mg, 25 mg, 50 mg, 100 mg. Intramuscular or intravenous: 20 mg/mL. 166, 168

Hydrea (Antivir, Chemo, Derm, Hem).   Antimetabolite chemotherapy drug with antiviral activity used to treat AIDS; used to treat head and neck cancer; used to treat severe psoriasis; used to treat thrombocytothemia.   For dosage, see *hydroxyurea*. [hy-DREE-ah]. 87, 189, 326, 341

hydrochlorothiazide (HCTZ) (Esidrix, HydroDIURIL, Microzide, Oretic) (Uro).   Thiazide diuretic. Capsule: 12.5 mg. Liquid: 50 mg/5 mL. Tablet: 25 mg, 50 mg, 100 mg. [hy-droh-klohr-oh-THY-eh-zide]. 103

hydrocodone (Hycodan) (ENT).   Narcotic antitussive drug. Tablet: 5 mg. [hy-droh-KOH-dohn]. 210

hydrocortisone (A-Hydrocort, Cortef, Hydrocortone, Solu-Cortef) (Endo).   Corticosteroid anti-inflammatory drug used to treat severe inflammation in various body systems. Tablet: 5 mg, 10 mg, 20 mg. Liquid: 10 mg/5 mL. Intramuscular, intravenous, or subcutaneous: 50 mg/mL, 100 mg/2 mL, 250 mg/2 mL, 500 mg/4 mL, 1000 mg/8 mL. [hy-droh-KOHR-teh-zohn]. 232

hydrocortisone (Anusol-HC, Anusol-HC-1, Cort-Dome High Potency, Proctocort, ProctoCream-HC) (GI).   Topical corticosteroid anti-inflammatory drug used to treat hemorrhoids. Cream: 1%, 2.5%. Ointment: 1%. Suppository: 25 mg, 30 mg. [hy-droh-KOHR-teh-zohn]. 133

hydrocortisone (Cortaid Intensive Therapy, Cortaid with Aloe, Cort-Dome, Cortizone-5, Cortizone-10, Dermacort, Dermolate, Hycort, Hytone, Lanacort 5, Lanacort 10, Locoid, Maximum Strength Bactine, Maximum Strength Caldecort, Maximum Strength Cortaid, Maximum Strength KeriCort-10, Pandel, Scalpicin, T/Scalp, Westcort) (Derm).   Topical corticosteroid anti-inflammatory drug. Cream: 0.1%, 0.2%, 0.5%, 1%, 2.5%. Liquid: 0.1%, 1%. Gel: 1%. Lotion: 0.25%, 0.5%, 1%, 2%, 2.5%. Ointment: 0.1%,

0.2%, 0.5%, 1%, 2.5%. Spray: 1%. [hy-droh-KOHR-teh-zohn]. 92

hydrocortisone (Cortenema, Cortifoam) (GI). Topical corticosteroid anti-inflammatory drug used to treat ulcerative colitis. Retention enema: 100 mg/60 mL. Rectal aerosol foam: 90 mg/applicator. [hy-droh-KOHR-teh-zohn]. 126

hydrocortisone (Hydrocortone) (Ortho). Corticosteroid anti-inflammatory drug injected into a joint to treat osteoarthritis and rheumatoid arthritis; injected near a joint to treat bursitis and tenosynovitis. Intra-articular or periarticular: 25 mg/mL, 50 mg/mL. [hy-droh-KOHR-teh-zohn]. 141

Hydrocortone (Endo). Corticosteroid anti-inflammatory drug used to treat severe inflammation in various body systems. For dosage, see *hydrocortisone*. [hy-droh-KOHR-tohn]. 232

Hydrocortone (Ortho). Corticosteroid anti-inflammatory drug injected into a joint to treat osteoarthritis and rheumatoid arthritis; also injected near a joint to treat bursitis and tenosynovitis. For dosage, see *hydrocortisone*. [hy-droh-KOHR-tohn]. 141

HydroDIURIL (Uro). Thiazide diuretic. For dosage, see *hydrochlorothiazide*. [hy-droh-DY-your-ihl]. 103

hydroflumethiazide (Diucardin) (Uro). Thiazide diuretic. Tablet: 50 mg. 103

hydrogen peroxide (Orabase HCA, Peroxyl) (ENT). Topical antiseptic for the mouth. Gel: 1.5%. Paste: 0.5%.

hydromorphone (Dilaudid, Dilaudid-5, Dilaudid HP) (Analges). Narcotic analgesic used to treat moderate-to-severe pain. (Schedule II drug). Liquid: 5 mg/5 mL. Tablet: 2 mg, 4 mg, 8 mg. Suppository: 3 mg. Subcutaneous, intramuscular, or intravenous: 1 mg/mL, 2 mg/mL, 4 mg/mL, 10 mg/mL. [hy-droh-MOHR-fohn]. 297

Hydromox (Uro). Thiazide diuretic. For dosage, see *quinethazone*. [HY-droh-mawks]. 103

(Hydropres) (Cardio). No longer on the market. (Generic names *reserpine, hydrochlorothiazide*; combination antihypertensive and diuretic drug).

hydroquinone (Esoterica, Melanex, Porcelana) (Derm). Topical drug used to lighten areas of hyperpigmentated skin. Cream: 1.5%, 2%, 4%. Gel: 2%, 3%, 4%. Liquid: 3%. [hy-droh-KWY-nohn]. 99

hydroxocobalamin (Cardio). Vitamin B$_{12}$ used to treat pernicious anemia. Intramuscular: 1000 mcg/mL. [hy-drawk-soh-koh-BAWL-eh-meen]. 173

hydroxyamphetamine (Paredrine) (Oph). Topical mydriatic drug. Ophthalmic solution: 1%. [hy-drawk-see-ehm-FEH-tah-meen]. 223

hydroxychloroquine (Plaquenil) (Ortho). Used to treat rheumatoid arthritis and systemic lupus erythematosis; it was originally used (and still is used)

to treat malaria. Tablet: 200 mg. [hy-drawk-see-KLOH-roh-kwihn]. 142, 148

hydroxyprogesterone (Hylutin) (OB/GYN). Progestins hormone drug used to treat amenorrhea. Intramuscular: 125 mg/mL, 250 mg/mL. [hy-drawk-see-proh-JEHS-teh-rohn]. 253

hydroxyurea (Hydrea, Mylocel) (Antivir, Chemo, Derm, Hem). Antimetabolite chemotherapy drug with antiviral activity used to treat AIDS; used to treat head and neck cancer; used to treat severe psoriasis; used to treat thrombocytothemia. Capsule: 500 mg. Tablet: 1000 mg. [hy-drawk-see-your-REE-ah]. 87, 189, 326, 341

hydroxyzine (Atarax, Atarax 100, Vistaril) (Derm). Drug used to treat severe itching. Capsule: 25 mg, 50 mg, 100 mg. Liquid: 25 mg/5 mL. Tablet: 10 mg, 25 mg, 50 mg, 100 mg. Syrup: 10 mg/5 mL. Intramuscular: 25 mg/mL, 50 mg/mL. [hy-DRAWK-seh-zeen].

hydroxyzine (Atarax, Atarax 100, Vistaril) (Psych). Drug used to treat anxiety and neurosis; used to treat hysteria; used to treat alcohol withdrawal. Capsule: 25 mg, 50 mg, 100 mg. Tablet: 10 mg, 25 mg, 50 mg, 100 mg. Syrup: 10 mg/5 mL. Suspension: 25 mg/5 mL. Intramuscular: 25 mg/mL, 50 mg/mL. [hy-DRAWK-seh-zeen]. 282

hydroxyzine (Vistaril) (Anes). Drug used preoperatively to produce sedation and relieve anxiety. Intramuscular: 25 mg/mL, 50 mg/mL. [hy-DRAWK-seh-zeen]. 371

hydroxyzine (Vistaril) (GI). Drug used to treat severe nausea and vomiting. Intramuscular: 25 mg/mL, 50 mg/mL. [hy-DRAWK-seh-zeen]. 127

Hygroton (Uro) Thiazide-like diuretic. For dosage, see *chlorthalidone*. [hy-GROH-tehn]. 103

Hylorel (Cardio). Blocks the release of norepinephrine from the adrenal medulla; used to treat hypertension. For dosage, see *guanadrel*. 166

Hylutin (OB/GYN). Progestins hormone drug used to treat amenorrhea. For dosage, see *hydroxyprogesterone*. [hy-LOO-tihn]. 253

hyoscyamine. See *L-hyoscyamine*.

hyperactivity. See *attention-deficit/hyperactivity disorder*.

hyperalimentation solution (I.V.). Total parenteral nutrition. 376

hypercholesterolemia, drugs used to treat. 168

hypericin (Chemo). Chemotherapy drug used to treat brain cancer; used to treat cutaneous T-cell lymphoma. Orphan drug. 347

hyperlipidemia, drugs used to treat. 168

Hypermune (Antivir). Immunoglobulin used to treat respiratory syncytial virus. Intravenous. 331.

Hyperstat (Cardio). Peripheral vasodilator used to treat hypertensive crisis. For dosage, see *diazoxide*. 167

hypertension, drugs used to treat. 161

hypertensive crisis, drugs used to treat. 167

hyperthyroidism, drugs used to treat. 229

hypertriglyceridemia, drugs used to treat. 168

Hypnos (father of Morpheus, the Greek god of dreams).

hypnotics (Neuro). Class of drugs used to produce sedation and sleep. 272

hypodermic. 63

HypoTears, HypoTears PF (Oph). Artificial tears. Drops.

hypothyroidism, drugs used to treat. 229

(HypRho-D) (OB/GYN). No longer on the market. (Generic name *immunoglobulin*; given to Rh-negative mother with Rh-positive baby).

Hyskon (OB/GYN). Dextran fluid used intraoperatively to facilitate visualization of uterus. [HIHS-kawn].

Hytone (Derm) (generic *hydrocortisone*). Topical corticosteroid anti-inflammatory drug. Cream: 1%, 2.5%. Lotion: 1%, 2.5%. Ointment: 1%, 2.5%. 92

Hytrin (Cardio, Uro). Alpha$_1$-receptor blocker used to treat hypertension; used to treat benign prostatic hypertrophy. For dosage, see *terazosin.* 109, 165

Hyzaar (Cardio) (generic *losartan, hydrochlorothiazide*). Combination angiotensin II receptor blocker antihypertensive and diuretic drug. Tablet: 50 mg/12.5 mg, 100 mg/25 mg. [HY-zahr]. 177

I&O (abbreviation for *intake and output*, measurements of fluid intake via diet and intravenous fluids and output via urine).

Iberet (Misc). Multivitamin nutritional supplement. Filmtab.

Iberet-500, Iberet-Folic-500 (Misc). Multivitamin with iron and folic acid nutritional supplement. Liquid. Filmtab.

ibuprofen (Advil, Advil Migraine, Children's Advil, Children's Motrin, Haltran, Infants' Motrin, Junior Strength Advil, Junior Strength Motrin, Midol Maximum Strength Cramp Formula, Motrin, Motrin IB, Motrin Migraine Pain, Pediatric Advil Drops, PediaCare Fever) (Analges, OB/GYN, Ortho). Nonsteroidal anti-inflammatory drug used to treat fever and pain in children and adults; used to treat migraine headaches; used to treat dysmenorrhea; used to treat osteoarthritis and rheumatoid arthritis. Capsule/Liqui-Gel: 200 mg. Chewable tablet: 50 mg, 100 mg. Drops: 40 mg/mL. Liquid: 100 mg/2.5 mL, 100 mg/5 mL. Tablet: 100 mg, 200 mg, 400 mg, 600 mg, 800 mg. [ii-byoo-PROH-fehn]. 139, 255, 304, 307

ibutilide (Corvert) (Cardio). Used to treat atrial arrhythmias. Intravenous: 0.1 mg/mL. [ii-BYOO-tih-lide].

Icy Hot, Icy Hot Arthritis Therapy, Icy Hot Balm (Ortho). Topical irritant drug used to mask the pain of arthritis and muscle aches. Cream. Ointment.

Idamycin, Idamycin PFS (Chemo). Chemotherapy antibiotic used to treat leukemia. For dosage, see *idarubicin.* [ii-dah-MY-sihn]. 342

idarubicin (Idamycin, Idamycin PFS) (Chemo). Chemotherapy antibiotic used to treat leukemia. Intravenous: 1 mg/mL, (powder to be reconstituted) 5 mg, 10 mg, 20 mg. [ii-dah-ROO-beh-sihn]. 342

idiosyncratic reaction to a drug. 55

(idoxuridine) (Oph). No longer on the market. (Trade name *Herplex*; topical drug for herpes infection of eye).

Ifex (Chemo). Alkylating chemotherapy drug used to treat testicular cancer, lung cancer, breast cancer, ovarian cancer, pancreatic cancer, gastric cancer, leukemia, and non-Hodgkin's lymphoma. For dosage, see *ifosfamide.* [II-fecks]. 341

ifosfamide (Ifex) (Chemo). Alkylating chemotherapy drug used to treat testicular cancer, lung cancer, breast cancer, ovarian cancer, pancreatic cancer, gastric cancer, leukemia, and non-Hodgkin's lymphoma. Intravenous (powder to be reconstituted): 1 g, 3 g. [ii-foh-FAWS-fah-mide]. 341

Iletin II Regular (Diab). Rapid-acting regular insulin. Subcutaneous: 100 units/mL. [II-leh-tihn]. 238

Ilopan (GI). Gastric stimulant used to treat paralytic ileus. For dosage, see *dexpanthenol.* [II-loh-pehn]. 126

(Ilosone) (Antbio). No longer on the market. (Generic name *erythromycin*; antibiotic).

Ilotycin (Antibio). Macrolide antibiotic used to treat a variety of infections, including *Streptococcus, H. influenzae*, gonorrhea, syphilis, *Chlamydia*, and Legionnaire's disease; used to prevent subacute bacterial endocarditis. For dosage, see *erythromycin.* [ii-loh-TY-sihn]. 319

Ilotycin (Oph). Topical antibiotic used to treat bacterial eye infections; used to prevent gonorrhea-caused blindness in newborn infants. For dosage, see *erythromycin.* [ii-loh-TY-sihn]. 214

I.M. or IM (abbreviation for *intramuscular*). 41

imatinib (Gleevec) (Chemo). Chemotherapy drug used to treat leukemia. Capsule: 100 mg.

Imdur (Cardio). Nitrate drug used to prevent and treat angina pectoris. For dosage, see *isosorbide mononitrate.* 156

imiglucerase (Cerezyme) (GI). An enzyme drug used to treat Gaucher's disease. Intravenous (powder to be reconstituted): 200 units. [eh-mee-GLOO-seh-race].

imipramine (Tofranil, Tofranil-PM) (Analges, Diab, Neuro, Ortho). Tricyclic antidepressant used to treat migraines; used to treat diabetic neuropathy; used to treat postherpetic neuralgia; used to treat phantom limb pain. Capsule: 75 mg, 100 mg, 125 mg, 150 mg. Tablet: 10 mg, 25 mg, 50 mg. [eh-MIH-prah-meen]. 147, 241, 276, 307

imipramine (Tofranil, Tofranil-PM) (Psych, Uro). Tricyclic antidepressant used to treat depression; used to treat panic disorder; used to treat anorexia nervosa and bulimia nervosa; used to treat childhood bedwetting. Capsule: 75 mg, 100 mg, 125 mg, 150 mg. Tablet: 10 mg, 25 mg, 50 mg. [eh-MIH-prah-meen]. 111, 286, 289, 291

imiquimod (Aldara) (OB/GYN). Topical drug used to treat genital/venereal warts or condyloma acuminatum. Cream: 5%. [ih-MIH-kwih-mawd]. 259

imatinib (Gleevec) (Chemo). Used to treat chronic myeloid leukemia. Capsule: 100 mg. [ih-MEH-tih-nib]. 348

Imitrex (Analges). Serotonin receptor agonist drug used to treat migraine headaches and cluster headaches. For dosage, see *sumatriptan*. [IHM-eh-trehks]. 306

ImmTher (Chemo). Chemotherapy drug used to treat metastases in patients with colon or rectal cancer. Orphan drug. 361

Immuno-C (Antivir). Cow immunoglobulin used to treat *Cryptosporidium parvum* gastrointestinal tract infection in patients with AIDS. For dosage, see *bovine immunoglobulin*. 331

immunosuppresant drugs for organ transplantation. 110

Immupath (Antivir). Used to treat AIDS. Orphan drug. 326

Imodium, Imodium A-D (GI). Nonnarcotic antidiarrheal drug. For dosage, see *loperamide*. 123

Imogam Rabies-HT (Antivir). Immunoglobulin used to treat patients exposed to rabies. Intramuscular: 150 IU/mL.

Impact (GI). Liquid nutritional supplement. Liquid.

Imuran (Uro). Immunosuppressant drug given after kidney transplantation to prevent rejection of the donor kidney. For dosage, see *azathioprine*. 110

Imuthiol (Antivir). Used to treat AIDS. Orphan drug. 326

Imuvert (Chemo). Chemotherapy drug used to treat brain cancer. Orphan drug. 348

inamrinone (Cardio). Used to treat congestive heart failure. Intravenous: 5 mg/mL. [ih-NEH-rih-nohn]. 154

Inapsine (Anes). Preoperative drug used to produce sedation; also used to induce and maintain general anesthesia. For dosage, see *droperidol*. [ih-NEHP-seen]. 369

inch (drug measurement). 70

indapamide (Lozol) (Uro). Thiazide diuretic. Tablet: 1.25 mg, 2.5 mg. [ihn-DEH-pah-mide]. 103

indecainide (Decabid) (Cardio). Antiarrhythmic drug. Investigational drug. 173

In Depth features
ACE inhibitors. 163
beta receptors/beta-blockers. 161
calcium channel blockers. 157
cardiac glycosides. 152
chronic myeloid leukemia. 358
cervical ripening. 247
corticosteroids. 93
COX-1 and COX-2 enzymes. 140
dopamine. 268
low molecular weight heparins. 186
MAO inhibitors and food interactions. 287
MTC. 362
tardive dyskinesia. 284

Inderal, Inderal LA (Analges, GI, Neuro, Ortho, Psych). Nonselective beta-blocker used to treat migraine headaches; used to prevent rebleeding of esophageal varices in patients with cirrhosis and gastric bleeding in patients with portal hypertension; used to treat the tremors of Parkinson's disease; used to treat essential familial tremors; used to treat the side effects of muscle restlessness from antipsychotic drugs; used to prevent performance anxiety. For dosage, see *propranolol*. [IHN-deh-rawl]. 134, 146, 269, 290, 294, 306

Inderal, Inderal LA (Cardio). Nonselective beta-blocker used to treat angina pectoris, hypertension, and ventricular arrhythmias; used to prevent repeat myocardial infarction. For dosage, see *propranolol*. [IHN-deh-rawl]. 155, 157, 158, 160, 162

Inderide 40/25, Inderide 80/20, Inderide LA 80/50, Inderide LA 120/50, Inderide LA 160/50 (Cardio) (generic *propranolol, hydrochlorothiazide*). Combination beta-blocker antihypertensive and diuretic drug. Capsule: 80 mg/50 mg, 120 mg/50 mg, 160 mg/50 mg. Tablet: 40 mg/25 mg, 80 mg/25 mg. [IHN-deh-ride]. 167

index, therapeutic (TI). 27, 152

indinavir (Crixivan) (Antivir). Protease inhibitor drug used to treat AIDS. Capsule: 200 mg, 400 mg. [ihn-DIH-nah-veer]. 325

Indocin, Indocin SR (Analges, Ortho). Nonsteroidal anti-inflammatory drug used to treat the pain of bursitis, gout, osteoarthritis, rheumatoid arthritis, and tendinitis. For dosage, see *indomethacin*. [IHN-doh-sihn]. 139, 146, 304

Indocin I.V. (Cardio). Nonsteroidal anti-inflammatory drug used to close a patent ductus arteriosus in premature newborn infants. For dosage, see *indomethacin*. [IHN-doh-sihn]. 173

indocyanine green (Cardio-Green) (Oph). Dye used during angiography of the eye. Intravenous (powder to be reconstituted): 25 mg, 50 mg. [ehn-doh-SY-ah-neen].

indomethacin (Indocin, Indocin SR) (Analges, Ortho). Nonsteroidal anti-inflammatory drug used to treat the pain of bursitis, gout, osteoarthritis, rheumatoid arthritis, and tendinitis. Capsule: 25 mg, 50 mg, 75 mg. Liquid: 25 mg/5 mL. Suppository: 50 mg. [ihn-doh-MEH-thah-sihn]. 139, 146, 304

indomethacin (Indocin I.V.) (Cardio). Nonsteroidal anti-inflammatory drug used to close a patent ductus arteriosus in premature newborn infants. Intravenous (powder to be reconstituted): 1 mg. [ihn-doh-MEH-thah-sihn]. 173

induction of anesthesia. 369

inert ingredients in drugs. 30

Infalyte (GI). Given to children to replace water and electrolytes lost from vomiting and diarrhea. Liquid. 133

Infants' Drops Panadol, see *Panadol*.

Infants' Drops Tylenol, see *Tylenol*.

Infants' Feverall (Analges). Nonnarcotic nonaspirin analgesic drug used to treat fever and pain in children. For dosage, see *acetaminophen*. 301

Infants' Motrin, see *Motrin*.

Infasurf (Resp). Natural lung surfactant used to prevent and treat respiratory distress syndrome in newborn infants. For dosage, see *calfactant*. [IHN-fah-sehrf].

Infatab. Part of the trade name of drug, indicating a chewable tablet in pediatric dose. 63

Infergen (GI). Antiviral drug used to treat hepatitis C. For dosage, see *interferon alfacon-1*. 133

infertility, drugs used to treat. 244

Inflamase Forte, Inflamase Mild (Oph). Topical corticosteroid used to treat inflammation of the eyes. For dosage, see *prednisolone*. 219

inflammation, drugs used to treat.
topical. 92
systemic. 232

infliximab (Remicade) (GI, Ortho). Monoclonal antibody used to treat Crohn's disease; used to treat rheumatoid arthritis. Intravenous: 100 mg/20 mL. [ihn-FLIHK-sih-mehb]. 133, 142

influenza, drugs used to treat or prevent. 330

influenza vaccine (FluShield, Fluvirin, Fluzone) (Antivir, Resp). Vaccine to prevent influenza A infection. Intramuscular (whole virus, part of the virus, or surface antigen): 0.5 mL. 330

Infumorph (Analges, Anes, Cardio, OB/GYN). Narcotic analgesic drug used to treat moderate-to-severe

pain; used as a preoperative drug to sedate and supplement anesthesia; used to treat dyspnea from congestive heart failure; used to treat the pain of childbirth. (Schedule II drug). For dosage, see *morphine*. [IHN-fyoo-mohrf]. 173, 297

INH (abbreviation for the chemical name of isoniazid).

inhalation, administration of drugs by. 40

inhaler. See *metered-dose inhaler*.

Inhibace (Cardio) (generic *cilazapril*). Angiotensin-converting enzyme inhibitor used to treat hypertension and congestive heart failure. Investigational drug. 172

Innohep (Hem). Low molecular weight heparin anticoagulant. For dosage, see *tinzaparin*.

(Innovar) (Anes). No longer on the market. (Generic name *droperidol, fentanyl*; used to decrease anxiety and motor activity during procedures in which the patient is conscious).

(Inocor) (Cardio). No longer on the market. (Generic name *amrinone*; used to treat congestive heart failure).

INOmax (Resp). Inhaled gas used to treat persistent pulmonary hypertension in newborns in respiratory failure on the ventilator. For dosage, see *nitric oxide*.

inosine pranobex (Isoprinosine) (Neuro). Used to treat sclerosing panencephalitis. Orphan drug.

inotropic effect.

insomnia, drugs used to treat. 272

isoxicam (Maxicam) (Ortho). Nonsteroidal anti-inflammatory drug used to treat osteoarthritis or rheumatoid arthritis. Investigational drug.

Insta-Glucose (Diab). Used to treat hypoglycemia. For dosage, see *glucose*.

insulin. 237

insulin, beef/pork. Focus on Healthcare Issues feature. 240

insulin aspart (Novolog) (Diab). Rapid-acting human recombinant DNA aspart insulin. Subcutaneous: 100 units/mL. 238

insulin glargine (Lantus) (Diab). Long-acting human recombinant DNA glargine insulin. Subcutaneous: 100 units/mL. 238

insulin lispro (Humalog) (Diab). Rapid-acting human recombinant DNA lispro insulin. Subcutaneous: 100 units/mL. 238

insulin pump. 239

insulin syringe. 63, 239

Intal (Resp). Mast cell stabilizer used to prevent acute asthma attacks. For dosage, see *cromolyn*. [IHN-tawl]. 197

Integrilin (Cardio, Hem). Platelet aggregation inhibitor used to prevent blood clots in patients with unstable angina or myocardial infarction, or who are undergoing angioplasty or atherectomy. For dosage, see *eptifibatide*. 173, 187

interaction.
drug–drug. 56
drug–food. 56

interferon alfa-2a (Roferon-A) (Antivir, Chemo). Antiviral drug used to treat hepatitis C, cytomegalovirus, and herpes eye infections; chemotherapy drug used to treat leukemia, bladder cancer, non-Hodgkin's lymphoma, cutaneous T-cell lymphoma, and Kaposi's sarcoma. Subcutaneous or intramuscular: 3 million IU/mL, 6 million IU/mL, 9 million IU/mL, 36 million IU/mL. [ihn-tehr-FEHR-awn]. 133, 330, 346

interferon alfa-2a (Roferon-A) (Derm, OB/GYN). Antiviral drug used to treat condyloma acuminatum/genital warts. Intralesional injection: 3 million IU/mL, 6 million IU/mL, 9 million IU/mL. [ihn-tehr-FEHR-awn].

interferon alfa-2b (Intron A) (Chemo, GI). Antiviral drug used to treat hepatitis C; chemotherapy drug used to treat leukemia, malignant melanoma, bladder cancer, cutaneous T-cell lymphoma, non-Hodgkin's lymphoma, and Kaposi's sarcoma. Subcutaneous or intramuscular: 3 million IU/0.5 mL, 5 million IU/0.5 mL, 10 million IU/mL, (powder to be reconstituted) 18 million IU/mL, 25 million IU/mL, 50 million IU/mL. [ihn-tehr-FEHR-awn]. 133, 346

interferon alfa-2b (Intron A) (Derm, OB/GYN). Antiviral drug used to treat genital/venereal warts or condyloma acuminatum. Intralesional injection: 3 million IU/mL, 5 million IU/mL, 10 million IU/mL. [ihn-tehr-FEHR-awn]. 259

interferon alfa-n3 (Alferon LDO, Alferon N) (Antivir, Derm, OB/GYN). Antiviral drug used to treat genital/venereal warts or condyloma acuminatum; investigational drug used to treat AIDS. Intralesional injection: 5 million IU/mL. [ihn-tehr-FEHR-awn]. 259, 326

interferon alfacon-1 (Infergen) (GI). Antiviral drug used to treat hepatitis C. Subcutaneous: 9 mcg/0.3 mL, 15 mcg/0.5 mL. [ihn-tehr-FEHR-awn]. 133

interferon beta-1a (Avonex) (Antivir, Chemo, GI, Neuro, OB/GYN). Used to treat AIDS; used to treat brain cancer, malignant melanoma, and cutaneous T-cell lymphoma; used to treat Kaposi's sarcoma; used to treat non-A, non-B hepatitis; used to treat multiple sclerosis; used to treat genital herpes simplex type 2 infection. Intramuscular (powder to be reconstituted): 33 mcg (6.6 million IU). [ihn-tehr-FEHR-awn]. 133, 148, 276, 326, 330, 346

interferon beta-1a (Rebif) (Antivir, Neuro). Used to treat AIDS; used to treat multiple sclerosis and juve-nile rheumatoid arthritis. Orphan drug. [ihn-tehr-FEHR-awn]. 148, 326

interferon beta-1b (Betaseron) (Antivir, Chemo, GI, Neuro, OB/GYN). Used to treat AIDS; used to treat brain cancer, malignant melanoma, and cutaneous T-cell lymphoma; used to treat Kaposi's sarcoma; used to treat hepatitis; used to treat multiple sclerosis; used to treat genital herpes simplex type 2 infection. Subcutaneous (powder to be reconstituted): 0.3 mg (9.6 million IU). [ihn-tehr-FEHR-awn]. 276, 326, 330

interferon gamma-1b (Actimmune) (Chemo, Derm). Used to treat renal cancer; used to treat the skin infections of chronic granulomatous disease. Subcutaneous: 100 mcg/0.5 mL (2 million IU/0.5 mL). [ihn-tehr-FEHR-awn]. 99, 346

interleukin-1 (Antril) (Chemo, Ortho). Used to prevent or treat graft-versus-host disease; used to treat juvenile rheumatoid arthritis. Orphan drug. 148, 361

interleukin-2. See *aldesleukin* and *teceleukin*.

interleukin-10 (Tenovil) (Antivir). Used to treat AIDS. Investigational drug. 326

intra-arterial route, administration of drugs by the. 42

intra-articular route, administration of drugs by the. 42

intracardiac route, administration of drugs by the. 42, 179

intradermal route, administration of drugs by the. 43

IntraDose (Chemo) (generic *cisplatin, epinephrine*). Combination chemotherapy drug and epinephrine used to treat head and neck cancer; used to treat malignant melanoma. Orphan drug. 361

Intralipid 10%, Intralipid 20% (I.V.). Intravenous fat solution. 378

intramuscular route, administration of drugs by the. 41

IntraSite (Derm). Topical drug used to absorb drainage from burns, skin ulcers, and wounds. Gel: 2%. 96

intrathecal route, administration of drugs by the. 43

intravenous (I.V.).
bag/bottle. 42, 374
bolus. 42, 374
continuous infusion. 374
dextrose. 375
drip. 42, 374
fluids. 375
heparin lock. 374
hyperalimentation solution. 376
KVO. 374
lactated Ringer's. 375
line. 42, 374
normal saline. 375
piggyback. 42, 374

port. 42, 374

push. 42, 374

total parenteral nutrition. 376

intravenous (I.V.) route, administration of drugs by the. 42, 179, 374

intravenous lipids (Intralipid 10%, Intralipid 20%, Liposyn II 10%, Liposyn II 20%, Liposyn III 10%, Liposyn III 20%) (I.V.). Intravenous fat solution. 378

intravenous multivitamins (Berocca Parenteral Nutrition, Cernevit-12, M.V.I.-12) (I.V.). Intravenous combination drug of nine water-soluble and three fat-soluble vitamins. 378

Introlite (GI). Liquid nutritional supplement. Liquid. 131

Intron A (Chemo, GI). Antiviral drug used to treat hepatitis C; chemotherapy drug used to treat leukemia, malignant melanoma, bladder cancer, cutaneous T-cell lymphoma, non-Hodgkin's lymphoma, and Kaposi's sarcoma. For dosage, see *interferon alfa-2b*. [IHN-trawn]. 133, 346

Intron A (Derm, OB/GYN). Antiviral drug used to treat genital/venereal warts or condyloma acuminatum. For dosage, see *interferon alfa-2b*. [IHN-trawn]. 259

Intropin (Cardio, Emerg, Resp). Vasopressor used to treat decompensated congestive heart failure; used to treat hypotension during emergency resuscitation; used to treat chronic obstructive pulmonary disease; used to treat respiratory distress syndrome in infants. For dosage, see *dopamine*. [ihn-TROH-pihn]. 173, 181

Invanz (Antibio). Carbapenem antibiotic used to treat a variety of infections. For dosage, see *ertapenem*. 317

Inversine (Cardio, Psych). Antihypertensive drug only used to treat severe hypertension; used to treat Tourette's syndrome. For dosage, see *mecamylamine*. 166, 293

Investigational New Drug (IND). 27

Invirase (Antibio). Protease inhibitor drug used to treat AIDS. For dosage, see *saquinavir*. [ihn-VEER-ace]. 325

in vitro drug testing. 27

in vivo drug testing. 27

Iocare Balanced Salt (Oph). Irrigating solution used during eye surgery. For dosage, see *balanced salt solution*.

iodinated glycerol (ENT). Expectorant. Liquid: 60 mg/5 mL. Tablet: 30 mg.

iodoquinol (Yodoxin) (Antibio, GI). Used to treat intestinal amebiasis. Tablet: 210 mg, 650 mg.

Iodotope (Endo). Radioactive drug used to treat hyperthyroidism and thyroid cancer. For dosage, see *radioactive sodium iodide 131*. [ii-OH-doh-tohp].

Iopidine (Oph). Topical alpha-agonist drug used to treat glaucoma. For dosage, see *apraclonidine*. [ii-OH-peh-deen]. 222

ipecac syrup (Emerg, GI). Used to induce vomiting to treat poisoning and drug overdose. Syrup: 15 mL, 30 mL. [IH-peh-kack]. 133, 182

ipratropium (Atrovent) (ENT, Resp). Used to treat allergic rhinitis; bronchodilator. Aerosol inhaler: 18 mcg/puff. Liquid for nebulizer: 0.02% (500 mcg/2.5 mL). Nasal spray: 0.03%, 0.06%. [ih-prah-TROH-pee-uhm]. 193, 214

Ipstyl (Endo). Used to treat acromegaly. For dosage, see *lanreotide*. 230

irbesartan (Avapro) (Cardio). Angiotensin II receptor blocker used to treat hypertension. Tablet: 75 mg, 150 mg, 300 mg. 164

irinotecan (Camptosar) (Chemo). Mitosis inhibitor chemotherapy drug used to treat colon or rectal cancer. Intravenous: 20 mg/mL. [ii-ree-noh-TEE-kehn]. 344

iron sucrose (Venofer) (Hem, Uro). Used to treat iron deficiency anemia in hemodialysis patients. Intravenous: 100 mg/5 mL.

Ismelin (Cardio, Neuro). Blocks the release of norepinephrine from the adrenal medulla; used to treat hypertension; used to treat sympathetic dystrophy and causalgia. For dosage, see *guanethidine*. [EHZ-meh-lihn]. 166, 276

ISMO (Cardio). Nitrate drug used to prevent and treat angina pectoris. For dosage, see *isosorbide mononitrate*.

Isocal, Isolcal HCN, Isocal HN (GI). Liquid nutritional supplement. Liquid.

isocarboxazid (Marplan) (Psych). Monoamine oxidase inhibitor used to treat depression. Tablet: 10 mg. [ii-soh-kahr-BAWK-sah-zihd]. 288

isoetharine (Resp). Bronchodilator. Liquid for nebulizer: 1%. 193

isoflurane (Forane) (Anes). Used to induce and maintain general anesthesia. Inhaled gas. [ii-soh-FLOH-rayn]. 370

isomer. 63

Isomil DF (GI). Infant soy formula for infants with diarrhea. Liquid.

Isomil, Isomil SF (GI). Infant soy formula for infants with allergies. Liquid. Powder (to be reconstituted).

isoniazid (INH) (Nydrazid) (Resp). Bactericidal antibiotic used only to treat tuberculosis. Liquid: 50 mg/5 mL. Tablet: 50 mg, 100 mg, 300 mg. Intramuscular: 100 mg/mL. [ii-soh-NY-ah-zihd]. 197

Isoprinosine (Antivir) (Neuro). Used to treat AIDS; used to treat sclerosing panencephalitis. For dosage, see *inosine pranobex*. [ii-soh-PRIH-noh-seen].

(isopropramide) (GI). No longer on the market. (Trade name *Darbid*; GI antispasmodic drug).

isoproterenol (Isuprel) (Cardio, Emerg). Nonselective beta-blocker used to treat heart block; vasopressor used to treat hypotension during cardiac resuscitation. Intracardiac, intramuscular, or intravenous: 1:50,000 (0.02 mg/mL), 1:5000 (0.2 mg/mL). [ii-soh-proh-TEH-reh-nawl]. 173, 180, 181

isoproterenol (Isuprel) (Resp). Bronchodilator. Intravenous: 1:5000 (0.2 mg/mL), 1:50,000 (0.02 mg/mL). [ii-soh-proh-TEH-reh-nawl]. 193

Isoptin, Isoptin SR (Cardio). Calcium channel blocker used to treat angina pectoris, congestive heart failure, hypertension, and atrial and ventricular arrhythmias. For dosage, see *verapamil*. [ii-SAWP-tihn] 154, 157, 160, 163

Isopto Atropine (Oph). Topical mydriatic drug. For dosage, see *atropine*. [ii-SAWP-toh EH-troh-peen]. 223

Isopto Carbachol (Oph). Topical miotic drug used to treat glaucoma. For dosage, see *carbachol*. [ii-SAWP-toh-KAHR-bah-kawl]. 221

Isopto Carpine (Oph). Topical miotic drug used to treat glaucoma. For dosage, see *pilocarpine*. [ii-SAWP-toh-KAHR-peen]. 221

Isopto Homatropine (Oph). Topical mydriatic drug. For dosage, see *homatropine*. [ii-SAWP-toh hoh-mah-TROH-peen]. 223

Isopto Hyoscine (Oph). Topical mydriatic drug. For dosage, see *scopolamine*. [ii-SAWP-toh HY-oh-seen]. 223

Isopto Plain, Isopto Tears (Oph). Artificial tears. Drops.

Isordil, Isordil Titradose, Isordil Tembids (Cardio). Nitrate drug used to prevent and treat angina pectoris. For dosage, see *isosorbide dinitrate*. 156

isosorbide dinitrate (Isordil, Isordil Titradose, Isordil Tembids, Sorbitrate) (Cardio). Nitrate drug used to prevent and treat angina pectoris. Capsule: 40 mg. Chewable tablet: 5 mg, 10 mg. Sublingual tablet: 2.5 mg, 5 mg, 10 mg. Tablet: 5 mg, 10 mg, 20 mg, 30 mg, 40 mg. [ii-soh-SOHR-bide dy-NY-trayt]. 156

isosorbide mononitrate (Imdur, ISMO) (Cardio). Nitrate drug used to prevent and treat angina pectoris. Tablet: 10 mg, 20 mg, 30 mg, 60 mg, 120 mg. [ii-soh-SOHR-bide maw-noh-NY-trayt]. 156

Isosource, Isosource HN (GI). Liquid nutritional supplement. Liquid.

Isotein HN (GI). Liquid nutritional supplement. Powder (to be reconstituted).

isotretinoin (Accutane) (Derm). Oral vitamin A-type drug used to treat severe cystic acne vulgaris. Capsule: 10 mg, 20 mg, 40 mg. [ii-soh-tree-teh-NOH-ihn]. 84

Isovorin (Chemo). Cytoprotective drug used to prevent toxicity in patients receiving fluorouracil and methotrexate chemotherapy. For dosage, see *L-leucovorin*. 350

isoxicam (Maxicam) (Ortho). Used to treat osteoarthritis and rheumatoid arthritis. Investigational drug. 148

isoxsuprine (Vasodilan) (Cardio). Peripheral vasodilator used to treat peripheral vascular disease and Raynaud's disease. Tablet: 10 mg, 20 mg. [ii-SAWK-suh-preen]. 168, 173

isradipine (DynaCirc, DynaCirc CR) (Cardio). Calcium channel blocker used to treat hypertension. Capsule: 2.5 mg, 5 mg. Tablet: 5 mg, 10 mg. [ihs-REH-dih-peen]. 163

Isuprel (Cardio, Emerg). Nonselective beta-blocker used to treat heart block; vasopressor used to treat hypotension during cardiac resuscitation. For dosage, see *isoproterenol*. [II-soo-prehl]. 173, 180, 181

Isuprel (Resp). Bronchodilator. For dosage, see *isoproterenol*. [II-soo-prehl]. 193

itching, drugs used to treat. 92

itraconazole (Sporanox) (Antifung). Used to treat severe topical and systemic fungal and yeast infections. Capsule: 100 mg. Liquid: 10 mg/mL. Intravenous: 10 mg/mL. [ih-trah-KAW-neh-zohl]. 90, 334, 335

IU (abbreviation for *International Unit*).

I.V. (abbreviation for *intravenous*). See *intravenous, intravenous route*.

Iveegam immunoglobulin (Antivir). AIDS drug. Intravenous (powder to be reconstituted): 5%.

jejunostomy tube, administration of drugs by. 40

Jenest-28 (OB/GYN) (generic *norethindrone, ethinyl estradiol*). Biphasic combination progestins and estrogen oral contraceptive. Tablet: 0.5 mg/35 mcg then 1 mg/35 mcg. [JEH-nehst]. 250

Jevity (GI). Liquid nutritional supplement. Liquid.

jock itch, drugs used to treat. 89

Junior Strength Advil, see *Advil*.

Junior Strengh Feverall (Analges). Nonnarcotic nonaspirin analgesic drug used to treat fever and pain in children. For dosage, see *acetaminophen*.

Junior Strength Motrin, see *Motrin*.

Junior Strength Panadol, see *Panadol*.

K (chemical symbol for *potassium*).

(Kabikinase) (Cardio, Hem). No longer on the market. (Generic name *streptokinase*; thrombolytic enzyme used to dissolve blood clots after myocardial infarction).

Kadian (Analges, Anes, Cardio, OB/GYN). Narcotic analgesic drug used to treat moderate-to-severe pain; used as a preoperative drug to sedate and supplement anesthesia; used to treat dyspnea from congestive heart failure; used to treat the pain of childbirth. (Schedule II drug). For dosage, see *morphine*. [KAY-dee-ehn]. 173, 297

Kaletra (Antivir) (generic *lopinavir, ritonavir*). Combination of two protease inhibitor drugs used to treat AIDS. Capsule: 133.3 mg/33.3 mg. Liquid: 80 mg/20 mg per mL. 325

kanamycin (Kantrex) (Antibio, GI). Aminoglycoside antibiotic used to treat various bacterial infections, including *E. coli* and *Klebsiella*; used to treat *Mycobacterium avium-intracellulare* in AIDS patients; used to treat hepatic coma. Capsule: 500 mg. Intramuscular or intravenous: 75 mg, 500 mg, 1 g. [keh-nah-MY-sihn]. 316

Kantrex (Antibio, GI). Aminoglycoside antibiotic used to treat various bacterial infections, including *E. coli* and *Klebsiella*; used to treat *Mycobacterium avium-intracellulare* in AIDS patients; used to treat hepatic coma. For dosage, see *kanamycin*. [KEHN-trehks]. 316

Kaodene Non-Narcotic (GI) (generic *bismuth, kaolin, pectin*). Combination antibacterial and antidiarrheal drug used to treat diarrhea. Liquid: 30 mg/3.9 mg/194.4 mg. 124

Kaolin with Pectin (GI). Antidiarrheal drug. For dosage, see *attapulgite*. 124

Kaon, Kaon-Cl 20% (Uro). Potassium supplement used to replace potassium loss caused by diuretics. Liquid: 20 mEq/15 mL, 40 mEq/15 mL. 104

Kaon-Cl 10 (Uro). Potassium supplement used to replace potassium loss caused by diuretics. Tablet: 10 mEq. 104

Kaopectate Advanced Formula, Kaopectate Maximum Strength (GI). Antidiarrheal drug. For dosage, see *attapulgite*. 124

Kaopectate II (GI). Nonnarcotic antidiarrheal drug. For dosage, see *loperamide*. 123

Kapseal. Part of the trade name of drug, indicating a time-release capsule. 63

K + Care, K + Care ET (Uro). Potassium supplement used to replace potassium loss caused by diuretics. Effervescent tablet: 20 mEq, 25 mEq. Powder to be reconstituted with water: 15 mEq, 20 mEq. 104

Kay Ciel (Uro). Potassium supplement used to replace potassium loss caused by diuretics. Liquid: 20mEq/15 ml. Powder (to be reconstituted): 20 mEq. 104

Kayexalate (Cardio). Used to treat hyperkalemia. Liquid (oral, nasogastric tube, or rectal): Powder to be reconstituted. [kay-EHK-sah-layt].

KCl (chemical symbol for *potassium chloride*).

K-Dur 10, K-Dur 20 (Uro). Potassium supplement used to replace potassium loss caused by diuretics. Tablet: 10 mEq, 20 mEq. 105

Kefauver–Harris Amendment. 15

Keflex (Antibio). Cephalosporin antibiotic used to treat a variety of bacterial infections, including *Streptococcus, Staphylococcus, E. coli*, and *H. influenzae*. For dosage, see *cephalexin*. [KEH-flehks]. 315

(Keflin) (Antibio). No longer on the market. (Generic name *cephalothin*; cephalosporin antibiotic).

Keftab (Antibio). Cephalosporin antibiotic used to treat a variety of bacterial infections, including *Streptococcus, Staphylococcus, E. coli*, and *H. influenzae*. For dosage, see *cephalexin*. [KEHF-tehb]. 315

Kefurox (Antibio). Cephalosporin antibiotic used to treat various types of infections, including *Streptococcus, Staphylococcus, H. influenzae, E. coli*, and gonorrhea. For dosage, see *cefuroxime*. [KEH-fyoor-awks]. 316

Kefzol (Antibio). Cephalosporin antibiotic used to treat a variety of bacterial infections, including *Streptococcus, Staphylococcus, E. coli*, and *H. influenzae*. For dosage, see *cefazolin*. [KEHF-zohl]. 315

K + 8 (Uro). Potassium supplement used to replace potassium loss caused by diuretics. Tablet: 8 mEq. 104

Kemadrin (Neuro). Anticholinergic drug used to treat Parkinson's disease. For dosage, see *procyclidine*. [KEH-mah-drehn]. 269

Kenacort (Chemo, Endo). Corticosteroid anti-inflammatory drug used to treat leukemia and lymphoma; used to treat severe inflammation in various body systems; used to treat Addison's disease. For dosage, see *triamcinolone*. [KEHN-ah-kohrt]. 93, 232, 233, 351

Kenalog, Kenalog-H (Derm) (generic *triamcinolone*). Topical corticosteroid anti-inflammatory drug. Cream: 0.025%, 0.1%, 0.5%. Lotion: 0.025%, 0.1%. Ointment: 0.025%, 0.1%, 0.5%. Spray. [KEHN-ah-lawg]. 92

Kenalog-40 (Endo, Ortho). Injected corticosteroid anti-inflammatory drug used to treat severe inflammation in various body systems; injected into a joint to treat osteoarthritis and rheumatoid arthritis. For dosage, see *triamcinolone*. [KEHN-ah-lawg]. 141, 233

Kenalog in Orabase (ENT). Topical corticosteroid drug used to treat ulcers and inflammation in the mouth. Paste: 0.1%. [KEHN-ah-lawg in OHR-ah-bays].

Kenalog-10 (Derm). Corticosteroid anti-inflammatory drug injected into skin lesions. For dosage, see *triamcinolone*. [KEHN-ah-lawg 10]. 92

Keppra (Neuro).   Anticonvulsant drug used to treat partial seizures.   For dosage, see *levetiracetam*. 265

Kerlone (Cardio).   Cardioselective beta-blocker drug used to treat hypertension.   For dosage, see *betaxolol*. [KUHR-lohn]. 162

Kestrone 5 (Chemo, OB/GYN).   Hormonal chemotherapy drug used to treat prostate cancer; hormone replacement therapy used to treat the symptoms of menopause.   For dosage, see *estrone*. [KEHS-trohn]. 252, 343

Ketalar (Anes).   Used to induce and maintain general anesthesia.   For dosage, see *ketamine*. [KEH-teh-lawr]. 369

ketamine (Ketalar) (Anes).   Used to induce and maintain general anesthesia. Intramuscular and intravenous: 10 mg/mL, 50 mg/mL, 100 mg/mL. [KEH-tah-meen]. 369

Ketek (Antibio, Resp).   Ketolide antibiotic used to treat community-acquired pneumonia.   For dosage, see *telithromycin*.

ketoconazole (Nizoral) (Antifung, Derm, ENT). Used to treat severe topical and systemic fungal and yeast infections. Tablet: 200 mg. [kee-toh-KAW-neh-zohl]. 334, 335

ketoconazole (Nizoral) (Cardio, GI, Uro).   Used to prevent toxicity to the kidney in patients with organ transplants who receive cyclosporine. Orphan drug.

ketoconazole (Nizoral, Nizoral A-D) (Derm).   Topical antifungal and antiyeast drug. Cream: 2%. Shampoo: 1%, 2%. [kee-toh-KAW-neh-zohl]. 89, 90

ketoprofen (Orudis, Orudis KT, Oruvail) (Analges, OB/GYN, Ortho).   Nonsteroidal anti-inflammatory drug used to treat pain; used to treat migraine headaches; used to treat dysmenorrhea; used to treat osteoarthritis and rheumatoid arthritis. Capsule: 25 mg, 50 mg, 75 mg, 100 mg, 150 mg, 200 mg. Tablet: 12.5 mg. [kee-toh-PROH-fehn]. 139, 255, 304, 307

ketorolac (Acular) (Oph).   Topical nonsteroidal anti-inflammatory drug used to treat inflammation of the eyes. Ophthalmic solution: 0.5%. [kee-TOHR-oh-lack]. 219

ketorolac (Toradol) (Analges).   Nonsteroidal anti-inflammatory drug used to treat pain; used to treat migraine headaches. Tablet: 10 mg. Intramuscular or intravenous: 15 mg/mL, 30 mg/mL. [kee-TOHR-oh-lack]. 304, 307

ketotifen (Zaditor) (Oph).   Topical mast cell stabilizer used to treat allergy symptoms in the eyes. Ophthalmic solution: 0.025%. [kee-toh-TIF-fehn]. 220

kg (abbreviation for *kilogram*). 69

Kindercal (GI).   Liquid nutritional supplement. Liquid.

Kineret (Ortho).   Interleukin-1 drug used to treat rheumatoid arthritis.   For dosage, see *anakinra*.

Klonopin (Neuro, Psych).   Benzodiazepine drug used to treat absence seizures; used to treat Lennox–Gastaut syndrome; used to treat the muscular symptoms of Parkinson's disease; used to treat neuralgia; used to treat schizophrenia; used to treat the manic phase of manic-depressive disorder. (Schedule IV drug).   For dosage, see *clonazepam*. [KLAW-neh-pihn]. 264, 270, 283, 288

K-Lor (Uro).   Potassium supplement used to replace potassium loss caused by diuretics. Powder to be reconstituted with water: 20 mEq. 105

Klor-Con, Klor-Con 8, Klor-Con 10, Klor-Con/EF, Klor-Con/25 (Uro).   Potassium supplement used to replace potassium loss caused by diuretics. Effervescent tablet: 25 mEq. Tablet: 8 mEq, 10 mEq. Powder to be reconstituted with water: 20 mEq, 25 mEq. 105

Klorvess (Uro).   Potassium supplement used to replace potassium loss caused by diuretics. Effervescent tablet: 20 mEq. Powder to be reconstituted with water: 20 mEq. [KLOHR-vehs]. 105

Klotrix (Uro).   Potassium supplement used to replace potassium loss caused by diuretics. Tablet: 10 mEq. [KLOH-trihks]. 105

K-Lyte, K-Lyte/Cl, K-Lyte/Cl 50, K-Lyte DS (Uro). Potassium supplement used to replace potassium loss caused by diuretics. Effervescent tablet: 25 mEq, 50 mEq. Powder to be reconstituted in water: 25 mEq. 105

Koate-HP (Hem).   Used to treat clotting Factor VIII deficiency in hemophiliac patients. Intravenous: 10 mg/mL.

Kogenate (Hem).   Used to treat clotting Factor VIII deficiency in hemophiliac patients. Intravenous: 10 mg/mL.

(Komed) (Derm).   No longer on the market. (Generic name *salicylic acid*; topical keratolytic for acne vulgaris).

Konyne 80 (Hem).   Used to treat clotting Factor IX deficiency in hemophiliac patients; also includes Factors II, VI, and X.

K-Phos M.F., K-Phos Neutral, K-Phos No. 2, K-Phos Original (Uro).   Combination potassium and phosphorus drug used to acidify the urine to prevent calcium kidney stones. Tablet: 500 mg. 111

K-Tab (Uro).   Potassium supplement used to replace potassium loss caused by diuretics. Tablet: 10 mEq. 105

K + 10 (Uro).   Potassium supplement used to replace potassium loss caused by diuretics. Tablet: 10 mEq. 104

KVO (abbreviation for *keep vein open*).   See *intravenous*.

(Kwell) (Derm). No longer on the market. (Generic name *lindane*; topical drug used to treat scabies and pediculosis).

Kytril (GI). Antiemetic drug; used to treat nausea and vomiting caused by chemotherapy. For dosage, see *granisetron*. 128

LA (abbreviation for *long-acting*). Part of the trade name of a drug. See *tablet*.

labetalol (Normodyne, Trandate) (Cardio). Alpha$_1$ and nonselective beta-receptor blocker used to treat hypertension and hypertensive crisis. Tablet: 100 mg, 200 mg, 300 mg. Intravenous: 5 mg/mL. [lah-BAY-toh-lawl]. 165, 168

labetalol (Normodyne, Trandate) (Endo). Alpha$_1$ and nonselective beta-receptor blocker used to treat hypertension caused by a pheochromocytoma. Tablet: 100 mg, 200 mg, 300 mg. Intravenous: 5 mg/mL. [lah-BAY-toh-lawl].

labor, drugs used to induce. 246

labor, drugs used to treat premature/preterm. 246

lacidipine (Lacipil) (Cardio). Calcium channel blocker used to treat hypertension. Investigational drug. 173

Lacipil (Cardio) (generic *lacidipine*). Calcium channel blocker used to treat hypertension. Investigational drug. 173

Lacri-Lube NP, Lacri-Lube S.O.P. (Oph). Artificial tears lubricating ointment for the eyes. Ophthalmic ointment.

Lacrisert (Oph). Artificial tear pellet inserted in conjunctival sac of eye. Pellet.

lactated Ringer's (LR) (I.V.). Intravenous fluid of dextrose, sodium, potassium, calcium, chloride, and lactate. 376

lactic acid (Aphthaid) (Antivir). Used to treat aphthous stomatitis in AIDS patients. Orphan drug. 331

lactobin (Antivir). Used to treat diarrhea in AIDS patients. Orphan drug. 328

lactulose (Cephulac) (GI). Used to decrease blood ammonia in patients with liver disease and encephalopathy. Liquid: 10 g/15 mL. [LEHK-tyoo-lohs]. 133

lactulose (Chronulac) (GI). Laxative. Liquid: 10 g/15 mL. [LEHK-tyoo-lohs]. 125

Lamictal, Lamictal Chewable Dispersible Tablets (Diab, Neuro). Anticonvulsant drug used to treat partial seizures; used to treat Lennox–Gestaut syndrome; used to treat diabetic neuropathy. For dosage, see *lamotrigine*. [leh-MIHK-tehl]. 241, 265

Lamisil AT, Lamisil DermGel (Derm) (generic *terbinafine*). Topical antifungal drug. Cream: 1%. Gel: 1%. Spray: 1%. [LEH-meh-sihl]. 89

Lamisil (Antifung). Oral drug used to treat severe topical fungal infections. For dosage, see *terbinafine*. [LEH-meh-sihl]. 334

lamivudine (3TC) (Epivir, Epivir-HBV) (Antivir, GI). Nucleoside reverse transcriptase inhibitor drug used to treat AIDS; used to treat hepatitis B. Tablet: 100 mg, 150 mg. Liquid: 5 mg/mL, 10 mg/mL. [leh-MIH-vyoo-deen]. 324

lamotrigine (Lamictal, Lamictal Chewable Dispersible Tablets) (Diab, Neuro). Anticonvulsant drug used to treat partial seizures; used to treat Lennox–Gestaut syndrome; used to treat diabetic neuropathy. Chewable tablet: 2 mg, 5 mg, 25 mg. Tablet: 25 mg, 100 mg, 150 mg, 200 mg. [leh-MOH-trih-jeen]. 241, 265

Lanacane (Derm) (generic *benzocaine*). Topical anesthetic. Cream: 6%. Spray: 20%. 94

Lanacort 5, Lanacort 5 Creme, Lanacort 10 Creme (Derm) (generic *hydrocortisone*). Topical corticosteroid anti-inflammatory drug. Cream: 0.5%, 1%. Ointment: 0.5%. 92

Landsteiner, Karl. 378

(Laniazid) (Resp). No longer on the market. (Generic name *isoniazid;* used to treat tuberculosis).

lanolin. 7

Lanoxicaps (Cardio). Cardiac glycoside drug used to treat atrial flutter/fibrillation and congestive heart failure. For dosage, see *digoxin*. [leh-NAWK-see-kehps]. 152, 160

Lanoxin (Cardio). Cardiac glycoside drug used to treat atrial flutter/fibrillation and congestive heart failure. For dosage, see *digoxin*. [leh-NAWK-sihn.] 152, 160

lanreotide (Ipstyl) (Endo). Used to treat acromegaly. Orphan drug. 230

lansoprazole (Prevacid) (GI). Proton pump inhibitor used to treat peptic ulcers, gastroesophageal reflux disease, and *H. pylori* infections. Capsule: 15 mg, 30 mg. 119, 121

Lantus (Diab). Long-acting human recombinant DNA glargine insulin. Subcutaneous: 100 units/mL. [LEHN-tuhs]. 238

(Largon) (Neuro). No longer on the market. (Generic name *propiomazine*; nonbarbiturate used to treat insomnia).

Larodopa (Neuro). Used to treat Parkinson's disease. For dosage, see *levodopa*. [leh-roh-DOH-pah]. 268

(Lasan) (Derm). No longer on the market. (Generic name *anthralin*; topical drug used to treat psoriasis).

Lasix (Endo, Uro). Loop diuretic; also used to treat syndrome of inappropriate antidiuretic hormone. For dosage, see *furosemide*. [LAY-sicks]. 104, 231

L-asparaginase (Chemo). See *aspariginase*.

latanoprost (Xalatan) (Oph). Topical drug used to treat glaucoma. Ophthalmic solution: 0.005%. [leh-TEH-noh-prawst]. 222

laughing gas. 366

law, drug. See *legislation, drug*.

laxative.
  bulk-producing. 125
  irritant. 124
  magnesium. 124
  mechanical. 125
  stool softener. 125

laxatives (GI). Class of drugs used to treat constipation. 124

L-baclofen (Neuralgon) (ENT, Ortho). Skeletal muscle relaxant used to treat trigeminal neuralgia; used to treat severe muscle spasticity associated with multiple sclerosis, cerebral palsy, stroke, or spinal cord injury. Orphan drug. 145, 276

L-dopa (Neuro). Used to treat Parkinson's disease. For dosage, see *levodopa*. 268

lead poisoning, drugs used to treat.

(Ledercillin VK) (Antibio). No longer on the market. (Generic name *penicillin*; antibiotic).

leflunomide (Arava) (Cardio, GI, Ortho, Uro). Used to treat rheumatoid arthritis; an orphan drug used to prevent rejection of a transplanted heart, liver, or kidney. Tablet: 10 mg, 20 mg, 100 mg.

Legionnaire's disease, drugs used to treat. 198

legislation, drug. 12

(Lente Iletin I) (Diab). No longer on the market. (Generic name *insulin*; intermediate-acting insulin).

Lente Iletin II (Diab). Intermediate-acting lente insulin. Subcutaneous: 100 units/mL. [LEHN-tay Il-leh-tihn]. 238

(Lente L) (Diab). No longer on the market. (Generic name *insulin*).

lepirudin (Refludan) (Hem). Used to treat heparin-induced thrombocytopenia. Intravenous (powder to be reconstituted): 50 mg.

Lescol, Lescol XL (Cardio). HMG-CoA reductase inhibitor drug used to treat hypercholesterolemia. For dosage, see *fluvastatin*. [LEHS-cawl]. 170

letrazuril (Antivir). Used to treat AIDS-related diarrhea. Investigational drug. 328

letrozole (Femara) (Chemo). Hormonal chemotherapy drug used to treat breast cancer. Tablet: 2.5 mg. [LEH-troh-zohl]. 343

Leucomax (Antivir). Granulocyte macrophage colony-stimulating factor used to treat neutropenia in AIDS patients; used to treat neutropenia in patients taking ganciclovir. For dosage, see *molgramostim*. [LOO-koh-mehks].

leucovorin (Wellcovorin) (Chemo). Cytoprotective drug used to prevent toxicity in patients receiving high-dose methotrexate. Tablet: 5 mg, 15 mg, 25 mg. Intravenous: 3 mg/mL, 10 mg/mL, (powder to be reconstituted) 50 mg, 100 mg, 350 mg. [loo-koh-VOHR-ehn]. 350

leucovorin rescue. 350

(Leukeran) (Chemo). No longer on the market. (Generic name *chlorambucil*; alkylating chemotherapy drug).

Leukine (Antivir, Chemo). Granulocyte macrophage colony-stimulating factor used to increase white blood cell count in AIDS patients receiving zidovudine; used to stimulate white blood cell count after chemotherapy or with bone marrow transplant. For dosage, see *sargramostim*.

leukotriene receptor blockers (Resp). Class of drugs used to treat asthma. 195

leuprolide (Eligard, Lupron, Lupron Depot, Lupron Depot-Ped, Lupron Depot-4 Month, Lupron Depot-3 Month, Viadur) (Chemo, Endo, OB/GYN). Hormonal chemotherapy drug used to treat prostatic cancer; used to treat precocious puberty; used to treat endometrosis and uterine leiomyomata. Subcutaneous or intramuscular: 5 mg/mL, 3.75 mg (microspheres), 7.5 mg (microspheres), 11.25 mg (microspheres), 15 mg (microspheres), 22.5 mg (microspheres), 30 mg (microspheres). Implant: 1 every 12 months. [LOO-proh-lide]. 248, 343

Leustatin (Chemo). Purine antagonist chemotherapy drug used to treat leukemia, non-Hodgkin's lymphoma, and cutaneous T-cell lymphoma. For dosage, see *cladribine*. [loo-STEH-tihn]. 339

Leuvectin (Chemo). Chemotherapy drug used to treat kidney cancer. Orphan drug. 348

levalbuterol (Xopenex) (Resp). Bronchodilator. Nebulizer: 0.63 mg/3 mL, 1.25 mg/3 mL. [lee-vehl-BYOO-teh-rawl]. 193

levamisole (Ergamisol) (Chemo). Chemotherapy drug used to treat colon cancer. Tablet: 50 mg. [lee-VAH-meh-sohl]. 348

Levaquin (Antibio). Fluoroquinolone antibiotic used to treat a variety of infections, including *Streptococcus*, *H. influenzae*, *Staphylococcus*, *E. coli*, community-acquired pneumonia, and Legionnaire's disease. For dosage, see *levofloxacin*. [LEH-vah-kwihn]. 105, 198, 318

Levatol (Cardio). Nonselective beta-blocker used to treat hypertension. For dosage, see *penbutolol*. 162

Levbid (GI, Uro). Antispasmodic drug used to treat spasm of the smooth muscle of the bowel and bladder. For dosage, see *L-hyoscyamine*. 122

levetiracetam (Keppra) (Neuro). Anticonvulsant drug used to treat partial seizures. Tablet: 250 mg, 500 mg, 750 mg. 265

Levlen (OB/GYN) (generic *levonorgestrel, ethinyl estradiol*). Monophasic combination progestins and estrogen oral contraceptive. Tablet: 0.15 mg/30 mcg. [LEHV-lehn]. 249

Levlite (OB/GYN) (generic *levonorgestrel, ethinyl estradiol*). Monophasic combination progestins and estrogen oral contraceptive. Tablet: 0.1 mg/20 mcg.

levobetaxolol (Betaxon) (Oph). Topical beta-receptor blocker drug used to treat glaucoma. Ophthalmic suspension: 0.5%. [lee-voh-beh-TACK-soh-lawl]. 221

levobunolol (Betagan Liquifilm) (Oph). Topical beta-receptor blocker used to treat glaucoma. Ophthalmic solution: 0.25%, 0.5%. [lee-voh-BUH-noh-lawl]. 221

levocabastine (Livostin) (Oph). Topical antihistamine used to treat allergy symptoms in the eyes; also an orphan drug used to treat vernal keratoconjunctivitis. Ophthalmic suspension: 0.05%. [lee-voh-kah-BEH-steen]. 220

levocarnitine (Carnitor) (Antivir). Used to protect against toxicity in patients receiving zidovudine. Orphan drug. 331

levodopa (L-dopa) (Larodopa) (Neuro). Used to treat Parkinson's disease. Tablet: 100 mg, 250 mg, 500 mg. [lee-voh-DOH-pah]. 268

Levo-Dromoran (Analges, Anes). Narcotic analgesic drug used to treat moderate-to-severe pain; preoperative drug used to produce sedation. (Schedule II drug). For dosage, see *levorphanol*. [lee-voh-DROH-mohr-ehn]. 297, 371

levofloxacin (Levaquin) (Antibio). Fluoroquinolone antibiotic used to treat a variety of infections, including *Streptococcus, H. influenzae, Staphylococcus, E. coli,* community-acquired pneumonia, and Legionnaire's disease. Tablet: 250 mg, 500 mg, 750 mg. Intravenous: 5 mg/mL, 25 mg/mL. [lee-voh-FLAWK-sah-sihn]. 105, 198, 318

levofloxacin (Quixin) (Oph). Topical antibiotic used to treat bacterial eye infections. Ophthalmic solution: 0.5%. [lee-voh-FLAWK-sah-sihn].

levomethadyl (Orlaam) (Analges). Narcotic used to manage heroin and narcotic dependence and withdrawal. (Schedule II drug). Liquid: 10 mg/mL. [lee-voh-MEH-thah-dill]. 308

Levophed (Emerg). Vasopressor used to treat hypotension during emergency resuscitation. For dosage, see *norepinephrine*. [LEE-voh-fehd]. 181

(Levoprome) (Analges). No longer on the market. (Generic name *methotrimeprazine*; nonnarcotic analgesic).

Levora 0.15/30 (OB/GYN) (generic *levonorgestrel, ethinyl estradiol*). Monophasic combination progestins and estrogen oral contraceptive. Tablet: 0.15 mg/30 mcg. [lee-VOHR-ah].

levorotary. 64

levorphanol (Levo-Dromoran) (Analges, Anes). Narcotic analgesic drug used to treat moderate-to-severe pain; preoperative drug used to produce sedation. (Schedule II drug). Tablet: 2 mg. [lee-VOHR-fah-nawl]. 297, 371

Levo-T (Endo). Thyroid hormone replacement. For dosage, see *levothyroxine*. 229

Levothroid (Endo). Thyroid hormone replacement. For dosage, see *levothyroxine*. [LEE-voh-throyd]. 229

levothyroxine (Levo-T, Levothroid, Synthroid, Unithroid) (Endo). Thyroid hormone replacement. Tablet: 0.025 mg, 0.05 mg, 0.075 mg, 0.088 mg, 0.1 mg, 0.112 mg, 0.125 mg, 0.137 mg, 0.15 mg, 0.175 mg, 0.2 mg, 0.3 mg. Intravenous (powder to be reconstituted): 200 mcg/10 mL, 500 mcg/10 mL. [lee-voh-thy-RAWK-zeen]. 229

Levsin, Levsin Drops, Levsin/SL (GI, Uro). Antispasmodic drug used to treat spasm of the smooth muscle of the bowel and bladder. For dosage, see *L-hyoscyamine*. 122

Levsinex Timecaps (GI, Uro). Antispasmodic drug used to treat spasm of the smooth muscle of the bowel and bladder. For dosage, see *L-hyoscyamine*. [LEH-sih-nehks]. 122

Levulan Kerastick (Derm) (generic *aminolevulinic acid*). Topical drug used to treat actinic keratoses. Liquid: 20%. [LEH-vyoo-lehn]. 98

Lexxel Extended-Release Tablet (Cardio) (generic *enalapril, felodipine*). Combination of two antihypertensive drugs. Tablet: 5 mg/2.5 mg, 2 mg/5 mg. 166

L-hyoscyamine (Anaspaz, Cystospaz, Cystospaz-M, Gastrosed, Levbid, Levsin, Levsin Drops, Levsin/SL, Levsinex Timecaps) (GI, Uro). Antispasmodic drug used to treat spasm of the smooth muscle of the bowel and bladder. Capsule: 0.375 mg. Elixir: 0.125 mg/5 mL. Liquid: 0.125 mg/mL. Tablet: 0.125 mg, 0.15mg, 0.375 mg. Sublingual tablet: 0.125 mg. Subcutaneous, intramuscular, or intravenous: 0.5 mg/mL. [hy-oh-SY-ah-meen]. 107, 122

Librax (GI, Psych) (generic *chlordiazepoxide, clidinium*). Combination antianxiety and antispasmodic drug. Capsule: 5 mg/2.5 mg. [LIH-bracks]. 122, 293

Librum (Anes, Neuro, Psych). Benzodiazepine drug used as a preoperative medication to relieve anxiety and provide sedation; used to treat anxiety and neurosis; used to treat alcohol withdrawal and prevent seizures. (Schedule IV drug). For dosage, see *chlordiazepoxide*. [LEH-bree-uhm]. 267

lice, drugs used to treat. 95

Lidakol (Antivir). Antiviral drug used to treat AIDS. Investigational drug. 326

Lidex, Lidex-E (Derm) (generic *fluocinonide*). Topical corticosteroid anti-inflammatory drug. Cream: 0.05%. Gel: 0.05%. Liquid: 0.05%. Ointment: 0.05%. [LY-dehks]. 92

lidocaine (Anestacon, Xylocaine) (Uro). Topical anesthetic applied to the urethra prior to cystoscopic procedures. Jelly: 2%. [LY-doh-kayn]. 111

lidocaine (Dentipatch, Xylocaine, Xylocaine 10% Oral, Xylocaine Viscous) (ENT). Topical dental and oral anesthetic. Dental patch. Oral liquid: 2%, 4%. Spray: 10%. [LY-doh-kayn].

lidocaine (Lidoderm Patch) (Derm, Neuro). Topical anesthetic used to treat the pain of herpes zoster lesions (shingles) and postherpetic neuralgia. Orphan drug. Patch: 5% (patch can be cut into pieces). [LY-doh-kayn]. 91, 276

lidocaine (LidoPen Auto-Injector) (Cardio). Self-injected drug used by the patient to treat cardiac arrhythmias. Intramuscular: 300 mg/3 mL. [LY-doh-kayn]. 159

lidocaine (Solarcaine Aloe Extra Burn Relief, Xylocaine, Unguentine Plus, Zilactin-L) (Derm). Topical anesthetic. Cream: 0.5%, 2%. Gel: 0.5%. Liquid: 2.5%, 5%. Ointment: 2.5%, 5%. Spray: 0.5%. [LY-doh-kayn]. 94

lidocaine (Xylocaine) (Oph). Anesthetic injected into the eye during surgery to produce corneal anesthesia and akinesis. Retrobulbar injection: 4%. [LY-doh-kayn].

lidocaine (Xylocaine HCl IV for Cardiac Arrhythmias) (Cardio, Emerg). Used to treat ventricular arrhythmias. Endotracheal or intravenous: 0.2%, 0.4%, 0.8%, 1%, 2%, 4%, 10%, 20%, 2 mg/mL, 4 mg/mL, 8 mg/mL, 10 mg/mL, 20 mg/mL, 40 mg/mL, 100 mg/mL, 200 mg/mL. [LY-doh-kayn]. 159, 180

lidocaine (Xylocaine, Xylocaine MPF) (Anes). Local, regional nerve block, epidural, and spinal anesthetic. Injection: 0.5%; 0.5% with 1:200,000 epinephrine; 1.0%; 1.0% with 1:100,000 epinephrine; 1.0% with 1:200,000 epinephrine; 1.5%; 1.5% with 1:200,000 epinephrine; 2%; 2% with 1:50,000 epinephrine; 2% with 1:100,000 epinephrine; 2% with 1:200,000 epinephrine; 4%. [LY-doh-kayn]. 367, 368

Lidoderm Patch (Derm, Neuro) (generic *lidocaine*). Topical anesthetic used to treat the pain of herpes zoster lesions (shingles) and postherpetic neuralgia. Orphan drug. Patch: 5% (patch can be cut into pieces). [LY-doh-dehrm]. 91, 276

LidoPen Auto-Injector (Emerg). Self-administered injectable lidocaine used to treat ventricular arrhythmias. Intramuscular: 10% (300 mg/3 mL). [LY-doh-pehn]. 159

Limbitrol DS 10-25 (Psych) (generic *amitriptyline, chlordiazepoxide*). Combination antidepressant and antianxiety drug. Tablet: 12.5 mg/5 mg, 25 mg/10 mg. [LIHM-beh-trawl]. 292

Lincocin (Antibio). Antibiotic used to treat serious infections, including *Staphylococcus, Streptococcus,* and *Pneumococcus.* For dosage, see *lincomycin.* [LIHN-koh-sihn]. 319

lincomycin (Lincocin) (Antibio). Antibiotic used to treat serious infections, including *Staphylococcus, Streptococcus,* and *Pneumococcus.* Capsule: 500 mg. Intramuscular or intravenous: 300 mg/mL. [lihn-koh-MY-sihn]. 319

lindane (Derm). Topical drug used to treat scabies (mites) and pediculosis (lice). Lotion: 1%. Shampoo: 1%. 95

linezolid (Zyvox) (Antibio). Antibiotic used to treat a variety of bacterial infections, including *Staphylococcus, Streptococcus,* and community-acquired pneumonia; used to treat methicillin-resistant *Staphylococcus aureus* (MRSA); used to treat vancomycin-resistant *Enterococcus.* Tablet: 400 mg, 800 mg. Intravenous (powder to be reconstituted): 100 mg/5 mL. 319

Linomide (Chemo). Used to treat leukemia patients who have undergone bone marrow transplantation. For dosage, see *roquinimex.* 362

Lioresal (GI, Neuro, Ortho, Psych). Skeletal muscle relaxant used to treat intractable hiccoughs; used to treat trigeminal neuralgia/tic douloureux; used to treat severe muscle spasticity associated with multiple sclerosis, cerebral palsy, stroke, or spinal cord injury; used to treat tardive dyskinesia caused by antipsychotic drugs. For dosage, see *baclofen.* [lee-OH-reh-sawl]. 132, 145, 275, 284

liothyronine (Cytomel, Triostat) (Endo). Thyroid hormone replacement. Tablet: 5 mcg, 25 mcg, 50 mcg. Intravenous: 10 mcg/mL. [ly-oh-THY-roh-neen]. 229

liotrix (Thyrolar) (Endo). Thyroid hormone replacement used to treat hypothyroidism. Tablet: 15 mg (1/4 grain), 30 mg (1/2 grain), 60 mg (1 grain), 120 mg (2 grains), 180 mg (3 grains). [LY-oh-trihks]. 229

lipase inhibitors (GI). Class of drugs used to treat obesity. 129

lipids, intravenous. See *intravenous lipids.*

Lipisorb (GI). Liquid nutritional supplement. Powder (to be reconstituted). 131

Lipitor (Cardio). HMG-CoA reductase inhibitor drug used to treat hypercholesterolemia. For dosage, see *atorvastatin.* 170

Liposyn II 10%, Liposyn II 20%, Liposyn III 10%, Liposyn III 20% (I.V.). Intravenous fat solution. 378

liquid nutritional supplements. 130

Liquifilm Tears (Oph). Artificial tears.

(Liquiprin) (Analges). No longer on the market. (Generic name *acetaminophen*; nonnarcotic non-aspirin analgesic drug).

lisinopril (Prinivil, Zestril) (Cardio). Angiotensin-converting enzyme inhibitor drug used to treat congestive heart failure and hypertension; used to improve survival rate after myocardial infarction. Tablet: 2.5 mg, 5 mg, 10 mg, 20 mg, 40 mg. [ly-SIH-noh-prihl]. 154, 158, 163

lispro (Humalog) (Endo). Human recombinant DNA insulin. Dose: Units. [LIHS-proh].

lithium (Eskalith, Eskalith CR, Lithobid) (Analges, Antivir, Chemo, Endo). Antipsychotic drug used to prevent cluster headaches; used to treat neutropenia in AIDS patients receiving zidovudine; used to treat chemotherapy-induced neutropenia; used to treat syndrome of inappropriate antidiuretic hormone. Capsule: 150 mg, 300 mg, 600 mg. Tablet: 300 mg, 450 mg. Syrup: 8 mEq/5 mL (300 mg/5 mL). [LIH-thee-uhm]. 231, 331, 362

lithium (Eskalith, Eskalith CR, Lithobid) (Psych). Antipsychotic drug used to treat the mania of manic-depressive disorder; used to treat tardive dyskinesia, a side effect of antipsychotic drugs; used to treat bulimia nervosa. Capsule: 150 mg, 300 mg, 600 mg. Tablet: 300 mg, 450 mg. Syrup: 8 mEq/5 mL. [LIH-thee-uhm]. 284, 288, 291

Lithobid (Psych). Antipsychotic drug used to treat the mania of manic-depressive disorder; used to treat tardive dyskinesia, a side effect of antipsychotic drugs; used to treat bulimia nervosa. For dosage, see *lithium*. [LIH-thoh-bihd]. 284, 288, 291

Lithobid (Analges, Antivir, Chemo, Endo). Antipsychotic drug used to prevent cluster headaches; used to treat neutropenia in AIDS patients receiving zidovudine; used to treat chemotherapy-induced neutropenia; used to treat syndrome of inappropriate antidiuretic hormone. For dosage, see *lithium*. [LIH-thoh-bihd]. 231, 331, 362

Lithostat (Uro). Used to treat urinary tract infections caused by urea-splitting bacteria. For dosage, see *acetohydroxamic acid*. 106

(Lithotabs) (Antivir, Chemo, Psych). No longer on the market. (Generic name *lithium*; used to treat manic-depressive disorder; used to treat neutropenia in AIDS and chemotherapy patients).

Livial (OB/GYN). Steroid that stimulates estrogen, progesterone, and androgen receptors; used to treat menopause in women who cannot or will not take estrogen hormone replacement therapy. Investigational drug. 253

Livostin (Oph). Topical antihistamine used to treat allergy symptoms in the eyes. For dosage, see *levocabastine*. [LIH-voh-stihn]. 220

L-glutathione (Cachexon) (Antivir). Used to treat AIDS wasting syndrome. Orphan drug.

L-leucovorin (Isovorin) (Chemo). Cytoprotective drug used to prevent toxicity in patients receiving fluorouracil and methotrexate chemotherapy. Orphan drug. 350

loading dose. 64

LoCHOLEST, LoCHOLEST Light (Cardio, Emerg). Bile acid sequestrant drug used to treat hypercholesterolemia; used to treat digitalis toxicity; used to treat thyroid hormone overdose or pesticide poisoning. For dosage, see *cholestyramine*. 153, 169

Locoid (Derm) (generic *hydrocortisone*). Topical corticosteroid anti-inflammatory drug. Cream: 0.1%. Liquid: 0.1%. Ointment: 0.1%. [LOH-koyd]. 92

Lodine, Lodine XL (Analges, Ortho). Nonsteroidal anti-inflammatory drug used to treat pain; used to treat bursitis, gout, osteoarthritis, rheumatoid arthritis, and tendinitis. For dosage, see *etodolac*. [LOH-deen]. 139, 304

Lodosyn (Neuro). Used to treat Parkinson's disease. For dosage, see *carbidopa*. [loh-DOH-sihn]. 268

lodoxamide (Alomide) (Oph). Topical mast cell stabilizer used to treat allergy symptoms in the eyes; used to treat vernal keratoconjunctivitis. Ophthalmic solution: 0.1%. [loh-DAWK-sah-mide]. 220

Loestrin Fe 1/20, Loestrin Fe 1.5/30, Loestrin 21 1/20, Loestrin 21 1.5/30 (OB/GYN) (generic *norethindrone, ethinyl estradiol*). Monophasic combination progestins and estrogen oral contraceptive. Tablet: 1 mg/20 mcg, 1.5 mg/30 mcg. [loh-EHS-trihn]. 249

Lofenalac (GI). Infant formula for infants with phenylketonuria. Powder (to be reconstituted).

lofexidine (Analges). Used to treat narcotic withdrawal. Investigational drug. 308

lomefloxacin (Maxaquin) (Antibio). Fluoroquinolone antibiotic used to treat a variety of infections, including *E. coli, H. influenzae,* and *Pseudomonas*; used to treat Legionnaire's disease. Tablet: 400 mg. [loh-mee-FLAWK-sah-sihn]. 105, 198, 318

Lomotil (GI). Narcotic antidiarrheal drug. For dosage, see *diphenoxylate*. [loh-MOH-tihl]. 123

lomustine (CeeNu) (Chemo). Alkylating chemotherapy drug used to treat brain cancer and Hodgkin's disease. Capsule: 10 mg, 40 mg, 100 mg. Dose pack: 100 mg (2 capsules), 40 mg (2 capsules), 10 mg (2 capsules). [loh-MUH-steen]. 341

Loniten (Cardio). Vasodilator. For dosage, see *minoxidil*. 166

Lonalac (GI). Liquid nutritional supplement. Powder (to be reconstituted). 131

loop diuretics (Uro). Class of diuretics that acts directly at the loop of Henle to excrete sodium and water.

loop of Henle.

Lo/Ovral (OB/GYN) (generic *norgestrel, ethinyl estradiol*). Monophasic combination progestins and estrogen oral contraceptive. Tablet: 0.3 mg/30 mcg. [loh-OHV-rawl]. 249

loperamide (Imodium A-D, Kaopectate II, Pepto Diarrhea Control) (GI). Nonnarcotic antidiarrheal drug. Capsule: 2 mg. Liquid: 1 mg/mL, 1 mg/5 mL. Tablet: 2 mg. 123

Lopid (Cardio). Used to treat hypertriglyceridemia by decreasing serum triglyercides and very low-density lipoprotein levels. For dosage, see *gemfibrozil*. 171

Lopressor (Analges, Ortho, Psych). Cardioselective beta-blocker used to treat migraine headaches; used to treat essential familial tremors; used to treat the side effects of muscle restlessness from antipsychotic drugs. For dosage, see *metoprolol*. [loh-PREH-sohr]. 146, 294, 306

Lopressor (Cardio). Cardioselective beta-blocker used to treat angina pectoris, congestive heart failure, hypertension, and ventricular arrhythmias; used to prevent repeat myocardial infarction. For dosage, see *metoprolol*. [loh-PREH-sohr]. 157, 158, 160, 162

Lopressor HCT 50/25, Lopressor HCT 100/25, Lopressor HCT 100/50 (Cardio) (generic *metoprolol, hydrochlorothiazide*). Combination beta-blocker antihypertensive and diuretic drug. Tablet: 50 mg/25 mg, 100 mg/25 mg, 100 mg/50 mg. [loh-PREH-sohr]. 167

Loprox (Derm) (generic *ciclopirox*). Topical antifungal drug. Cream: 0.77%. Lotion: 0.77%. [LOH-prawks]. 89

Lorabid (Antibio). Cephalosporin antibiotic used to treat a variety of bacterial infections, including *Streptococcus, Staphylococcus*, and *H. influenzae*. For dosage, see *loracarbef*. [LOH-rah-bihd]. 316

loracarbef (Lorabid) (Antibio). Cephalosporin antibiotic used to treat a variety of bacterial infections, including streptococci, staphylococci, and *H. influenzae*. Capsule/Pulvule: 200 mg, 400 mg. Liquid: 100 mg/5 mL, 200 mg/5 mL. [lohr-ah-KAHR-behf]. 316

loratadine (Claritin, Claritin Reditabs) (Derm, ENT). Antihistamine used to treat allergic rhinitis and allergic reactions with hives and itching. Liquid: 1 mg/mL. Syrup: 10 mg/10 mL. Tablet: 10 mg. [lohr-EH-teh-deen]. 207

lorazepam (Ativan) (Anes, Neuro, Psych). Benzodiazepine drug used as a preoperative medication to decrease anxiety and produce sedation; used to treat status epilepticus; used to treat chronic insomnia; used to treat anxiety and neurosis; used to treat alcohol withdrawal. (Schedule IV drug). Tablet: 0.5 mg, 1 mg, 2 mg. Liquid: 2 mg/mL. Intramuscular or intravenous: 4 mg/mL. [lohr-EH-zeh-pehm]. 267, 272, 281, 371

Lorcet-HD, Lorcet Plus (Analges) (generic *hydrocodone, acetaminophen*). Combination narcotic and nonnarcotic analgesic drug. (Schedule III drug). Capsule: 5 mg/500 mg. Tablet: 7.5 mg/650 mg. [LOHR-seht]. 302

Lortab, Lortab 2.5/500, Lortab 5/500, Lortab 7.5/500, Lortab 10/500, Lortab 10/650 (Analges) (generic *hydrocodone, acetaminophen*). Combination narcotic and nonnarcotic analgesic drug. (Schedule III drug). Liquid: 2.5 mg/167 mg. Tablet: 2.5 mg/500 mg, 5 mg/500 mg, 7.5 mg/500 mg, 10 mg/500 mg, 10 mg/650 mg. [LOHR-tehb]. 303

Lortab ASA (Analges) (generic *hydrocodone, aspirin*). Combination narcotic and nonnarcotic analgesic drug. (Schedule III drug). Tablet: 5 mg/500 mg. [LOHR-tehb]. 302

losartan (Cozaar) (Cardio). Angiotensin II receptor blocker used to treat hypertension. Tablet: 25 mg, 50 mg, 100 mg. [loh-SAWR-tehn]. 164

Lotemax (Oph). Topical corticosteroid used to treat inflammation of the eyes. For dosage, see *loteprednol*. 219

Lotensin (Cardio). Angiotensin-converting enzyme inhibitor used to treat hypertension. For dosage, see *benazepril*. [loh-TEH-sihn]. 163

Lotensin 5/6.25, Lotensin HCT 10/12.5, Lotensin HCT 20/12.5, Lotensin HCT 20/25 (Cardio) (generic *benazepril, hydrochlorothiazide*). Combination angiotensin-converting enzyme inhibitor antihypertensive and diuretic drug. Tablet: 5 mg/6.25 mg, 10 mg/12.5 mg, 20 mg/12.5 mg, 20 mg/25 mg. [loh-TEH-sihn]. 167

loteprednol (Alrex, Lotemax) (Oph). Topical corticosteroid used to treat inflammation of the eyes. Ophthalmic suspension: 0.2%, 0.5%. [loh-teh-PREHD-nawl]. 219

lotion. 35

Lotrel (Cardio) (generic *amlodipine, benazepril*). Combination of two antihypertensive drugs. Capsule: 2.5 mg/10 mg, 5 mg/10 mg, 5 mg/20 mg. 166

Lotrimin, Lotrimin AF 1% (Derm) (generic *clotrimazole*). Topical antifungal and antiyeast drug. Cream: 1%. Liquid: 1%. Lotion: 1%. [LOH-treh-mihn]. 89

Lotrimin AF 2% (Derm) (generic *miconazole*). Topical antifungal drug. Powder: 2%. Spray: 2%. [LOH-treh-mihn]. 89

Lotrisone (Derm) (generic *betamethasone, clotrimazole*). Topical combination corticosteroid and antifungal/antiyeast drug. Cream: 0.05%/1%. [LOH-trih-zohn]. 89, 90

Lotronex (GI). Used to treat diarrhea in women with irritable bowel syndrome. For dosage, see *alosetron*.

lovastatin (Mevacor) (Cardio). HMG-CoA reductase inhibitor drug used to treat hypercholesterolemia. Tablet: 10 mg, 20 mg, 40 mg. [loh-vah-STEH-tihn]. 170

Lovenox (Hem). Low molecular weight heparin anticoagulant; used to prevent deep venous thrombosis in patients with restricted mobility. For dosage, see *enoxaparin*. [LAH-veh-nawks].

low molecular weight heparins. In Depth feature.

loxapine (Loxitane, Loxitane C) (Psych). Drug used to treat psychosis. Capsule: 5 mg, 10 mg, 25 mg, 50 mg. Liquid: 25 mg/mL. Intramuscular: 50 mg/mL. [LAWK-sah-peen]. 284

Loxitane, Loxitane C (Psych). Drug used to treat psychosis. For dosage, see *loxapine*. [LAWK-seh-tayhn]. 284

Lozol (Uro). Thiazide diuretic. For dosage, see *indapamide*. [LOH-zawl]. 103

lozenge. 35

L-PAM. See *melphalan*.

LR. See *lactated Ringer's*.

LSD (abbreviation for *lysergic acid diethylamide*). 16

L-threonin (Threostat) (Neuro). Used to treat spasticity associated with amyotrophic lateral sclerosis. Orphan drug. 276

(Ludiomil) (Psych). No longer on the market. (Generic name *maprotiline*; tetracyclic antidepressant).

Lufyllin, Lufyllin-400 (Resp). Bronchodilator. For dosage, see *dyphylline*. [LAH-fih-lihn]. 193

Lufyllin-EPG (Resp) (generic *dyphylline, ephedrine, guaifenesin, phenobarbital*). Combination drug with two bronchodilators, an expectorant, and a sedative. Liquid: 150 mg/24 mg/300 mg/24 mg. Tablet: 100 mg/16 mg/200 mg/16 mg. [LAH-fih-lihn]. 195

Lufyllin-GG (Resp) (generic *dyphylline, guaifenesin*). Combination bronchodilator and expectorant drug. Liquid: 100 mg/100 mg. Tablet: 200 mg/200 mg. [LAH-fih-lihn]. 195

Lugol's Solution (Endo). Combination iodine and potassium antithyroid drug given prior to thyroidectomy. Drops: 5% iodine/10% potassium. [LOO-gawlz soh-LOO-shun]. 230

Lumigan (Oph). Topical drug used to treat glaucoma. For dosage, see *bimatoprost*. [LOO-meh-gehn]. 222

Luminal (Neuro). Barbiturate used to treat tonic-clonic and partial seizures; used to treat status epilepticus; used to treat the seizures of eclampsia during pregnancy; used to treat insomnia. (Schedule IV drug). For dosage, see *phenobarbital*. [LOO-meh-nawl]. 264, 267, 272

Lunelle (OB/GYN) (generic *medroxyprogesterone, estradiol*). Monophasic combination progestins and estrogen one-month contraceptive. Intramuscular: 25 mg/5 mg per 0.5 mL. [loo-NELL]. 250

Lupron, Lupron Depot, Lupron Depot-Ped, Lupron Depot-4 Month, Lupron Depot-3 Month (Chemo, Endo, OB/GYN). Hormonal chemotherapy drug used to treat prostatic cancer; used to treat precocious puberty; used to treat endometrosis and uterine leiomyomata. For dosage, see *leuprolide*. [LOO-prawn]. 248, 343

Lutrepulse (OB/GYN). Pituitary gland hormone drug used to treat amenorrhea. For dosage, see *gonadorelin*. [LOO-treh-puhls]. 253

Luvox (Psych). (OB/GYN). Selective serotonin reuptake inhibitor antidepressant used to treat premenstrual dysphoric disorder. For dosage, see *fluvoxamine*. [LOO-vawks]. 255

Luvox (Psych). Selective serotonin reuptake inhibitor antidepressant used to treat depression; used to treat anxiety; used to treat obsessive-compulsive disorder; used to treat autism; used to treat social anxiety disorder; used to treat panic disorder; used to treat posttraumatic stress disorder. For dosage, see *fluvoxamine*. [LOO-vawks]. 282, 287, 289, 290

Luxiq (Derm) (generic *betamethasone*). Topical corticosteroid anti-inflammatory drug. Foam: 1.2 mg/g. [luhks-EEK]. 92

LymphoCide (Chemo). Monoclonal antibody used to treat non-Hodgkin's lymphoma. Orphan drug. 346

(lypressin) (Endo). No longer on the market. (Trade name *Diapid*; used to treat diabetes insipidus).

lysergic acid diethylamide (LSD) (Misc). Illegal drug with no medical use. (Schedule I drug).

Lysodase (GI). Used to treat Gaucher's disease. Orphan drug.

Lysodren (Chemo). Chemotherapy drug used to treat cancer of the adrenal cortex. For dosage, see *mitotane*. 348

Maalox Antacid Caplets (GI). Calcium-containing antacid. Tablet: 1000 mg. 116

Maalox Anti-Gas (GI). Antiflatulent drug. For dosage, see *simethicone*. 118

Maalox, Maalox Therapeutic Concentrate (GI) (generic *aluminum, magnesium*). Combination antacid. Suspension: 140 mg/175 mg, 225 mg/200 mg, 600 mg/300 mg. 117

Macrobid (Antibio, Uro). Antibiotic used only to treat urinary tract infections. For dosage, see *nitrofurantoin*. [MEH-kroh-bihd]. 106, 319

Macrodantin (Antibio, Uro). Antibiotic used only to treat urinary tract infections. For dosage, see *nitrofurantoin*. [meh-kroh-DEHN-tihn]. 106, 319

Macrodex (I.V.). Intravenous nonblood plasma volume expander. 382

macrolide antibiotics (Antibio). Class of antibiotics. 318

mafenide (Sulfamylon) (Derm). Topical antibiotic used to treat severe burns. Cream, liquid. 97

"magic bullet, the."

magnesium salicylate (Backache Maximum Strength Relief, Bayer Select Maximum Strength Backache Formula, Extra Strength Doan's) (Analges). Salicylate nonaspirin drug used to treat pain and inflammation. Caplet: 467 mg, 500 mg, 580 mg. Tablet: 545 mg, 600 mg. [mahg-NEE-see-umh sah-LIH-seh-layt]. 300

magnesium sulfate (Neuro, OB/GYN, Uro). Anticonvulsant drug used to prevent seizures in pregnant women in preeclampsia; used to treat nephritis. Intramuscular or intravenous: 12.5% (1 mEq/mL), 50% (4 mEq/mL). 267

magnetic targeted carrier (Chemo). 362

maintenance dose. 64

Maitec (Antivir). Antibiotic used to treat *Mycobacterium avium-intracellulare* in AIDS patients. For dosage, see *gentamicin liposomal*. 329

major tranquilizers. See *antipsychotic drugs*.

malathion (Ovide) (Derm). Topical drug used to treat pediculosis (lice). Lotion: 0.5%. [mah-LAY-thee-awn]. 95

(Mandelamine) (Uro). No longer on the market. (Generic name *methenamine*; urinary tract antibiotic).

Mandol (Antibio). Cephalosporin antibiotic used to treat a variety of bacterial infections, including *Streptococcus*, *Staphylococcus*, *E. coli*, and *H. influenzae*. For dosage, see *cefamandole*. [MEHN-dawl]. 315

manic-depressive disorder, drugs used to treat. 288

mannitol (Osmitrol) (Neuro, Oph, Uro). Diuretic used to decrease cerebral edema; used to decrease intraocular pressure; used to treat renal failure. Intravenous: 5%, 10%, 15%, 20%, 25%. [MEH-neh-tawl]. 112, 276

mannitol (Resectisol) (Uro). Used during urologic surgical procedures. Irrigation solution. [MEH-neh-tawl]. 112

Mantoux test (Aplisol, Tubersol) (Resp). Diagnostic test that uses purified protein derivative (PPD) from *Mycobacterium tuberculosis* injected under the skin to test for tuberculosis. Intradermal injection: 5 TU/0.1 mL. [mehn-TOO].

MAO (abbreviation for *monoamine oxidase inhibitors*). See *MAO inhibitors*.

MAO inhibitors. Historical Notes feature. 285

MAO inhibitors and food interactions. In Depth feature. 287

MAO inhibitors (Psych). Class of drugs that inhibits monoamine oxidase enzyme and acts as antidepressants. 287

Maolate (Ortho). Skeletal muscle relaxant used to treat minor muscle spasms associated with injuries. For dosage, see *chlorphenesin*. 144

maprotiline (Psych). Tetracyclic antidepressant. Tablet: 25 mg, 50 mg, 75 mg. [mah-PROH-teh-leen]. 286

Marax (Resp) (generic *theophylline, ephedrine*). Combination drug with two bronchodilators. Tablet: 130 mg/25 mg. [MEH-rehks]. 195

Marax-DF (Resp) (generic *theophylline, ephedrine, hydroxyzine*). Combination drug with two bronchodilators and an antihistamine. Liquid: 97.5 mg/18.75 mg/7.5 mg. [MEH-rehks]. 195

Marcaine (Anes). Local, regional nerve block, epidural, and spinal anesthetic. For dosage, see *bupivacaine*. {MAWR-kayn]. 368

Marcaine (Dental, Oph, Ortho). Local anesthetic used before dental procedures; used in eye surgery; used to treat osteoarthritis or rheumatoid arthritis. For dosage, see *bupivacaine*. [MAWR-kayn]. 147

Marezine (GI). Antiemetic; also used to treat motion sickness. For dosage, see *cyclizine*. [MEH-rehzeen]. 127, 128

marijuana (Antivir). Used to treat AIDS wasting syndrome. Orphan drug. 327

marijuana (*Cannabis sativa*), legalization of. Focus on Healthcare Issues feature. 17

marijuana. See *dronabinol*.

Marinol (Antivir, GI). Appetite stimulant used to treat AIDS patients; antiemetic drug used to treat nausea and vomiting caused by chemotherapy. For dosage, see *dronabinol*. [MEH-rih-nawl]. 128

marketing, drug. 21, 31

Marogen (Uro). Erythropoietin-type drug used to treat anemia in patients with end-stage renal disease. For dosage, see *epoetin beta*. [MEH-roh-jehn]. 111

Marplan (Psych). MAO inhibitor used to treat depression. For dosage, see *isocarboxazid*. [MAWR-plehn]. 288

(masoprocol) (Derm). No longer on the market. (Trade name *Actinex*; topical drug used to treat keratoses and basal cell carcinoma).

Massengill Medicated Douche (OB/GYN). Antibacterial povidone-iodine vaginal douche. Douche: 10%, 12%.

mast cell stabilizers (ENT, Oph, Resp). Class of drugs that inhibits release of histamine from mast cells in the lungs, nose and eyes. 196, 207

Matulane (Chemo). Chemotherapy drug used to treat Hodgkin's disease. For dosage, see *procarbazine*. [MEH-tyoo-layn]. 348

Mavik (Cardio). Angiotensin-converting enzyme inhibitor used to treat hypertension. For dosage, see *trandolapril*. 164

Maxair Autohaler, Maxair Inhaler (Resp). Bronchodilator. For dosage, see *pirbuterol*. 193

Maxalt, Maxalt-MLT (Analges). Serotonin receptor agonist drug used to treat migraine headaches. For dosage, see *rizatriptan*. [MACKS-uhlt]. 306

Maxamine (Chemo). Used to treat leukemia and malignant melanoma. For dosage, see *histamine*. 361

Maxaquin (Antibio). Fluoroquinolone antibiotic used to treat a variety of infections, including *E. coli*, *H. influenzae*, and *Pseudomonas*; used to treat Legionnaire's disease. For dosage, see *lomefloxacin*. [MACK-sah-kwihn]. 105, 198, 318

Maxicam (Ortho) (generic *isoxicam*). Nonsteroidal anti-inflammatory drug used to treat osteoarthritis or rheumatoid arthritis. Investigational drug. 148

Maxidex (Oph). Topical corticosteroid used to treat inflammation of the eyes. For dosage, see *dexamethasone*. [MACK-seh-dehks]. 219

Maxiflor (Derm) (generic *diflorasone*). Topical corticosteroid anti-inflammatory drug. Cream: 0.05%. Ointment: 0.05%. 92

Maximum Bayer Aspirin. See *Genuine Bayer Aspirin*.

Maximum Strength Acutrim II. See *Acutrim*.

Maximum Strength Anbesol. See *Anbesol*.

Maximum Strength Bactine (Derm) (generic *hydrocortisone*). Topical corticosteroid anti-inflammatory drug. Cream: 1%. [behk-TEEN]. 92

Maximum Strength Benadyl, Maximum Strength Benadryl Itch Relief. See *Benadryl*.

Maximum Strength Caldecort (Derm) (generic *hydrocortisone*). Topical corticosteroid anti-inflammatory drug. Cream: 1%. 92

Maximum Strength Comtrex (ENT) (generic *pseudoephedrine, chlorpheniramine, dextromethorphan, acetaminophen*). Combination decongestant, antihistamine, nonnarcotic antitussive, and analgesic drug. Caplet: 30 mg/2 mg/15 mg/500 mg.

(Maximum Strength Comtrex Liqui-Gels) (ENT). No longer on the market. (Combination drug with *phenylpropanolamine*; decongestant, antihistamine, nonnarcotic antitussive, and analgesic drug).

Maximum Strength Cortaid. See *Cortaid*.

Maximum Strength Dexatrim. See *Dexatrim*.

Maximum Strength Dristan Cold (ENT) (generic *pseudoephedrine, brompheniramine, acetaminophen*). Combination decongestant, antihistamine, and analgesic drug. Caplet: 30 mg/2 mg/500 mg.

Maximum Strength KeriCort-10 (Derm) (generic *hydrocortisone*). Topical corticosteroid anti-inflammatory drug. Cream: 1%. 92

Maximum Strength Sine-Aid (ENT) (generic *pseudoephedrine, acetaminophen*). Combination decongestant and analgesic drug. Caplet: 30 mg/500 mg. Gelcap: 30 mg/500 mg. Tablet: 30 mg/500 mg.

Maximum Strength Sinutab Without Drowsiness (ENT) (generic *pseudoephedrine, acetaminophen*). Combination decongestant and analgesic drug. Caplet: 30 mg/500 mg. Tablet: 30 mg/500 mg.

Maximum Strength Sudafed Sinus (ENT) (generic *pseudoephedrine, acetaminophen*). Combination decongestant and analgesic drug. Caplet: 30 mg/500 mg. Tablet: 30 mg/500 mg.

Maximum Strength Tylenol Allergy Sinus, Maximum Strength Tylenol Flu NightTime (ENT) (generic *pseudoephedrine, chlorpheniramine, acetaminophen*). Combination decongestant, antihistamine, and analgesic drug. Caplets: 30 mg/2 mg/500 mg. Gelcaps: 30 mg/2 mg/500 mg.

Maximum Strength Tylenol Sinus (ENT) (generic *pseudoephedrine, acetaminophen*). Combination decongestant and analgesic drug. Caplet: 30 mg/500 mg. Gelcap: 30 mg/500 mg. Geltab: 30 mg/500 mg. Tablet: 30 mg/500 mg.

Maximum Strength Unisom Sleep Gels (Neuro). Antihistamine drug sleep aid. For dosage, see *diphenhydramine*.

Maxipime (Antibio). Cephalosporin antibiotic used to treat a variety of bacterial infections, including *Streptococcus*, *Staphylococcus*, and *E. coli*. For dosage, see *cefepime*. [MACK-sih-peem]. 316

Maxitrol Ophthalmic Suspension (Oph) (generic *dexamethasone, neomycin, polymyxin B*). Topical combination corticosteroid and two antibiotic drugs. Ophthalmic suspension: 0.1%/0.35%/10,000 units. [MACK-sih-trawl].

Maxivate (Derm) (generic *betamethasone*). Topical corticosteroid anti-inflammatory drug. Cream: 0.05%. Lotion: 0.05%. Ointment: 0.05%. [MACK-sih-vayt]. 92

Maxivate (Uro) (generic *betamethasone*). Topical corticosteroid anti-inflammatory drug used to treat phimosis (nonretractable foreskin). Cream: 0.05%. [MACK-sih-vayt]. 111

Maxolon (GI). Gastric stimulant used to treat gastroesophageal reflux disease, diabetic gastroparesis, and paralytic ileus. Also used to treat nausea and vomiting caused by chemotherapy. For dosage, see *metoclopramide*. [MACK-soh-lawn]. 122, 126, 128

Maxzide (Uro) (generic *hydrochlorothiazide, triamterene*). Combination diuretic. Tablet: 25 mg/37.5 mg, 50 mg/75 mg. [MACK-side]. 104

mazindol (Sanorex) (Ortho). Used to treat Duchenne's muscular dystrophy. Orphan drug. 148

McCaughey septuplets.

mcg (abbreviation for *microgram*). 69

MCT (abbreviation for *medium-chain triglyceride*). See *medium-chain triglyceride oil.*

MDI (abbreviation for *metered-dose inhaler*). See *metered-dose inhaler.*

measurement, drug. 68

   apothecary. 69

   drops. 70

   household. 70

   inch. 70

   metric. 69

   milliequivalent. 70

   percentage. 70

   ratio. 70

   units. 70

Mebaral (Neuro). Barbiturate used to treat tonic-clonic and absence seizures. (Schedule IV drug). For dosage, see *mephobarbital*. [meh-BEH-rawl]. 264

mebendazole (Vermox) (Misc). Used to treat pinworms, roundworms, and hookworms. Chewable tablet: 100 mg. [meh-BEHN-dah-zohl].

mecamylamine (Inversine) (Cardio, Psych). Antihypertensive drug only used to treat severe hypertension; orphan drug used to treat the psychiatric disorder Tourette's syndrome. Tablet: 2.5 mg. [meh-kah-MIHL-ah-meen]. 166, 293

mecasermin (Myotrophin) (Endo, Neuro). Used to treat growth hormone insufficiency syndrome; used to treat amyotrophic lateral sclerosis. Orphan drug. 276

mechlorethamine (Mustargen) (Chemo). Alkylating chemotherapy drug used to treat leukemia, Hodgkin's disease, lung cancer, and cutaneous T-cell lymphoma. Intraperitoneal, intracardiac, intrapleural, or intravenous (powder to be reconstituted): 10 mg. [meh-klohr-EH-thah-meen]. 341

Meclan (Derm) (generic *meclocycline*). Topical antibiotic used to treat acne vulgaris. Cream: 1%. [MEH-klehn]. 84

meclizine (Antivert, Antivert/25, Antivert/50, Bonine) (ENT). Antiemetic drug used to treat motion sickness. Capsule: 25 mg, 30 mg. Chewable tablet: 25 mg. Tablet: 12.5 mg, 25 mg, 50 mg. [MEH-klih-zeen]. 128

meclocycline (Meclan) (Derm). Topical antibiotic used to treat acne vulgaris. Cream: 1%. [meh-kloh-SY-kleen]. 84

meclofenamate (Analges, OB/GYN, Ortho). Nonsteroidal anti-inflammatory drug used to treat pain; used to treat migraine headaches; used to treat dysmenorrhea; used to treat osteoarthritis and rheumatoid arthritis. Capsule: 50 mg, 100 mg. [meh-kloh- FEH-nah-mayt]. 139, 255, 304, 307

(Meclomen) (Analges, OB/GYN, Ortho). No longer on the market. (Generic name *meclofenamate*; nonsteroidal anti-inflammatory drug).

medication order. See *order.*

medicine.

   definition of. 2

   linguistic origin of. 2

   patent. 12

Medi-Flu (ENT) (generic *pseudoephedrine, pyrilamine, dextromethorphan, acetaminophen*). Combination decongestant, antihistamine, nonnarcotic antitussive, and analgesic drug. Liquid: 10 mg/0.67 mg/5 mg/167 mg.

(Medihaler-Epi) (Resp). No longer on the market. (Generic name *epinephrine*; bronchodilator).

(Medihaler Ergotamine) (Analges). No longer on the market. (Generic name *ergotamine*; used to treat migraine headaches).

(Medihaler-Iso) (Resp). No longer on the market. (Generic name *isoproterenol*; bronchodilator).

Medi-Quik (Derm) (generic *benzalkonium, lidocaine*). Topical combination antiseptic and anesthetic. Spray. 94

medium-chain triglyceride oil (MCT) (GI). Nutritional supplement that provides extra calories in an easily digested oil. Oil: 115 calories/15 mL. 133

Medrol (Derm, Endo). Corticosteroid anti-inflammatory used to treat severe inflammation in various body systems. For dosage, see *methylprednisolone*. [MEH-drawl]. 93, 232

medroxyprogesterone (Amen, Cycrin, Provera) (OB/GYN). Progestins hormone drug used to treat amenorrhea; used to treat abnormal uterine bleeding. Tablet: 2.5 mg, 5 mg, 10 mg. [meh-drawk-see-proh-JEHS-teh-rohn]. 253

medroxyprogesterone (Depo-Provera) (Chemo, OB/GYN). Hormonal chemotherapy drug used to treat breast cancer, uterine cancer, and kidney cancer; progestins-only three-month contraceptive. Intramuscular: 150 mg/mL, 400 mg/mL. [meh-drawk-see-proh-JEHS-teh-rohn]. 251, 343

medrysone (HMS) (Oph). Topical corticosteroid used to treat inflammation in the eyes. Ophthalmic suspension: 1%. 219

mefenamic acid (Ponstel) (Analges, OB/GYN). Nonsteroidal anti-inflammatory drug used to treat pain; used to treat migraine headaches; also used to treat dysmenorrhea. Capsule: 250 mg. [meh-feh-NAH-mihk EH-sihd]. 255, 304, 307

Mefoxin (Antibio). Cephalosporin antibiotic used to treat various types of bacterial infections, including *Streptococcus, Staphylococcus, E. coli, H. influenzae,* and gonorrhea. For dosage, see *cefoxitin.* [meh-FAWK-sihn]. 316

Megace (Antivir, Chemo). Hormonal chemotherapy drug used to treat AIDS wasting syndrome; used to treat breast cancer and uterine cancer. For dosage, see *megestrol.* [MEH-gays]. 327, 343

megestrol (Megace) (Antivir, Chemo). Hormonal chemotherapy drug used to treat AIDS wasting syndrome; used to treat breast cancer and uterine cancer. Tablet: 20 mg, 40 mg. [meh-GEHS-trawl]. 327, 343

Melacine (Chemo). Vaccine used to treat malignant melanoma. Orphan drug. 349

Melagesic PM (Neuro) (generic *acetaminophen, melatonin*). Combination analgesic and melatonin sleep aid. Tablet: 500 mg/1.5 mg. [mehl-ah-GEE-sihk]. 273

Melanex (Derm) (generic *hydroquinone*). Topical drug used to lighten areas of hyperpigmented skin. Liquid: 3%. 99

Melanocid (Chemo). Chemotherapy drug used to treat malignant melanoma. Orphan drug. 348

Melimmune (Chemo) (generic *indium 111, monoclonal antibody*). Combination radioisotope and monoclonal antibody chemotherapy drug used to treat non-Hodgkin's lymphoma. Orphan drug. 349

meloxicam (Mobic) (Analges, Ortho). Nonsteroidal anti-inflammatory drug used to treat osteoarthritis. Tablet: 7.5 mg, 15 mg. [meh-LAWK-seh-kehm]. 139, 304

Mellaril, Mellaril-S (Psych). Phenothiazine drug used to treat psychosis; used to treat anxiety; used as short-term treatment for explosive, impulsive behavior and mood lability in children; used to treat attention-deficit/hyperactivity disorder. For dosage, see *thioridazine.* [MEHL-ah-rihl]. 283, 292

melphalan (Alkeran) (Chemo). Alkylating chemotherapy drug used to treat ovarian cancer, malignant melanoma, and multiple myeloma. Tablet: 2 mg. Intravenous (powder to be reconstituted): 50 mg. [MEHL-fah-lehn]. 341

memantine (Antivir). Used to treat AIDS dementia. Investigational drug. 331

Menest (Chemo, OB/GYN, Ortho). Hormonal chemotherapy drug used to treat breast and prostate carcinoma; hormone replacement therapy used to treat the symptoms of menopause; used to prevent and treat osteoporosis. [MEH-nehst]. 252, 343

menopause, drugs used to treat. 252

menotropins (Humegon, Pergonal, Repronex) (OB/GYN). Ovulation-stimulating drug used to treat infertility. Intramuscular (powder to be reconstituted): 75 IU, 150 IU. [men-noh-TROH-pihns]. 244

(Menrium) (OB/GYN). No longer on the market. (Generic name *estrogen, meprobamate*; estrogen replacement therapy and antianxiety drug for menopause).

menstruation, drugs used to treat abnormal. 253

Mentane (Neuro). Cholinesterase inhibitor used to treat Alzheimer's disease. Generic: *velnacrine.* Investigational drug. 271

Mentax (Derm) (generic *butenafine*). Topical antifungal drug. Cream: 1%. [MEHN-tehks]. 89

mepenzolate (Cantil) (GI). Antispasmodic drug used to treat spasm of the smooth muscle of the bowel. Tablet: 25 mg. [meh-PEHN-zoh-layt]. 122

Mepergan Fortis (Analges) (generic *meperidine, promethazine*). Combination narcotic and antihistamine analgesic and sedative drug. (Schedule II drug). Capsule: 50 mg/25 mg. [MEH-pehr-gehn FOHR-tihs]. 303

meperidine (Demerol) (Analges, Anes, OB/GYN). Narcotic analgesic used to treat moderate-to-severe pain; given preoperatively to produce sedation and relieve pain; used for pain relief during childbirth. (Schedule II drug). Tablet: 50 mg, 100 mg. Syrup: 50 mg/5 mL. Intramuscular and intravenous: 10 mg/mL, 25 mg/mL, 50 mg/mL, 75 mg/mL, 100 mg/mL. [meh-PEH-reh-deen]. 297, 371

mephentermine (Wyamine) (Anes). Vasopressor used to treat hypotension that occurs with spinal anesthesia. Intramuscular or intravenous: 30 mg/mL. [meh-FEHN-tehr-meen]. 371

mephenytoin (Mesantoin) (Neuro). Anticonvulsant drug used to treat tonic-clonic and simple and complex partial seizures. Tablet: 100 mg. [meh-FEHN-toh-ehn]. 264

mephobarbital (Mebaral) (Neuro). Barbiturate used to treat tonic-clonic and absence seizures. (Schedule IV drug). Tablet: 32 mg, 50 mg, 100 mg. [meh-foh-BAWR-beh-tawl]. 264

Mephyton (Hem). Used to treat patients with clotting factor deficiency; used to restore normal blood clotting times in patients who have had an overdose of anticoagulants other than heparin; given prophylactically to newborns to prevent hemorrhagic disease of the newborn.   For dosage, see *vitamin K.* 189

mepivacaine (Carbocaine, Polocaine, Polocaine MPF) (Anes).   Local, regional nerve block, and epidural anesthetic drug. Injection: 1%, 1.5%, 2%, 3%. [meh-PIH-vah-kayn]. 368

meprobamate.   Historical Notes feature.

meprobamate (Equanil, Miltown) (Psych).   Drug used to treat anxiety and neurosis. (Schedule IV drug). Tablet: 200 mg, 400 mg. [meh-proh-BEH-mayt]. 282

Mepron (Antivir).   Used to treat *Pneumocystis carinii* pneumonia in AIDS patients.   For dosage, see *atovaquone.* [MEH-prawn]. 328

(Meprospan) (Psych).   No longer on the market. (Generic name *meprobamate*; antianxiety drug). 70

mEq (abbreviation for *milliequivalent*).

mercaptopurine (Purinethol) (Chemo).   Purine antagonist chemotherapy drug used to treat leukemia. Tablet: 50 mg. [muhr-kehp-toh-PYOUR-een]. 339

Meridia (GI).   Appetite suppressant used to treat obesity. (Schedule IV drug).   For dosage, see *sibutramine.* 129

Meritene (GI).   Liquid nutritional supplement. Powder (to be reconstituted). 131

meropenem (Merrem IV) (Antibio).   Carbapenem antibiotic used to treat ruptured appendicitis and peritonitis; used to treat bacterial meningitis. Intravenous (powder to be reconstituted): 500 mg, 1 g. [mehr-oh-PEH-nehm]. 133, 276, 317

Merrem IV (Antibio).   Carbapenem antibiotic used to treat ruptured appendicitis and peritonitis; used to treat bacterial meningitis.   For dosage, see *meropenem.* [MEHR-ehm]. 133, 276, 317

mesalamine (Asacol, Canasa, Pentasa, Rowasa) (GI).   Anti-inflammatory-type drug used to treat ulcerative colitis. Capsule: 250 mg. Tablet: 400 mg. Rectal liquid: 4 g/60 mL. Suppository: 500 mg. Enema. 126

Mesantoin (Neuro).   Anticonvulsant drug used to treat tonic-clonic and simple and complex partial seizures.   For dosage, see *mephenytoin.* [meh-SEHN-toh-ehn] 264

mesna (Mesnex) (Chemo).   Cytoprotective drug used to prevent hemorrhagic cystitis in patients receiving ifosfamide chemotherapy. Intravenous: 100 mg/mL. [MEHS-nah]. 350

Mesnex (Chemo).   Cytoprotective drug used to prevent hemorrhagic cystitis in patients receiving ifosfamide chemotherapy.   For dosage, see *mesna.* [MEHS-nehks]. 350

mesoridazine (Serentil) (Psych).   Phenothiazine drug used to treat schizophrenia; used to treat behavioral problems in patients with mental retardation or

chronic brain syndrome; used to treat anxiety and depression in alcoholism; used to treat anxiety. Tablet: 10 mg, 25 mg, 50 mg, 100 mg. Liquid: 25 mg/mL. Intramuscular: 25 mg/mL. [meh-SOHR-eh-dah-zeen]. 283

Mestinon (Anes, Neuro).   Anticholinesterase drug used to reverse the action of neuromuscular blocking drugs during general anesthesia; used to treat myasthenia gravis.   For dosage, see *pyridostigmine.* [MEH-stih-nawn]. 271, 371

metabolic acidosis, drugs used to treat. 181

metabolism, drug. 47

metabolite. 47, 48

Metadate CD, Metadate ER (Neuro, Psych).   Central nervous system stimulant used to treat narcolepsy; used to treat attention-deficit/hyperactivity disorder. (Schedule II drug).   For dosage, see *methylphenidate.* [meh-tah-dayt]. 274, 292

Metahydrin (Uro).   Thiazide diuretic.   For dosage, see *trichlormethiazide.* [meh-tah-HY-drayt]. 103

Metamucil (GI).   Bulk-producing laxative.   For dosage, see *psyllium.* 125

(Metaprel) (Resp).   No longer on the market. (Generic name *metaproterenol*; bronchodilator).

metaproterenol (Alupent) (Resp).   Bronchodilator. Oral liquid: 10 mg/5 mL. Aerosol inhaler: 0.65 mg/puff. Liquid for nebulizer: 0.4%, 0.6%, 5%. Tablet: 10 mg, 20 mg. [meh-tah-proh-TEH-reh-nawl]. 193

metaraminol (Aramine) (Anes.) Vasopressor used to treat hypotension that occurs with spinal anesthesia. Subcutaneous, intramuscular, or intravenous: 10 mg/mL. [meh-tah-REH-mih-nawl]. 371

Metaret (Chemo).   Chemotherapy drug used to treat prostate cancer.   For dosage, see *suramin.* 348

Metastron (Chemo).   Radioactive strontium 89 isotope used to treat bone pain in cancer patients with bone metastases. There is preferential uptake of the drug by sites of active osteogenesis, primarily by the metastatic bone lesions. Intravenous: 4 mCi/mL. [MEH-tah-strawn]. 362

Metatensin #4 (Cardio) (generic *reserpine, trichlormethiazide*).   Combination antihypertensive and diuretic drug. Tablet: 0.1 mg/4 mg. [meh-tah-TEHN-sihn]. 167

metaxalone (Skelaxin) (Ortho).   Skeletal muscle relaxant used to treat minor muscle spasms associated with injuries. Tablet: 400 mg. [meh-TEHK-sah-lohn]. 144

metered-dose inhaler (MDI).

metformin (Glucophage, Glucophage XR) (Diab, OB/GYN).   Oral antidiabetic drug; used to treat the elevated insulin levels caused by polycystic ovary syndrome. Tablet: 500 mg, 625 mg, 850 mg, 1000 mg. [meht-FOHR-mihn]. 241

methacycline (Antibio). No longer on the market. (Trade name *Rondomycin*; tetracycline-type antibiotic).

methadone (Dolophine, Methadone Intensol, Methadose) (Analges). Narcotic analgesic used to treat severe pain; used to manage dependence and withdrawal from narcotics. (Schedule II drug). Liquid: 5 mg/5 mL, 10 mg/5 mL, 10 mg/mL. Tablet: 5 mg, 10 mg, 40 mg. Subcutaneous or intramuscular: 10 mg/mL. [MEH-thah-dohn]. 297, 308

Methadone Intensol (Analges). Narcotic analgesic used to treat severe pain; used to manage dependence and withdrawal from narcotics. (Schedule II drug). For dosage, see *methadone*. [MEH-thah-dohn]. 297, 308

Methadose (Analges). Narcotic analgesic used to treat severe pain; used to manage dependence and withdrawal from narcotics. (Schedule II drug). For dosage, see *methadone*. [MEH-thah-dohs]. 297, 308

methamphetamine (Desoxyn, Desoxyn Gradumet) (Neuro, Psych). Central nervous system stimulant used to treat narcolepsy; used to treat attention-deficit/hyperactivity disorder. (Schedule II drug). Tablet: 5 mg, 10 mg. [meth-ehm-FEH-tah-meen]. 274, 291

methantheline (Banthine) (GI). Antispasmodic drug used to treat spasm of the smooth muscle of the bowel. Tablet: 50 mg. [meh-THEHN-theh-leen]. 122

methazolamide (GlaucTabs, Neptazane) (Oph). Carbonic anhydrase inhibitor used to treat glaucoma. Tablet: 25 mg, 50 mg. [meh-thah-ZOH-lah-mide]. 221

(methdilazine) (GI). No longer on the market. (Trade name *Tacaryl*; antiemetic drug).

methenamine (Hiprex, Urex) (Antibio, Uro). Anti-infective drug only used to treat urinary tract infections. Tablet: 1 g. [meh-THEN-tah-meen]. 106, 319

Methergine (OB/GYN). Used to treat postpartum uterine bleeding. For dosage, see *methylergonovine*. [MEH-thuhr-jeen]. 248

(methicillin) (Antibio). No longer on the market. (Trade name *Staphcillin*; penicillin-type antibiotic).

methimazole (Tapazole) (Endo). Antithyroid drug used to treat hyperthyroidism. Tablet: 5 mg, 10 mg. [meh-THEM-ah-zohl]. 230

Methitest (Chemo, Endo). Male sex hormone used to treat breast cancer in women; used to treat the lack of production of testosterone due to absence, injury, or malfunction of the testes or malfunction of the pituitary gland; used to treat delayed puberty in boys. For dosage, see *methyltestosterone*. [MEH-theh-tehst].

methocarbamol (Robaxin, Robaxin-750) (Ortho). Skeletal muscle relaxant used to treat minor muscle spasms associated with injuries. Tablet: 500 mg, 750 mg. Intramuscular or intravenous: 100 mg/mL. [meh-thoh-KAWR-bah-mawl]. 144

methohexital (Brevital) (Anes). Barbiturate used to induce and maintain general anesthesia. Intravenous: 500 mg/50 mL. [meh-thoh-HEHK-sih-tawl]. 369

methotrexate (Methotrexate LPF, Rheumatrex Dose Pack) (Chemo). Folic acid antagonist chemotherapy drug used to treat breast cancer, ovarian cancer, head and neck cancer, lung cancer, osteosarcoma, leukemia, cutaneous T-cell lymphoma, and non-Hodgkin's disease. Tablet: 2.5 mg. Intramuscular or intravenous: 2.5 mg/mL, 25 mg/mL, (powder to be reconstituted) 20 mg, 50 mg, 1 g. [meh-thoh-TREHK-sayt]. 340

methotrexate (Rheumatrex, Rheumatrex Dose Pack) (Derm, Ortho). Folic acid antagonist chemotherapy drug used to treat severe, disabling psoriasis; used to treat severe, active rheumatoid arthritis. Tablet: 2.5 mg. Intramuscular or intravenous: 2.5 mg/mL, 25 mg/mL, (powder to be reconstituted) 20 mg, 50 mg, 1 g. [meh-thoh-TREHK-sayt]. 87, 142

Methotrexate LPF (Chemo). Folic acid antagonist chemotherapy drug used to treat breast cancer, ovarian cancer, head and neck cancer, lung cancer, osteosarcoma, leukemia, cutaneous T-cell lymphoma, and non-Hodgkin's disease. For dosage, see *methotrexate*. [meh-thoh-TREHK-sayt]. 340

(methotrimeprazine) (Analges). No longer on the market. (Trade name *Levoprome*; nonnarcotic analgesic).

methoxamine (Vasoxyl) (Anes). Vasopressor used to treat hypotension that occurs with spinal anesthesia. Intramuscular or intravenous: 20 mg/mL. [meh-THAWK-sah-meen]. 371

methoxsalen (Oxsoralen) (Derm). Topical drug used with ultraviolet light to treat vitiligo. Lotion: 1%. [meh-THAWK-say-lehn]. 99

methoxsalen (Oxsoralen-Ultra, 8-MOP) (Derm). Oral drug used to treat severe, disabling psoriasis. Capsule: 10 mg. [meh-THAWK-say-lehn]. 87

methoxsalen (Uvadex) (Chemo). Topical drug used in conjunction with ultraviolet light to treat cutaneous T-cell lymphoma. Liquid: 20 mcg/mL. [meh-THAWK-sah-lehn].

methoxyflurane (Penthrane) (Anes). Used to induce and maintain general anesthesia. Inhaled gas. [meh-thawk-see-FLOO-rayn]. 370

methscopolamine (Pamine) (GI, Uro). Antispasmodic drug used to treat spasm of the smooth muscle of the bowel. Tablet: 2.5 mg. [meth-skoh-PAW-lah-meen]. 122

methsuximide (Celontin) (Neuro). Anticonvulsant drug used to treat absence seizures. Capsule: 150 mg, 300 mg. [meth-SUHK-seh-mide]. 264

methyclothiazide (Aquatensen, Enduron) (Uro). Thiazide diuretic. Tablet: 2.5 mg, 5 mg. [meh-ee-kloh-THY-eh-zide]. 103

methylcellulose (Citrucel) (GI). Bulk-producing laxative. Powder: 2 g/Tbsp. 125

methylcellulose (Gonak, Goniosol, OcuCoat) (Oph). Injected into the eye during surgery to keep the anterior chamber expanded and replace intraocular fluid. Injection (anterior chamber): 2%, 2.5%. [meh-thul-SELL-yoo-lohs].

methyldopa (Aldomet) (Cardio). Alpha-receptor blocker used to treat hypertension. Liquid: 50 mg/mL. Tablet: 125 mg, 250 mg, 500 mg. Injection: 50 mg/mL. [meh-thul-DOH-pah]. 165

methylene blue (Urolene Blue) (Emerg, Uro). Used to treat cyanide poisoning; used to treat oxalate kidney stones. Tablet: 65 mg. Intravenous: 10 mg/mL. [MEH-thul-leen bloo]. 112

methylergonovine (Methergine) (OB/GYN). Used to treat postpartum uterine bleeding. Tablet: 0.2 mg. Intramuscular or intravenous: 0.2 mg/mL. [meh-thul-ehr-goh-NOH-veen]. 248

Methylin ER (Neuro, Psych). Central nervous system stimulant used to treat narcolepsy; used to treat attention-deficit/hyperactivity disorder. (Schedule II drug). For dosage, see *methylphenidate*. [MEH-thuhl-ehn]. 274, 292

methylphenidate (Concerta, Metadate CD, Metadate ER, Methylin ER, Ritalin, Ritalin-SR) (Neuro). Central nervous system stimulant used to treat narcolepsy. Capsule: 20 mg. Capsule: Opened and sprinkled on applesauce. Tablet: 5 mg, 10 mg, 18 mg, 20 mg, 36 mg, 54 mg. [meh-thuhl-FEH-neh-dayt]. 274

methylphenidate (Concerta, Metadate CD, Metadate ER, Methylin ER, Ritalin, Ritalin-SR) (Neuro, Psych). Central nervous system stimulant used to treat narcolepsy; used to treat attention-deficit/hyperactivity disorder. (Schedule II drug). Capsule: 20 mg. Capsule: Opened and sprinkled on applesauce. Tablet: 5 mg, 10 mg, 18 mg, 20 mg, 36 mg, 54 mg. [meh-thuhl-FEH-neh-dayt]. 274, 292

methylprednisolone (A-Methapred, Medrol, Solu-Medrol) (Derm, Endo). Corticosteroid anti-inflammatory used to treat severe inflammation in various body systems. Dosepak 21. Tablet: 2 mg, 4 mg, 8 mg, 16 mg, 24 mg, 32 mg. Intramuscular or intravenous (powder to be reconstituted): 40 mg, 125

mg, 500 mg, 1 g, 2 g. [meh-thul-prehd-NIH-soh-lohn]. 93, 232

methylprednisolone (Depo-Medrol, Depopred-40, Depopred-80) (Derm, Endo, Ortho). Corticosteroid anti-inflammatory drug used to treat Addison's disease and rheumatoid arthritis; injected into a joint to treat osteoarthritis and rheumatoid arthritis; injected near a joint to treat bursitis and tenosynovitis; injected into skin lesions. Intra-articular, periarticular, intradermal, or intramuscular: 20 mg/mL, 40 mg/mL, 80 mg/mL. [meh-thul-prehd-NIH-soh-lohn]. 92, 141, 232

methyltestosterone (Android, Methitest, Testred, Virilon, Virilon IM) (Chemo, Endo). Male sex hormone used to treat breast cancer in women; used to treat the lack of production of testosterone due to absence, injury, or malfunction of the testes or malfunction of the pituitary gland; used to treat delayed puberty in boys. Capsule: 10 mg. Tablet: 10 mg, 25 mg. Buccal tablet: 10 mg. Intramuscular: 200 mg/mL. [meh-thul-tehs-TAW-steh-rohn]. 343

(methyprylon) (Neuro). No longer on the market. (Trade name *Noludar*; nonbarbiturate used to treat insomnia).

methysergide (Sansert) (Analges). Used to treat migraine headaches. Tablet: 2 mg. [meh-thee-SEHR-jide]. 307

Meticorten (Chemo, Endo). Corticosteroid anti-inflammatory drug used to treat severe inflammation in various body systems; used as part of chemotherapy treatment. For dosage, see *prednisone*. [meh-tee-KOHR-tehn]. 232, 351

Metimyd, Metimyd Suspension (Oph) (generic name *prednisolone, sulfacetamide*). Topical combination corticosteroid and sulfa anti-infective drug. Ophthalmic ointment: 0.5%/10%. Ophthalmic suspension: 0.5%/10%. [MEH-tih-mihd].

metipranolol (OptiPranolol) (Oph). Topical beta receptor blocker used to treat glaucoma. Ophthalmic solution: 0.3%. [meh-tee-PRAH-noh-lawl]. 221

metoclopramide (Maxolon, Reglan) (GI). Gastric stimulant used to treat gastroesophageal reflux disease, diabetic gastroparesis, and paralytic ileus. Also used to treat nausea and vomiting caused by chemotherapy. Tablet: 5 mg, 10 mg. Syrup: 5 mg/5 mL. Intramuscular or intravenous: 5 mg/mL. 122, 126, 128

metocurine (Anes). Muscle-relaxing drug used during surgery. Intravenous: 2 mg/mL. 370

metolazone (Mykrox, Zaroxolyn) (Uro). Thiazide-like diuretic. Tablet: 0.5 mg, 2.5 mg, 5 mg, 10 mg. [meh-TOHL-ah-zohn]. 103

metoprolol (Lopressor, Toprol-XL) (Analges, Ortho, Psych). Cardioselective beta-blocker used to treat migraine headaches; used to treat essential familial tremor; used to treat the side effects of muscle restlessness from antipsychotic drugs. Tablet: 25 mg, 50 mg, 100 mg, 200 mg. Intravenous: 1 mg/mL. [meh-TOH-proh-lawl]. 146, 294, 306

metoprolol (Lopressor, Toprol-XL) (Cardio). Cardioselective beta-blocker used to treat angina pectoris, congestive heart failure, hypertension, and ventricular arrhythmias; used to prevent repeat myocardial infarction. Tablet: 50 mg, 100 mg, 200 mg. Intravenous: 1 mg/mL. [meh-TOH-proh-lawl]. 157, 158, 160, 162

Metric Conversion Act of 1975. 69

metric system of drug measurement. 69

Metrodin (OB/GYN). Used to stimulate ovulation in infertility. Orphan drug. 244

MetroGel (Derm) (generic *metronidazole*). Topical antibacterial and antiprotozoal drug used to treat acne rosacea. Gel: 0.75%. [MEH-troh-jell]. 85

MetroGel-Vaginal (OB/GYN) (generic *metronidazole*). Topical antibiotic drug used to treat bacterial vaginal infections. Gel: 0.75%. [MEH-troh-jell]. 256

MetroLotion (Derm) (generic *metronidazole*). Topical antibacterial and antiprotozoal drug used to treat acne rosacea. Lotion: 0.75%. 85

metronidazole (Flagyl, Flagyl 375, Protostat) (GI, OB/GYN). Antibacterial and antiprotozoal drug used to treat intestinal amebiasis; used to treat *Trichomonas vaginalis* vaginal infection, a sexually transmitted disease. Capsule: 375 mg. Tablet: 250 mg, 500 mg. [meh-troh-NY-dah-zohl].

metronidazole (Flagyl, Flagyl ER, Flagyl 375, Flagyl IV, Flagyl IV RTU, Protostat) (Antibio, GI). Antibacterial and antiprotozoal drug used to treat a variety of infections, including *Bacteroides*, Crohn's disease, and *H. pylori* infections of the gastrointestinal tract. Capsule: 375 mg. Tablet: 250 mg, 500 mg, 750 mg. Intravenous (powder to be reconstituted): 500 mg. [meh-troh-NY-dah-zohl]. 120

metronidazole (MetroGel, MetroGel-Vaginal, MetroLotion) (Derm, OB/GYN). Topical antibacterial and antiprotozoal drug used to treat acne rosacea; used to treat bacterial vaginal infections. Cream: 1%. Gel: 0.75%. Lotion: 0.75%. Vaginal gel: 0.75%. [meh-troh-NY-dah-zohl]. 85, 256

(Metubine) (Anes). No longer on the market. (Generic name *metocurine*; muscle relaxant used during surgery).

metyrosine (Demser) (Endo). Inhibits the enzyme that helps produce epinephrine and norepinephrine. Used to treat the hypertension caused by excessive epinephrine and norepinephrine produced by a pheochromocytoma of the adrenal medulla. Capsule: 250 mg. [meh-TY-roh-seen].

Mevacor (Cardio). HMG-CoA reductase inhibitor drug used to treat hypercholesterolemia. For dosage, see *lovastatin*. [MEH-vah-kohr]. 170

mexiletine (Mexitil) (Cardio). Used to treat ventricular arrhythmias. Capsule: 150 mg, 200 mg, 250 mg. [mehk-SIH-leh-teen]. 159

Mexitil (Cardio). Used to treat ventricular arrhythmias. For dosage, see *mexiletine*. [MEHK-sih-tihl]. 159

(Mezlin) (Antibio). No longer on the market. (Generic name *mezlocillin*; penicillin-type antibiotic).

(mezlocillin) (Antibio). No longer on the market. (Trade name *Mezlin*; penicillin-type antibiotic).

mg (abbreviation for *milligram*). 69

mg/kg/day (abbreviation for *milligrams of drug per kilograms* of body weight *per day*). 72

mg/m² (abbreviation for *milligrams per meter squared* of body surface area). 72

Miacalcin (Ortho). Calcium-regulating hormone used to prevent and treat osteoporosis; used to treat Paget's disease. For dosage, see *calcitonin*. [mee-ah-KEHL-sihn]. 143

(mibefradil) (Cardio). No longer on the market. (Trade name *Posicor*; calcium channel blocker used to treat angina and hypertension).

Micanol (Derm) (generic *anthralin*). Topical drug used to treat psoriasis. Cream: 1%. [MY-keh-nawl]. 87

Micardis (Cardio). Angiotensin II receptor blocker used to treat hypertension. For dosage, see *telmisartan*. [my-KAWR-dihs]. 164

Micardis HCT (Cardio) (generic *telmisartan, hydrochlorothiazide*). Combination angiotensin II receptor blocker antihypertensive and diuretic drug. Tablet: 40 mg/12.5 mg, 80 mg/12.5 mg. [my-KAWR-dihs]. 167

Micatin (Derm) (generic *miconazole*). Topical antifungal drug. Cream: 2%. Powder: 2%. Spray: 2%. [MIH-kah-tihn]. 89

miconazole (Lotrimin AF 2%, Micatin, Monistat-Derm, Prescription Strength Desenex, Ting) (Derm). Topical antifungal and antiyeast drug. Cream: 2%. Liquid: 2%. Powder: 2%. Spray: 2%. [my-KAW-neh-zohl]. 89, 90

miconazole (Monistat, Monistat 3, Monistat 7) (OB/GYN). Topical antifungal drug used to treat vaginal yeast infections. Vaginal cream: 2%. Vaginal suppository: 100 mg, 200 mg. [my-KAW-neh-zohl]. 256

miconazole (Monistat-Derm) (OB/GYN). Topical antifungal drug used to treat vaginal yeast infections. Cream: 2%. [my-KAW-neh-zohl].

MICRhoGAM (OB/GYN). Immunoglobulin given after abortion, amniocentesis, or chorionic villus sampling to treat Rh-negative mother with an Rh-positive baby to prevent hemorrhagic disease of the newborn in a subsequent pregnancy. Intramuscular: 5%. [my-kroh-ROH-gehm].

microgram (mcg). 69

Micro-K Extencaps, Micro-K LS, Micro-K 10 Extencaps (Uro). Potassium supplement used to replace potassium loss caused by diuretics. Capsule: 8 mEq, 10 mEq. Powder to be reconstituted with water: 20 mEq. 105

Micronase (Diab). Oral antidiabetic drug. For dosage, see *glyburide*. [MY-kroh-nays]. 240

microNefrin (Resp). Bronchodilator. For dosage, see *epinephrine*. [my-kroh-NEH-frihn]. 193

Micronor (OB/GYN) (generic *norethindrone*). Progestins-only oral contraceptive. Tablet: 0.35 mg. [MY-kroh-nohr]. 251

Microzide (Uro). Thiazide diuretic. For dosage, see *hydrochlorothiazide*. [MY-kroh-zide]. 103

Micturin (Uro) (generic *terodiline*). Used to treat urinary incontinence. Investigational drug. 112

Midamor (Uro). Potassium-sparing diuretic. For dosage, see *amiloride*. [MIH-dah-mohr]. 104

midazolam (Versed) (Anes, Resp). Preoperative drug used to produce sedation; used to induce and maintain general anesthesia; used to sedate patients who are intubated and on a ventilator. Oral liquid: 2 mg/mL. Intramuscular and intravenous: 1 mg/mL, 5 mg/mL. [mih-DEH-zoh-lehm]. 199, 369

midodrine (ProAmatine) (Cardio). Alpha$_1$-receptor stimulator used to treat orthostatic hypotension. Tablet: 2.5 mg, 5 mg. [MY-doh-drihn]. 173

Midol Maximum Strength Cramp Formula (OB/GYN). Nonsteroidal anti-inflammatory drug used to treat dysmenorrhea. For dosage, see *ibuprofen*. [MY-dawl].

Midol Maximum Strength Menstrual (OB/GYN) (generic *acetaminophen, pyrilamine*). Combination analgesic and antihistamine to treat premenstrual dysphoric disorder and dysmenorrhea. Caplet/Gelcap: 500 mg/15 mg. [MY-dawl].

Midol Maximum Strength PMS (OB/GYN) (generic *acetaminophen, pamabrom*). Combination analgesic and diuretic used to treat premenstrual dysphoric disorder and dysmenorrhea. Caplet/Gelcap: 500 mg/25 mg. [MY-dawl].

Midol PM (Neuro). Antihistamine drug sleep aid. For dosage, see *diphenhydramine*. [MY-dawl]. 273

Midol Teen Maximum Strength (OB/GYN) (generic *acetaminophen, pamabrom*). Combination analgesic and diuretic used to treat premenstrual dysphoric disorder and dysmenorrhea. Caplet: 500 mg/25 mg. [MY-dawl].

Midrin (Analges) (generic *isometheptene, dichloralphenazone, acetaminophen*). Combination vasoconstrictor, sedative, and analgesic used to treat migraine headaches. Capsule: 65 mg/100 mg/325 mg. [MIH-drihn]. 307

Mifeprex (OB/GYN). Used to produce abortion. For dosage, see *mifepristone*. [MIH-feh-prehks]. 255

mifepristone (Mifeprex) (OB/GYN). Used to produce abortion. Tablet: 200 mg. [mih-feh-PRIHS-tohn]. 255

miglitol (Glyset) (Diab). Oral antidiabetic drug. Tablet: 25 mg, 50 mg, 100 mg. [MIH-glih-tawl]. 241

migraine headaches, drug used to treat. 306

Migranal (Analges). Used to treat migraine headaches. For dosage, see *dihydroergotamine*. [MY-greh-nawl]. 307

Miles Nervine (Neuro). Antihistamine drug sleep aid. For dosage, see *diphenhydramine*. 273

milk of magnesia (M.O.M.) (Phillips' Milk of Magnesia, Concentrated Phillips' Milk of Magnesia) (GI). Magnesium-containing antidiarrheal drug. Suspension: 400 mg/5 mL, 800 mg/5 mL. 124

milliequivalent (mEq). 70

milligram (mg). 69

milliliter (mL). 69

Milontin (Neuro). Anticonvulsant drug used to treat absence seizures. For dosage, see *phensuximide*. [mih-LAWN-tihn]. 264

milrinone (Primacor) (Cardio). Nondigitalis drug used to treat congestive heart failure. Intravenous: 1 mg/mL. [MIHL-rih-nohn]. 154

Miltown (Psych). Drug used to treat anxiety and neurosis. (Schedule IV drug). For dosage, see *meprobamate*. [MILL-town]. 282

mineral oil (GI). Laxative. Oral liquid. 125

minim. 69

Minipress (Cardio, Uro). Alpha$_1$-receptor blocker used to treat congestive heart failure and hypertension; used to treat benign prostatic hypertrophy. For dosage, see *prazosin*. 109, 155, 165

Minitran (Cardio). Nitrate drug used to prevent and treat angina pectoris. For dosage, see *nitroglycerin*. 156

Minizide 1, Minizide 2, Minizide 5 (Cardio) (generic *prazosin, polythiazide*). Combination alpha$_1$-receptor blocker antihypertensive and diuretic drug. Capsule: 1 mg/0.5 mg, 2 mg/0.5 mg, 5 mg/0.5 mg. 167

Minocin, Minocin IV (Antibio). Tetracycline-type antibiotic used to treat a variety of infections, including acne vulgaris, gonorrhea, syphilis, and *Chlamydia*; used to treat malignant pleural effusion. For dosage, see *minocycline*. [MIH-noh-sihn]. 84, 317, 362 minocycline (Arestin) (ENT). Topical drug used to treat periodontal disease. Placed in the pockets between the gums and teeth. Microspheres: 1 mg. [mih-noh-SY-kleen].

minocycline (Dynacin, Minocin, Minocin IV, Vectrin) (Antibio). Tetracycline-type antibiotic used to treat a variety of infections, including acne vulgaris, gonorrhea, syphilis, and *Chlamydia*; used to treat malignant pleural effusion. Capsule: 50 mg, 75 mg, 100 mg. Liquid: 50 mg/5 mL. Intravenous (powder to be reconstituted): 100 mg. [mih-noh-SY-kleen]. 84, 317, 362

minor tranquilizers. See *antianxiety drugs.*

minoxidil (Loniten) (Cardio). Peripheral vasodilator used to treat hypertension. Tablet: 2.5 mg, 10 mg. [mih-NAWK-sih-dihl]. 166

minoxidil (Rogaine, Rogaine Extra Strength) (Derm). Topical vasodilator drug used to treat male and female pattern baldness. Liquid: 2%, 5%. [mih-NAWK-sih-dihl]. 99

Miochol-E (Oph). Miotic drug only used during eye surgery. For dosage, see *acetylcholine.* [MY-oh-kawl].

Miostat (Oph). Miotic drug used only during eye surgery. For dosage, see *carbachol.* [MY-oh-steht].

miotics (Oph). Class of drugs that constricts the pupil; used to treat glaucoma.

Miradon (Hem). Anticoagulant. For dosage, see *anisindione.* [MEER-ah-dawn]. 186

MiraLax (GI) (generic *polyethylene glycol*). Bowel evacuant/bowel prep. Oral liquid (powder to be reconstituted). [MEER-ah-lehks]. 126

Mirapex (Neuro). Used to treat Parkinson's disease. For dosage, see *pramipexole.* [MEER-ah-pehks]. 268

Mircette (OB/GYN) (generic *desogestrel, ethinyl estradiol*). Biphasic combination progestins and estrogen oral contraceptive. Tablet: 0.15 mg/20 mcg then 0.01 mg. [meer-SEHT]. 250

Mirena (OB/GYN) (generic *levonorgestrel*). Progestins-only five-year contraceptive. Intrauterine T-shaped implant. 52 mg. [meer-EE-nah]. 251

mirtazapine (Remeron, Remeron SolTab) (Psych). Tetracyclic antidepressant. Tablet: 15 mg, 30 mg, 45 mg. Orally disintegrating tablet: 15 mg, 30 mg, 45 mg. [meer-TEH-zah-peen]. 286

misoprostol (Cytotec) (GI, OB/GYN). Used to prevent ulcers in patients taking aspirin or NSAIDs; used to induce labor; used to assist in abortion. Tablet: 100 mcg, 200 mcg. [mee-soh-PRAW-stohl]. 119, 148, 255, 309

mites, drugs used to treat. 95

Mithracin (Chemo). Chemotherapy antibiotic used to treat testicular cancer. For dosage, see *plicamycin.* [MIH-thrah-sihn]. 342

mithramycin. See *plicamycin.*

mitoguazone (Zyrkamine) (Chemo). Chemotherapy drug used to treat non-Hodgkin's lymphoma. Orphan drug. 348

mitolactol (Chemo). Chemotherapy drug used to treat brain cancer and cervical cancer. [mih-toh-LACK-tawl]. 348

mitomycin (Mutamycin) (Chemo). Chemotherapy antibiotic used to treat stomach cancer, pancreatic cancer, and bladder cancer. Intravenous (powder to be reconstituted): 5 mg, 20 mg, 40 mg. [mih-toh-MY-sihn]. 342

mitomycin-C. See *mitomycin.*

mitosis inhibitor chemotheraphy drugs (Chemo). Class of chemotherapy drugs. 344

mitotane (Lysodren) (Chemo). Chemotherapy drug used to treat cancer of the adrenal cortex. Tablet: 500 mg. [MIH-toh-tayn]. 348

mitoxantrone (Novantrone) (Chemo, Neuro). Chemotherapy antibiotic used to treat leukemia and prostate cancer; used to treat multiple sclerosis. Intravenous: 2 mg/mL. [meh-TAWK-sehn-trohn]. 276, 341

Mitran (Anes, Neuro, Psych). Benzodiazepine drug used as a preoperative medication to relieve anxiety and provide sedation; used to treat anxiety and neurosis; used to treat alcohol withdrawal and prevent seizures. (Schedule IV drug). For dosage, see *chlordiazepoxide.* [MIH-trehn]. 281

Mitrolan (GI). Bulk-producing laxative. For dosage, see *polycarbophil.* [MIH-troh-lehn]. 125

Mivacron (Anes, Resp). Muscle relaxant drug used during surgery; used to treat patients who are intubated and on the ventilator. For dosage, see *mivacurium.* [MIH-vah-krawn]. 199, 370

mivacurium (Mivacron) (Anes, Resp). Muscle relaxant drug used during surgery; used to treat patients who are intubated and on the ventilator. Intravenous: 0.5 mg/mL, 2 mg/mL. [mih-vah-KYOUR-ee-uhm]. 199, 370

Mixtard 70/30 (Endo). 70% NPH and 30% regular insulin.

mL (abbreviation for *milliliter*). 69

Moban (Psych). Drug used to treat psychosis. For dosage, see *molindone.* [MOH-behn]. 284

Mobic (Analges, Ortho). Nonsteroidal anti-inflammatory drug used to treat osteoarthritis. For dosage, see *meloxicam.* [MOH-bihk]. 139, 304

Mobigesic (Analges) (generic *magnesium salicylate, phenyltoloxamine*). Combination salicylate analgesic and sedative drug. Tablet: 325 mg/30 mg. [moh-bih-GEE-sihk]. 301

Moctanin (GI). Used to dissolve gallstones. For dosage, see *monoctanin.* 129

modafinil (Provigil) (Neuro).   Central nervous system stimulant used to treat narcolepsy. (Schedule IV drug). Tablet: 100 mg, 200 mg. [moh-DAH-feh-nill]. 274

Modane (GI).   Irritant/stimulant laxative.   For dosage, see *bisacodyl*. 124

Modane Bulk (GI).   Bulk-producing laxative.   For dosage, see *psyllium*. 125

Modane Soft (GI).   Stool softener laxative.   For dosage, see *docusate*. 125

Modicon (OB/GYN) (generic *norethindrone, ethinyl estradiol*).   Monophasic combination progestins and estrogen oral contraceptive. Tablet: 0.5 mg/35 mcg. [MOH-dih-kawn]. 249

Moduretic (Uro) (generic *amiloride, hydrochlorothiazide*). Combination diuretic. Tablet: 5 mg/50 mg. [maw-dyour-EH-tihk]. 104

moexipril (Univasc) (Cardio).   Angiotensin-converting enzyme inhibitor used to treat hypertension. Tablet: 7.5 mg, 15 mg. [moh-EHK-sih-prihl]. 163

Mogadon (Neuro).   Used to treat epilepsy. Generic: *nitrazepam*. Investigational drug. 265

Moisture Drops (Oph).   Aritificial tears. Drops.

Moisture Eyes PM (Oph).   Artificial tears lubricating ointment for the eyes. Ophthalmic ointment.

molecular pharmacology. 1

molgramostim (Leucomax) (Antivir).   Granulocyte macrophage colony-stimulating factor used to treat neutropenia in AIDS patients; used to treat neutropenia in patients taking ganciclovir. Orphan drug. 331

molindone (Moban) (Psych).   Drug used to treat psychosis. Tablet: 5 mg, 10 mg, 25 mg, 50 mg, 100 mg. Liquid: 20 mg/mL. [MOH-lihn-dohn]. 284

M.O.M. (abbreviation for *milk of magnesia*).   See *milk of magnesia*.

mometasone (Elocon) (Derm).   Topical corticosteroid anti-inflammatory drug. Cream: 0.1%. Lotion: 0.1%. Ointment: 0.1%. [moh-MEE-tah-zohn]. 92

mometasone (Nasonex) (ENT).   Topical intranasal corticosteroid used to treat allergic rhinitis. Spray: 50 mcg/spray. [moh-MEE-tah-zohn]. 208

Monistat, Monistat 3, Monistat 7 (OB/GYN) (generic *miconazole*).   Topical antiyeast drug used to treat vaginal yeast infections. Vaginal cream: 2%. Vaginal suppository: 100 mg, 200 mg. [MAW-neh-steht]. 256

Monistat 1 (OB/GYN) (generic *tioconazole*).   Topical antiyeast drug used to treat vaginal yeast infections. Vaginal ointment: 6.5%. [MAW-nih-steht]. 256

Monistat-Derm (Derm) (generic *miconazole*).   Topical antifungal and antiyeast drug. Cream: 2%. [MAW-nih-steht]. 89

(Monistat i.v.) (Antifung).   No longer on the market. (Generic name *miconazole*; used to treat fungal and yeast infections).

monoamine oxidase (MAO) inhibitors (Psych). Class of antidepressant drugs. 287

monobactams (Antibio).   Class of antibiotics. 317

Mono-Chlor (Derm) (generic *monochloroacetic acid*). Topical drug used to treat warts. Liquid: 80%. [MAW-noh-klohr]. 91

monochloroacetic acid (Mono-Chlor) (Derm).   Topical drug used to treat warts. Liquid: 80%. [maw-noh-klohr-oh-ah-SEE-tihk EH-sihd]. 91

Monocid (Antibio).   Cephalosporin antibiotic used to treat a variety of bacterial infections, including *Staphylococcus, Streptococcus, E. coli,* and *H. influenzae.* For dosage, see *cefonicid*. [MAW-noh-sihd]. 316

monoclonal antibodies (Chemo).   Class of chemotherapy drugs. 346

monoctanoin (Moctanin) (GI).   Used to dissolve gallstones. Liquid (continuous perfusion via catheter or T-tube into the common bile duct). [maw-nawk-tah-NOH-ihn]. 129

(Monodox) (Antibio).   No longer on the market. (Generic name *doxycycline*; tetracycline antibiotic).

monophasic oral contraceptives. 249

Monopril (Cardio).   Angiotensin-converting enzyme inhibitor used to treat congestive heart failure and hypertension.   For dosage, see *fosinopril*. [MAW-noh-prihl]. 154, 163

montelukast (Singulair) (Resp).   Leukotriene receptor blocker used to prevent and treat asthma. Chewable tablet: 4 mg, 5 mg. Tablet: 10 mg. 196

Monurol (Uro).   Urinary anti-infective drug.   For dosage, see *fosfomycin*. [mawn-YOUR-ohl]. 106

mood-elevating drugs.   See *antidepressants*.

moricizine (Ethmozine) (Cardio).   Used to treat ventricular arrhythmias. Tablet: 200 mg, 250 mg, 300 mg. [moh-RIH-sih-zeen]. 159

Morpheus (Greek god of dreams).

morphine.   Historical Notes feature.

morphine (Astramorph PF, Duramorph, Duramorph PF, Infumorph, Kadian, MS Contin, MSIR, OMS Concentrate, Oramorph SR, RMS, Roxanol, Roxanol 100, Roxanol Rescudose, Roxanol T) (Analges, Anes, Cardio, OB/GYN).   Narcotic analgesic drug used to treat moderate-to-severe pain; used as a preoperative drug to sedate and supplement anesthesia; used to treat dyspnea in patients with congestive heart failure; used to treat the pain of childbirth. (Schedule II drug). Capsule: 15 mg, 20 mg, 30 mg, 50 mg, 100 mg. Liquid: 10 mg/2.5 mL, 10 mg/5 mL, 20 mg/mL, 20 mg/5 mL, 100 mg/5 mL. Tablet: 15 mg, 30 mg, 60 mg, 100 mg, 200 mg. Suppository: 5 mg, 10 mg, 20 mg, 30 mg. Subcutaneous, intramuscular, intravenous, intraspinal: 0.5 mg/mL, 1 mg/mL, 2 mg/mL, 4 mg/mL, 5 mg/mL, 8 mg/mL, 10 mg/mL, 15 mg/mL, 25 mg/mL, 50 mg/mL. [MOHR-feen]. 173, 297, 298

morphine sulfate (MS). See *morphine.*

morrhuate (Scleromate) (Cardio, GI). Sclerosing drug used to treat varicose veins; also used to stop bleeding from esophageal varices. Intravenous (injection into the varicose vein or esophageal varix): 50 mg/mL. [MOHR-yoo-ate]. 133, 173

Morton, William. 366

Motilium (GI) (generic *domperidone*). Antiemetic drug; used to treat nausea and vomiting caused by chemotherapy. Investigational drug. 128

motion sickness, drugs used to treat. 128

Motofen (GI). Narcotic antidiarrheal drug. For dosage, see *difenoxin*. [MOH-toh-fehn]. 123

Motrin, Motrin IB, Motrin Migraine Pain, Children's Motrin, Infants' Motrin, Junior Strength Motrin (Analges, OB/GYN, Ortho). Nonsteroidal anti-inflammatory drug used to treat fever and pain in children and adults; used to treat migraine headaches; used to treat dysmenorrhea; used to treat osteoarthritis and rheumatoid arthritis. For dosage, see *ibuprofen*. 139, 304, 307

Motrin IB Sinus (ENT) (generic *pseudoephedrine, ibuprofen*). Combination decongestant and analgesic drug. Caplet: 30 mg/200 mg.

moxifloxacin (Avelox) (Antibio). Fluoroquinolone antibiotic used to treat a variety of infections, including *S. aureus* and *H. influenzae*. Tablet: 400 mg. [mawk-see-FLAWK-sah-sihn]. 318

M-oxy (Analges, Neuro). Narcotic analgesic used to treat moderate-to-severe pain; used to treat neuralgia from herpes zoster infection (shingles). (Schedule II drug). For dosage, see *oxycodone*. [ehm-AWK-see]. 276, 297

MPF (abbreviation for *methylparaben free*). 368

MRSA (abbreviation for *methicillin-resistant Staphylococcus aureus*). [MEHR-sah]. 88, 319

MS Contin (Analges). Narcotic analgesic drug used to treat moderate-to-severe pain. (Schedule II drug). For dosage, see *morphine*. [M-S-kawn-tihn]. 173, 297

MSIR (Analges, Anes, Cardio, OB/GYN). Narcotic analgesic drug used to treat moderate-to-severe pain; used as a preoperative drug to sedate and supplement anesthesia; used to treat dyspnea from congestive heart failure; used to treat the pain of childbirth. (Schedule II drug). For dosage, see *morphine*. 173, 397

MTC. See *mitomycin* and *magnetic targeted carrier.*

MTC-DOX (Chemo) (generic *doxorubicin, iron particles*). Combination chemotherapy drug and iron particles used to treat liver cancer. MTC stands for *magnetic targeted carrier*. The drug-coated iron particles are in-

jected and then pulled into the liver by a magnet positioned above the abdomen outside the body. 342, 362

MTX. See *methotrexate.*

Mucomyst (Emerg, Resp). Mucolytic drug used to break apart thick mucus secretions in patients with pulmonary disease and cystic fibrosis; used to treat acetaminophen overdose. For dosage, see *acetylcysteine*. [MYOO-koh-mihst]. 183, 200, 308

Multikine (Antivir). Used to treat AIDS. Investigational drug. 326

multiple sclerosis, drugs used to treat.

Multi-Symptom Tylenol Cold (ENT) (generic *pseudoephedrine, chlorpheniramine, dextromethorphan, acetaminophen*). Combination decongestant, antihistamine, nonnarcotic antitussive, and analgesic drug. Caplet: 30 mg/2 mg/15 mg/325 mg. Tablet: 30 mg/2 mg/15 mg/325 mg.

Multi-Symptom Tylenol Cough (ENT) (generic *dextromethorphan, acetaminophen*). Combination nonnarcotic antitussive and analgesic drug. Liquid: 10 mg/216.7 mg.

multivitamins, intravenous. See *intravenous multivitamins.*

mupirocin (Bactroban) (Derm, ENT). Topical antibiotic used to treat bacterial infections of the skin and methicillin-resistant *Staphylococcus aureus* (MRSA) infections of the nose. Cream: 2%. Ointment: 2%. [myoo-PEER-oh-sihn]. 88

Murine (Oph). Artificial tears. Drops.

Murine Ear (ENT). Topical drug used to soften hardened cerumen in the ear. Drops. [MYOUR-een].

Murine Plus (Oph). Topical decongestant/vasoconstrictor used to treat irritation and allergy symptoms in the eyes. For dosage, see *tetrahydrozoline*. [MYOUR-een].

Muro 128 (Oph). Topical drug to reduce corneal edema after eye surgery. Ophthalmic ointment: 5%. Ophthalmic solution: 2%, 5%.

Murocell (Oph). Artificial tears. Drops.

Murocoll-2 (Oph). Topical combination mydriatic and ophthalmic decongestant drug; used to lyse synechiae. Ophthalmic solution: 0.3%/10%. [MUHR-oh-kawl]. 223

muromonab-CD3 (Orthoclone OKT3) (Cardio, GI, Uro). Immunosuppressant monoclonal antibody given after organ transplantation to prevent rejection of the donor heart, liver, or kidney. Intravenous: 5 mg/5 mL. [muhr-oh-MAW-nahb]. 110, 133, 173

muscle relaxant drugs.

musculoskeletal diseases, drugs used to treat. 137

Muse (Uro). Used to treat impotence due to erectile dysfunction. Pellet inserted into urethra: 125 mcg, 250 mcg, 500 mcg, 1000 mcg. 109

Mustargen (Chemo). Alkylating chemotherapy drug used to treat leukemia, Hodgkin's disease, lung cancer, and cutaneous T-cell lymphoma. For dosage, see *mechlorethamine*. [MUH-stahr-jehn]. 341

Musterole Deep Strength Rub (Ortho). Topical irritant drug used to mask the pain of arthritis and muscle aches. Liquid. 148

Mutamycin (Chemo). Chemotherapy antibiotic used to treat stomach cancer, pancreatic cancer, and bladder cancer. For dosage, see *mitomycin*. [myoo-tah-MY-sihn]. 342

M-Vax (Chemo). Chemotherapy drug vaccine used to treat melanoma. Orphan drug. 349

M.V.I.-12 (I.V.). Intravenous combination drug of nine water-soluble and three fat-soluble vitamins. 378

Myambutol (Resp). Bactericidal antibiotic used only to treat tuberculosis. For dosage, see *ethambutol*. [my-EHM-byoo-tawl]. 197

myasthenia gravis, drugs used to treat. 271

(Mycelex) (Derm). No longer on the market. (Generic *clotrimazole*; topical antifungal skin drug).

Mycelex (ENT). Topical antiyeast drug used to treat yeast infections in the mouth. For dosage, see *clotrimazole*. [MY-seh-lehks]. 211

Mycelex-3 (OB/GYN) (generic *butoconazole*). Topical antiyeast drug used to treat vaginal yeast infections. Vaginal cream: 2%. [MY-seh-lehks]. 256

Mycelex-7 (OB/GYN) (generic *clotrimazole*). Topical antiyeast drug used to treat vaginal yeast infections. Vaginal cream: 1%, 2%. Vaginal suppository: 100 mg, 200 mg. [MY-seh-lehks]. 256

(Mycelex-G) (OB/GYN). No longer on the market. (Generic name *clotrimazole*; topical drug for vaginal yeast infections).

(Mycifradin) (Antibio). No longer on the market. (Generic name *neomycin*; aminoglycoside antibiotic).

Myciguent (Derm) (generic *neomycin*). Topical antibiotic used to treat bacterial infections. Cream, ointment. 88

Mycinaire Saline Nasal Mist (ENT). Topical saline nasal moisturizing drug. Mist.

Mycinettes (ENT) (generic *benzocaine*). Topical anesthetic used to treat sore throats. Lozenge: 15 mg.

Mycitracin Triple Antibiotic (Derm) (generic *bacitracin, neomycin, polymyxin B*). Topical combination antibiotic drug. Ointment. [my-seh-TRAY-sihn]. 88

Mycobacterium avium-intracellulare (MAC), drugs used to treat. 329

Mycobacterium tuberculosis, drugs used to treat.

Mycobutin (Antivir). Used to prevent *Mycobacterium avium-intracellulare* infection in AIDS patients. For dosage, see *rifabutin*. [my-koh-BYOO-tihn]. 329

Mycolog-II (Derm) (generic *nystatin, triamcinolone*). Topical combination corticosteroid and antiyeast drug. Cream, ointment: 100,000 units/0.1%. [MY-koh-lawg]. 90

mycophenolate (CellCept) (Cardio, GI, Uro). Immunosuppressant drug given after organ transplantation to prevent rejection of the donor heart, liver, or kidney. Capsule: 250 mg, 500 mg. Intravenous: 500 mg/20 mL. [my-koh-FEH-noh-layt]. 110, 133, 174

Mycostatin (Derm) (generic *nystatin*). Topical antiyeast drug. Cream, ointment, powder. [my-koh-STEH-tihn]. 90

Mycostatin, Mycostatin Pastilles (ENT). Topical drug used to treat yeast infections in the mouth. For dosage, see *nystatin*. [my-koh-STEH-tihn]. 211, 331

Mydfrin (Oph). Topical miotic drug used to treat irritation and allergy symptoms in the eyes; used to treat uveitis; used to treat glaucoma; used as a mydriatic during eye surgery. For dosage, see *phenylephrine*. [MID-frehn]. 221, 223

Mydriacyl (Oph). Topical mydriatic drug. For dosage, see *tropicamide*. [meh-DRY-ah-sill]. 223

mydriatics (Oph). Class of drugs that dilate the pupils. 64, 222

Mykrox (Uro). Thiazide-like diuretic. For dosage, see *metolazone*. [MY-krawks]. 103

Mylanta Double Strength, Mylanta Tablet (GI) (generic *aluminum, magnesium, simethicone*). Combination antacid and anti-gas drug. Liquid: 400 mg/400 mg/40 mg. Tablet: 200 mg/200 mg/20 mg, 400 mg/400 mg/40 mg. 117

Mylanta Gelcaps, Mylanta Supreme (GI) (generic *calcium, magnesium*). Combination antacid. Gelcap: 311 mg/232 mg, 400 mg/135 mg. 117

Mylanta Liquid (GI) (generic *aluminum, simethicone*). Combination antacid and anti-gas drug. Liquid: 200 mg/20 mg. 117

Mylanta Lozenge (GI). Calcium-containing antacid. Lozenge: 600 mg. 116

Myleran (Chemo). Alkylating chemotherapy drug used to treat leukemia. For dosage, see *busulfan*. [MY-leh-rehn]. 341

Mylicon (GI). Antiflatulent. For dosage, see *simethicone*. [MY-lih-kawn]. 118

Mylinax (Neuro). Purine antagonist chemotherapy drug used to treat multiple sclerosis. For dosage, see *cladribine*. [MY-lih-nacks]. 275

Mylocel (Antivir, Chemo, Derm, Hem). Antimetabolite chemotherapy drug with antiviral activity used to treat AIDS; used to treat head and neck cancer; used to treat severe psoriasis; used to treat thrombocytothemia. For dosage, see *hydroxyurea*. [MY-loh-sell]. 87, 189, 326, 341

Mylotarg (Chemo) Monoclonal antibody used to treat leukemia. For dosage, see *gemtuzumab*. [MY-loh-tawrg]. 346

Myobloc (Ortho). Used to treat the muscle contractions and abnormal head position of cervical dystonia. For dosage, see *botulinum toxin type B*. 147

myocardial infarction, drugs used to prevent a second.

(Myochrysine) (Ortho). No longer on the market. (Generic name *gold sodium thiomalate*; gold compound used to treat rheumatoid arthritis).

Myotonachol (Uro). Antispasmodic drug used to treat urinary frequency and urgency. For dosage, see *bethanechol*. [my-oh-TOH-nah-kawl]. 107

Myotrophin (Endo, Neuro). Used to treat growth hormone insufficiency syndrome; used to treat amyotrophic lateral sclerosis. For dosage, see *mecasermin*. [my-oh-TROH-fihn]. 276

Mysoline (Neuro). Anticonvulsant drug used to treat tonic-clonic and simple and complex partial seizures. For dosage, see *primidone*. [MY-soh-leen]. 265

Mytelase (Neuro). Anticholinesterase drug used to treat myasthenia gravis. For dosage, see *ambenonium*. [MY-teh-lace]. 271

Mytrex (Derm) (generic *nystatin, triamcinolone*). Topical combination antiyeast and corticosteroid drug. Cream, ointment. [MY-trehks]. 90

N₂O (chemical symbol for *nitrous oxide*). See *nitrous oxide*.

N_2O (chemical symbol for *nitrous oxide*). See *nitrous oxide*.

Na (chemical symbol for *sodium*).

nabumetone (Relafen) (Analges, Ortho). Nonsteroidal anti-inflammatory drug used to treat osteoarthritis and rheumatoid arthritis. Tablet: 500 mg, 750 mg. [nah-BYOO-meh-tohn]. 139, 304

NaCl (chemical symbol for *sodium chloride*).

nadolol (Corgard) (Analges, GI, Ortho, Neuro, Psych). Nonselective beta-blocker used to treat migraine headaches; used to prevent rebleeding from esophageal varices in patients with cirrhosis; used to treat essential familial tremor; used to treat the tremors of Parkinson's disease; used to treat aggressive behavior; used to treat the side effects of muscle tremor and restlessness from antipsychotic drugs; used to treat performance anxiety. Tablet: 20 mg, 40 mg, 80 mg, 120 mg, 160 mg. [NEH-doh-lawl]. 134, 146, 269, 306

nadolol (Corgard) (Cardio). Nonselective beta-blocker used to treat angina pectoris, hypertension, and ventricular arrhythmias. Tablet: 20 mg, 40 mg, 80 mg, 120 mg, 160 mg. [NEH-doh-lawl]. 157, 160, 162

nafarelin (Synarel) (Endo, OB/GYN). Hormonal drug used to treat precocious puberty in boys and girls; used to treat endometriosis. Nasal spray: 2 mg/mL. [neh-fah-RAY-lihn]. 248

Nafazair (Oph). Topical decongestant/vasoconstrictor used to treat irritation and allergy symptoms in the eyes. For dosage, see *naphazoline*. [NEH-fah-zayr]. 220

nafcillin (Unipen) (Antibio). Penicillin-type antibiotic used to treat a variety of bacterial infections, including staphylococci. Capsule: 250 mg. [NEHF-sill-ehn]. 313

naftifine (Naftine) (Derm). Topical antifungal drug. Cream: 1%. Gel: 1%. 89

Naftin (Derm) (generic *naftifine*). Topical antifungal drug. Cream: 1%. Gel: 1%. 89

nalbuphine (Nubain) (Analges, OB/GYN). Narcotic analgesic drug used to treat moderate-to-severe pain; used to treat pain during labor and delivery. Intravenous: 10 mg/mL, 20 mg/mL. [nehl-BYOO-feen]. 297

(Naldecon, Naldecon Pediatric) (ENT). No longer on the market. (Combination drug with *phenylpropanolamine*; decongestant and antihistamine).

(Naldecon CX Adult) (ENT). No longer on the market. (Combination drug with *phenylpropanolamine*; decongestant, narcotic antitussive, and expectorant drug).

(Naldecon DX Adult, Naldecon DX Children's, Naldecon DX Pediatric) (ENT). No longer on the market. (Combination drug with *phenylpropanolamine*; decongestant, nonnarcotic antitussive, and expectorant drug).

(Naldecon EX Children's Syrup, Naldecon EX Pediatric Drops) (ENT). No longer on the market. (Combination drug with *phenylpropanolamine*; decongestant and expectorant).

Naldecon Senior DX (ENT) (generic *dextromethorphan, guaifenesin*). Combination nonnarcotic antitussive and expectorant drug. Liquid: 10 mg/200 mg. [NEHL-de-kawn].

Naldecon Senior EX (ENT). Expectorant. For dosage, see *guaifenesin*. [NEHL-de-kawn]. 210

Nalfon Pulvules (Analges, Ortho). Nonsteroidal anti-inflammatory drug used to treat pain and migraine headaches; used to treat osteoarthritis and rheumatoid arthritis. For dosage, see *fenoprofen*. 139, 304, 307

nalidixic acid (NegGram) (Antibio). Quinolone antibiotic used only to treat urinary tract infections. Capsule: 250 mg, 500 mg, 1 g. Liquid: 250 mg/5 mL. [neh-lih-dihk-sihk EH-sihd]. 105, 318

(Nallpen) (Antibio). No longer on the market. (Generic name *nafcillin*; penicillin-type antibiotic).

nalmefene (Revex) (Analges, Emerg). Narcotic antagonist used to reverse the effects of narcotic overdose. Subcutaneous, intramuscular, intravenous: 100 mcg/mL, 1 mg/mL. [NEHL-meh-feen]. 182, 308

naloxone (Narcan) (Analges, Emerg). Narcotic antagonist used to reverse the effects of narcotic overdose; used to reverse narcotic dependence in babies born to addicts; used to reverse the effects of narcotics used during surgery. Endotracheal, subcutaneous, intramuscular, or intravenous: 0.02 mg/mL, 0.4 mg/mL, 1 mg/mL. [nah-LAWK-zohn]. 182, 308

naloxone (Narcan) (Neuro, Psych). Narcotic antagonist used to treat Alzheimer's dementia, alcoholic coma, and schizophrenia. Endotracheal, subcutaneous, intramuscular, or intravenous: 0.02 mg/mL, 0.4 mg/mL, 1 mg/mL. [nah-LAWK-zohn].

naltrexone (ReVia, Trexan) (Analges). Narcotic antagonist used to block the effect of narcotics, ongoing treatment for former narcotic-dependent patients; used to treat alcohol dependence. Tablet: 50 mg. [nehl-TREHK-sohn]. 182, 308

names, drug. 22

nandrolone (Deca-Durabolin) (Chemo, Endo, Hem). Anabolic steroid used to treat metastatic breast cancer; used to increase red blood cell production to treat anemia; also used illegally by athletes. Intramuscular: 100 mg/mL, 200 mg/mL. [NEHN-droh-lohn]. 234

naphazoline (Albalon, Allerest Eye Drops, Nafazair, Naphcon, Naphcon Forte, VasoClear, VasoClear A Solution, Vasocon Regular) (Oph). Topical decongestant/vasoconstrictor used to treat irritation and allergy symptoms in the eyes. Ophthalmic drops: 0.012%. Ophthalmic solution: 0.012%, 0.02%, 0.03%, 0.1%. [neh-FEH-zoh-leen]. 220

naphazoline (Privine) (ENT). Decongestant. Drops: 0.05%. Spray: 0.05%. [neh-FEH-zoh-leen]. 206

Naphcon, Naphcon Forte (Oph). Topical decongestant/vasoconstrictor used to treat irritation and allergy symptoms in the eyes. For dosage, see *naphazoline*. [NEHF-kawn]. 220

Naphcon-A Solution (Oph) (generic *naphazoline, pheniramine*). Topical combination decongestant and antihistamine. Ophthalmic solution: 0.025%/0.3%. [NEHF-kawn].

Naprosyn, EC-Naprosyn (Analges, OB/GYN, Ortho). Nonsteroidal anti-inflammatory drug used to treat pain; used to treat migraine headaches; used to treat dysmenorrhea; used to treat bursitis, gout, osteoarthritis, rheumatoid arthritis, and tendinitis. For dosage, see *naproxen*. [NEH-proh-sihn]. 139, 146, 255, 304, 307

naproxen (Aleve, Anaprox, Anaprox DS, EC-Naprosyn, Naprosyn) (Analges, OB/GYN, Ortho). Non-

steroidal anti-inflammatory drug used to treat pain; used to treat migraine headaches; used to treat dysmenorrhea; used to treat bursitis, gout, osteoarthritis, rheumatoid arthritis, and tendinitis. Liquid: 125 mg/5 mL. Tablet: 200 mg, 250 mg, 375 mg, 500 mg. [nah-PRAWK-sihn]. 139, 146, 255, 304, 307

Naqua (Uro). Thiazide diuretic. For dosage, see *trichlormethiazide*. [NEH-kwah]. 103

naratriptan (Amerge) (Analges). Serotonin receptor agonist drug used to treat migraine headaches. Tablet: 1 mg, 2.5 mg. [neh-rah-TRIP-tehn]. 306

Narcan (Analges, Emerg). Narcotic antagonist used to reverse the effects of narcotic overdose; used to reverse narcotic dependence in babies born to addicts. For dosage, see *naloxone*. [NAWR-kehn]. 182, 308

Narcan (Neuro, Psych). Narcotic antagonist used to treat Alzheimer's dementia, alcoholic coma, and schizophrenia. For dosage, see *naloxone*. [NAWR-kehn]. 275

narcotic addiction and overdose, drugs used to treat. 182, 307

narcotics (Analges). Class of addictive drugs derived from opium that are used to treat pain. 297

Nardil (Psych). MAO inhibitor used to treat depression. For dosage, see *phenelzine*. [NAWR-dihl]. 288

Naropin (Anes). Local, regional nerve block, and epidural anesthetic. For dosage, see *ropivacaine*. [neh-ROH-pihn]. 368

Nasacort, Nasacort AQ (ENT). Topical intranasal corticosteroid used to treat allergic rhinitis. For dosage, see *triamcinolone*. [NAY-seh-kohrt]. 208

NasalCrom, Children's NasalCrom (ENT). Topical mast cell stabilizer used to treat allergic rhinitis. For dosage, see *cromolyn*. [NAY-suhl-krawm]. 208

Nasalide (ENT). Topical intranasal corticosteroid used to treat allergic rhinitis. For dosage, see *flunisolide*. [NAY-sah-lide]. 208

Nascobal (Hem). Vitamin B_{12} used to treat pernicious anemia. Intranasal gel. [NEHS-koh-bawl]. 172

nasogastric tube, administration of drugs by. 39

Nasonex (ENT). Topical intranasal corticosteroid used to treat allergic rhinitis. For dosage, see *mometasone*. [NAY-soh-nehks]. 208

Natacyn (Oph). Topical drug used to treat fungal infection of the eyes. For dosage, see *natamycin*. [NEH-tah-sihn]. 219

natamycin (Natacyn) (Oph). Topical drug used to treat fungal infection of the eyes. Ophthalmic suspension: 5%. [neh-tah-MY-sihn]. 219

nateglinide (Starlix) (Diab). Oral antidiabetic drug. Tablet: 60 mg, 120 mg. [neh-TEHG-lih-nide]. 240

National Formulary *(NF)*. 14

Natrecor (Cardio). A human B-type natriuretic peptide (hBNP) drug used to treat severely decompensated congestive heart failure. For dosage, see *nesiritide*. [NAY-treh-kohr]. 155

Naturetin (Uro). Thiazide diuretic. For dosage, see *bendroflumethiazide*. [nay-tyour-EE-tihn]. 103

nausea and vomiting, drugs used to treat. 127

Navane (Psych). Used to treat psychosis. For dosage, see *thiothixene*. [NEH-vayn]. 284

NAVEL (abbreviation for *naloxone/Narcan, atropine, Valium, epinephrine, lidocaine*). See *emergency resuscitation drugs*. 179

Navelbine (Chemo). Mitosis inhibitor chemotherapy drug used to treat lung cancer, breast cancer, uterine cancer, and Kaposi's sarcoma. For dosage, see *vinorelbine*. 344

nebacumab (Centoxin) (Antibio). Used to treat gram-negative bacteremia and shock. Orphan drug. 321

Nebcin, Nebcin Pediatric (Antibio). Aminoglycoside antibiotic used to treat a variety of bacterial infections, including *Staphylococcus, E. coli, Pseudomonas,* and *Klebsiella*; used to treat cystic fibrosis patients with *Pseudomonas* infection. For dosage, see *tobramycin*. [NEHB-sihn]. 317

NebuPent (Antivir). Used to treat *Pneumocystis carinii* infection in AIDS patients. For dosage, see *pentamidine*. [NEH-byoo-pehnt]. 328

Necon 0.5/35, Necon 1/35, Necon 1/50 (OB/GYN) (generic *norethindrone, ethinyl estradiol* or *mestranol*). Monophasic combination progestins and estrogen oral contraceptive. Tablet: 0.5 mg/35 mcg, 2 mg/35 mcg, 1 mg/50 mcg. [NEE-kawn]. 249

Necon 10/11 (OB/GYN) (generic *norethindrone, ethinyl estradiol*). Biphasic combination progestins and estrogen oral contraceptive. Tablet: 0.5 mg/35 mcg then 1 mg/35 mcg. [NEE-kawn]. 250

nedocromil (Alocril) (Oph). Topical mast cell stabilizer used to treat allergy symptoms in the eyes. Ophthalmic solution: 2%. [neh-DOH-kroh-mihl]. 220

nedocromil (Tilade) (Resp). Mast cell stabilizer used to prevent acute asthma attacks. Aerosol inhaler: 1.75 mg/puff. [neh-DOH-kroh-mihl]. 197

needle.
bore of. 62
butterfly. 64
gauge of. 63

nefazodone (Serzone) (Psych). Antidepressant. Tablet: 50 mg, 100 mg, 150 mg, 200 mg, 250 mg. [neh-FEH-zoh-dohn]. 288

NegGram (Antibio). Quinolone antibiotic used only to treat urinary tract infections. For dosage, see *nalidixic acid*. [NEH-grehm]. 105, 318

nelfinavir (Viracept) (Antivir). Protease inhibitor drug used to treat AIDS. Tablet: 250 mg. Powder: 50 mg/g. [nehl-FIHN-ah-veer]. 325

Nelova 1/35E, Nelova 1/50M (OB/GYN) (generic *norethindrone, ethinyl estradiol* or *mestranol*). Monophasic combination progestins and estrogen oral contraceptive. Tablet: 35 mcg/1 mg, 50 mcg/1 mg. [neh-LOH-vah]. 249

(Nelova 10/11) (OB/GYN). No longer on the market. (Oral contraceptive).

Nembutal (Anes, Neuro). Barbiturate used to provide preoperative sedation; used for short-term treatment of insomnia. (Schedule II drug). For dosage, see *pentobarbital*. [NEHM-byoo-tawl]. 272, 371

(Neocaf) (Resp). No longer on the market. (Generic name *caffeine*; used to prevent apnea in premature infants).

(Neo-Cortef) (Derm). No longer on the market. (Generic name *hydrocortisone, neomycin*; combination topical corticosteroid and antibiotic drug).

NeoDecadron Ophthalmic Solution (Oph) (generic *dexamethasone, neomycin*). Topical combination corticosteroid and antibiotic drug. Ophthalmic solution: 0.1%, 0.35%. [nee-oh-DEHK-ah-drawn].

Neomark (Chemo). Radiation sensitizer drug used to treat brain tumors. For dosage, see *broxuridine*. 361

(Neo-Medrol) (Derm). No longer on the market. (Generic name *methylprednisolone, neomycin*; combination topical corticosteroid and antibiotic drug).

neomycin (Antibio, GI). Aminoglycoside antibiotic; used before gastrointestinal surgery to inhibit bacteria in the gastrointestinal tract. Tablet: 500 mg. Liquid: 125 mg/5 mL. [nee-oh-MY-sihn]. 316

neomycin (Myciguent) (Derm). Topical antibiotic used to treat bacterial infections. Cream, ointment. [nee-oh-MY-sihn]. 88

Neopap (Analges). Nonnarcotic nonaspirin analgesic drug used to treat fever and pain in children. For dosage, see *acetaminophen*. [NEE-oh-pehp]. 301

Neoral (Cardio, GI, Uro). Immunosuppressant drug given after organ transplantation to prevent rejection of the donor heart, liver, or kidney. For dosage, see *cyclosporine*. [nee-OHR-awl]. 110, 132, 173

Neoral (Derm, Ortho). Immunosuppressant drug used to treat severe, disabling psoriasis and rheumatoid arthritis. For dosage, see *cyclosporine*. [nee-OHR-awl]. 87, 110

Neosar (Chemo, Uro). Alkylating chemotherapy drug used to treat Hodgkin's disease, non-Hodgkin's lymphomas, multiple myeloma, leukemia, brain cancer, eye cancer, cutaneous T-cell lymphoma, and cancer of the breast and ovary; used to treat pediatric nephrotic syndrome. For dosage, see *cyclophosphamide*. [NEE-oh-sawr]. 111, 341

Neosporin, Maximum Strength Neosporin (Derm) (generic *bacitracin, neomycin, polymyxin B*). Topical combination antibiotic drug. Cream, ointment. [nee-oh-SPOHR-ehn]. 88

Neosporin Ophthalmic Ointment (Oph) (generic *bacitracin, neomycin, polymyxin B*). Topical combination antibiotic drug. Ophthalmic ointment: 400 units/10,000 units/3.5 mg per g. [nee-oh-SPOHR-ehn].

Neosporin Ophthalmic Solution (Oph) (generic *gramicidin, neomycin, polymyxin B*). Topical combination antibiotic drug. Ophthalmic solution: 0.025 mg/1.75 mg/10,000 units per mL. [nee-oh-SPOHR-ehn].

neostigmine (Prostigmin) (Neuro). Anticholinesterase drug used to treat myasthenia gravis. Intramuscular, intravenous, or subcutaneous: 1:1000 solution (1 mg/mL), 1:2000 solution (0.5 mg/mL), 1:4000 solution (0.25 mg/mL). [nee-oh-STIHG-meen]. 271

neostigmine (Prostigmin) (Uro). Urinary antispasmodic drug; used to treat postoperative urinary retention. Intramuscular: 1:1000 solution (1 mg/mL), 1:2000 solution (0.5 mg/mL), 1:4000 solution (0.25 mg/mL). [nee-oh-STIHG-meen]. 107

Neo-Synephrine (ENT). Decongestant. For dosage, see *phenylephrine*. 206

Neo-Synephrine (Oph). Topical miotic drug used to treat uveitis; used to treat glaucoma; used as a mydriatic during eye surgery. For dosage, see *phenylephrine*. [nee-oh-sih-NEH-frehn]. 221, 223

(Neotricin) (Oph). No longer on the market. (Combination corticosteroid and antibiotic drug for the eye).

NephrAmine 5.4% (I.V.). Intravenous fluids used for total parenteral nutrition, especially for patients with renal failure. 378

nephrotoxicity. 53, 317

Nepro (GI). Liquid nutritional supplement. Liquid. 131

Neptazane (Oph). Carbonic anhydrase inhibitor used to treat glaucoma. For dosage, see *methazolamide*. [NEHP-tah-zayn]. 221

Nesacaine, Nesacaine MPF (Anes). Local, regional nerve block, and epidural anesthetic. For dosage, see *chloroprocaine*. [NEH-seh-kayn]. 368

nesiritide (Natrecor) (Cardio). A human B-type natriuretic peptide (hBNP) drug used to treat severely decompensated congestive heart failure. Intravenous: 1.5 mg/mL. [neh-SEER-eh-tide]. 155

netilmicin (Netromycin) (Antibio). Aminoglycoside antibiotic used to treat various bacterial infections,

including *E. coli, Klebsiella, Pseudomonas*, and *Staphylococcus*. Intramuscular or intravenous: 100 mg/mL. [neh-tihl-MY-sihn]. 317

Netromycin (Antibio). Aminoglycoside antibiotic used to treat various bacterial infections, including *E. coli, Klebsiella, Pseudomonas*, and *Staphylococcus*. For dosage, see *netilmicin*. [neh-troh-MY-sihn]. 317

Neumega (Chemo). Used to prevent thrombocytopenia in patients undergoing chemotherapy. For dosage, see *oprelvekin*. [noo-MEH-gah]. 189, 362

Neupogen (Antivir, Chemo, Hem). Granulocyte colony-stimulating factor used to treat neutropenia in AIDS patients; used with chemotherapy and bone marrow transplants; used to treat aplastic anemia. For dosage, see *filgrastim*. [NOO-poh-jehn]. 331, 361

Neuralgon (ENT, Ortho). Skeletal muscle relaxant used to treat trigeminal neuralgia; used to treat severe muscle spasticity associated with multiple sclerosis, cerebral palsy, stroke, or spinal cord injury. For dosage, see *L-baclofen*. [nyour-EHL-gawn]. 145, 276

Neurelan (Neuro). Used to treat multiple sclerosis. For dosage, see *fampridine*. [NYOUR-eh-lawn]. 275

NeuroCell-HD (Neuro). Fetal pig nerve cells that are surgically implanted in the cerebrum to produce GABA, one of the chemical compounds lacking in patients with Huntington's chorea. Orphan drug. 276

NeuroCell-PD (Neuro). Fetal pig neuron cells that are surgically implanted in the cerebrum to replace nerve cells lost because of Parkinson's disease. Orphan drug. 270

neuroleptics (Psych). See *antipsychotic drugs*.

neurological drugs. 262

neuromuscular blocking drugs. Historical Notes feature. 367

neuromuscular blocking drugs (Anes). Class of drugs that produce muscle relaxation during surgery. 370

Neurontin (Analges, Derm, Neuro, Psych). Used to treat migraine headaches; used to treat postherpetic neuralgia; used to treat partial seizures of epilepsy; used to treat multiple sclerosis and amyotrophic lateral sclerosis; used to treat manic-depressive disorder. For dosage, see *gabapentin*. [nyour-AWN-tihn]. 265, 276

neurosis, drugs used to treat. 280

neurotransmitter. 47

NeuTrexin (Antivir, Chemo). Used to treat *Pneumocystis carinii* pneumonia in AIDS patients; chemotherapy drug used to treat bone cancer, head and neck cancer, colon and rectal cancer, pancreatic cancer, and lung cancer. For dosage, see *trimetrexate*. [noo-TREHK-sihn]. 328, 348

Neutrogena Acne Mask (Derm) (generic *benzoyl peroxide*). Used to treat acne vulgaris. Mask: 5%. 83

Neutrogena T/Derm, Neutrogena T/Gel (Derm) (generic *coal tar*). Topical drug used to treat psoriasis. Oil: 5%. Shampoo: 2%. [noo-troh-GEE-nah]. 86

nevirapine (Viramune) (Antivir). Nonnucleoside reverse transcriptase inhibitor drug used to treat AIDS. Tablet: 200 mg. Liquid: 50 mg/5 mL. [neh-VEER-ah-peen]. 325

Nexium (GI). Proton pump inhibitor drug used to treat heartburn, gastroesophageal reflux disease, and *H. pylori* infection. For dosage, see *esomeprazole*. [NEHK-see-uhm]. 121

NF (abbreviation for *National Formulary*). See *National Formulary.*

NG (nasogastric) tube. See *nasogastric tube.*

niacin (Niaspan) (Cardio). Vitamin B used to treat hypercholesterolemia and hypertriglyceridemia. Tablet: 500 mg, 750 mg, 1000 mg. [NY-ah-sihn]. 171

Niaspan (Cardio). Vitamin B used to treat hypercholesterolemia and hypertriglyceridemia. For dosage, see *niacin*. [NY-ah-spehn]. 171

nicardipine (Cardene, Cardene I.V., Cardene SR) (Cardio). Calcium channel blocker used to treat angina pectoris, congestive heart failure, and hypertension; used to treat hypertensive crisis. Capsule: 20 mg, 30 mg, 45 mg, 60 mg. Intravenous: 2.5 mg/mL. [ny-KAWR-dih-peen]. 154, 157, 163, 168

Nicoderm CQ (Resp, Psych). Nicotine drug used to stop smoking; used to treat Tourette's syndrome. Transdermal patch: 7 mg/24 hr, 14 mg/24 hr, 21 mg/24 hr. [NIH-koh-dehrm]. 199, 294

(Nicolar) (Cardio). No longer on the market. (Generic name *niacin*; used to treat hyperlipidemia).

Nicorette, Nicorette DS (Resp). Nicotine drug used to stop smoking. Chewing gum: 2 mg/piece, 4 mg/piece. [nih-koh-REHT]. 199

nicotine (Habitrol, Nicoderm CQ, Nicorette, Nicotrol, Nicotrol Inhaler, Nicotrol NS) (Resp, Psych). Used to stop smoking; used to treat Tourette's syndrome. Chewing gum: 2 mg/piece, 4 mg/piece. Nasal spray: 0.5 mg/spray. Inhaler: 4 mg/inhalation. Transdermal patch: 7 mg/24 hr, 14 mg/24 hr, 15 mg/24 hr, 21 mg/24 hr. [NIH-koh-teen]. 199, 294

nicotinic acid (Cardio). Used to treat hyperlipidemia. For dosage, see *niacin*. [nih-koh-TIH-nihk EH-sihd].

Nicotrol, Nicotrol Inhaler, Nicotrol NS (Resp). Nicotine drug used to stop smoking. Nasal spray: 0.5 mg/spray. Inhaler: 4 mg/inhalation. Transdermal patch: 15 mg/24 hr. [NIH-koh-trawl]. 199

nifedipine (Adalat, Procardia) (Analges). Calcium channel blocker used to treat migraine headaches. Capsule: 10 mg, 20 mg. Tablet: 30 mg, 60 mg, 90 mg. [ny-FEH-deh-peen]. 306

nifedipine (Adalat, Adalat CC, Procardia, Procardia XL) (Cardio). Calcium channel blocker used to treat angina pectoris, congestive heart failure, and hypertension; used to treat hypertensive crisis; used to treat Raynaud's disease. Capsule: 10 mg, 20 mg. Tablet: 30 mg, 60 mg, 90 mg. [ny-FEH-deh-peen]. 154, 157, 163

Nighttime Pamprin (Neuro) (generic *acetaminophen, diphenhydramine*). Combination analgesic and antihistamine sleep aid. Powder to be reconstituted: 650 mg/50 mg. 273

NightTime TheraFlu (ENT) (generic *pseudoephedrine, chlorpheniramine, dextromethorphan, acetaminophen*). Combination decongestant, antihistamine, nonnarcotic antitussive, and analgesic drug. Powder (to be mixed with water): 60 mg/4 mg/30 mg/1000 mg.

Nilandron (Chemo). Hormonal chemotherapy drug used to treat prostatic cancer. For dosage, see *nilutamide*. [NIH-lehn-drohn]. 344

Nilstat (Derm) (generic *nystatin*). Topical antiyeast drug. Cream, ointment. 90

Nilstat (ENT). Topical drug used to treat yeast infections in the mouth. For dosage, see *nystatin*. 211, 331

nilutamide (Nilandron) (Chemo). Hormonal chemotherapy drug used to treat prostatic cancer. Tablet: 50 mg, 150 mg. [nih-LOO-tah-mide]. 344

Nimbex (Anes, Resp). Muscle relaxant drug used during surgery; used to treat patients who are intubated and on the ventilator. For dosage, see *cisatracurium*. 199, 370

nimodipine (Nimotop) (Analges, Neuro). Calcium channel blocker used to treat migraine headaches; also used to increase blood flow to improve neurological deficits after subarachnoid hemorrhage. Capsule: 30 mg. [nih-MOH-deh-peen]. 276, 306

Nimotop (Analges, Neuro). Calcium channel blocker used to treat migraine headaches; also used to improve neurological deficits after subarachnoid hemorrhage. For dosage, see *nimodipine*. [NIH-moh-tawp]. 276, 306

Nipent (Chemo). Purine antagonist chemotherapy drug used to treat leukemia and cutaneous T-cell lymphoma; investigational drug used to treat non-Hodgkin's lymphoma. For dosage, see *pentostatin*. [NY-pehnt]. 339

nisoldipine (Sular) (Cardio). Calcium channel blocker used to treat hypertension. Tablet: 10 mg, 20 mg, 30 mg, 40 mg. [nih-SOHL-deh-peen]. 163

nitazoxanide (NTZ) (Cryptaz) (Antivir, GI). Used to treat protozoal diarrhea in the general population or *Cryptosporidium parvum* parasite diarrhea in AIDS patients. Capsule: 500 mg. [ny-tah-ZAWK-seh-nide]. 134, 331

nitrates (Cardio).   Class of drugs used to prevent or treat angina pectoris. 156

nitrazepam (Mogadon) (Neuro).   Used to treat epilepsy. Investigational drug. 265

nitrendipine (Baypress) (Cardio).   Calcium channel blocker used to treat hypertension. Investigational drug. 174

nitric oxide (INOmax) (Resp).   Used to treat persistent pulmonary hypertension in newborns in respiratory failure on the ventilator. Inhaled gas: 100 ppm, 800 ppm.

Nitro-Bid, Nitro-Bid IV (Cardio).   Nitrate drug used to prevent and treat angina pectoris; used to treat hypertensive crisis.   For dosage, see *nitroglycerin*. 156, 168

Nitrodisc (Cardio).   Nitrate drug used to prevent and treat angina pectoris.   For dosage, see *nitroglycerin*. 156

Nitro-Dur (Cardio).   Nitrate drug used to prevent and treat angina pectoris.   For dosage, see *nitroglycerin*. 156

nitrofurantoin (Furadantin, Macrobid, Macrodantin) (Antibio, Uro).   Antibiotic used only to treat urinary tract infections. Capsule: 25 mg, 50 mg, 100 mg. Liquid: 25 mg/5 mL. [ny-troh-fyour-EHN-toh-ehn]. 106, 319

nitrofurazone (Furacin) (Derm).   Topical antibiotic used to treat severe burns. Cream: 0.2%. Liquid: 0.2%. Ointment: 0.2%. [ny-troh-FYOUR-eh-zohn]. 97

Nitrogard (Cardio).   Nitrate drug used to prevent and treat angina pectoris.   For dosage, see *nitroglycerin*. 156

nitrogen mustard.   Historical Notes feature. 341

nitrogen mustard.   See *mechlorethamine*.

nitroglycerin (Deponit, Minitran, Nitro-Bid, Nitro-Bid IV, Nitrodisc, Nitro-Dur, Nitrogard, Nitrol, Nitrolingual, Nitrong, Nitrostat, Transderm-Nitro, Tridil) (Cardio).   Nitrate drug used to prevent and treat angina pectoris; used to treat hypertensive crisis (intravenous form). Capsule: 2.5 mg, 6.5 mg, 9 mg, 13 mg. Buccal tablet: 2 mg, 3 mg. Sublingual tablet: 0.3 mg, 0.4 mg, 0.6 mg. Tablet: 2.5 mg, 6.5 mg, 9 mg. Translingual spray: 0.5 mg/spray. Ointment: 2% (1 inch = 15 mg). Transdermal: 9 mg, 12.5 mg, 20 mg. Intravenous: 0.5 mg/mL, 5 mg/mL, 25 mg/250 mL, 50 mg/250 mL, 50 mg/500 mL, 100 mg/250 mL, 200 mg/500 mL. [ny-troh-GLIH-seh-rihn]. 156, 168

Nitrol (Cardio).   Nitrate drug used to prevent and treat angina pectoris.   For dosage, see *nitroglycerin*. [NY-trawl]. 156

Nitrolingual (Cardio).   Nitrate drug used to prevent and treat angina pectoris.   For dosage, see *nitroglycerin*. [ny-troh-LIHNG-gwal]. 156

Nitrong (Cardio).   Nitrate drug used to prevent and treat angina pectoris.   For dosage, see *nitroglycerin*. [NY-trawng]. 156

Nitropress (Cardio).   Peripheral vasodilator used to treat hypertensive crisis.   For dosage, see *nitroprusside*. [NY-troh-prehs]. 168

nitroprusside (Nitropress) (Cardio).   Peripheral vasodilator used to treat hypertensive crisis. Intravenous (powder to be reconstituted): 50 mg. [ny-troh-PRUH-side]. 168

Nitrostat (Cardio).   Nitrate drug used to prevent and treat angina pectoris.   For dosage, see *nitroglycerin*. [NY-troh-steht]. 156

nitrous oxide (N$_2$O) (Anes).   Used to induce and maintain general anesthesia. Inhaled gas. [NY-truhs AWK-side]. 366, 370

nits.   See *lice*.

Nix (Derm) (generic *permethrin*).   Topical drug used to treat scabies (mites) and pediculosis (lice). Liquid (creme rinse): 1%. 95

nizatidine (Axid AR, Axid Pulvules) (GI).   H$_2$ blocker used to treat peptic ulcers and *H. pylori* infection. Capsule: 150 mg, 300 mg. Tablet: 75 mg. [ny-ZEH-tih-deen]. 118

Nizoral (Antifung, Derm, ENT).   Used to treat severe topical and systemic fungal and yeast infections. For dosage, see *ketoconazole*. [ny-ZOHR-awl]. 334, 335

Nizoral (Cardio, GI, Uro).   Used to prevent toxicity to the kidney in patients with organ transplants who receive cyclosporine. Orphan drug.

Nizoral, Nizoral A-D (Derm) (generic *ketoconazole*). Topical drug used to treat fungal and yeast infections. Cream: 2%. Shampoo: 1%, 2%. [ny-ZOHR-awl]. 89, 90

NKDA (abbreviation for *no known drug allergies*). 55

(Noctec) (Neuro).   No longer on the market. (Generic name *chloral hydrate*; nonbarbiturate used to treat insomnia).

No Drowsiness Allerest (ENT) (generic *pseudoephedrine, acetaminophen*).   Combination decongestant and analgesic drug. Tablet: 30 mg/500 mg.

No Drowsiness Sinarest (ENT) (generic *pseudoephedrine, acetaminophen*).   Combination decongestant and analgesic drug. Tablet: 30 mg/500 mg.

Nolahist (ENT).   Antihistamine used to treat allergic rhinitis.   For dosage, see *phenindamine*. 207

nolatrexed (Thymitaq) (Chemo).   Chemotherapy drug used to treat head and neck cancer, lung cancer, gastric cancer, pancreatic cancer, and colon cancer. Investigational drug. 348

(Noludar) (Neuro). No longer on the market. (Generic name *methyprylon*; nonbarbiturate used to treat insomnia).

Nolvadex (Chemo, Endo). Hormonal chemotherapy drug used to treat breast cancer; used to treat gynecomastia in men. For dosage, see *tamoxifen*. [NOHL-vah-dehks]. 343

nonnarcotic drugs (Analges). Class of drugs that do not contain a narcotic and are used to treat mild-to-moderate pain. 299

nonnucleoside reverse transcriptase inhibitors (Antivir). Class of drugs used to treat HIV/AIDS. 325

nonselective beta-blockers. Subclass of beta-blocker drugs. See *beta-blockers*. 162

nonsteroidal anti-inflammatory drugs (NSAIDs) (Analges, OB/GYN, Ortho). Class of drugs that reduce pain and inflammation. 139, 304

Norcuron (Anes, Resp). Muscle relaxant drug used during surgery; used to treat patients who are intubated and on the ventilator. For dosage, see *vecuronium*. [NOHR-kyour-awn]. 199, 370

Nordette (OB/GYN) (generic *levonorgestrel, ethinyl estradiol*). Monophasic combination progestins and estrogen oral contraceptive. Tablet: 0.15 mg/30 mcg. [nohr-DEHT]. 249

Norditropin (Endo, OB/GYN). Growth hormone replacement for adults and children with growth failure; used to treat growth failure of infants who are small for gestational age; orphan drug used to stimulate ovulation in infertility. For dosage, see *somatropin*. [nohr-deh-TROH-pihn]. 230, 244

norepinephrine (Levophed) (Emerg). Vasopressor used to treat hypotension during emergency resuscitation. Intravenous: 1 mg/mL. [nohr-eh-pih-NEH-frihn]. 181

(Norethin) (OB/GYN). No longer on the market. (Oral contraceptive).

norethindrone (Aygestin) (OB/GYN). Progestins hormone drug used to treat amenorrhea; used to treat abnormal uterine bleeding; used to treat endometriosis. Tablet: 5 mg. [nohr-EH-thihn-drohn]. 248, 254

Norflex (Ortho). Skeletal muscle relaxant used to treat minor muscle spasms associated with injuries. For dosage, see *orphenadrine*. [NOHR-flehks]. 144

norfloxacin (Chibroxin) (Oph). Topical antibiotic used to treat bacterial eye infections. Ophthalmic solution: 0.3%. [nohr-FLAWK-sah-sihn].

norfloxacin (Noroxin) (Antibio). Fluoroquinolone antibiotic used to treat urinary tract infections and gonorrhea. Tablet: 400 mg. [nohr-FLAWK-sah-sihn]. 105, 318

Norgesic (Ortho) (generic *aspirin, orphenadrine*). Combination analgesic and skeletal muscle relaxant drug. Tablet: 385 mg/25 mg. [nohr-JEE-sihk]. 146

(Norgesic Forte) (Ortho). No longer on the market. (Generic name *aspirin, orphenadrine*; skeletal muscle relaxant).

Norinyl 1 + 35, Norinyl 1 + 50 (OB/GYN) (generic *norethindrone, ethinyl estradiol* or *mestranol*). Monophasic combination progestins and estrogen oral contraceptive. Tablet: 35 mcg/1 mg, 50 mcg/1 mg. [NOHR-eh-nill]. 249

normal saline (NS) (0.9% NaCl) (I.V.). Intravenous fluid of sodium and water at the same concentration as tissue fluids. 375

(Normiflo) (Hem). No longer on the market. (Generic name *ardeparin*; anticoagulant).

Normix (Neuro). Used to treat hepatic encephalopathy. For dosage, see *rifaximin*. 277

Normodyne (Cardio). Alpha$_1$ and nonselective beta-receptor blocker used to treat hypertension and hypertensive crisis. For dosage, see *labetalol*. [NOHR-moh-dine]. 165, 168

Normodyne (Endo). Alpha$_1$ and nonselective beta-receptor blocker used to treat hypertension caused by a pheochromocytoma of the adrenal medulla. For dosage, see *labetalol*. [NOHR-moh-dine].

Normosang (Chemo). Chemotherapy drug used to treat myelodysplastic syndrome. Orphan drug. 348

Noroxin (Antibio). Fluoroquinolone antibiotic used to treat urinary tract infections and gonorrhea. For dosage, see *norfloxacin*. [noh-RAWK-sihn]. 105, 318

Norpace, Norpace CR (Cardio). Used to treat ventricular arrhythmias. For dosage, see *disopyramide*. 159

Norplant System (OB/GYN) (generic *levonorgestrel*). Progestins-only five-year implant contraceptive. Subdermal capsules (in upper arm): 6 capsules (36 mg each). [NOHR-plant]. 251

Norpramin (Analges, Derm, Diab, Neuro, Ortho). Tricyclic antidepressant used to treat migraines; used to treat urticaria; used to treat diabetic neuropathy; used to treat postherpetic neuralgia; used to treat phantom limb pain. For dosage, see *desipramine*. [NOHR-prah-mihn]. 98, 147, 241, 254, 275, 307

Norpramin (OB/GYN, Psych). Tricyclic antidepressant used to treat depression; used to treat panic disorder; used to treat anorexia nervosa and bulimia nervosa; used to treat the symptoms of cocaine withdrawal; used to treat premenstrual dysphoric disorder. For dosage, see *desipramine*. [NOHR-prah-mihn]. 285, 289

Nor-Q.D. (OB/GYN) (generic *norethindrone*). Progestins-only oral contraceptive. Tablet: 0.35 mg. 250

nortriptyline (Aventyl, Aventyl Pulvules, Pamelor) (Analges, Derm, Diab, Neuro, Ortho). Tricyclic antidepressant used to treat migraines; used to treat urticaria; used to treat diabetic neuropathy; used to treat postherpetic neuralgia; used to treat phantom limb pain. Capsule: 10 mg, 25 mg, 50 mg, 75 mg. Liquid: 10 mg/5 mL. [nohr-TRIP-teh-leen]. 99, 147, 241, 276, 307

nortriptyline (Aventyl, Aventyl Pulvules, Pamelor) (OB/GYN, Psych). Tricyclic antidepressant used to treat depression; used to treat panic disorder; used to treat premenstrual dysphoric disorder. Capsule: 10 mg, 25 mg, 50 mg, 75 mg. Liquid: 10 mg/5 mL. [nohr-TRIP-teh-leen]. 255, 286, 289

Norvasc (Cardio). Calcium channel blocker used to treat angina pectoris and hypertension. For dosage, see *amlodipine*. [NOHR-vehsk]. Aventyl Pulvules, 157, 163

Norwich Extra-Strength (Analges, Ortho). Salicylate drug used to relieve fever and pain; used to treat the pain and inflammation of osteoarthritis and rheumatoid arthritis. For dosage, see *aspirin*. 300

Nostril, Children's Nostril (ENT). Decongestant. For dosage, see *phenylephrine*.

Nostrilla (ENT). Decongestant. For dosage, see *oxymetazoline*. [noh-STRIH-lah].

Novafed A (ENT) (generic *pseudoephedrine, chlorpheniramine*). Combination decongestant and antihistamine drug. Capsule: 120 mg/8 mg. [NOH-vah-fehd].

Novahistine DMX (ENT) (generic *pseudoephedrine, dextromethorphan, guaifenesin*). Combination decongestant, nonnarcotic antitussive, and expectorant drug. Liquid: 30 mg/10 mg/100 mg. [noh-vah-HIH-steen].

Novamine, Novamine 15% (I.V.). Intravenous fluids for total parenteral nutrition. [NOH-vah-meen]. 378

Novantrone (Chemo, Neuro). Chemotherapy antibiotic used to treat leukemia and prostate cancer; used to treat multiple sclerosis. For dosage, see *mitoxantrone*. [noh-VEHN-trohn]. 276, 341

Novir (Antivir). Protease inhibitor drug used to treat AIDS. For dosage, see *ritonavir*. 325

(novobiocin) (Antibio). No longer on the market. (Trade name *Albamycin*; antibiotic).

Novocain (Anes). Local, regional nerve block, and spinal anesthetic. For dosage, see *procaine*. [NOH-voh-kayn]. 367, 368

Novolin L (Diab). Intermediate-acting lente insulin. Subcutaneous: 100 units/mL. [NOH-voh-lihn]. 238

Novolin N, Novolin N PenFill (Diab). Intermediate-acting NPH insulin. Subcutaneous: 100 units/mL. [NOH-voh-lihn]. 238

Novolin R, Novolin R PenFill (Diab). Fast-acting regular insulin. Subcutaneous: 100 units/mL. [NOH-voh-lihn]. 238

Novolin 70/30, Novolin 70/30 PenFill (Diab) (generic *human recombinant DNA NPH and regular insulins*). Combination of intermediate-acting and fast-acting insulin. Subcutaneous: 70 units/30 units per mL. [NOH-voh-lihn]. 239

NovoLog (Diab). Rapid-acting human recombinant DNA aspart insulin; indicated for use with an external insulin pump. Subcutaneous: 100 units/mL. [NOH-voh-lawg]. 238

NovoSeven (Hem). Clotting factor used to treat hemophiliac patients. Intravenous (powder to be reconstituted): 1.2 mg, 4.8 mg.

NPH Iletin II (Diab). Intermediate-acting NPH insulin. Subcutaneous: 100 units/mL. [II-leh-tihn]. 238

NPO or **n.p.o.** (abbreviation meaning *nothing by mouth*).

NS (abbreviation for *normal saline*).

NSAIDs (abbreviation for *nonsteroidal anti-inflammatory drugs*). [EHN-sayds]. See *nonsteroidal anti-inflammatory drugs*.

NTZ (abbreviation for *nitazoxanide*). See *nitazoxanide*.

Nubain (Analges, OB/GYN). Narcotic analgesic drug used to treat moderate-to-severe pain; used to treat pain during labor and delivery. For dosage, see *nalbuphine*. [NOO-bayn]. 297

nucleoside reverse transcriptase inhibitors (Antivir). Class of drugs used to treat AIDS. 324

nucleotide reverse transcriptase inhibitors (Antivir). Class of drugs used to treat AIDS. Similar to nucleoside reverse transcriptase inhibitors, but chemically preactivated so they work more quickly. 324, 325

NuLytely (GI) (generic *polyethylene glycol, electrolyte solution*). Bowel evacuant/bowel prep. Oral liquid (powder to be reconstituted). 125

Numorphan (Analges, Anes, Cardio). Narcotic analgesic drug used to treat moderate-to-severe pain; used as a preoperative medication; used to treat dyspnea in patients with congestive heart failure. (Schedule II drug). For dosage, see *oxymorphone*. [noo-MOHR-fehn]. 297, 371

Numzit Teething (ENT) (generic *benzocaine*). Topical anesthetic drug for the mouth. Gel: 7.5%. Lotion: 0.2%.

Nupercainal (Derm) (generic *dibucaine*). Topical anesthetic drug. Cream: 0.5%. Ointment: 1%. [noo-pehr-KAY-nawl]. 94

Nupercainal (GI) (generic *zinc oxide*). Topical drug used to treat hemorrhoids. Suppository. [noo-pehr-KAY-nawl]. 135

(Nuprin) (Analges, OB/GYN, Ortho). No longer on the market. (Generic name *ibuprofen*; nonsteroidal anti-inflammatory drug used to treat pain).

Nuromax (Anes, Resp).   Muscle relaxant drug used during surgery; used to treat patients who are intubated and on the ventilator.   For dosage, see *doxacurium*. [NYOUR-oh-mehks]. 199, 370

Nursoy (GI).   Infant soy formula. Liquid, powder (to be reconstituted).

Nu-Tears, Nu-Tears II (Oph).   Artificial tears. Drops.

Nutramigen (GI).   Infant formula for infants with allergies. Liquid, powder (to be reconstituted). [noo-TREH-mih-jehn].

Nutropin, Nutropin AQ, Nutropin Depot (Endo). Growth hormone replacement for adults and children with growth failure; used to treat growth failure of infants who are small for gestational age. For dosage, see *somatropin*. [noo-TROH-pihn]. 230

NuvaRing (OB/GYN) (generic *etonogestrel, ethinyl estradiol*).   Monophasic combination progestins and estrogen contraceptive. Vaginal ring: Three-inch ring, 0.12 mcg/0.015 mg per 24 hours. [NOO-vah]. 250

Nydrazid (Resp).   Bactericidal antibiotic used only to treat tuberculosis.   For dosage, see *isoniazid*. [NY-drah-zihd]. 197

Nyotran (Antifung).   Used to treat invasive fungal infections.   For dosage, see *nystatin*. [NY-oh-trehn]. 335

NyQuil Hot Therapy, NyQuil Nighttime Cold/Flu Medicine (ENT) (generic *pseudoephedrine, doxylamine, dextromethorphan, acetaminophen*).   Combination decongestant, antihistamine, nonnarcotic antitussive, and analgesic drug. Powder (to be mixed with water): 60 mg/12.5 mg/30 mg/1000 mg. Liquid: 10 mg/1.25 mg/5 mg/167 mg. [NY-kwihl].

nystatin (Mycostatin, Nilstat) (Derm).   Topical antiyeast drug. Cream, ointment, powder. [ny-STEH-tihn]. 90

nystatin (Mycostatin, Mycostatin Pastilles, Nilstat) (ENT).   Topical drug used to treat yeast infections in the mouth. Liquid: 100,000 units/mL. Powder (to be reconstituted): 50 million units. Tablet: 500,000 units. Troche: 200,000 units. [ny-STEH-tihn]. 221, 331

nystatin (Nyotran) (Antifung).   Used to treat invasive fungal infections. Orphan drug. [ny-STEH-tihn]. 335

nystatin (OB/GYN).   Topical drug used to treat vaginal yeast infections. Vaginal tablet: 100,000 units. [ny-STEH-tihn]. 256

Nytol, Maximum Strength Nytol (Neuro).   Antihistamine drug sleep aid.   For dosage, see *diphenhydramine*. [NY-tawl]. 273

obesity, drugs used to treat. 129

OB/GYN drugs. 243

obsessive-compulsive disorder, drugs used to treat. 289

Ocean (ENT).   Topical saline nasal moisturizing drug. Drops. Mist. Spray.

OCL (GI) (generic *polyethylene glycol, electrolyte solution*). Bowel evacuant/bowel prep. Oral liquid. 125

Octicair (ENT) (generic *hydrocortisone, neomycin, polymyxin B*).   Combination topical corticosteroid and antibiotic drug for the ears. Drops: 1%/5 mg/ 10,000 units. [AWK-tih-kehr].

octreotide (Sandostatin, Sandostatin LAR Depot) (Endo).   Used to inhibit overproduction of growth hormone in adults with acromegaly. Subcutaneous or intravenous: 0.05 mg/mL, 0.1 mg/mL, 0.2 mg/mL, 0.5 mg/mL, 1 mg/mL. Intramuscular: 10 mg/5 mL, 20 mg/5 mL, 30 mg/5 mL. [awk-TREE-oh-tide]. 230

octreotide (Sandostatin, Sandostatin LAR Depot) (GI). Slows intestinal transit time; used to treat severe diarrhea caused by irritable bowel syndrome, AIDS, carcinoid tumors, VIPomas, short bowel syndrome, dumping syndrome, or chemotherapy. Subcutaneous or intravenous: 0.05 mg/mL, 0.1 mg/mL, 0.2 mg/mL, 0.5 mg/mL, 1 mg/mL. Intramuscular: 10 mg/5 mL, 20 mg/5 mL, 30 mg/5 mL. [awk-TREE-oh-tide]. 134, 328

OcuClear (Oph).   Topical decongestant/vasoconstrictor used to treat irritation and allergy symptoms in the eyes.   For dosage, see *oxymetazoline*. [AWK-yoo-kleer].

OcuCoat, Ocucoat PF (Oph).   Artificial tears. Drops.

OcuCoat Solution (Oph).   Injected into the eye during surgery to keep the anterior chamber expanded and replace intraocular fluid.   For dosage, see *methylcellulose*.

Ocufen (Oph).   Topical nonsteroidal anti-inflammatory drug used only to prevent miosis during eye surgery.   For dosage, see *flurbiprofen*. [AWK-yoo-fehn].

Ocuflox (Oph).   Topical antibiotic used to treat bacterial eye infections.   For dosage, see *ofloxacin*. [AWK-yoo-FLAWKS]. 218

Ocupress (Oph).   Topical beta-receptor blocker used to treat glaucoma.   For dosage, see *carteolol*. [AWK-yoo-prehs]. 221

Ocusulf-10 (Oph).   Topical sulfonamide anti-infective drug used to treat bacterial eye infections. For dosage, see *sulfacetamide*. [AWK-yoo-suhlf]. 218

O.D. or **OD** (abbreviation meaning *right eye*).

ODT (abbreviation for *orally disintegrating tablet*).

ofloxacin (Floxin) (Antibio).   Fluoroquinolone antibiotic used to treat a variety of infections, including *H. influenzae*, *E. coli*, and gonorrhea. Tablet: 200 mg, 300 mg, 400 mg. Intravenous: 400 mg/10 mL. [oh-FLAWK-sah-sihn]. 105, 318

ofloxacin (Ocuflox) (Oph). Topical antibiotic used to treat bacterial eye infections. Ophthalmic solution: 0.3%. [oh-FLAWK-sah-sihn].

Ogen (OB/GYN, Ortho). Hormone replacement therapy used to treat the symptoms of menopause; used to prevent or treat osteoporosis. For dosage, see *estropipate*. 252

ointment. 35

ointment, nitroglycerin. 156

olanzapine (Zyprexa, Zyprexa Zydis) (Neuro, Psych). Drug used to treat the dementia of Alzheimer's disease; used to treat psychosis and schizophrenia; used to treat the mania of manic-depressive disorder. Tablet: 2.5 mg, 5 mg, 7.5 mg, 10 mg, 15 mg, 20 mg. Orally disintegrating tablet: 5 mg, 10 mg. Intramuscular: (Pending). [oh-LEHN-zah-peen]. 271, 284, 288

olopatadine (Patanol) (Oph). Topical antihistamine used to treat allergy symptoms in the eyes. Ophthalmic solution: 0.1%. [oh-loh-PEH-tah-deen]. 220

olsalazine (Dipentum) (GI). Anti-inflammatory-type drug used to treat ulcerative colitis. Capsule: 250 mg. [ohl-SEH-lah-zeen].

Olux (Derm) (generic *clobetasol*). Topical corticosteroid anti-flammatory drug. Foam: 0.05%. [OH-luhks]. 92

omapatrilat (Vanlev) (Cardio). Drug that acts as an angiotensin-converting enzyme inhibitor but also inhibits NEP, another enzyme that regulates the blood pressure. [oh-mah-PEH-trih-leht]. 165

omega-3 fatty acids (Promega Pearls Softgels, Promega Softgels) (Cardio). Fish oil nutritional supplement used to treat hypertriglyceridemia. Capsule: 600 mg, 1000 mg. 171

omeprazole (Prilosec) (GI). Proton pump inhibitor used to treat peptic ulcers, gastroesophageal reflux disease, and *H. pylori* infections. Capsule: 10 mg, 20 mg, 40 mg. [oh-MEH-prah-zohl]. 119, 121

Omnicef (Antibio). Cephalosporin antibiotic used to treat a variety of bacterial infections, including *Streptococcus*, *Staphylococcus*, community-acquired pneumonia, and *H. influenzae*. For dosage, see *cefdinir*. [AWM-nih-sehf]. 316

(Omnipen-N) (Antibio). No longer on the market. (Generic name *ampicillin*; penicillin-type antibiotic).

OMS Concentrate (Analges, Anes, Cardio, OB/GYN). Narcotic analgesic drug used to treat moderate-to-severe pain; used as a preoperative drug to sedate and supplement anesthesia; used to treat dyspnea from congestive heart failure; used to treat the pain of childbirth. (Schedule II drug). For dosage, see *morphine*. 173, 297

Oncaspar (Chemo). Chemotherapy enzyme drug used to treat leukemia. For dosage, see *pegaspargase*. [AWN-kah-spawr]. 345

Oncolym (Chemo). Monoclonal antibody chemotherapy drug used to treat non-Hodgkin's lymphoma. Orphan drug. 346

Oncophage (Chemo, Uro) (generic *autologous tumor-derived gp96 heatshock protein-peptide complex [HSPPC-96]*). Vaccine for renal cell carcinoma. Investigational drug. 112, 349

(Oncovin) (Chemo). No longer on the market. (Generic name *vincristine*; mitosis inhibitor chemotherapy drug).

ondansetron (Zofran, Zofran ODT) (GI). Antiemetic drug; used to treat nausea and vomiting caused by chemotherapy. Tablet: 4 mg, 8 mg, 24 mg. Orally disintegrating tablets: 4 mg, 8 mg. Liquid: 4 mg/5 mL. Intravenous: 2 mg/mL, 32 mg/50 mL. [awn-DEHN-seh-trawn].

Onkolox (Chemo). Chemotherapy drug used to treat renal cancer. For dosage, see *coumarin*. [AWN-koh-lawks]. 347

Ontak (Chemo). Chemotherapy recombinant DNA drug that combines interleukin-2 and diphtheria toxin protein; kept frozen until thawed for use; used to treat cutaneous T-cell lymphoma. For dosage, see *denileukin*. 347

Onxol (Chemo, Uro). Mitosis inhibitor chemotherapy drug used to treat breast cancer, ovarian cancer, lung cancer, head and neck cancer, gastrointestinal tract cancer, pancreatic cancer, prostatic cancer, non-Hodgkin's lymphoma, and Kaposi's sarcoma; used to treat polycystic kidney disease. For dosage, see *paclitaxel*. 344

onychomycosis, drugs used to treat. 89

Opcon-A Solution (Oph) (generic *naphazoline, pheniramine*). Topical combination decongestant and antihistamine. Ophthalmic solution: 0.025%/0.3%. [AWP-kawn].

Ophthaine (Oph). Topical anesthetic for the eyes. For dosage, see *proparacaine*. [AWP-thayn]. 222

Ophthalgan (Oph). Topical drug used to treat corneal edema. For dosage, see *glycerin*. [awp-THAHL-gehn].

ophthalmic drugs. 217

Ophthetic (Oph). Topical anesthetic for the eyes. For dosage, see *proparacaine*. [awp-THEH-tick]. 222

Ophthocort (Oph) (generic *chloramphenicol, hydrocortisone, polymyxin B*). Topical combination corticosteroid and antibiotic drug. Ophthalmic ointment: 1%/0.5%/10,000 units. [AWP-thoh-kohrt].

opium. See *paregoric*.

opportunistic infections. 335

oprelvekin (Neumega) (Chemo). Used to prevent thrombocytopenia in patients undergoing chemotherapy. Subcutaneous (powder to be reconstituted): 5 mg.

Opticrom (Oph). Orphan drug used to treat keratoconjunctivitis. For dosage, see *cromolyn*. [AWP-teh-krawm].

Optigene 3 (Oph). Topical decongestant/vasoconstrictor used to treat irritation and allergy symptoms in the eyes. For dosage, see *tetrahydrozoline*. [AWP-teh-jeen].

Optimental (GI). Liquid nutritional supplement. Liquid. [awp-tih-MEH-tuhl].

Optimine (Derm, ENT). Antihistamine used to treat allergic rhinitis and allergic reactions with hives and itching. For dosage, see *azatadine*. [AWP-tih-meen]. 207

Optimmune (Oph). Used to treat Sjogren's syndrome. For dosage, see *cyclosporine*. [AWP-tih-myoon].

Optimoist (ENT). Artificial saliva used to treat dry mouth due to salivary gland dysfunction. Liquid.

OptiPranolol (Oph). Topical beta-receptor blocker used to treat glaucoma. For dosage, see *metipranolol*. [awp-teh-PREH-noh-lawl]. 221

Optivar (Oph). Topical antihistamine used to treat allergy symptoms in the eyes. For dosage, see *azelastine*. [AWP-tih-vawr]. 220

Orabase-B, Orabase Baby, Orabase Gel, Orabase Lip (ENT) (generic *benzocaine*). Topical anesthetic for mouth. Cream: 5%. Gel: 7.5%, 15%. Paste: 20%. [OHR-ah-bays].

Orabase HCA (ENT) (generic *hydrogen peroxide*). Topical antiseptic for the mouth. Paste: 0.5%.

Oracit (Ortho) (generic *sodium citrate, citric acid*). Used to treat gout. Liquid: 490 mg/640 mg per 5 mL. [OHR-ah-siht].

oral contraceptives. See *contraceptives*.

oral route, administration of drugs by the. 38

Oramorph SR (Analges, Anes, Cardio, OB/GYN). Narcotic analgesic drug used to treat moderate-to-severe pain; used as a preoperative drug to sedate and supplement anesthesia; used to treat dyspnea in patients with congestive heart failure; used to treat the pain of childbirth. (Schedule II drug). For dosage, see *morphine*. [OHR-ah-mohrf]. 173, 297

Orap (Psych). Antipsychotic drug used to treat Tourette's syndrome but not psychosis. For dosage, see *pimozide*. [OHR-ehp]. 294

Orapred (Endo, Neuro, Ortho). Corticosteroid anti-inflammatory drug used to treat severe inflammation in various body systems; used to treat multiple sclerosis; injected into a joint to treat osteoarthritis

and rheumatoid arthritis; injected near a joint to treat bursitis and tenosynovitis. For dosage, see *prednisolone*. [OHR-ah-prehd]. 232, 277

Orasone (Chemo, Endo). Corticosteroid anti-inflammatory drug used to treat severe inflammation in various body systems; used as part of chemotherapy treatment. For dosage, see *prednisone*. [OHR-ah-sohn]. 232, 351

orBec (Chemo). Used to prevent graft-versus-host disease. For dosage, see *beclomethasone*. [OHR-behk].

order.
automatic stop. 76
medication. 75–80
prescription. 75
standing. 76
telephone. 76
verbal. 76

Oretic (Uro). Thiazide diuretic. For dosage, see *hydrochlorothiazide*. [ohr-EH-tihk]. 103

(Oreton) (Chemo). No longer on the market. (Generic name *methyltestosterone;* hormonal chemotherapy drug).

Organidin NR (ENT). Expectorant. For dosage, see *guaifenesin*. [ohr-GEH-nih-dihn]. 210

Orgaran (Hem). Low molecular weight heparin-like anticoagulant. For dosage, see *danaparoid*.

Original Alka-Seltzer. See *Extra Strength Alka-Seltzer*.

Orinase (Diab). Oral antidiabetic drug. For dosage, see *tolbutamide*. [OHR-ih-nays]. 240

Orlaam (Analges). Narcotic used to manage heroin and narcotic dependence and withdrawal. For dosage, see *levomethadyl*. 308

orlistat (Xenical) (GI). Lipase inhibitor used to treat obesity. Capsule: 120 mg. [OHR-li-steht]. 129

(Ornade Spansules) (ENT). No longer on the market. (Combination drug with *phenylpropanolamine;* decongestant and antihistamine).

Ornidyl (Antivir). Used to treat *Pneumocystis carinii* pneumonia in AIDS patients. For dosage, see *eflornithine*. [OHR-neh-dill]. 328

orphan drug. 18

Orphan Drug Act of 1983, The. 18

orphenadrine (Norflex) (Ortho). Skeletal muscle relaxant used to treat minor muscle spasms associated with injuries. Tablet: 100 mg. Intramuscular or intravenous: 30 mg/mL. [ohr-FEH-nah-deen].

Ortho-Cept (OB/GYN) (generic *desogestrel, ethinyl estradiol*). Monophasic combination progestins and estrogen oral contraceptive. Tablet: 0.15 mg/30 mcg. [OHR-thoh-sehpt]. 249

Orthoclone OKT3. (Cardio, GI, Uro). Immunosuppressant monoclonal antibody given after organ transplantation to prevent rejection of the donor heart, liver, or kidney. For dosage, see *muro-monab-CD3*. [OHR-thoh-klohn]. 110, 133, 173

Ortho-Cyclen (OB/GYN) (generic *norgestimate, ethinyl estradiol*). Monophasic combination progestins and estrogen oral contraceptive. Tablet: 0.25 mg/35 mcg. [ohr-thoh-SY-klehn]. 249

Ortho Dienestrol Vaginal Cream (OB/GYN). Topical hormone replacement therapy used to treat atrophic vaginitis of menopause. Cream: 0.01%. [OHR-thoh dy-eh-NEHS-trawl]. 252

Ortho-Est (OB/GYN, Ortho). Hormone replacement therapy used to treat the symptoms of menopause; used to prevent or treat osteoporosis. For dosage, see *estropipate*. 252

Ortho Evra (OB/GYN) (generic *norelgestromin, ethinyl estradiol*). Monophasic combination progestins and estrogen transdermal contraceptive. Transdermal patch: 150 mcg/20 mcg per 24 hours. [OHR-thoh EHV-rah]. 250

Ortho-Novum 1/35, Ortho-Novum 1/50 (OB/GYN) (generic *norethindrone, ethinyl estradiol* or *mestranol*). Monophasic combination progestins and estrogen oral contraceptive. Tablet: 35 mcg/1 mg, 50 mcg/1 mg. [ohr-thoh-NOH-vuhm]. 249

Ortho-Novum 7/7/7 (OB/GYN) (generic *norethindrone, ethinyl estradiol*). Triphasic combination progestins and estrogen oral contraceptive. Tablet: 0.5 mg/35 mcg then 0.75 mg/35 mcg then 1 mg/35 mcg. [ohr-thoh-NOH-vuhm]. 251

Ortho-Novum 10/11 (OB/GYN) (generic *norethindrone, ethinyl estradiol*). Biphasic combination progestins and estrogen oral contraceptive. Tablet: 0.5 mg/35 mcg then 1 mg/35 mcg. [ohr-thoh-NOH-vuhm]. 250

Ortho-Prefest (OB/GYN, Ortho) (generic *norgestimate, estradiol*). Combination progestins and estrogen drug used to treat symptoms of menopause; used to prevent or treat postmenopausal osteoporosis. [OHR-thoh-PREE-fehst]. 253

Ortho Tri-Cyclen (OB/GYN) (generic *norgestimate, ethinyl estradiol*). Triphasic combination progestins and estrogen oral contraceptive. Tablet: 0.18 mg/35 mcg then 0.215 mg/35 mcg then 0.25 mg/35 mcg. [ohr-thoh-try-SY-klehn]. 251

Orudis, Orudis KT (Analges, OB/GYN, Ortho). Nonsteroidal anti-inflammatory drug used to treat pain; used to treat migraine headaches; used to treat dysmenorrhea; used to treat osteoarthritis and rheumatoid arthritis. For dosage, see *ketoprofen*. [oh-ROO-dihs]. 139, 255, 304, 307

Oruvail (Analges, OB/GYN, Ortho). Nonsteroidal anti-inflammatory drug used to treat pain; used to treat migraine headaches; used to treat dysmenorrhea; used to treat osteoarthritis and rheumatoid

arthritis. For dosage, see *ketoprofen*. [OH-roo-vayl]. 139, 255, 304, 307

O.S. or **OS** (abbreviation meaning *left eye*).

oseltamivir (Tamiflu) (Antivir). Antiviral drug used to prevent and treat influenza A virus infections. Capsule: 75 mg. Liquid: 12 mg/mL. [oh-sehl-TEH-mih-veer]. 330

Osmitrol (Neuro, Oph, Uro). Diuretic used to decrease cerebral edema; used to decrease intraocular pressure; used to treat renal failure. For dosage, see *mannitol*. [AWS-meh-trawl]. 112, 276

Osmolite, Osmolite HN (GI). Liquid nutritional supplement. Liquid.

osteoarthritis, drugs used to treat. 138

osteoporosis, drugs used to treat. 143

OTC (abbreviation *for over-the-counter*). See *over-the-counter drugs*.

OTC Drugs Advisory Committee. 18

Otic Domeboro (ENT). Topical antibacterial Burow's solution for the ear. Drops.

(Otic Tridesilon) (ENT). No longer on the market. (Generic names *desonide, acetic acid*; topical corticosteroid and antiseptic for the ear).

OtiTricin (ENT) (generic *hydrocortisone, neomycin, polymyxin B*). Combination topical corticosteroid and two antibiotics for the ears. Drops: 1%/5 mg/10,000 units.

Otobiotic Otic (ENT) (generic *hydrocortisone, polymyxin B*). Combination topical drug with a corticosteroid and an antibiotic for the ears. Drops: 0.5%/10,000 units. [oh-toh-by-AW-tihk OH-tihk].

ototoxicity. 53, 317

Otrivin, Otrivin Pediatric Nasal Drops (ENT). Decongestant. For dosage, see *xylometazoline*. [OH-trih-vihn]. 206

O.U. or **OU** (abbreviation meaning *both eyes*).

OvaRex (Chemo). Monoclonal antibody chemotherapy drug used to treat ovarian cancer. [OH-veh-rehks]. 346

Ovastat (Chemo). Chemotherapy drug used to treat ovarian cancer. For dosage, see *treosulfan*. [OH-vah-steht]. 348

O-Vax (Chemo). Chemotherapy vaccine used to treat ovarian cancer. Orphan drug. 348

Ovcon-35, Ovcon-50 (OB/GYN) (generic *norethindrone, ethinyl estradiol*). Monophasic combination progestins and estrogen oral contraceptive. Tablet: 35 mcg/0.4 mg, 50 mcg/1 mg. [AWV-kawn]. 250

overdose, drugs used to treat. 182, 307
   acetaminophen. 183, 308
   narcotics. 182, 308
   tricyclic antidepressants. 182

over-the-counter drugs (OTC). 18

Ovide (Derm) (generic *malathion*). Topical drug used to treat pediculosis (lice). Lotion: 0.5%. [OH-vide]. 95

Ovidrel (OB/GYN). Ovulation-stimulating drug. For dosage, see *choriogonadotropin alfa*. 244

Ovral-28 (OB/GYN) (generic *ethynodiol, norgestrel*). Monophasic combination progestins and estrogen oral contraceptive. Tablet: 0.5 mg/50 mcg. [OHV-rawl]. 250

Ovrette (OB/GYN) (generic *norgestrel*). Progestins-only oral contraceptive. Tablet: 0.075 mg. [ohv-REHT]. 251

ovulation-stimulating drugs. Focus on Healthcare Issues feature. 245

ovulation-stimulating drugs (OB/GYN). Class of drugs used to treat infertility. 244

oxacillin (Antibio). Penicillin-type antibiotic used to treat a variety of bacterial infections, including staphylococci. Capsule: 250 mg, 500 mg. Liquid: 250 mg/5 mL. Intramuscular or intravenous: 250 mg, 500 mg, 1 g, 2 g, 4 g. [awk-sah-SIH-lihn]. 313

oxaliplatin (Eloxatin) (Chemo). Chemotherapy platinum drug used to treat ovarian cancer and colon cancer. Orphan drug. [awk-sah-lih-PLEH-tihn]. 345

Oxandrin (Antivir, Chemo, Endo, Ortho). Anabolic steroid used to treat AIDS wasting syndrome; used to promote weight gain following extensive surgery or trauma; used to treat metastatic breast cancer; used to treat lack of growth in Turner's syndrome; used to treat muscular dystrophy; also used illegally by athletes. For dosage, see *oxandrolone*. [awk-SEHN-drihn]. 234, 327

oxandrolone (Oxandrin) (Antivir, Chemo, Endo). Anabolic steroid used to treat AIDS wasting syndrome; used to promote weight gain following extensive surgery or trauma; used to treat metastatic breast cancer; used to treat lack of growth in Turner's syndrome; used to treat muscular dystrophy; also used illegally by athletes. Tablet: 2.5 mg. [awk-SEHN-droh-lohn]. 234, 327

oxaprozin (Daypro) (Analges, Ortho). Nonsteroidal anti-inflammatory drug used to treat osteoarthritis and rheumatoid arthritis. Caplet: 600 mg. Tablet: 600 mg. [awk-sah-PROH-zihn]. 139, 304

oxazepam (Serax) (Psych). Benzodiazepine drug used to treat anxiety and neurosis; used to treat alcohol withdrawal. (Schedule IV drug). Capsule: 10 mg, 15 mg, 30 mg. Tablet: 15 mg. [awk-SAY-zeh-pehm]. 281

oxcarbazepine (Trileptal) (Neuro). Anticonvulsant used to treat partial seizures. Tablet: 150 mg, 300 mg, 600 mg. Liquid: 300 mg/5 mL. [awks-kar-BEH-seh-peen]. 265

oxiconazole (Oxistat) (Derm). Topical antifungal drug. Cream: 1%. Lotion: 1%. [awk-see-KAW-neh-zohl]. 89

Oxistat (Derm) (generic *oxiconazole*). Topical antifungal drug. Cream: 1%. Lotion: 1%. [AWK-see-steht]. 89

Oxsodrol (Cardio, GI, Uro). Used to treat a transplanted donor heart, liver, or kidney. Orphan drug.

Oxsoralen (Derm) (generic *methoxsalen*). Topical drug used with ultraviolet light to treat vitiligo. Lotion: 1%. [awk-soh-RAY-lehn]. 99

Oxsoralen-Ultra (Derm). Psoralen drug used with ultraviolet light to treat severe psoriasis. For dosage, see *methoxsalen*. [awk-soh-RAY-lehn]. 87

oxtriphylline (Choledyl SA) (Resp). Bronchodilator. Tablet: 100 mg, 200 mg, 400 mg, 600 mg. Liquid: 50 mg/5 mL, 100 mg/5 mL. 193

oxybate (Xyrem) (Neuro). Used to treat narcolepsy. Orphan drug. 274

oxybutynin (Ditropan, Ditropan XL) (Uro). Antispasmodic drug used to treat urinary urgency and frequency. Syrup: 5 mg/5 mL. Tablet: 5 mg, 10 mg, 15 mg. Transdermal patch: 1.3 mg/day, 3.9 mg/day. [awk-see-BYOO-tih-nihn]. 107

Oxycel (Hem). Topical hemostatic drug used to control bleeding during surgery. Pad. Pledget. Strip. [AWK-see-sehl].

oxychlorosene (Chlorpactin WCS-90) (Derm). Topical antibacterial, antifungal, and antiviral drug used to irrigate wounds. Powder to be reconstituted to a solution. [awk-see-KLOHR-oh-seen]. 99

oxycodone (Endocodone, M-oxy, OxyContin, OxyFast, OxyIR, Percolone, Roxicodone, Roxicodone Intensol) (Analges, Neuro). Narcotic analgesic used to treat moderate-to-severe pain; used to treat neuralgia from herpes zoster infection (shingles). (Schedule II drug). Capsule: 5 mg. Liquid: 5 mg/5 mL, 20 mg/mL. Tablet: 5 mg, 10 mg, 15 mg, 20 mg, 30 mg, 40 mg, 80 mg, 160 mg. [awk-see-KOH-dohn]. 276, 297

OxyContin (Analges, Neuro). Narcotic analgesic used to treat moderate-to-severe pain; used to treat neuralgia from herpes zoster infection (shingles). (Schedule II drug). For dosage, see *oxycodone*. [awk-see-KAWN-tihn]. 276, 297

OxyContin as a drug of abuse. Focus on Healthcare Issues feature. 298

OxyFast (Analges, Neuro). Narcotic analgesic used to treat moderate-to-severe pain; used to treat neuralgia from herpes zoster infection (shingles). (Schedule II drug). For dosage, see *oxycodone*. [awk-see-FEHST]. 276, 297

Oxy 10 Maximum Strength Advanced Formula, Oxy 10 Wash (Derm) (generic *benzoyl peroxide*). Topical antibacterial drug used to treat acne vulgaris. Gel: 10%. Liquid: 10%.

OxyIR (Analges, Neuro). Narcotic analgesic used to treat moderate-to-severe pain; used to treat neuralgia from herpes zoster infection (shingles). (Schedule II drug). For dosage, see *oxycodone*. 276, 297

oxymetazoline (OcuClear, Visine L.R.) (Oph). Topical decongestant/vasoconstrictor used to treat irritation and allergy symptoms in the eyes. Ophthalmic solution: 0.025%. [awk-see-meh-tah-ZOH-leen].

oxymetazoline (Afrin, Afrin Children's Nose Drops, Afrin Sinus, Allerest 12 Hour Nasal, Cheracol Nasal, Dristan 12 Hr Nasal, Duramist Plus, Duration, 4-Way Long Lasting Nasal, Nostrilla, Sinarest 12 Hour, Vicks Sinex 12-Hour) (ENT). Decongestant. Drops: 0.025%, 0.05%. Spray: 0.05%. [awk-see-meh-teh-ZOH-leen].

oxymetholone (Anadrol-50) (Chemo, Endo, Hem). Anabolic steroid used to treat anemia caused by chemotherapy drugs; used to increase red blood cell production to treat anemia; also used illegally by athletes. Tablet: 50 mg. [awk-see-MEH-thoh-lohn]. 234

oxymorphone (Numorphan) (Analges, Anes, Cardio). Narcotic analgesic drug used to treat moderate-to-severe pain; used as a preoperative medication; used to treat dyspnea in patients with congestive heart failure. (Schedule II drug). Suppository: 5 mg. Subcutaneous, intramuscular, or intravenous: 1 mg/mL, 1.5 mg/mL. [awk-see-MOHR-fohn]. 298, 371

(oxyphencyclimine) (GI). No longer on the market. (Trade name *Daricon*; GI antispasmodic drug).

OxyIR (Analges, Neuro). Narcotic analgesic used to treat moderate-to-severe pain; used to treat neuralgia from herpes zoster infection (shingles). (Schedule II drug). For dosage, see *oxycodone*. [awk-sehl-R].

oxytetracycline (Terramycin IM, Uri-Tet) (Antibio, OB/GYN). Tetracycline antibiotic used to treat a variety of infections, including gonorrhea, syphilis, and *Chlamydia*. Capsule: 250 mg. Intramuscular and intravenous: 50 mg/mL, 125 mg/mL. [awk-see-teh-trah-SY-kleen]. 317

oxytocin (Pitocin, Syntocinon) (OB/GYN). Used to stimulate uterine contractions; used to treat postpartum uterine bleeding; used to treat incomplete abortion. Intramuscular or intravenous: 10 units/mL. [awk-see-TOH-sihn]. 246, 248

P_1E_1, P_2E_1, P_3E_1, P_4E_1, P_6E_1 (Oph) (generic *pilocarpine, epinephrine*). Topical combination miotic and alpha/beta-receptor agonist drug used to treat glaucoma. Ophthalmic solution: 1%/1%, 2%/1%, 4%/1%, 6%/1%. 222

Pacis (Chemo). Chemotherapy drug used to treat bladder cancer. For dosage, see *BCG*. 347

packed red blood cells (PRBCs) (I.V.). Intravenous blood cellular product. 379

paclitaxel (Onxol, Taxol) (Chemo, Uro). Mitosis inhibitor chemotherapy drug used to treat breast cancer, ovarian cancer, lung cancer, head and neck cancer, gastrointestinal tract cancer, pancreatic cancer, prostatic cancer, non-Hodgkin's lymphoma, and Kaposi's sarcoma; used to treat polycystic kidney disease. Intravenous: 6 mg/mL. [pehk-lih-TEHK-suhl]. 112, 344

palivizumab (Synagis) (Antivir). Monoclonal antibody used to treat respiratory syncytial virus. Intramuscular (powder to be reconstituted): 50 mg, 100 mg. [peh-lih-VIH-zoo-mehb].

Pamelor (Analges, Derm, Diab, Neuro, Ortho). Tricyclic antidepressant used to treat migraines; used to treat urticaria; used to treat diabetic neuropathy; used to treat postherpetic neuralgia; used to treat phantom limb pain. For dosage, see *nortriptyline*. [PEH-meh-lohr]. 99, 147, 241, 276, 307

Pamelor (OB/GYN, Psych). Tricyclic antidepressant used to treat depression; used to treat panic disorder; used to treat premenstrual dysphoric disorder. For dosage, see *nortriptyline*. [PEH-meh-lohr]. 255, 286, 289

pamidronate (Aredia) (Chemo, OB/GYN, Ortho). Inhibits the breakdown of bone; used to treat hypercalcemia of malignancy; used to treat the metastatic bone lesions of breast cancer and multiple myeloma; used to prevent and treat postmenopausal osteoporosis; used to treat Paget's disease. Intravenous (powder to be reconstituted): 30 mg, 90 mg. [peh-MIH-droh-nayt]. 144, 148, 362

Pamine (GI, Uro). Antispasmodic drug used to treat spasm of the smooth muscle of the bowel. For dosage, see *methscopolamine*. [PEH-meen]. 122

Pamisyl (GI). Used to treat ulcerative colitis. For dosage, see *4-aminosalicylic acid*. [PEH-mih-sihl].

Pamprin Maximum Pain Relief (OB/GYN) (generic *magnesium salicylate, pamabrom*). Combination analgesic and diuretic used to treat premenstrual dysphoric disorder and dysmenorrhea. Caplet: 250 mg/25 mg. [PEHM-prihn].

Pamprin Multi-Symptom Maximum Strength (OB/GYN) (generic *acetaminophen, pamabrom*). Combination analgesic and diuretic used to treat premenstrual dysphoric disorder and dysmenorrhea. Caplet/Tablet: 500 mg/25 mg. [PEHM-prihn].

Panadol, Children's Panadol, Infants' Drops Panadol, Junior Strength Panadol (Analges, Ortho). Non-narcotic nonaspirin analgesic drug used to treat fever and pain in children and adults; used to treat osteoarthritis in adults. For dosage, see *acetaminophen*.

Panafil (Derm) (generic *papain*). Topical enzyme drug used to debride burns and wounds. Ointment. 96

Panavir (Antivir). Antiviral drug used to treat AIDS. For dosage, see *probucol*. 326

Pancrease, Pancrease MT4, Pancrease MT 10, Pancrease MT 16, Pancrease MT 20, Pancrease MT 25 (GI) (generic *amylase, lipase, protease*). Combination drug replacement therapy for digestive enzymes. Capsule, tablet: 12,000 units/4500 units/12,000 units; 20,000 units/4500 units/25,000 units; 30,000 units/10,000 units/30,000 units; 48,000 units/16,000 units/48,000 units; 56,000 units/20,000 units/44,000 units; 75,000 units/25,000 units/75,000 units. [PEHN-kree-ace].

pancuronium (Pavulon) (Anes, Resp). Muscle relaxant drug used during surgery; used to treat patients who are intubated and on the ventilator. Intravenous: 1 mg/mL, 2 mg/mL. [pehn-kyour-OH-nee-uhm]. 199, 370

Pandel (Derm) (generic *hydrocortisone*). Topical corticosteroid anti-inflammatory drug. Cream: 0.1%, 1%. 92

Panhematin (Misc). Used to treat acute intermittent porphyria. For dosage, see *hemin*.

panic disorder, drugs used to treat. 289

Panmycin (Antibio). Antibiotic used to treat a variety of infections, including acne vulgaris, *H. pylori* of the gastrointestinal tract, *Chlamydia*, gonorrhea, and syphilis. For dosage, see *tetracycline*. [pehn-MY-sihn]. 84, 120, 317

Panorex (Chemo). Monoclonal antibody chemotherapy drug used to treat pancreatic cancer. Orphan drug. 346

Panretin (Chemo, Oph). Chemotherapy drug used to treat leukemia; used to prevent retinal detachment in patients with proliferative retinopathy. Orphan drug. 348

Panretin (Chemo, Derm) (generic *alitretinoin*). Topical vitamin A-type drug used to treat the cancerous skin ulcers of Kaposi's sarcoma. Gel: 0.1%. [pehn-REH-tihn]. 97

Panthoderm (Derm) (generic *dexpanthenol*). Topical antipruritic drug. Cream: 2%. [PEHN-thoh-dehrm]. 95

(Pantopon) (Analges, GI). No longer on the market. (Generic name *opium*; narcotic antidiarrheal drug).

pantoprazole (Protonix, Protonix I.V.) (GI). Proton pump inhibitor used to treat gastroesophageal reflux disease; used to treat Zollinger-Ellison syndrome. Tablet: 40 mg. Intravenous (powder to be reconstituted): 40 mg. [pehn-TAW-preh-zohl]. 121

Panzem (Chemo). Angiogenesis inhibiting drug used to treat multiple myeloma. Orphan drug.

papain (Accuzyme, Panafil) (Derm). Topical enzyme drug used to debride burns and wounds. Ointment. [peh-PAYN]. 96

papaverine (Cardio, Neuro). Vasodilator used to treat blood vessel spasms of the coronary arteries; used to treat peripheral vascular disease and cerebrovascular disease. Capsule: 150 mg. Intravenous: 30 mg/mL. 168, 174

(Paradione) (Neuro). No longer on the market. (Generic name *paramethadione*; used to treat absence seizures).

Paraflex (Ortho). Skeletal muscle relaxant used to treat minor muscle spasms associated with injuries. For dosage, see *chlorzoxazone*. [PEH-rah-flehks]. 144

Parafon Forte DSC (Ortho). Skeletal muscle relaxant used to treat minor muscle spasms associated with injuries. For dosage, see *chlorzoxazone*. [PEH-rah-fawn FOHR-tay]. 144

Paral (Psych). Nonbarbiturate used to provide sedation during alcohol withdrawal. For dosage, see *paraldehyde*. 294

paraldehyde (Paral) (Psych). Nonbarbiturate used to provide sedation during alcohol withdrawal. Oral liquid: 30 mL. Rectal liquid: 30 mL. [pah-REHL-deh-hide]. 294

(paramethadione) (Neuro). No longer on the market. (Trade name *Paradione*; used to treat absence seizures).

Paraplatin (Chemo). Chemotherapy platinum drug used to treat ovarian cancer. For dosage, see *carboplatin*. [peh-rah-PLEH-tihn]. 345

Paredrine (Oph). Topical mydriatic drug. For dosage, see *hydroxyamphetamine*. [PEH-reh-dreen]. 223

paregoric (Analges, GI). Narcotic used to treat pain; narcotic side effect of constipation used to treat diarrhea. (Schedule III drug). Liquid: 10%, 2 mg/5 mL. [peh-rah-GOHR-ihk]. 123, 297

(Paremyd) (Oph). No longer on the market. (Combination mydriatic drug).

parenteral route, administration of drugs by the. 40

Parepectolin (GI). Antidiarrheal drug. For dosage, see *attapulgite*. [peh-rah-PEHK-toh-lihn]. 124

Parkinson's disease, drugs used to treat. 267

Parlodel, Parlodel Snap Tabs (Neuro). Used to treat Parkinson's disease. For dosage, see *bromocriptine*. [PAWR-loh-dell]. 268

Parnate (Psych). MAO inhibitor used to treat depression. For dosage, see *tranylcypromine*. [PAWR-nayt]. 288

paromomycin (Humatin) (Antibio, GI). Aminoglycoside antibiotic and amebicide used to treat intestintal amebiasis and hepatic coma. Capsule: 250 mg. [peh-roh-moh-MY-sihn]. 134, 317

paroxetine (Paxil, Paxil CR) (Diab). Selective serotonin reuptake inhibitor antidepressant used to treat diabetic peripheral neuropathy. Capsule: (Pending).

Tablet: 10 mg, 12.5 mg, 20 mg, 25 mg, 30 mg, 37.5 mg, 40 mg. Liquid: 10 mg/5 mL. [peh-RAWK-seh-teen].

paroxetine (Paxil, Paxil CR) (OB/GYN). Selective serotonin reuptake inhibitor antidepressant used to treat premenstrual dysphoric disorder. Capsule: (Pending). Tablet: 10 mg, 12.5 mg, 20 mg, 25 mg, 30 mg, 37.5 mg, 40 mg. Liquid: 10 mg/5 mL. [peh-RAWK-seh-teen]. 255

paroxetine (Paxil, Paxil CR) (Ortho, Uro). Selective serotonin reuptake inhibitor antidepressant used to treat fibromyalgia; used to treat premature ejaculation. Capsule: (Pending). Tablet: 10 mg, 12.5 mg, 20 mg, 25 mg, 30 mg, 37.5 mg, 40 mg. Liquid: 10 mg/5 mL. [peh-RAWK-seh-teen]. 112, 148

paroxetine (Paxil, Paxil CR) (Psych). Selective serotonin reuptake inhibitor antidepressant used to treat depression; used to treat anxiety; used to treat manic-depressive disorder; used to treat obsessive-compulsive disorder; used to treat social anxiety disorder; used to treat panic disorder; used to treat posttraumatic stress disorder. Capsule: (Pending). Tablet: 10 mg, 12.5 mg, 20 mg, 25 mg, 30 mg, 37.5 mg, 40 mg. Liquid: 10 mg/5 mL. [peh-RAWK-seh-teen]. 282, 287, 289, 290

(Parsidol) (Neuro). No longer on the market. (Generic name *ethopropazine*; used to treat Parkinson's disease).

Paser Granules (Resp). Used to treat tuberculosis. For dosage, see *aminosalicylic acid*. 197

pastille (drug form). 35

Patanol (Oph). Topical antihistamine used to treat allergy symptoms in the eyes. For dosage, see *olopatadine*. [PEH-teh-nawl]. 220

patch, transdermal. 38

patent drugs/medicines. 13

patent on new drugs. 29

Pathilon (GI). Antispasmodic drug used to treat spasm of smooth muscle of the bowel. For dosage, see *tridihexethyl*. [PEH-thih-lawn]. 122

Pathocil (Antibio). Penicillin-type antibiotic used to treat a variety of bacterial infections, including staphylococci. For dosage, see *dicloxacillin*. [PEH-thoh-sill]. 313

pathogen. 65

Pavulon (Anes, Resp). Muscle relaxant drug used during surgery; used to treat patients who are intubated and on the ventilator. For dosage, see *pancuronium*. [PEH-vyoo-lawn]. 199, 370

Paxarel (Anes, OB/GYN, Neuro, Psych). Nonbarbiturate sedative/hypnotic drug used for preoperative sedation; used to treat premenstrual dysphoric disorder; used to treat insomnia; used to treat anxiety. For dosage, see *acecarbromal*. [PEHK-sah-rehl]. 254, 272, 282, 370

Paxil, Paxil CR (Diab). Selective serotonin reuptake inhibitor antidepressant used to treat diabetic peripheral neuropathy. For dosage, see *paroxetine*. [PEHK-sihl].

Paxil, Paxil CR (OB/GYN). Selective serotonin reuptake inhibitor antidepressant used to treat premenstrual dysphoric disorder. For dosage, see *paroxetine*. [PEHK-sihl]. 255

Paxil (Ortho, Uro). Selective serotonin reuptake inhibitor antidepressant used to treat fibromyalgia; used to treat premature ejaculation. For dosage, see *paroxetine*. [PEHK-sihl]. 112, 148

Paxil, Paxil CR (Psych). Selective serotonin reuptake inhibitor antidepressant used to treat depression; used to treat anxiety; used to treat manic-depressive disorder; used to treat obsessive-compulsive disorder; used to treat social anxiety disorder; used to treat panic disorder; used to treat post-traumatic stress disorder. For dosage, see *paroxetine*. [PEHK-sihl]. 282, 287, 289, 290

(Paxipam) (Psych). No longer on the market. (Generic name *halazepam*; benzodiazepine antianxiety drug).

p.c. (abbreviation meaning *after meals*).

PCE Dispertab (Antibio). Macrolide antibiotic used to treat a variety of infections, including *Streptococcus*, *H. influenzae*, gonorrhea, syphilis, *Chlamydia*, and Legionnaire's disease; used to prevent subacute bacterial endocarditis. For dosage, see *erythromycin*. 319

PCN (abbreviation for *penicillin*). See *penicillin*.

PCP (abbreviation for *phencyclidine* and *Pneumocystis carinii pneumonia*).

PediaCare Fever (Analges). Nonsteroidal anti-inflammatory drug used to treat fever and pain. For dosage, see *ibuprofen*.

PediaCare Infants' Decongestant (ENT). Decongestant. For dosage, see *pseudoephedrine*.

Pedialyte Solution, Pedialyte Freezer Pops (GI). Given to children to replace water and electrolytes lost from vomiting and diarrhea. Liquid. Frozen pop.

Pediapred (Endo). Corticosteroid anti-inflammatory used to treat severe inflammation in various body systems. For dosage, see *prednisolone*. [PEE-dee-ah-prehd]. 232

PediaSure (GI). Infant formula. Liquid.

Pediatric Advil Drops, see *Advil*.

Pediatric Vicks 44d Dry Hacking Cough and Head Congestion (ENT). Nonnarcotic antitussive drug. For dosage, see *dextromethorphan*.

Pediazole (Antibio) (generic *erythromycin, sulfisoxazole*). Combination erythromycin and sulfonamide anti-infective drug used to treat otitis media. Liquid (granules to be reconstituted): 200 mg/600 mg per 5 mL. [PEE-dee-ah-zohl]. 320

pediculosis (lice), drugs used to treat. 95

Pediotic (ENT) (generic *hydrocortisone, neomycin, polymyxin B*). Combination topical corticosteroid and antibiotic drug for the ears. Drops: 1%/5 mg/10,000 units.

PEG (abbreviation for *polyethylene glycol*). See *bowel prep/enema*.

pegademase bovine (Adagen). Replacement therapy used to treat adenosine deaminase (ADA) deficiency. Orphan drug.

Peganone (Neuro). Anticonvulsant drug used to treat tonic-clonic and psychomotor seizures. For dosage, see *ethotoin*. [PEH-gah-nohn]. 264

pegaspargase (Oncaspar) (Chemo). Chemotherapy enzyme drug used to treat leukemia. Intramuscular or intravenous: 750 IU/mL. 345

Pegasys (Chemo). Chemotherapy drug used to treat renal cancer and leukemia. For dosage, see *peginterferon alfa-2a*. [PEH-gah-sihs]. 346

peginterferon alfa-2a (Pegasys) (Chemo). Chemotherapy drug used to treat renal cancer and leukemia. Orphan drug. 346

peginterferon alfa-2b (PEG-Intron) (Chemo, GI). Chemotherapy drug used to treat renal cancer; antiviral drug used to treat hepatitis C. Subcutaneous: 100 mcg/mL, 160 mcg/mL, 240 mcg/mL, 300 mcg/mL. [pehg-ihn-tehr-FEER-awn]. 134, 346

PEG-Intron (Chemo, GI). Chemotherapy drug used to treat renal cancer; antiviral drug used to treat hepatitis C. For dosage, see *peginterferon alfa-2b*. 134, 346

pellet (drug form). 38

PemADD, PemADD CT (Neuro, Psych). Central nervous system stimulant used to treat narcolepsy; used to treat attention-deficit/hyperactivity disorder. (Schedule IV drug). For dosage, see *pemoline*. 274, 292

pemirolast (Alamast) (Oph). Topical mast cell stabilizer used to treat allergy symptoms in the eyes. Ophthalmic solution: 0.1%. [peh-MEER-oh-lehst]. 220

pemoline (Cylert, PemADD, PemADD CT) (Neuro, Psych). Central nervous system stimulant used to treat narcolepsy; used to treat attention-deficit/hyperactivity disorder. (Schedule IV drug). Tablet: 18.75 mg, 37.5 mg, 75 mg. [PEH-moh-leen]. 274, 292

penbutolol (Levatol) (Cardio). Nonselective beta-blocker used to treat hypertension. Tablet: 20 mg. [pehn-BYOO-toh-lawl]. 162

penciclovir (Denavir) (Derm, ENT). Topical drug used to treat herpes simplex virus type 1 lesions (cold sores). Cream: 10 mg/g. [pehn-SIH-kloh-veer]. 91

Penetrex (Antibio). Fluoroquinolone antibiotic used to treat urinary tract infections and gonorrhea. For dosage, see *enoxacin*. [PEH-neh-trehks]. 105, 318

penicillin discovered. Historical Notes feature. 314

penicillin G (Pfizerpen) (Antibio). Penicillin antibiotic used to treat various types of bacterial infections, including gonorrhea, syphilis, and Lyme disease. Intramuscular or intravenous (powder to be reconstituted): 1,00,000 units, 2,000,000 units, 3,000,000 units, 5,000,000 units. [peh-neh-SILL-ehn]. 313

penicillin G benzathine (Bicillin L-A, Permapen) (Antibio). Penicillin antibiotic used to treat various types of bacterial infections, including *Streptococcus* and syphilis; used prophylactically to prevent subacute bacterial endocarditis in at-risk patients undergoing dental or surgical procedures. Intramuscular: 300,000 units, 600,000 units, 1,200,000 units, 2,400,000 units. [peh-neh-SILL-ehn]. 313

(penicillin G potassium) (Antibio). No longer on the market. (Trade name *Pentids*; penicillin antibiotic).

penicillin G procaine (Wycillin) (Antibio). Penicillin antibiotic used to treat various types of bacterial infections, including *Streptococcus, Pneumococcus, Staphylococcus*, gonorrhea, and syphilis; used to treat cutaneous and inhaled anthrax from bioterrorism. Intramuscular: 1,200,000 units, 2,400,000 units. [peh-neh-SILL-ehn]. 313

penicillin V (Beepen-VK, Penicillin VK, Pen-Vee K, Veetids) (Antibio). Penicillin antibiotic used to treat a variety of bacterial infections, including *Streptococcus, Staphylococcus, Pneumococcus*, and Lyme disease. Tablet: 250 mg, 500 mg. Liquid: 125 mg/5 mL, 250 mg/5 mL. [peh-neh-SILL-ehn]. 313

Penicillin VK (Antibio). Penicillin antibiotic used to treat a variety of bacterial infections, including *Streptococcus, Staphylococcus, Pneumococcus*, and Lyme disease. For dosage, see *penicillin V*. 313

penicillinase. 313

penicillins (Antibio). Class of drugs that kill bacteria. 312

Penlac Nail Lacquer (Derm) (generic *ciclopirox*). Topical antifungal drug. Liquid nail solution: 8%. 89

Pentam 300 (Antivir). Used to treat *Pneumocystis carinii* pneumonia in AIDS patients; used to treat leishmaniasis. For dosage, see *pentamidine*. [PEHN-tehm]. 328

pentamidine (NebuPent, Pentam 300, Pneumopent) (Antivir). Used to treat *Pneumocystis carinii* pneumonia in AIDS patients; used to treat leishmaniasis. Intramuscular or intravenous (powder to be reconstituted): 300 mg. Respirgard II nebulizer aerosol: 300 mg. [pehn-TEH-mih-deen]. 328

Pentasa (GI).   Anti-inflammatory-type drug used to treat ulcerative colitis.   For dosage, see *mesalamine*. [pehn-TAH-sah]. 126

pentazocine (Talwin) (Analges, Anes).   Narcotic analgesic drug used to treat moderate-to-severe pain; used as a preoperative drug to sedate. (Schedule IV drug). Subcutaneous, intramuscular, or intravenous: 30 mg/mL. [pehn-teh-ZOH-seen]. 298, 371

Penthrane (Anes).   Used to induce and maintain general anesthesia. Inhaled gas. [PEHN-thrayn]. 370

(Pentids) (Antibio).   No longer on the market. (Generic name *penicillin G potassium*; penicillin antibiotic).

pentobarbital (Nembutal) (Anes, Neuro).   Barbiturate used to provide preoperative sedation; used for short-term treatment of insomnia. (Schedule II drug). Capsule: 100 mg. Liquid: 20 mg/5 mL. Suppository: 30 mg, 120 mg. Intramuscular or intravenous: 50 mg/mL. [pehn-toh-BAR-beh-tawl]. 272, 371

Pentolair (Oph).   Topical mydriatic drug.   For dosage, see *cyclopentolate*. [PEHN-toh-lehr]. 223

pentostatin (Nipent) (Chemo).   Purine antagonist chemotherapy drug used to treat leukemia and cutaneous T-cell lymphoma; investigational drug used to treat non-Hodgkin's lymphoma. Intravenous (powder to be reconstituted): 10 mg. [pehn-toh-STEH-tihn]. 339

pentosan (Elmiron) (Uro).   Urinary tract analgesic. Capsule: 100 mg. [PEHN-toh-sehn]. 107

Pentothal (Anes).   Barbiturate used to induce and maintain general anesthesia.   For dosage, see *thiopental*. [PEHN-toh-thawl]. 367, 369

pentoxifylline (Trental) (Cardio).   Used to improve circulation in the legs of patients with peripheral vascular disease by decreasing blood viscosity. Tablet: 400 mg. [pehn-tawk-sih-FIH-lihn].

Pen-Vee K (Antibio).   Penicillin antibiotic used to treat various types of bacterial infections, including *Streptococcus*, *Staphylococcus*, *Pneumococcus*, and Lyme disease.   For dosage, see *penicillin V*. 313

Pepcid, Pepcid AC, Pepcid AC Acid Controller, Pepcid RPD (GI).   H₂ blocker used to treat peptic ulcers and *H. pylori* infection.   For dosage, see *famotidine*. 118

Pepcid Complete (GI) (generic *calcium, famotidine, magnesium*).   Combination H₂ blocker and antacid drug used to treat peptic ulcers and *H. pylori* infection. Chewable tablet: 800 mg/10 mg/165 mg. 118

Peptamen (GI).   Liquid supplemental nutrition formulated for patients with gastrointestinal problems. Liquid.

peptic ulcer disease, drugs used to treat. 116

Pepto-Bismol, Pepto-Bismol Maximum Strength (GI). Antidiarrheal drug.   For dosage, see *bismuth*. 124

Pepto Diarrhea Control (GI).   Nonnarcotic antidiarrheal drug.   For dosage, see *loperamide*. 123

percentage (drug measurement). 70

Percocet (Analges) (generic *oxycodone, acetaminophen*). Combination narcotic and nonnarcotic analgesic drug. (Schedule II drug). Tablet: 2.5 mg/325 mg, 5 mg/325 mg, 7.5 mg/500 mg, 10 mg/650 mg. [PEHR-koh-seht]. 303

Percodan, Percodan-Demi (Analges) (generic *oxycodone, aspirin*).   Combination narcotic and nonnarcotic analgesic drug. (Schedule II drug). Tablet: 2.25 mg/325 mg, 4.5 mg/325 mg. [PEHR-koh-dehn]. 302

Percogesic (ENT) (generic *phenyltoloxamine, acetaminophen*).   Combination antihistamine and analgesic drug. Tablet: 30 mg/325 mg. 213

Percolone (Analges, Neuro).   Narcotic analgesic used to treat moderate-to-severe pain; used to treat neuralgia from herpes zoster infection (shingles). (Schedule II drug).   For dosage, see *oxycodone*. [PEHR-koh-lohn]. 276, 297

Perdiem Fiber Therapy (GI).   Bulk-producing laxative.   For dosage, see *psyllium*. [pehr-DEE-uhm]. 125

Perdiem Overnight Relief (GI) (generic *psyllium, senna*).   Combination bulk-producing and irritant/stimulant laxative. Granules. [pehr-DEE-uhm]. 125

performance anxiety, drugs used to treat. 290

pergolide (Permax) (Neuro, Psych).   Used to treat Parkinson's disease; orphan drug used to treat the psychiatric disorder of Tourette's syndrome. Tablet: 0.05 mg, 0.25 mg, 1 mg. [PEHR-goh-lide]. 268, 294

Pergonal (OB/GYN).   Ovulation-stimulating drug used to treat infertility.   For dosage, see *menotropins*. [PEHR-goh-nawl]. 244

Periactin (Antivir) (Derm, ENT).   Antihistamine used to treat AIDS wasting syndrome; used to treat allergic rhinitis and allergic reactions with hives and itching.   For dosage, see *cyproheptadine*. [peh-ree-EHK-tihn]. 207, 367

Peri-Colace (GI) (generic *docusate, casanthranol*). Stool softener and irritant/stimulant laxative. Capsule. [peh-ree-KOH-lays]. 125

Peridex (ENT).   Topical mouthwash drug used to treat oral mucositis in chemotherapy patients; used to treat gingivitis.   For dosage, see *chlorhexidine*.

perindopril (Aceon) (Cardio).   Angiotensin-converting enzyme inhibitor used to treat hypertension. Tablet: 2 mg, 4 mg, 8 mg. [peh-RIHN-doh-prihl]. 163

PerioGard (ENT).   Topical mouthwash drug used to treat gingivitis.   For dosage, see *chlorhexidine*.

Periostat (Antibio, ENT). Used to treat periodontal disease. For dosage, see *doxycycline*.

peripheral vasodilators (Cardio). Class of drugs used to treat hypertension.

Permapen (Antibio). Penicillin antibiotic used to treat various types of bacterial infections, including *Streptococcus* and syphilis; used prophylactically to prevent subacute bacterial endocarditis in at-risk patients undergoing dental or surgical procedures. For dosage, see *penicillin G benzathine*. [PEHR-mah-pehn]. 313

Permax (Neuro, Psych). Used to treat Parkinson's disease; used to treat Tourette's syndrome. For dosage, see *pergolide*. [PEHR-macks]. 268, 294

permethrin (Acticin, Elimite, Nix) (Derm). Topical drug used to treat scabies (mites) and pediculosis (lice). Cream: 5%. Liquid (creme rinse): 1%. [pehr-MEE-thrihn]. 95

Permitil (Psych). Phenothiazine drug used to treat psychosis and schizophrenia. For dosage, see *fluphenazine*. [pehr-MIH-tuhl]. 283

pernicious anemia, drugs used to treat.

Pernox Lathering Abradant Scrub (Derm) (generic *salicylic acid*). Topical keratolytic drug used to treat acne vulgaris. Lotion. 83

Peroxyl (ENT) (generic *hydrogen peroxide*). Topical antiseptic for the mouth. Gel: 1.5%.

perphenazine (Trilafon) (GI). Phenothiazine drug used to treat nausea and vomiting; used to treat intractable hiccoughs. Liquid: 16 mg/5 mL. Tablet: 2 mg, 4 mg, 8 mg, 16 mg. Intramuscular or intravenous: 5 mg/mL. [pehr-PHEN-ah-zeen]. 127

perphenazine (Trilafon) (Psych). Phenothiazine drug used to treat psychosis. Tablet: 2 mg, 4 mg, 8 mg, 16 mg. Intramuscular: 5 mg/mL. [pehr-PHEN-ah-zeen]. 283

Persantine (Cardio). Coronary artery vasodilator used diagnostically to provoke angina in patients with coronary artery disease who cannot tolerate exercise stress testing; a platelet aggregation inhibitor used to prevent blood clot after cardiac valve replacement surgery. For dosage, see *dipyridamole*. [pehr-SEHN-teen]. 173, 187

Pertussin CS, Pertussin ES (ENT). Nonnarcotic antitussive drug. For dosage, see *dextromethorphan*. 210

Pfizerpen (Antibio). Penicillin antibiotic used to treat various types of bacterial infections, including gonorrhea, syphilis, and Lyme disease. For dosage, see *penicillin G*. [FY-zehr-pehn]. 313

phantom limb pain, drugs used to treat. 147

pharmaceutical milestones. 9

pharmacist. 8, 76

pharmacodynamics. 1

pharmacokinetics. 1

pharmacology.
  ancient. 5
  Aztec Indian. 5
  Chinese. 6
  definition of. 1
  Egyptian. 5
  history of. 5
  linguistic origin of. 1
  medieval. 6
  molecular. 1
  Sumarian. 5

pharmacology in the 1500s. 6

pharmacology in the 1800s. 7

pharmacology in the 1900s. 7

Phazyme, Phazyme 95, Phazyme 125 (GI). Antiflatulent. For dosage, see *simethicone*. [FAY-zime]. 118

(phenacemide) (Neuro). No longer on the market. (Trade name *Phenurone*; used to treat complex partial seizures).

Phenaphen with Codeine No. 3 (Analges) (generic *acetaminophen, codeine*). Combination narcotic and nonnarcotic analgesic drug. (Schedule III drug). Capsule: 30 mg/325 mg. [FEHN-ah-fehn]. 303

Phenaphen with Codeine No. 4 (Analges) (generic *acetaminophen, codeine*). Combination narcotic and nonnarcotic analgesic drug. (Schedule III drug). Capsule: 60 mg/325 mg. [FEHN-ah-fehn]. 303

phenazopyridine (Pyridium, Urogesic) (Uro). Urinary tract analgesic. Tablet: 95 mg, 97.2 mg, 100 mg, 150 mg, 200 mg. [peh-neh-zoh-PY-rih-deen}. 107

phencyclidine (PCP) (Misc). Illegal Schedule I drug. 16

phendimetrazine (Plegine, Prelu-2) (GI). Appetite suppressant used to treat obesity. (Schedule III drug). Capsule: 35 mg, 105 mg. Tablet: 35 mg. [fen-dih-MEH-trah-zeen]. 129

phenelzine (Nardil) (Psych). Monoamine oxidase inhibitor used to treat depression. Tablet: 15 mg. [FEH-nehl-zeen]. 288

Phenergan, Phenergan Fortis, Phenergan Plain (Derm, ENT). Antihistamine used to treat allergic rhinitis and allergic reactions with hives and itching. For dosage, see *promethazine*. [FEH-nehr-gehn]. 207

Phenergan (GI). Antiemetic drug; used to treat motion sickness. For dosage, see *promethazine*. [FEH-nehr-gehn]. 128

Phenergan VC (ENT) (generic *phenylephrine, promethazine*). Combination decongestant and antihistamine drug. Syrup: 5 mg/6.25 mg. [FEH-nehr-gehn].

Phenergan VC with Codeine (ENT) (generic *phenylephrine, promethazine, codeine*). Combination decongestant, antihistamine, and narcotic antitussive drug. Syrup: 5 mg/6.25 mg/10 mg.

Phenergan with Codeine (ENT) (generic *promethazine, codeine*). Combination antihistamine and narcotic antitussive drug. Syrup: 6.25 mg/10 mg.

Phenergan with Dextromethorphan (ENT) (generic *promethazine, dextromethorphan*). Combination antihistamine and nonnarcotic antitussive drug. Syrup: 6.25 mg/15 mg.

Phenex-1 (GI). Infant formula for infants with phenylketonuria. Powder (to be reconstituted).

Phenex-2 (GI). Liquid nutritional supplement formulated for patients with phenylketonuria. Powder (to be reconstituted).

phenindamine (Nolahist) (ENT). Antihistamine used to treat allergic rhinitis. Tablet: 25 mg. [feh-NIHN-dah-meen]. 207

phenobarbital. Historical Notes feature.

phenobarbital (Luminal, Solfoton) (Neuro, OB/GYN). Barbiturate used to treat tonic-clonic and partial seizures; used to treat status epilepticus; used to treat insomnia; used to treat the seizures of eclampsia during pregnancy. (Schedule IV drug). Tablet: 15 mg, 16 mg, 30 mg, 60 mg, 90 mg, 100 mg. Capsule: 16 mg. Liquid: 15 mg/5 mL, 20 mg/5 mL. Intramuscular: 30 mg/mL, 60 mg/mL, 65 mg/mL, 130 mg/mL. [fee-noh-BAR-beh-tawl]. 264, 267, 272

(Phenolax) (GI). No longer on the market. (Irritant/stimulant laxative).

phensuximide (Milontin Kapseals) (Neuro). Anticonvulsant drug used to treat absence seizures. Capsule: 500 mg. [fehn-SUHK-seh-mide]. 264

phentermine (Fastin) (GI). Appetite suppressant used to treat obesity. (Schedule IV drug). Capsule: 15 mg, 30 mg. Tablet: 8 mg, 30 mg. [FEHN-tehr-meen]. 129

phentolamine (Regitine) (Cardio, Endo). Alpha-adrenergic blocker drug used to treat hypertensive crisis; used to treat hypertension caused by pheochromocytoma of the adrenal medulla. Intramuscular or intravenous (powder to be reconstituted): 5 mg. [fehn-TOHL-ah-meen]. 168

(Phenurone) (Neuro). No longer on the market. (Generic name *phenacemide*; used to treat complex partial seizures).

(phenylbutazone) (Ortho). No longer on the market. (Trade name *Butazolidin*; anti-inflammatory drug).

phenylbutyrate (Chemo). Chemotherapy drug used to treat leukemia. Orphan drug. 348

phenylephrine (Children's Nostril, Neo-Synephrine, Nostril, Rhinall, Sinex) (ENT). Decongestant. Chewable tablet: 10 mg. Drops: 0.125%, 0.16%, 0.25%, 0.5%, 1%. Spray: 0.25%, 0.5%, 1%. [fee-nuhl-EH-frihn]. 206

phenylephrine (Mydfrin, Neo-Synephrine) (Oph). Topical miotic drug used to treat uveitis; used to treat glaucoma; used as a mydriatic during eye surgery. Ophthalmic solution: 2.5%, 10%. [fee-nuhl-EH-frehn]. 221, 223

phenylephrine (Prefrin Liquifilm, Relief, Zincfrin) (Oph). Topical decongestant/vasoconstrictor used to treat irritation and allergy symptoms in the eyes. Ophthalmic solution: 0.12%. [fee-nuhl-EH-frehn].

(phenylpropanolamine) (ENT, GI). No longer on the market. (Trade name Propagest, also in many trade name combination drugs; appetite suppressant and ENT decongestant). Historical Notes feature.

phenytoin (Dilantin Infatabs, Dilantin Kapseals, Dilantin-125) (Neuro). Anticonvulsant drug used to treat tonic-clonic and complex partial seizures; used to treat status epilepticus. Capsule: 30 mg, 100 mg. Chewable tablet: 50 mg. Liquid: 125 mg/5 mL. Intramuscular: 50 mg/mL. [feh-nih-TOH-ihn]. 264, 267

Phillips' Liqui-Gels (GI). Stool softener laxative. For dosage, see *docusate*. 125

Phillips' Milk of Magnesia, Concentrated Phillips' Milk of Magnesia (GI). For dosage, see *milk of magnesia*. 116, 124

pHisoDerm (Derm). Topical soapless skin cleanser. Liquid. 99

pHisoHex (Derm) (generic *hexachlorophene*). Topical antibacterial cleanser. Liquid: 3%. 99

Phospholine Iodide (Oph). Topical cholinesterase inhibitor drug used to treat glaucoma. For dosage, see *echothiophate*. [FAHS-foh-leen II-oh-dide].

phosphorated carbohydrate solution (Emetrol) (GI). Antiemetic drug. Liquid. 127

Photofrin (Chemo). Chemotherapy photosensitizing drug used to treat esophageal cancer and lung cancer. This drug sensitizes tumor cells to light, then laser light causes the release of free radicals that destroy the tumor cells. For dosage, see *porfimer*. [FOH-toh-frihn]. 348

Phyllocontin (Resp). Bronchodilator; used to prevent apnea in premature infants. For dosage, see *aminophylline*. [fy-loh-KAWN-tihn]. 193

physostigmine (Antilirium) (Emerg, Neuro, Psych). Tricylic antidepressant antagonist used as an antidote to reverse an overdose of a tricyclic antidepressant; used as an orphan drug to treat ataxia. Intramuscular or intravenous: 1 mg/mL. [fy-soh-STIG-meen]. 183, 277, 294

(Pilagan) (Oph). No longer on the market. (Generic name *pilocarpine*; topical drug used to treat glaucoma).

Pilocar (Oph). Topical miotic drug used to treat glaucoma. For dosage, see *pilocarpine*. [PY-loh-kawr]. 221

pilocarpine (Salagen) (ENT, Oph). Used to treat dry mouth due to salivary gland dysfunction after radiation for head and neck cancer; an orphan drug used to treat Sjogren's syndrome. Tablet: 5 mg. Orphan drug.

pilocarpine (Akarpine, Isopto Carpine, Pilocar, Pilopine HS) (Oph). Topical drug used to treat glaucoma. Ophthalmic gel: 4%. Ophthalmic solution: 0.25%, 0.5%, 1%, 2%, 3%, 4%, 5%, 6%, 8%, 10%. Ophthalmic insert (in cul-de-sac of eye): 20 mcg/hr for one week, 40 mcg/hr for one week. [py-loh-KAWR-peen]. 221

Pilopine HS (Oph). Topical miotic drug used to treat glaucoma. For dosage, see *pilocarpine*. [PY-loh-peen]. 221

(Pilostat) (Oph). No longer on the market. (Generic name *pilocarpine*; topical drug used to treat glaucoma).

pimecrolimus (Elidel) (Derm). Topical nonsteroidal anti-inflammatory drug used to treat infant eczema. Cream. 95

pimozide (Orap) (Psych). Antipsychotic drug used to treat Tourette's syndrome but not psychosis. Tablet: 1 mg, 2 mg. [PIHM-oh-zide]. 294

pinacidil (Pindac) (Cardio). Vasodilator used to treat hypertension. Investigational drug. 174

Pindac (Cardio) (generic *pinacidil*). Vasodilator used to treat hypertension. Investigational drug. 174

pindolol (Visken) (Cardio). Nonselective beta-blocker used to treat hypertension and ventricular arrhythmias. Tablet: 5 mg, 10 mg. [PIHN-doh-lawl]. 160, 162

Pin-Rid, Pin-X (Misc). Used to treat pinworms and roundworms. For dosage, see *pyrantel*.

pioglitazone (Actos) (Endo, OB/GYN). Oral antidiabetic drug; used to treat the elevated insulin levels caused by polycystic ovary syndrome. Tablet: 15 mg, 30 mg, 45 mg. [pee-oh-GLIH-tah-zohn]. 240

pipecuronium (Arduan) (Anes). Muscle relaxant drug used during surgery. Intravenous (powder to be reconstituted): 10 mg. 370

piperacillin (Pipracil) (Antibio). Penicillin-type antibiotic used to treat various types of bacterial infections, including *Streptococcus*, *E. coli*, *Pseudomonas*, and gonorrhea. Intramuscular or intravenous (powder to be reconstituted): 42.5 mg, 2 g, 3 g. [pih-pehr-ah-sill-ihn]. 313

Pipracil (Antibio). Penicillin-type antibiotic used to treat various types of bacterial infections, including streptococci, *E. coli*, *Pseudomonas*, and gonorrhea. For dosage, see *piperacillin*. [PIP-rah-sill]. 313

pirbuterol (Maxair Autohaler, Maxair Inhaler) (Resp). Bronchodilator. Aerosol inhaler: 0.2 mg/puff [peer-BYOO-teh-rawl]. 193

pirenzepine (Gastrozepine) (GI). Used to treat peptic ulcers. Investigational drug. 134

piritrexim (Antivir). Used to treat *Pneumocystis carinii*, *Mycobacterium avium-intracellulare*, and *Toxoplasma gondii* infections in AIDS patients. Orphan drug. 328, 329, 332

piroxicam (Feldene) (Analges, OB/GYN, Ortho). Nonsteroidal anti-inflammatory drug used to treat dysmenorrhea; used to treat osteoarthritis and rheumatoid arthritis. Capsule: 10 mg, 20 mg. [pih-RAWK-sih-kehm]. 139, 255, 304

Pitocin (OB/GYN). Used to stimulate uterine contractions; used to treat postpartum uterine bleeding; used to treat incomplete abortion. For dosage, see *oxytocin*. [pih-TOH-sihn]. 246, 248

Pitressin (Endo). Antidiuretic hormone replacement used to treat diabetes insipidus. For dosage, see *vasopressin*. [pih-TREH-sihn]. 231

pituitary gland dysfunction, drugs used to treat. 230

placebo. 28, 65

(Placidyl) (Neuro). No longer on the market. (Generic name *ethchlorvynol*; nonbarbiturate used to treat insomnia).

Plan B (OB/GYN) (generic *levonorgestrel*). Progestins-only drug taken after intercourse to prevent pregnancy. Tablet: 0.75 mg. 251

Plaquenil (Ortho). Used to treat rheumatoid arthritis and systemic lupus erythematosis; it was originally used (and still is used) to treat malaria. For dosage, see *hydroxychloroquine*. [PLEH-kwih-nihl]. 142, 148

Plasbumin-5, Plasbumin-25 (I.V.). Intravenous blood product that contains no cellular components and is used to replace plasma protein. [plehs-BYOO-mihn]. 381

plasma (I.V.). Intravenous blood product that contains no cellular components and is used to replace plasma proteins and clotting factors.
fresh frozen. 381
plasma protein fraction. 381

Plasmanate (I.V.). Intravenous blood product that contains no cellular components and is used to replace plasma proteins.

plasmapheresis. Historical Notes feature.

plasmapheresis (I.V.). The process of removing plasma, plasma proteins, and clotting factors from the cellular components of blood.

Plasma-Plex (I.V.). Intravenous blood product that contains no cellular components and is used to replace plasma proteins.

plasma protein fraction (PPF) (Plasmanate, Plasma-Plex, Plasmatein, Protenate) (I.V.). Intravenous blood product that contains no cellular components and is used to replace plasma proteins.

plasma proteins. 46

Plasmatein (I.V.). Intravenous blood product that contains no cellular components and is used to replace plasma proteins.

plasma volume expanders (I.V.). Plasma and synthetic substances given intravenously.

platelet aggregation inhibitors. 187

platelets (I.V.). Intravenous blood cellular product. 380

Platinol-AQ (Chemo). Chemotherapy platinum drug used to treat ovarian cancer, testicular cancer, and bladder cancer. For dosage, see *cisplatin*. [PLEH-tih-nawl]. 345

platinum chemotherapy drugs (Chemo). Class of chemotherapy drugs. 344

Plavix (Cardio, Hem, Neuro). Platelet aggregation inhibitor used to prevent blood clots and reduce the risk of myocardial infarction or stroke in patients with atherosclerosis and previous history of myocardial infarction or stroke. For dosage, see *clopidogrel*. [PLEH-vicks]. 172, 187, 275

Plegine (GI). Appetite suppressant used to treat obesity. (Schedule III drug). For dosage, see *phendimetrazine*. [PLEH-jeen]. 129

Plegisol (Cardio). Electrolyte solution injected at the beginning of open heart surgery to induce cardiac arrest. Intra-arterial (into the aortic root). [PLEH-jeh-sawl]. 172

Plendil (Cardio). Calcium channel blocker used to treat congestive heart failure, hypertension, and Raynaud's disease. For dosage, see *felodipine*. [PLEHN-dihl]. 154, 163

Pletal (Cardio). Vasodilator used to treat peripheral vascular disease. For dosage, see *cilostazol*. 172

plicamycin (Mithracin) (Chemo). Chemotherapy antibiotic used to treat testicular cancer. Intravenous (powder to be reconstituted): 2500 mcg. [ply-kah-MY-sihn]. 342

(PMB) (OB/GYN). No longer on the market. (Generic name *estrogen, meprobamate*; estrogen replacement therapy and antianxiety drug for menopause).

PMDD (abbreviation for *premenstrual dysphoric disorder*). See *premenstrual dysphoric disorder*.

pneumococcal vaccine (Pneumovax 23, Pnu-Imune 23) (Resp). Vaccine used to protect the elderly and others against the 23 most common strains of pneumococcal pneumonia. Subcutaneous or intramuscular: 25 mcg of each different strain/0.5 mL.

pneumococcal vaccine (Prevnar) (Resp). Vaccine used to protect infants against the seven most prevalent strains of *Streptococcus pneumoniae*. Intramuscular: 2–4 mcg of each different strain/0.5 mL.

Pneumocystis carinii **pneumonia,** drugs used to treat. 328

Pneumopent (Antivir) (generic *pentamidine*). Used to treat *Pneumocystis carinii* pneumonia in AIDS patients. Orphan drug. 328

Pneumovax 23 (Resp). Vaccine used to protect the elderly and others against the 23 most common strains of pneumococcal pneumonia. For dosage, see *pneumococcal vaccine*.

Pnu-Imune 23 (Resp). Vaccine used to protect the elderly and others against the 23 most common strains of pneumococcal pneumonia. For dosage, see *pneumococcal vaccine*.

PO or **p.o.** (abbreviation meaning *by mouth*).

Podocon-25 (Derm, OB/GYN) (generic *podophyllum*). Topical drug used to treat keratoses and genital warts. Liquid: 25%. [POH-doh-kawn]. 259

podofilox (Condylox) (OB/GYN). Topical drug used to treat genital/venereal warts or condyloma acuminatum. Gel: 0.5%. Liquid: 0.5%. [poh-DAW-fih-lawks]. 259

podophyllum (Podocon-25) (Derm, OB/GYN). Topical drug used to treat genital/veneral warts or condyloma acuminatum; used to treat keratoses. Liquid: 25%. [poh-DAW-fih-luhm]. 259

Polaramine, Polaramine Repetabs (Derm, ENT). Antihistamine used to treat allergic rhinitis and allergic reactions with hives and itching. For dosage, see *dexchlorpheniramine*. [poh-LEH-rah-meen]. 207

Polaramine Expectorant (ENT) (generic *pseudoephedrine, dexchlorpheniramine, guaifenesin*). Combination decongestant, antihistamine, and expectorant drug. Liquid: 20 mg/2 mg/100 mg. [poh-LEH-rah-meen].

Polocaine, Polocaine MPF (Anes). Local, regional nerve block, and epidural anesthetic drug. For dosage, see *mepivacaine*. 368

poloxamer 331 (Protox) (Antivir). Used to treat toxoplasmosis in AIDS patients. Orphan drug. 332

polycarbophil (FiberCon, Mitrolan) (GI). Bulk-producing laxative. Chewable tablets: 500 mg. Tablet: 625 mg. [paw-lee-KAWR-boh-fihl]. 125

(Polycillin-N) (Antibio). No longer on the market. (Generic name *ampicillin*; penicillin-type antibiotic).

Polycitra, Polycitra-LC (Ortho, Uro) (generic *potassium citrate, sodium citrate*). Combination drug used to prevent the formation of uric acid kidney stones in patients with gout. Liquid: 550 mg/500 mg. Syrup: 550 mg/500 mg. 112, 146

Polycitra-K (Ortho, Uro). Used to prevent the formation of uric acid kidney stones in patients with gout. For dosage, see *potassium citrate*. 112, 146

(polyestradiol) (Chemo). No longer on the market. (Trade name *Estradurin*; hormonal chemotherapy drug).

PolyHeme (I.V.). Polymerized hemoglobin in solution that is transfused when no other blood products are available. Units. 380

Poly-Histine (Derm, ENT) (generic *pheniramine, phenyltoloxamine, pyrilamine*). Combination antihistamine drug used to treat allergic rhinitis and allergic reactions with hives and itching. Liquid: 4 mg/4 mg/4 mg per 5 mL.

(Poly-Histine-D Ped Caps) (ENT). No longer on the market. (Combination drug with *phenylpropanolamine*; decongestant and antihistamines).

polymyxin B (Antibio). Antibiotic used to treat serious infections including *E. coli, H. influenzae,* and *Klebsiella.* Intravenous: 500,000 units. [paw-lee-MICK-sehn bee]. 319

polymyxin B (Derm, Oph). Topical antibiotic used to treat bacterial eye infections; also an ingredient in many topical drugs used to treat bacterial skin infections. Ophthalmic solution (powder to be reconstituted): 500,000 units. [paw-lee-MICK-sehn bee].

polypharmacy. 56

Poly-Pred Liquifilm Ophthalmic Suspension (Oph) (generic *neomycin, polymyxin B, prednisolone*). Topical combination corticosteroid and antibiotic drug. Ophthalmic suspension: 0.35%/10,000 units/0.5%.

Polysporin (Derm) (generic *bacitracin, polymyxin B*). Topical combination antibiotic drug used to treat bacterial skin infections. Ointment. Powder. [paw-lee-SPOHR-ihn]. 88

Polysporin Ophthalmic Ointment (Oph) (generic *bacitracin, polymyxin B*). Topical combination antibiotic drug. Ophthalmic ointment: 500 units/10,000 units per g. [paw-lee-SPOHR-ihn].

polythiazide (Renese) (Uro). Thiazide diuretic. Tablet: 1 mg, 2 mg, 4 mg. [paw-lee-THY-oh-zide]. 103

Polytrim Ophthalmic Solution (Oph) (generic *polymyxin B, trimethoprim*). Topical combination antibiotic drug. Ophthalmic solution: 10,000 units/1 mg per mL.

(Pondimin) (GI). No longer on the market. (Generic name *fenfluramine*; appetite suppressant used to treat obesity).

Ponstel (Analges, OB/GYN). Nonsteroidal anti-inflammatory drug used to treat pain; used to treat migraine headaches; used to treat dysmenorrhea. For dosage, see *mefenamic acid*. [PAWN-stehl]. 255, 304, 307

Pontocaine (Anes). Spinal/epidural anesthetic drug. For dosage, see *tetracaine*. [PAWN-toh-kayn]. 368

Pontocaine (Derm) (generic *tetracaine*). Topical anesthetic. Ointment: 1%. [PAWN-toh-kayn]. 94

Pontocaine (ENT, GI, Resp) (generic *tetracaine*). Topical anesthetic applied to the throat prior to performing laryngoscopy, esophagoscopy, and bronchoscopy. Liquid: 2%. [PAWN-toh-kayn].

Pool, Judith. 381

poractant alfa (Curosurf) (Resp). Natural lung surfactant used to prevent and treat respiratory distress syndrome in newborn infants; used to treat respiratory distress syndrome in adults. Endotracheal: 120 mg/1.5 mL, 240 mg/3 mL. [pohr-ack-tehnt EHL-fah].

Porcelana (Derm) (generic *hydroquinone*). Topical drug used to treat hyperpigmented areas of skin. Cream: 1.5%. [pohr-seh-LAW-nah].

porfimer (Photofrin) (Chemo). Chemotherapy photosensitizing drug used to treat esophageal cancer and lung cancer. This drug sensitizes tumor cells to light, then laser light causes the release of free radicals that destroy the tumor cells. Intravenous (powder to be reconstituted): 75 mg. [POHR-fih-mehr]. 348

porfiromycin (Promycin) (Chemo). Chemotherapy drug used to treat head and neck cancer and cervical cancer of the uterus. Orphan drug. 348

port.

Portagen (GI). Liquid nutritional supplement. Powder (to be reconstituted).

(Posicor) (Cardio). No longer on the market. (Generic name *mibefradil*; calcium channel blocker used to treat angina and hypertension).

postpartum bleeding, drugs used to treat. 247

postpartum depression. See *depression*.

posttraumatic stress disorder, drugs used to treat. 290

potassium citrate (Polycitra-K, Urocit-K) (Ortho, Uro). Used to prevent the formation of uric acid kidney stones in patients with gout. Crystals (to be reconstituted): 3300 mg. Liquid: 1100 mg/5 mL. Tablet: 5 mEq, 10 mEq. 112, 146

potassium iodide (SSKI) (ENT). Expectorant. Liquid: 1 g/mL. 210

potassium-sparing diuretics (Uro). Class of diuretics that cause sodium and water, but less potassium than usual, to be excreted in the urine.

potassium supplements (K + 8, K + 10, K + Care, K + Care ET, Kaon, Kaon Cl-10, Kaon-Cl-20%, Kay Ciel, K-Dur 10, K-Dur 20, K-Lor, Klor-Con, Klor-Con 8, Klor-Con 10, Klor-Con/EF, Klor-Con/25, Klorvess, Klotrix, K-Lyte, K-Lyte/Cl, K-Lyte/Cl 50, K-Lyte DS, K-Tab, Micro-K Extencaps, Micro-K LS, Micro-K

10 Extencaps, Slow-K, Ten-K, Tri-K) (Uro).   Class of drugs used to replace potassium loss caused by diuretics. Capsule: 8 mEq, 10 mEq. Tablet: 8 mEq, 10 mEq, 20 mEq. Effervescent tablet: 20 mEq, 25 mEq, 50 mEq. Liquid: 20 mEq/15 mL, 30 mEq/15 mL, 40 mEq/15 mL, 45 mEq/15 mL. Powder (to be reconstituted): 15 mEq, 20 mEq, 25 mEq. 104

potassium-wasting diuretics (Uro).   Class of diuretics that cause potassium to be lost in the urine. 103

povidone iodine, see *ACU-dyne* and *Betadine*.

powder (drug form). 35

PPD (abbreviation for *purified protein derivative*).   See *Mantoux test, tine test*.

PPF (abbreviation for *plasma protein fraction*).   See *plasma protein fraction*.

pralidoxime (Protopam) (Emerg, Neuro).   Used to reverse the effect of pesticide poisoning; used to reverse an overdose of an anticholinergic drug used to treat myasthenia gravis. Intramuscular, intravenous, or subcutaneous: 600 mg, 1 g. [preh-lih-DAWK-zeem]. 183, 277

pramipexole (Mirapex) (Neuro).   Used to treat Parkinson's disease. Tablet: 0.125 mg, 0.25 mg, 0.5 mg. 1 mg, 1.5 mg. [preh-mee-PECK-sawl]. 268

pramiracetam (Psych).   Used to treat symptoms of mental dysfunction following electroshock therapy. Orphan drug. 294

pramlintide (Symlin) (Diab).   Given to patients with type I and type II diabetes mellitus to delay gastric emptying and improve blood sugar control. Subcutaneous. Investigational drug.

pramoxine (Tronothane) (Derm).   Topical anesthetic. Cream: 1%. [preh-MAWK-seen]. 94

pramoxine (Anusol, ProctoFoam NS, Tronolane) (GI). Topical anesthetic used to treat hemorrhoids. Cream: 1%. Foam: 1%. Ointment: 1%. [preh-MAWK-seen]. 134

Prandin (Diab).   Oral antidiabetic drug.   For dosage, see *repaglinide*. [PREHN-dihn]. 240

Pravachol (Cardio).   HMG-CoA reductase inhibitor drug used to treat hypercholesterolemia.   For dosage, see *pravastatin*. [PREH-vah-kawl]. 170

pravastatin (Pravachol) (Cardio).   HMG-CoA reductase inhibitor drug used to treat hypercholesterolemia. Tablet: 10 mg, 20 mg, 40 mg. [preh-vah-STEH-tihn]. 170

(prazepam) (Psych).   No longer on the market. (Trade name *Centrax*; benzodiazepine antianxiety drug).

prazosin (Minipress) (Cardio, Uro).   Alpha₁-receptor blocker used to treat congestive heart failure and hypertension; used to treat benign prostatic hypertrophy. Capsule: 1 mg, 2 mg, 5 mg. [PRAY-zoh-sihn]. 109, 155, 165

PRBC (abbreviation for *packed red blood cells*).   See *packed red blood cells*.

Precedex (Anes, Resp).   Nonbarbiturate drug used as a preoperative sedative; used to sedate patients who are intubated and on the ventilator.   For dosage, see *dexmedetomidine*. [PREH-seh-decks]. 371

Precose (Diab).   Oral antidiabetic drug.   For dosage, see *acarbose*. 241

Predalone 50 (Derm, Endo, Neuro, Ortho).   Corticosteroid anti-inflammatory drug injected into skin lesions; used to treat severe inflammation in various body systems; used to treat multiple sclerosis; injected into a joint to treat osteoarthritis and rheumatoid arthritis; injected near a joint to treat bursitis and tenosynovitis.   For dosage, see *prednisolone*. [PREH-dah-lohn]. 92, 141, 232, 277

Pred Forte, Pred Mild (Oph).   Topical corticosteroid used to treat inflammation of the eyes.   For dosage, see *prednisolone*. 219

Pred-G Ophthalmic Suspension, Pred-G S.O.P. (Oph) (generic *gentamicin, prednisolone*).   Topical combination antibiotic and corticosteroid drug. Ophthalmic suspension: 0.3%/1%. Ophthalmic ointment: 0.3%/0.6%.

prednicarbate (Dermatop) (Derm).   Topical corticosteroid anti-inflammatory drug. Cream: 0.1%. [prehd-nih-KAWR-bayt]. 92

prednimustine (Sterecyt) (Chemo).   Chemotherapy drug used to treat non-Hodgkin's lymphoma. Orphan drug.

Prednisol TBA (Ortho).   Corticosteroid anti-inflammatory drug injected into a joint to treat osteoarthritis and rheumatoid arthritis; injected near a joint to treat bursitis and tenosynovitis.   For dosage, see *prednisolone*. [PREHD-neh-sawl]. 141

prednisolone (Hydeltrasol, Orapred, Pediapred, Predalone 50, Prednisol TBA, Prelone) (Derm, Endo, Neuro, Ortho).   Corticosteroid anti-inflammatory injected into skin lesions; used to treat severe inflammation in various body systems; used to treat multiple sclerosis; injected into a joint to treat osteo- arthritis and rheumatoid arthritis; injected near a joint to treat bursitis and tenosynovitis. Liquid: 5 mg/mL, 15 mg/5 mL. Tablet: 5 mg. Syrup: 5 mg/5 mL, 15 mg/5 mL. Intra-articular, periarticular, intradermal, intramuscular, or intravenous: 20 mg/mL, 25 mg/mL, 50 mg/mL. [prehd-NIH-soh-lohn]. 92, 141, 232, 277

prednisolone (Econopred, Econopred Plus, Inflamase Forte, Inflamase Mild, Pred Forte, Pred Mild) (Oph). Topical corticosteroid used to treat inflammation of the eyes. Ophthalmic suspension: 0.12%, 0.125%, 1%. Ophthalmic solution: 0.125%, 1%. [prehd-NIH-soh-lohn]. 219

prednisone (Deltasone, Meticorten, Orasone, Prednisone Intensol Concentrate) (Chemo, Endo). Corticosteroid anti-inflammatory drug used to treat severe inflammation in various body systems; used as part of chemotherapy treatment. Tablet: 1 mg, 2.5 mg, 5 mg, 10 mg, 20 mg, 50 mg. Liquid: 5 mg/mL, 5 mg/5 mL. Syrup: 5 mg/5 mL. [PREHD-nih-sohn]. 232, 351

Prednisone Intensol Concentrate (Chemo, Endo). Corticosteroid anti-inflammatory drug used to treat severe inflammation in various body systems; used as part of chemotherapy treatment. For dosage, see *prednisone*. [PREHD-nih-sohn ihn-TEHN-sawl]. 232, 351

Prefrin Liquifilm (Oph). Topical decongestant/vasoconstrictor used to treat irritation and allergy symptoms in the eyes. For dosage, see *phenylephrine*. [PREHF-rihn].

Pregestimil (GI). Infant formula for infants with gastrointestinal malabsorption disorders. Powder (to be reconstituted).

pregnancy, drugs used during. 245

Pregnyl (Endo, OB/GYN). Ovulation-stimulating drug used to treat infertility; used to treat undescended testicles and hypogonadism in men. For dosage, see *human chorionic gonadotropin*. [PREHG-nill]. 244

preload (Cardio). 155

Prelone (Endo, Neuro). Corticosteroid anti-inflammatory used to treat severe inflammation in various body systems; used to treat multiple sclerosis. For dosage, see *prednisolone*. [PREH-lohn]. 232, 277

Prelu-2 (GI). Appetite suppressant used to treat obesity. (Schedule III drug). For dosage, see *phendimetrazine*. 129

Premarin, Premarin Intravenous (Chemo, OB/GYN, Ortho). Estrogen used to treat breast and prostate carcinoma; hormone replacement therapy used to treat the symptoms of menopause; used to treat abnormal uterine bleeding; used to prevent and treat osteoporosis. For dosage, see *conjugated estrogens*. [PREH-meh-rihn]. 252, 254, 343

Premarin Vaginal Cream (OB/GYN). Topical hormone replacement therapy used to treat atrophic vaginitis of menopause. Cream: 0.625 mg. [PREH-meh-rihn]. 252

premature/preterm labor, drugs used to treat. 246

premenstrual dysphoric disorder (PMDD), drugs used to treat. 254

Premphase (OB/GYN, Ortho) (generic *medroxyprogesterone, conjugated estrogens*). Combination progestins and estrogen drug used to treat symptoms of menopause; used to prevent or treat postmenopausal osteoporosis. Tablet: 5 mg/0.625 mg. [PREHM-fays]. 253

Prempro (OB/GYN, Ortho) (generic *medroxyprogesterone, conjugated estrogens*). Combination progestins and estrogen drug used to treat symptoms of menopause; used to prevent or treat postmenopausal osteoporosis. Tablet: 2.5 mg, 5 mg/0.625 mg. [PREHM-proh]. 253

Premsyn PMS (OB/GYN) (generic *acetaminophen, pamabrom*). Combination analgesic and diuretic used to treat premenstrual dysphoric disorder and dysmenorrhea. Caplet: 500 mg/25 mg.

Preparation H (GI) (generic *cocoa butter, shark liver oil*). Topical drug used to treat hemorrhoids. Cream, ointment, suppository. 134

Preparation H Cooling Gel (GI) (generic *witch hazel*). Topical drug used to treat hemorrhoids. Gel: 50%. 134

Prepidil (OB/GYN). Prostaglandin drug used to ripen the cervix for delivery. For dosage, see *dinoprostone*. [PREH-pih-dill].

prescription. 6, 74–80

prescription drugs. 18

prescription drugs changed to OTC drugs. Focus on Healthcare Issues feature. 19

prescription forms, steps to prevent theft of. 75

Prescription Strength Desenex (Derm) (generic *miconazole*). Topical antifungal drug. Spray: 2%. 89

Presley, Elvis. 56

Prevacid (GI). Proton pump inhibitor used to treat peptic ulcers, gastroesophageal reflux disease, and *H. pylori* infections. For dosage, see *lansoprazole*. 119, 121

Prevalite (Cardio, Emerg). Bile acid sequestrant drug used to treat hypercholesterolemia; used to treat digitalis toxicity; used to treat thyroid hormone overdose or pesticide poisoning. For dosage, see *cholestyramine*. 153, 169

Preven (OB/GYN) (generic *levonorgestrel*). Progestins-only drug taken after intercourse to prevent pregnancy. Tablet: 0.25 mg. [PREH-vehn]. 251

Prevnar (Resp). Vaccine used to protect infants against the seven most prevalent strains of *Streptococcus pneumoniae*. For dosage, see *pneumococcal vaccine*.

Prevpac (GI) (generic *amoxicillin, clarithromycin, lansoprazole*). Combination antibiotic and proton pump inhibitor used to treat peptic ulcers caused by *H. pylori* infection. Each daily pack contains four Trimox capsules (500 mg), two Biaxin tablets (500 mg), and two Prevacid capsules (30 mg). 120

Priftin (Antivir, Resp). Antibiotic used to treat tuberculosis; orphan drug used to treat *Mycobacterium avium-intracellular* in AIDS patients. For dosage, see *rifapentine*. [PRIHF-tihn]. 197, 329

prilocaine (Citanest) (ENT). Local and regional nerve block anesthetic for dental procedures. Injection: 4%, 4% with 1:200,000 epinephrine. [PRY-loh-kayn].

Prilosec (GI). Proton pump inhibitor used to treat peptic ulcers, gastroesophageal reflux disease, and *H. pylori* infections. For dosage, see *omeprazole*. [PRY-loh-sehk]. 119, 121

Primacor (Cardio). Nondigitalis drug used to treat congestive heart failure. For dosage, see *milrinone*. [PRY-mah-kohr]. 154

primaquine (Antivir). Used to treat *Pneumocystis carinii* pneumonia in AIDS patients. Orphan drug. 328

Primatene (ENT) (generic *ephedrine, guaifenesin*). Combination decongestant and expectorant drug. Tablet: 12.5 mg/200 mg. [PRY-mah-teen].

Primatene Dual Action (Resp) (generic *theophylline, ephedrine, guaifenesin*). Combination bronchodilator and expectorant drug. Tablet: 60 mg/12.5 mg/100 mg. [PRY-mah-teen]. 195

Primatene Mist (Resp). Bronchodilator. For dosage, see *epinephrine*. [PRY-mah-teen]. 193

Primaxin I.M., Primaxin I.V. (Antibio) (generic *imipenem, cilastatin*). Combination drug containing a carbapenem antibiotic and a drug that inhibits an enzyme in the kidney that normally breaks down the antibiotic. Intramuscular or intravenous (powder to be reconstituted): 250 mg/250 mg, 500 mg/500 mg, 750 mg/750 mg. [pry-MACK-sihn]. 320

primidone (Mysoline) (Neuro). Anticonvulsant drug used to treat tonic-clonic and simple and complex partial seizures. Tablet: 50 mg, 250 mg. Liquid: 250 mg/5 mL. [PRIH-meh-dohn]. 265

Primsol (Antibio, Uro). Antibiotic used to treat urinary tract and other types of infections. For dosage, see *trimethoprim*. [PRIHM-sawl].

Princess Diana. 56

Principen (Antibio). Penicillin-type antibiotic used to treat various types of bacterial infections, including *E. coli* and gonorrhea; used to prevent subacute bacterial endocarditis. For dosage, see *ampicillin*. [PRIHN-sih-pehn]. 313

Prinivil (Cardio). Angiotensin-converting enzyme inhibitor drug used to treat congestive heart failure and hypertension; used to improve survival rate after myocardial infarction. For dosage, see *lisinopril*. [PRIH-nih-vihl]. 154, 158, 163

Prinzide, Prinzide 12.5, Prinzide 25 (Cardio) (generic *lisinopril, hydrochlorothiazide*). Combination angiotensin-converting enzyme inhibitor antihypertensive

and diuretic drug. Tablet: 10 mg/12.5 mg, 20 mg/12.5 mg, 20 mg/25 mg. 167

Priscoline (Cardio). Used to treat persistent pulmonary hypertension in newborns with persistent fetal circulation. For dosage, see *tolazoline*. [PRIHS-koh-leen]. 174

Privine (ENT). Decongestant. For dosage, see *naphazoline*. 206

p.r.n. (abbreviation meaning *as needed*).

ProAmatine (Cardio). Alpha$_1$-receptor stimulator used to treat orthostatic hypotension. For dosage, see *midodrine*. 173

Pro-Banthine (GI). Antispasmodic drug used to treat spasm of smooth muscle of the bowel. For dosage, see *propantheline*. [proh-BEHN-theen]. 122

probenecid (Antibio). Given in conjunction with ampicillin and cephalosporins to prolong therapeutic blood levels. Tablet: 0.5 g. [proh-BEH-neh-sihd]. 321

probenecid (Ortho). Used to treat gout. Tablet: 0.5 g. [proh-BEH-neh-sihd]. 146

probucol (Panavir) (Antivir). Antiviral drug used to treat AIDS. Investigational drug. 326

procainamide (Procanbid, Pronestyl, Pronestyl-SR) (Cardio). Used to treat ventricular arrhythmias. Capsule: 250 mg, 375 mg, 500 mg. Tablet: 250 mg, 375 mg, 500 mg, 750 mg, 1000 mg. Intramuscular or intravenous: 100 mg/mL, 500 mg/mL. [proh-KAY-neh-mide]. 159

procaine (Novocain) (Anes). Local, regional nerve block, and spinal anesthetic. Injection: 1%, 2%, 10%. [PROH-kayn]. 367, 368

ProcalAmine (I.V.). Intravenous fluids for total parenteral nutrition. [proh-KEHL-ah-meen]. 378

(Procan SR) (Cardio). No longer on the market. (Generic name *procainamide*; used to treat ventricular arrhythmias).

Procanbid (Cardio). Used to treat ventricular arrhythmias. For dosage, see *procainamide*. 159

procarbazine (Matulane) (Chemo). Chemotherapy drug used to treat Hodgkin's disease. Capsule: 50 mg. [proh-KAWR-bah-zeen]. 348

Procardia (Analges). Calcium channel blocker used to treat migraine headaches. For dosage, see *nifedipine*. [proh-KAWR-dee-ah]. 306

Procardia, Procardia XL (Cardio). Calcium channel blocker used to treat angina pectoris, congestive heart failure, and hypertension; used to treat hypertensive crisis; used to treat Raynaud's disease. For dosage, see *nifedipine*. [proh-KAWR-dee-ah]. 154, 157, 163

prochlorperazine (Compazine) (GI). Phenothiazine drug used to treat nausea and vomiting. Tablet: 5

mg, 10 mg, 15 mg, 25 mg. Syrup: 5 mg/5mL. Suppository: 2.5 mg, 5 mg, 25 mg. Intramuscular: 5 mg/mL. [proh-klohr-PEH-rah-zeen]. 127

prochlorperazine (Compazine) (Psych). Phenothiazine drug used to treat psychosis; used to treat anxiety. Tablet: 5 mg, 10 mg, 15 mg, 25 mg. Syrup: 5 mg/5mL. Suppository: 2.5 mg, 5 mg, 25 mg. Intramuscular: 5 mg/mL. [proh-klohr-PEH-rah-zeen]. 282, 283

Procrit (Antivir, Chemo, Hem, Uro).   Erythropoietin-type drug that stimulates red blood cell production in patients with AIDS, patients on chemotherapy, and patients with anemia or chronic renal failure. For dosage, see *epoetin alfa.* 111, 331, 361

Proctocort (GI) (generic *hydrocortisone*).   Topical corticosteroid anti-inflammatory drug used to treat hemorrhoids. Cream: 1%. Suppository: 30 mg. [PRAWK-toh-kohrt]. 133

ProctoCream-HC (GI) (generic *hydrocortisone*).   Topical corticosteroid anti-inflammatory drug used to treat hemorrhoids. Cream: 1%, 2.5%. 133

Proctofoam-HC (GI) (generic *hydrocortisone, pramoxine*). Combination topical corticosteroid anti-inflammatory and anesthetic drug. Foam: 1%/1%. 134

ProctoFoam NS (GI) (generic *pramoxine*).   Topical anesthetic drug used to treat hemorrhoids. Foam: 1%. 134

procyclidine (Kemadrin) (Neuro).   Anticholinergic drug used to treat Parkinson's disease. Tablet: 5 mg. [proh-SY-klih-deen]. 269

Procysteine (Resp, Neuro).   Used to treat adult respiratory distress syndrome; used to treat amyotrophic lateral sclerosis. Orphan drug.

Profasi (Endo, OB/GYN).   Ovulation-stimulating drug used to treat infertility; used to treat undescended testicles and hypogonadism in men.   For dosage, see *human chorionic gonadotropin.* 244

Profenal (Oph).   Topical nonsteroidal anti-inflammatory drug used only to prevent miosis during eye surgery.   For dosage, see *suprofen.* [PROH-feh-nawl].

Progestasert (OB/GYN) (generic *progesterone*).   Progestins-only one-year contraceptive. Intrauterine T-shaped implant: 38 mg. [proh-JEHS-tah-serht]. 251

progesterone (Crinone, Prometrium) (OB/GYN). Progestins hormone used to treat infertility; used to treat amenorrhea; used to treat functional uterine bleeding. Capsule: 100 mg. Intramuscular: 50 mg/mL. Vaginal gel: 4%, 8%. [proh-JEHS-teh-rohn]. 245, 254

Proglycem (Diab).   Used to treat hypoglycemia. For dosage, see *diazoxide.* [proh-GLY-sehm].

Prograf (Cardio, GI, Uro).   Immunosuppressant drug given after organ transplant to prevent rejection of the donor heart, liver, or kidney.   For dosage, see *tacrolimus.* 110, 135, 174

Prolastin (Resp).   Enzyme replacement therapy for emphysema patients with alpha$_1$-antitrypsin deficiency.   For dosage, see *alpha$_1$-proteinase inhibitor.*

Proleukin (Antivir, Chemo).   Interleukin-2 chemotherapy drug used to treat colon and rectal cancer, non-Hodgkin's lymphoma, and Kaposi's sarcoma; investigational drug used to treat Hodgkin's disease and AIDS.   For dosage, see *aldesleukin.* [proh-LOO-kihn]. 325, 347

Prolixin (Psych).   Phenothiazine drug used to treat psychosis and schizophrenia.   For dosage, see *fluphenazine.* [proh-LIHK-sihn]. 283

(Proloid) (Endo).   No longer on the market. (Generic name *thyroglobulin;* thyroid hormone replacement).

Proloprim (Antibio, Uro).   Antibiotic used to treat urinary tract and other types of infections.   For dosage, see *trimethoprim.* [PROH-loh-prihm].

(promazine) (Psych).   No longer on the market. (Trade name *Sparine;* phenothiazine antipsychotic drug).

Promega Pearls Softgels, Promega Softgels (Cardio). Fish oil nutritional supplement used to treat hypertriglyceridemia.   For dosage, see *omega-3 fatty acids.* 171

promethazine (Phenergan, Phenergan Fortis, Phenergan Plain) (Derm, ENT).   Antihistamine used to treat allergic rhinitis and allergic reactions with hives and itching. Liquid: 6.25 mg/5 mL, 25 mg/5 mL. Tablet: 12.5 mg, 25 mg, 50 mg. Intramuscular or intravenous: 50 mg/mL. [proh-MEH-thah-zeen]. 207

promethazine (Phenergan) (GI).   Antiemetic drug; used to treat motion sickness. Syrup: 6.25 mg/5 mL, 25 mg/5 mL. Tablet: 12.5 mg, 25 mg, 50 mg. Suppository: 12.5 mg, 25 mg, 50 mg. Intramuscular or intravenous: 50 mg/mL. 127, 128

Prometrium (OB/GYN).   Progestins hormone used to treat infertility; used to treat amenorrhea; used to treat functional uterine bleeding.   For dosage, see *progesterone.* [proh-MEE-tree-uhm]. 245, 254

Promit (I.V.).   Given intravenously before a dextran infusion to prevent an anaphylactic reaction.   For dosage, see *dextran 1.* 383

Promycin (Chemo).   Chemotherapy drug used to treat head and neck cancer and cervical cancer of the uterus.   For dosage, see *porfiromycin.* 348

Pronemia Hematinic Capsule (Cardio).   Combination iron, intrinsic factor, vitamin B$_{12}$, vitamin C, and folic acid drug used to treat iron deficiency anemia and pernicious anemia. Capsule: 115 mg/75 mg/15 mcg/150 mg/1 mg.

Pronestyl, Pronestyl-SR (Cardio). Used to treat ventricular arrhythmias. For dosage, see *procainamide*. [proh-NEHS-tuhl]. 159

propafenone (Rythmol) (Cardio). Used to treat ventricular arrhythmias. Tablet: 150 mg, 225 mg, 300 mg. 159

(Propagest) (ENT). No longer on the market. (Generic name *phenylpropanolamine*; decongestant).

propantheline (Pro-Banthine) (GI). Antispasmodic drug used to treat spasm of smooth muscle of the bowel. Tablet: 7.5 mg, 15 mg. [proh-PEHN-thah-leen]. 122

PROPApH Foaming Face Wash, PROPApH Peel-Off Acne Mask (Derm) (generic *salicylic acid*). Topical keratolytic used to treat acne vulgaris. Liquid: 2%. Mask: 2%.

proparacaine (Alcaine, Ophthaine, Ophthetic) (Oph). Topical anesthetic for the eyes. Ophthalmic solution: 0.5%. [proh-PEH-rah-kayn]. 222

Propecia (Derm). Oral drug used to treat male pattern baldness. For dosage, see *finasteride*. [proh-PEE-see-ah]. 98

prophylaxis. 65

Propine (Oph). Topical alpha/beta-agonist drug used to treat glaucoma. For dosage, see *dipivefrin*. [PROH-peen]. 222

(propiomazine) (Neuro). No longer on the market. (Trade name *Largon*; nonbarbiturate used to treat insomnia).

Proplex T (Hem). Used to treat clotting Factor IX deficiency in hemophiliac patients; also includes Factors II, VI, and X.

propofol (Diprivan) (Anes, Resp). Used to induce and maintain general anesthesia; used to sedate patients who are intubated and on the ventilator. Intravenous: 10 mg/mL. [PROH-poh-fawl]. 199, 369

(propoxycaine) (Anes). No longer on the market. (Local anesthetic).

propoxyphene (Darvon-N, Darvon Pulvules) (Analges). Narcotic analgesic drug used to treat mild-to-moderate pain. (Schedule IV drug). Capsule: 65 mg. Tablet: 100 mg. [proh-PAWK-see-feen]. 298

propranolol (Inderal, Inderal LA, Propranolol Intensol) (Analges, GI, Neuro, Ortho, Psych). Nonselective beta-receptor blocker used to treat migraine headaches; used to prevent rebleeding of esophageal varices in patients with cirrhosis and gastric bleeding in patients with portal hypertension; used to treat the tremors of Parkinson's disease; used to treat essential familial tremors; used to treat the side

effects of muscle restlessness from antipsychotic drugs; used to prevent performance anxiety. Capsule: 60 mg, 80 mg, 120 mg, 160 mg. Liquid: 4 mg/mL, 8 mg/mL, 80 mg/mL. Tablet: 10 mg, 20 mg, 40 mg, 60 mg, 80 mg, 90 mg. Intravenous: 1 mg/mL. [proh-PREH-noh-lawl]. 134, 146, 269, 290, 294, 306

propranolol (Inderal, Inderal LA, Propranolol Intensol) (Cardio). Nonselective beta-receptor blocker used to treat angina pectoris, hypertension, and ventricular arrhythmias; used to prevent repeat myocardial infarction. Capsule: 60 mg, 80 mg, 120 mg, 160 mg. Liquid: 4 mg/mL, 8 mg/mL, 80 mg/mL. Tablet: 10 mg, 20 mg, 40 mg, 60 mg, 80 mg, 90 mg. Intravenous: 1 mg/mL. [proh-PREH-noh-lawl]. 155, 157, 158, 160, 162

propranolol (Inderal, Inderal LA, Propranolol Intensol) (Endo). Nonselective beta-receptor blocker drug used to treat the hypertension caused by a pheochromocytoma of the adrenal medulla. Capsule: 60 mg, 80 mg, 120 mg, 160 mg. Liquid: 4 mg/mL, 8 mg/mL, 80 mg/mL. Tablet: 10 mg, 20 mg, 40 mg, 60 mg, 80 mg, 90 mg. Intravenous: 1 mg/mL. [proh-PREH-noh-lawl].

Propranolol Intensol (Analges, GI, Neuro, Ortho, Psych). Nonselective beta-receptor blocker used to treat migraine headaches; used to prevent rebleeding of esophageal varices in patients with cirrhosis and gastric bleeding in patients with portal hypertension; used to treat the tremors of Parkinson's disease; used to treat essential familial tremors; used to treat the side effects of muscle restlessness from antipsychotic drugs; used to prevent performance anxiety. For dosage, see *propranolol*. [proh-PREH-noh-lawl]. 269, 290, 294, 306

Propranolol Intensol (Cardio). Nonselective beta-receptor blocker used to treat angina pectoris, hypertension, and ventricular arrhythmias; used to prevent repeat myocardial infarction. For dosage, see *propranolol*. [proh-PREH-noh-lawl]. 157

Propranolol Intensol (Endo). Nonselective beta-receptor blocker drug used to treat the hypertension caused by a pheochromocytoma of the adrenal medulla. For dosage, see *propranolol*. [proh-PREH-noh-lawl].

(Propulsid) (GI). No longer on the market. (Generic name *cisapride*; gastric stimulant used to treat heartburn and gastroesophageal reflux disease).

propylthiouracil (Endo). Antithyroid drug used to treat hyperthyroidism. Tablet: 50 mg. [proh-pull-thy-oh-YOUR-ah-sill]. 230

Proscar (Uro). Used to treat benign prostatic hypertrophy. For dosage, see *finasteride*. [PROH-skawr]. 108

ProSobee (GI).   Infant soy formula for infants with allergies. Liquid, powder (to be reconstituted).

ProSom (Neuro).   Nonbarbiturate drug used to treat insomnia. (Schedule IV drug).   For dosage, see *estazolam*. [PROH-sawm]. 272

prostacyclin (beraprost) (Resp).   Used to treat pulmonary arterial hypertension. Orphan drug. 198

prostaglandin E1 (Cardio).   See *alprostadil*.

Prostat (GI).   Used to treat *Helicobacter pylori* infection.   For dosage, see *metronidazole*.

ProStep (Resp).   Nicotine drug used to stop smoking. Transdermal patch: 30 mg/7 cm^2, 15 mg/3.5 cm^2. 199

Prostigmin (Neuro, Uro).   Anticholinesterase drug used to treat myasthenia gravis; used to treat postoperative urinary retention.   For dosage, see *neostigmine*. [proh-STIHG-mihn].

Prostin E2 (OB/GYN).   Used to produce abortion. For dosage, see *dinoprostone*. 255

Prostin VR Pediatric (Cardio).   Used to keep the ductus arteriosus open until surgery can be performed in newborns with congenital heart defects.   For dosage, see *alprostadil*. [PRAW-stihn].

protamine sulfate (Hem).   Used to reverse the effects of heparin. Intravenous: 10 mg/mL. [PROH-tah-meen].

protease inhibitors (Antivir).   Class of drugs used to treat AIDS. 325

Protenate (I.V.).   Intravenous blood product that contains no cellular components and is used to replace plasma proteins. [PROH-teh-nayt].

Prothiaden (Psych).   Tricyclic antidepressant used to treat depression. Generic: *dothiepin*. Investigational drug. 285

protirelin (Neuro).   Used to treat amyotrophic lateral sclerosis. Orphan drug.

proton pump inhibitor drugs (GI).   Class of drugs used to treat peptic ulcer disease and gastroesophageal reflux disease. 119

Protonix, Protonix I.V. (GI).   Proton pump inhibitor used to treat gastroesophageal reflux disease; used to treat Zollinger–Ellison syndrome.   For dosage, see *pantoprazole*. [PROH-toh-nihks]. 121

Protopam (Emerg, Neuro).   Used to reverse the effects of pesticide poisoning; used to reverse the effects of an overdose of anticholinergic drugs used to treat myasthenia gravis.   For dosage, see *pralidoxime*. [PROH-toh-pehm]. 183, 277

Protopic (Derm) (generic *tacrolimus*).   Topical nonsteroidal anti-inflammatory drug used to treat eczema. Ointment: 0.03%, 0.1%. [proh-TAW-pihk]. 100

Protostat (Antibio, GI).   Antibacterial and antiprotozoal drug used to treat a variety of infections, including *Bacteroides*, Crohn's disease, and *H. pylori* infections of the gastrointestinal tract.   For dosage, see *metronidazole*. [PROH-toh-steht]. 120

Protostat (GI, OB/GYN).   Antibacterial and antiprotozoal drug used to treat intestinal amebiasis; used to treat *Trichomonas vaginalis* vaginal infection, a sexually transmitted disease.   For dosage, see *metronidazole*. [PROH-toh-steht].

Protox (Antivir).   Used to treat toxoplasmosis in AIDS patients.   For dosage, see *poloxamer 331*. 332

protriptyline (Vivactil) (Analges, Diab, Neuro, Ortho).   Tricyclic antidepressant used to treat migraines; used to treat diabetic neuropathy; used to treat postherpetic neuralgia; used to treat obstructive sleep apnea; used to treat phantom limb pain. Tablet: 5 mg, 10 mg. [proh-TRIP-teh-leen]. 147, 277, 307

protriptyline (Vivactil) (Psych).   Tricyclic antidepressant used to treat depression. Tablet: 5 mg, 10 mg. [proh-TRIP-teh-leen]. 241, 286

Protropin (Endo).   Growth hormone replacement. For dosage, see *somatrem*. [pro-TROH-pihn]. 230

Provenge (Chemo).   Cancer vaccine. Investigational drug. 349

Proventil, Proventil HFA, Proventil Repetabs (Resp). Bronchodilator.   For dosage, see *albuterol*. 193

Provera (OB/GYN).   Progestins hormone drug used to treat amenorrhea; used to treat abnormal uterine bleeding.   For dosage, see *medroxyprogesterone*. [proh-VEER-ah]. 253

Provigil (Neuro).   Central nervous system stimulant used to treat narcolepsy. (Schedule IV drug).   For dosage, see *modafinil*. [proh-VIH-juhl]. 274

Prozac, Prozac Weekly (Analges, Neuro).   Selective serotonin reuptake inhibitor used to treat migraine headaches; used to treat narcolepsy; used to treat levodopa-induced dyskinesia.   For dosage, see *fluoxetine*. [PROH-zack]. 270, 274, 307

Prozac, Prozac Weekly (Diab).   Selective serotonin reuptake inhibitor used to treat diabetic peripheral neuropathy.   For dosage, see *fluoxetine*. [PROH-zack].

Prozac, Prozac Weekly (Psych).   Selective serotonin reuptake inhibitor antidepressant used to treat depression; used to treat obsessive-compulsive disorder; used to treat bulimia nervosa and anorexia nervosa; used to treat attention-deficit/hyperactivity disorder; used to treat manic-depressive disorder; used to treat kleptomania; used to treat posttraumatic stress disorder; used to treat psychosis and schizophrenia; used to treat autism; used to treat social anxiety disorder/social phobias; used to treat panic disorder.   For dosage, see *fluoxetine*. [PROH-zack]. 284, 287, 289, 290, 291, 292

pruritus, drugs used to treat.

pseudoephedrine (Afrin, Drixoral Non-Drowsy Formula, Efidac/24, PediaCare Infants' Decongestant, Sudafed, Sudafed 12 Hour, Triaminic AM Decongestant Formula, Triaminic Infant Oral Decongestant) (ENT). Decongestant. Capsule: 60 mg. Drops: 7.5 mg/0.8 mL. Liquid: 15 mg/5 mL, 30 mg/5 mL. Tablet: 30 mg, 60 mg, 120 mg, 240 mg. [soo-doh-eh-FEH-drihn]. 206

psoralens (Derm). Class of drugs used with ultraviolet light to treat severe psoriasis. 87

Psorcon E (Derm) (generic *diflorasone*). Topical corticosteroid anti-inflammatory drug. Cream: 0.05%. Ointment: 0.05%. [SOHR-kawn]. 92

psoriasis, drugs used to treat. 86

Psorion (Derm) (generic *betamethasone*). Topical corticosteroid anti-inflammatory drug. Cream: 0.05%. [SOHR-ee-ehn]. 92

psychiatric drugs. 279

psychiatric drugs, history of. Historical Notes feature. 280, 281, 283

psychosis, drugs used to treat. 283

psyllium (Fiberall, Metamucil, Modane Bulk, Perdien Fiber Therapy) (GI). Bulk-producing laxative. Granules: 4.03 g/tsp. Powder: 3.5 g/tsp. [SIH-lee-uhm]. 125

Pulmicort Turbuhaler (Resp). Inhaled corticosteroid used to prevent acute asthma attacks. For dosage, see *budesonide*. 196

Pulmocare (GI). Liquid nutritional supplement formulated for patients with pulmonary disease. Liquid.

pulmonary arterial hypertension, drugs used to treat. 198

pulmonary drugs. 192

Pulmozyme (Resp). Enzyme that breaks apart the DNA in mucus and thins it in patients with cystic fibrosis. For dosage, see *dornase alfa*. [PUHL-moh-zime].

purine antagonists (Chemo). Class of chemotherapy drugs. 339

Purinethol (Chemo). Purine antagonist chemotherapy drug used to treat leukemia. For dosage, see *mercaptopurine*. [pyour-RIH-neh-thawl]. 339

Putnam, Tracy. 263

PUVA (abbreviation for *psoralen* drug and *ultraviolet* light wavelength *A*) (Derm). Combination therapy used to treat severe psoriasis. [POO-vah]. 88

pyrantel (Antiminth, Pin-Rid, Pin-X) (Misc). Used to treat pinworms and roundworms. Capsule: 180 mg. Liquid: 50 mg/mL.

pyrazinamide (Resp). Bactericidal antibiotic used only to treat tuberculosis. Tablet: 500 mg. [py-rah-ZIH-nah-mide]. 197

Pyridium (Uro). Urinary tract analgesic. For dosage, see *phenazopyridine*. [py-RIH-dee-uhm]. 107

Pyridium Plus (Uro) (generic *butabarbital, L-hyoscyamine, phenazopyridine*). Combination sedative, urinary tract antispasmodic, and analgesic drug. Tablet: 150 mg. [py-RIH-dee-uhm]. 107

pyridostigmine (Mestinon, Regonol) (Anes, Neuro). Anticholinesterase drug used to reverse the effects of neuromuscular blocking drugs during general anesthesia; used to treat myasthenia gravis. Liquid: 60 mg/5 mL. Tablet: 60 mg, 180 mg. [py-rih-doh-STIHG-meen]. 271, 371

pyrimidine antagonist (Chemo). Class of chemotherapy drugs. 339

q.d. (abbreviation meaning *every day*).

q.h. (abbreviation meaning *every hour*).

q.h.s. (abbreviation meaning *at bedtime*).

q.i.d. (abbreviation meaning *four times a day*).

q.o.d. (abbreviation meaning *every other day*).

Quadramet (Chemo). Radioactive samarium 153 isotope used to treat bone pain in cancer patients with bone metastases. There is preferential uptake of the drug by sites of active osteogenesis, primarily metastatic bone lesions. Intravenous: 50 mCi/mL. [KWAH-drah-meht]. 362

Quarzan (GI). Antispasmodic drug. For dosage, see *clidinium*. [KWAHR-zehn]. 122

quazepam (Doral) (Neuro). Nonbarbiturate benzodiazepine drug used to treat insomnia. (Schedule IV drug). Tablet: 7.5 mg, 15 mg. [KWAH-seh-pehm]. 272

Quelicin (Anes, Resp). Muscle relaxant drug used during surgery; used to treat patients who are intubated and on the ventilator. For dosage, see *succinylcholine*. [KWEH-lih-sihn]. 199, 370

Questran, Questran Light (Cardio, Emerg). Bile acid sequestrant drug used to treat hypercholesterolemia; used to treat digitalis toxicity; used to treat thyroid hormone overdose or pesticide poisoning. For dosage, see *cholestyramine*. [KWEHS-trehn]. 153, 169

quetiapine (Seroquel) (Psych). Drug used to treat psychosis and schizophrenia. Tablet: 25 mg, 100 mg, 200 mg, 300 mg. [kweh-TY-ah-peen]. 284

Quibron, Quibron-300 (Resp) (generic *theophylline, guaifenesin*). Combination bronchodilator and expectorant drug. Capsule: 150 mg/90 mg, 300 mg/180 mg. [KWIH-brawn]. 195

Quibron-T Dividose, Quibron-T/SR Dividose (Resp). Bronchodilator. For dosage, see *theophylline*. [KWIH-brawn]. 193

Quinaglute Dura-Tabs (Cardio). Used to treat atrial and ventricular arrhythmias. For dosage, see *quinidine*. [KWIH-nah-gloot]. 159

quinapril (Accupril) (Cardio). Angiotensin-converting enzyme inhibitor used to treat congestive heart failure and hypertension. Tablet: 5 mg, 10 mg, 20 mg, 40 mg. [KWIH-nah-prihl]. 154, 158, 164

(quinestrol) (OB/GYN). No longer on the market. (Trade name *Estrovis*; estrogen replacement for menopause).

quinethazone (Hydromox) (Uro). Thiazide diuretic. Tablet: 50 mg. [kwih-NEH-thah-zohn]. 103

Quinidex Extentabs (Cardio). Used to treat atrial and ventricular arrhythmias. For dosage, see *quinidine*. [KWIH-nih-dehks]. 159

quinidine (Quinaglute Dura-Tabs, Quinidex Extentabs) (Cardio). Used to treat atrial and ventricular arrhythmias. Tablet: 200 mg, 300 mg, 324 mg. Intramuscular or intravenous: 80 mg/mL. 159

quinolones (Antibio, Uro). Class of antibiotics. 318

Quixin (Oph). Topical antibiotic used to treat bacterial eye infections. For dosage, see *levofloxacin*. [KWIK-sehn]. 218

QVAR (Resp). Corticosteroid used to prevent acute asthma attacks. For dosage, see *beclomethasone*. 196

R & C (Derm). Topical drug used to treat pediculosis (lice). Shampoo. 95

rabeprazole (Aciphex) (GI). Proton pump inhibitor used to treat peptic ulcers and gastroesophageal reflux disease. Tablet: 20 mg. [rah-BEH-prah-zohl]. 119, 121

racemic. 65

radioactive sodium iodide 131 (Iodotope) (Endo). Radioactive antithyroid drug used to treat hyperthyroidism and thyroid cancer. Capsule: 8 mCi (millicuries), 15 mCi, 30 mCi, 50 mCi, 100 mCi. Liquid: 7.05 mCi/mL.

Raleigh, Sir Walter. 367

raloxifene (Evista) (OB/GYN, Ortho). Selective estrogen receptor modulator (SERM) used to prevent and treat osteoporosis after menopause. Tablet: 60 mg. [rah-LAWK-sih-feen]. 144

ramipril (Altace) (Cardio). Angiotensin-converting enzyme inhibitor used to treat hypertension and congestive heart failure; used to decrease the risk of myocardial infarction or stroke. Capsule: 1.25 mg, 2.5 mg, 5 mg, 10 mg. [REH-mih-prihl]. 154, 164

ranitidine (Zantac, Zantac 75, Zantac EFFERdose, Zantac GELdose) (GI). H_2 blocker used to treat peptic ulcers and *H. pylori* infection. Capsule: 150 mg, 300 mg. Effervescent tablet: 150 mg. Effervescent granules: 150 mg. Tablet: 75 mg, 150 mg, 300 mg. Syrup: 15 mg/mL. Intramuscular or intravenous: 0.5 mg/mL, 25 mg/mL. [reh-NIH-tih-deen]. 118

rapacuronium (Raplon) (Anes). Muscle relaxant drug used during surgery. Intravenous: 100 mg/5 mL, 200 mg/10 mL. [rah-peh-kyour-OH-nee-uhm]. 370

Rapamune (Derm). Immunsuppressant drug used to treat severe, disabling psoriasis. For dosage, see *sirolimus*. [REH-pah-myoon]. 87

Rapamune (Uro). Immunosuppressant drug given after kidney transplant to prevent rejection of the donor kidney. For dosage, see *sirolimus*. [REH-pah-myoon]. 110

Raplon (Anes). Muscle relaxant drug used during surgery. For dosage, see *rapacuronium*. 370

ratio (drug measurement). 70

Rauzide (Cardio) (generic *rauwolfia, bendroflumethiazide*). Combination antihypertensive and diuretic drug. Tablet: 50 mg/4 mg. 167

(Raxar) (Antibio). No longer on the market. (Generic name *grepafloxacin*; fluoroquinolone antibiotic).

RCF (GI). Infant soy formula. Liquid.

reaction.

allergic. 53

idiosyncratic. 55

Rebetol (GI). Used to treat hepatitis C. For dosage, see *ribavirin*.

Rebetron (GI) (generic *interferon alfa-2b, ribavirin*). Combination antiviral drug used to treat hepatitis C. Combination pack. Capsule: 200 mg. Injection: 3 million IU/0.5 mL.

Rebif (Antivir, Neuro). Used to treat AIDS; used to treat multiple sclerosis and juvenile rheumatoid arthritis. For dosage, see *interferon beta-1a*. [REE-bihf]

reboxetine (Vestra) (Psych). First drug of a new class of selective norepinephrine reuptake inhibitor (SNRI) antidepressants used to treat depression. Investigational drug.

Receptin (Antivir). Used to treat AIDS. For dosage, see *recombinant human CD4*. [re-SEHP-tihn].

receptor. 46, 55

adrenergic. 60

alpha. 165

beta$_1$. 161

beta$_2$. 161

cholinergic. 62

Recombinant DNA Advisory Committee. 26

recombinant DNA technology. 26

recombinant human CD4 (Receptin) (Antivir). Used to treat AIDS. Orphan drug. 326

Recombinate (Hem). Used to treat clotting Factor VIII deficiency in hemophiliac patients. Intravenous: 12.5 mg/mL. [re-KAWM-bih-nayt].

Recombivax HB (GI). Hepatitis B vaccine. For dosage, see *hepatitis B vaccine*. [re-KAWM-bih-vehks].

Rectagene, Rectagene Medicated Rectal Balm (GI) (generic *live yeast cells, shark liver oil*). Topical combination drug used to treat hemorrhoids. Ointment, suppository.

Rectagene II (GI) (generic *bismuth, zinc oxide*). Topical combination drug used to treat hemorrhoids. Suppository.

rectal route, administration of drugs by the. 40

(Redux) (GI). No longer on the market. (Generic name *dexfenfluramine*; appetite suppressant used to treat obesity).

ReFacto (Hem). Factor VIII used to treat hemophilia. Intravenous: 250 IU, 500 IU, 1000 IU.

Refludan (Hem). Used to treat heparin-induced thrombocytopenia. For dosage, see *lepirudin*.

Refresh, Refresh Plus, Refresh Tears (Oph). Artificial tears. Drops.

Refresh PM (Oph). Artificial tears lubricating ointment for the eyes. Ophthalmic ointment.

Regitine (Cardio, Endo). Alpha-adrenergic blocker drug used to treat hypertensive crisis; used to treat hypertension caused by a pheochromocytoma of the adrenal medulla. For dosage, see *phentolamine*. [REH-jah-teen]. 168

Reglan (GI). Gastric stimulant used to treat gastroesophageal reflux disease, diabetic gastroparesis, and paralytic ileus; used to treat nausea and vomiting caused by chemotherapy. For dosage, see *metoclopramide*. [REH-glehn]. 122, 126, 128

Regonol (Anes, Neuro). Anticholinesterase drug used to reverse the action of neuromuscular blocking drugs during general anesthesia; used to treat myasthenia gravis. For dosage, see *pyridostigmine*. [REH-goh-nawl]. 271, 371

Regranex (Derm) (generic *becaplermin*). Topical drug used to stimulate the formation of granulation tissue in skin ulcers. Gel. 97

(Regular Iletin I) (Diab). No longer on the market. (Fast-acting regular insulin).

Regular Iletin II (Diab). Fast-acting regular insulin. Subcutaneous: 100 units/mL.

regular insulin (Regular Iletin II, Humulin R, Novolin R, Velosulin Human BR) (Endo). Fast-acting insulin. Subcutaneous: Units.

Relafen (Analges, Ortho). Nonsteroidal anti-inflammatory drug used to treat osteoarthritis and rheumatoid arthritis. For dosage, see *nabumetone*. [REH-lah-fehn]. 139, 304

Relenza (Antivir). Antiviral drug used to treat influenza A virus infection. For dosage, see *zanamivir*. [reh-LEHN-zah]. 330

Relief (Oph). Topical decongestant/vasoconstrictor used to treat irritation and allergy symptoms in the eyes. For dosage, see *phenylephrine*.

Remeron, Remeron SolTab (Psych). Tetracyclic antidepressant. For dosage, see *mirtazapine*. [REH-mehr-awn]. 286

Remicade (GI, Ortho). Monoclonal antibody used to treat Crohn's disease; used to treat rheumatoid arthritis. For dosage, see *infliximab*. [REH-mih-kayd]. 133, 142

remifentanil (Ultiva) (Anes). Narcotic used to induce and maintain general anesthesia. (Schedule II drug). Intravenous: 1 mg/mL. [reh-mee-FEHN-tah-nill]. 369

Reminyl (Neuro). Cholinesterase inhibitor used to treat Alzheimer's disease. For dosage, see *galantamine*. [REH-mih-nill]. 271

remission of cancer. 339

Remodulin (Resp). Vasodilator used to treat pumonary arterial hypertension. For dosage, see *treprostinil*. [ree-MAW-dyoo-lihn]. 198

remoxipride (Roxiam) (Psych). Used to treat psychosis. Investigational drug. 284

Remune (Antivir). AIDS vaccine. Investigational drug. 327

Renacidin (Uro). Used to dissolve calcium and magnesium kidney stones. Irrigation solution (via nephrostomy tube and/or catheter). [ree-nah-SY-dihn]. 112

Renagel (Uro). Used to decrease serum phosphorus levels in hemodialysis patients with end-stage renal disease. For dosage, see *sevelamer*. 112

RenAmin (I.V.). Intravenous fluids for total parenteral nutrition, especially for patients in renal failure. 378

Renese (Uro). Thiazide diuretic. For dosage, see *polythiazide*. [REE-nees]. 103

Renese-R (Cardio) (generic *reserpine, polythiazide*). Combination antihypertensive and diuretic drug. Tablet: 0.25 mg/2 mg. 167

renin inhibitors (Cardio). Class of drugs used to treat hypertension. Investigational drugs. 166

(Renoquid) (Uro). No longer on the market. (Generic name *sulfacytine*; sulfonamide used to treat urinary tract infections).

Renova (Derm) (generic *tretinoin*). Topical vitamin A-type drug used to treat facial wrinkle lines and areas of hyperpigmentation. Cream: 0.02%, 0.05%. [reh-NOH-vah].

ReoPro (Cardio, Hem). Platelet aggregation inhibitor used to prevent blood clots in patients with unstable angina or myocardial infarction, or who are undergoing angioplasty or atherectomy. For dosage, see *abciximab*. 172, 187

repaglinide (Prandin) (Diab). Oral antidiabetic drug. Tablet: 0.5 mg, 1 mg, 2 mg. [reh-PEHG-lih-nide]. 240

Repetabs. Part of the trade name of drug, indicating a sustained-release tablet. 65

Replagal (Neuro). Used to replace a missing enzyme and improve cerebral blood flow in patients with Fabry's disease. For dosage, see *agalsidase alfa*. 275

Replete (GI). Liquid nutritional supplement. Liquid.

Reposans-10 (Anes, Neuro, Psych). Benzodiazepine drug used as a preoperative medication to relieve anxiety and provide sedation; used to treat anxiety and neurosis; used to treat alcohol withdrawal and prevent seizure. (Schedule IV drug). For dosage, see *chlordiazepoxide*. 281

Repronex (OB/GYN). Ovulation-stimulating drug used to treat infertility. For dosage, see *menotropins*. [REE-proh-nehks]. 244

Requip (Neuro). Used to treat Parkinson's disease. For dosage, see *ropinirole*. 269

Rescriptor (Antivir). Nonnucleoside reverse transcriptase inhibitor drug used to treat AIDS. For dosage, see *delavirdine*. [reh-SKRIHP-tohr]. 325

Rescula (Oph). Topical drug used to treat glaucoma. For dosage, see *unoprostone*. [REHS-kyoo-lah]. 222

Resectisol (Uro). Irrigation solution used during urologic surgical procedures. 112

reserpine (Cardio). Depletes the store of norepinephrine in the adrenal medulla; used to treat hypertension. Tablet: 0.1 mg, 0.25 mg. [reh-SEHR- peen]. 166

resistant bacteria. 319

Resource, Resource Plus (GI). Liquid nutritional supplement. Liquid.

Respalor (GI). Liquid nutritional supplement formulated for patients with pulmonary disease. Liquid.

Respbid (Resp). Bronchodilator. For dosage, see *theophylline*. 193

RespiGam (Antivir). Immunoglobulin used to treat respiratory syncytial virus. Intravenous: [REHS-pih-gehm].331

respiratory drugs. 192

respiratory syncytial virus, drugs used to treat. 331

respiratory syncytial virus immunoglobulin (Hypermune RSV, RespiGam) (Antivir). Used to treat respiratory syncytial virus infection. 50 mg/mL. Orphan drug. 331

Restoril (Neuro). Nonbarbiturate benzodiazepine drug used to treat insomnia. (Schedule IV drug). For dosage, see *temazepam*. [REHS-toh-rill]. 272

Retavase (Cardio, Hem). Tissue plasminogen activator used to dissolve blood clots from a myocardial infarction. For dosage, see *reteplase*. [REH-teh-vays]. 174, 188

reteplase (Retavase) (Cardio, Hem). Tissue plasminogen activator used to dissolve blood clots from a myocardial infarction. Intravenous (powder to be reconstituted): 10.8 IU. [REH-teh-plays]. 174, 188

Retin-A, Retin-A Micro (Derm) (generic *tretinoin*). Topical vitamin A-type drug used to treat acne vulgaris. Cream: 0.025%, 0.05%, 0.1%. Gel: 0.025%, 0.01%. Liquid: 0.05%. 84

Retrovir (Antivir). Nucleoside reverse transcriptase inhibitor drug used to treat AIDS. For dosage, see *zidovudine*. [REH-troh-veer]. 324

retrovirus. 327

Reversol (Neuro). Anticholinesterase drug used to diagnose (not treat) myasthenia gravis. For dosage, see *edrophonium*. 275

Revex (Analges, Emerg). Narcotic antagonist used to reverse the effects of narcotic overdose. For dosage, see *nalmefene*. [REH-vehks]. 182, 308

Rev-Eyes (Oph). Topical alpha-receptor blocker used to treat glaucoma. For dosage, see *dapiprazole*. 221

ReVia (Analges). Narcotic antagonist used to block the effect of narcotics as ongoing treatment for former narcotic-dependent patients; used to treat alcohol dependence. For dosage, see *naltrexone*. 182, 308

Revimid (Chemo). Chemotherapy drug used to treat multiple myeloma. Orphan drug. 348

Rexolate (Ortho). Salicylate nonaspirin drug used to treat gout. For dosage, see *sodium thiosalicylate*. [REHK-soh-layt]. 146

Reye's syndrome. 330

Rezipas (GI). Used to treat ulcerative colitis. For dosage, see *4-aminosalicylic acid*. 126

(Rezulin) (Diab). No longer on the market. (Generic name *troglitazone*; oral antidiabetic drug).

Rheaban Maximum Strength (GI). Antidiarrheal drug. For dosage, see *attapulgite*. 124

Rheomacrodex (I.V.). Intravenous plasma volume expander. [ree-oh-MEH-krah-dehks]. 382

rheumatoid arthritis, drugs used to treat. 141

Rheumatrex, Rheumatrex Dose Pack (Chemo, Derm, Ortho). Folic acid antagonist chemotherapy drug used to treat breast cancer, ovarian cancer, head and neck cancer, lung cancer, leukemia, cutaneous T-cell lymphoma, and non-Hodgkin's disease; used to treat severe, disabling psoriasis; used to treat severe, active rheumatoid arthritis. For dosage, see *methotrexate*. [ROO-mah-trehks]. 87, 142, 340

Rhinall (ENT). Decongestant. For dosage, see *phenylephrine*. [RY-nawl]. 206

Rhinocort, Rhinocort Aqua (ENT). Topical intranasal corticosteroid used to treat allergic rhinitis. For dosage, see *budesonide*. 208

RhoGAM (OB/GYN). Immunoglobulin used after delivery to treat Rh-negative mother with an Rh-positive baby to prevent hemorrhagic disease of the newborn in a subsequent pregnancy. Intramuscular: 5%. [ROH-gehm].

ribavirin (Rebetol) (GI). Used to treat hepatitis C. Capsule: 200 mg. [rih-bah-VEER-ihn]. 331

ribavirin (Virazole) (Antivir). Antiviral drug used to treat respiratory syncytial virus. Aerosol (powder to be reconstituted): 6 g. [rih-bah-VEER-ihn].

RID (Derm). Topical drug used to treat pediculosis (lice). Shampoo. 96

Ridaura (Ortho). Gold compound used to treat rheumatoid arthritis. For dosage, see *auranofin*. [rih-DAWR-ah]. 142

rifabutin (Mycobutin) (Antivir). Used to prevent *Mycobacterium avium-intracellulare* infection in AIDS patients. Capsule: 150 mg. [ry-fah-BYOO-tihn]. 329

Rifadin (Resp). Bactericidal antibiotic used to treat tuberculosis; used to treat Legionnaire's disease. For dosage, see *rifampin*. 197, 198

rifalazil (Antivir). Used to treat *Mycobacterium avium-intracellulare* infection in AIDS patients. Investigational drug. 329

Rifamate (Resp) (generic *isoniazid, rifampin*). Combination antibiotic drug used only to treat tuberculosis. Capsule: 150 mg/300 mg. 197

rifampin (Rifadin, Rimactane) (Resp). Bactericidal antibiotic used to treat tuberculosis; used to treat Legionnaire's disease. Capsule: 150 mg, 300 mg. Intravenous (powder to be reconstituted): 600 mg. [ry-FEHM-pihn]. 197, 198

rifapentine (Priftin) (Antivir, Resp). Antibiotic used to treat tuberculosis; orphan drug used to treat *Mycobacterium avium-intracellular* in AIDS patients. Tablet: 150 mg. [ry-fah-PEHN-tihn]. 197, 329

Rifater (Resp) (generic *isoniazid, pyrazinamide, rifampin*). Combination antibiotic drug used only to treat tuberculosis. Tablet: 50 mg/300 mg/120 mg. 197

rifaximin (Normix) (Neuro). Used to treat hepatic encephalopathy. Orphan drug. 277

Rilutek (Neuro). Used to treat amyotrophic lateral sclerosis and Huntington's chorea. For dosage, see *riluzole*. [RILL-yoo-tehk]. 277

riluzole (Rilutek) (Neuro). Used to treat amyotrophic lateral sclerosis and Huntington's chorea. Tablet: 50 mg. [RILL-yoo-zohl]. 277

Rimactane (Resp). Bactericidal antibiotic used to treat tuberculosis; used to treat Legionnaire's disease. For dosage, see *rifampin*. [rih-MACK-tayn]. 197, 198

Rimadyl (Analges, Ortho) (generic *carprofen*). Nonsteroidal anti-inflammatory drug for rheumatoid arthritis and osteoarthritis. Already approved for use by veterinarians in cats and dogs. Investigational drug for humans. 147, 304

rimantadine (Flumadine) (Antivir). Antiviral drug used to prevent and treat influenza A virus infection. Tablet: 100 mg. Syrup: 50 mg/5 mL. [rih-MEHN-teh-deen]. 330

rimexolone (Vexol) (Oph). Topical corticosteroid used to treat inflammation of the eyes. Ophthalmic suspension: 1%. [reh-MEHK-seh-lohn]. 219

Rimso-50 (Uro). Urinary tract analgesic solution instilled into the bladder. For dosage, see *dimethyl sulfoxide*. 107

Ringer's lactate (RL) (I.V.). Intravenous fluid of dextrose, sodium, calcium, chloride, and lactate. 376

ringworm, drugs used to treat. 89

Riopan (GI) (generic *aluminum-magnesium complex*). Combination antacid. Suspension: 540 mg/5 mL. [RY-oh-pehn]. 117

Riopan Plus, Riopan Plus Double Strength (GI) (generic *aluminum-magnesium complex, simethicone*). Combination antacid and anti-gas drug. Tablet: 480 mg/20 mg, 1080 mg/20 mg. Suspension: 540 mg/40 mg, 1080 mg/40 mg. [RY-oh-pehn]. 117

risedronate (Actonel) (OB/GYN, Ortho). Inhibits the breakdown of bone; used to prevent and treat postmenopausal osteoporosis; used to treat Paget's disease. Tablet: 5 mg, 30 mg (once daily). Tablet: 35 mg (once weekly). [rih-SEH-droh-nayt]. 144

Risperdal (Psych). Drug used to treat psychosis, manic-depressive disorder, schizophrenia, and dementia with psychosis. For dosage, see *risperidone*. [RIHS-pehr-dawl]. 284, 289

risperidone (Risperdal) (Psych). Drug used to treat psychosis, manic-depressive disorder, schizophrenia, and dementia with psychosis. Tablet: 0.25 mg, 0.5 mg, 1 mg, 2 mg, 3 mg, 4 mg. Liquid: 1 mg/mL. [rihs-PEHR-eh-dohn]. 284, 289

Ritalin and Prozac prescribed for preschoolers. Focus on Healthcare Issues feature.

Ritalin, Ritalin-SR (Neuro, Psych). Central nervous system stimulant used to treat narcolepsy; used to treat attention-deficit/hyperactivity disorder. (Schedule II drug). For dosage, see *methylphenidate*. [RIH-tah-lihn]. 274, 292

ritanserin (Neuro, Psych). Used to treat Parkinson's disease; used to treat anxiety, depression, schizophrenia, alcoholism, and drug abuse. Investigational drug. 270, 280, 284, 294

ritodrine (Yutopar) (OB/GYN). Used to stop preterm labor contractions. Intravenous: 10 mg/mL, 15 mg/mL. [RIH-toh-dreen]. 246

ritonavir (Norvir) (Antivir). Protease inhibitor drug used to treat AIDS. Capsule: 100 mg. Liquid: 80 mg/mL. 325

Rituxan (Chemo). Human monoclonal antibody used to treat non-Hodgkin's lymphoma. For dosage, see *rituximab*. [rih-TUHK-sehn]. 346

rituximab (Rituxan) (Chemo). Human monoclonal antibody used to treat non-Hodgkin's lymphoma. Intravenous: 10 mg/mL. [rih-TUHK-sih-mehb]. 346

rivastigmine (Exelon) (Neuro). Cholinesterase inhibitor used to treat Alzheimer's disease. Capsule: 1.5 mg, 3 mg, 4.5 mg, 6 mg. Liquid: 2 mg/mL. [rih-vah-STIG-meen]. 271

rizatriptan (Maxalt, Maxalt-MLT) (Analges). Serotonin receptor agonist drug used to treat migraine headaches. Tablet/orally disintegrating tablet: 5 mg, 10 mg. [ry-zah-TRIP-tehn]. 306

RL (abbreviation for *Ringer's lactate*). See *Ringer's lactate*.

RMS (Analges, Anes, Cardio, OB/GYN). Narcotic analgesic drug used to treat moderate-to-severe pain; used as a preoperative drug to sedate and supplement anesthesia; used to treat dyspnea from congestive heart failure; used to treat the pain of childbirth. (Schedule II drug). For dosage, see *morphine*. 173, 297

Robaxin, Robaxin-750 (Ortho). Skeletal muscle relaxant used to treat minor muscle spasms associated with injuries. For dosage, see *methocarbamol*. [roh-BEHK-sihn]. 144

Robaxisal (Ortho) (generic *aspirin, methocarbamol*). Combination analgesic and skeletal muscle relaxant drug. Tablet: 325 mg/400 mg. [roh-BEHK-sih-sawl]. 146

Robinul, Robinul Forte (GI). Antispasmodic drug. For dosage, see *glycopyrrolate*. [ROH-bih-nuhl]. 122

Robitussin (ENT, OB/GYN). Expectorant; used to thin cervical mucus to treat infertility. For dosage, see *guaifenesin*. [roh-bih-TUH-sihn]. 210

Robitussin A-C (ENT) (generic *codeine, guaifenesin*). Combination narcotic antitussive and expectorant drug. Syrup: 10 mg/100 mg. [roh-bih-TUH-sihn].

(Robitussin-CF) (ENT). No longer on the market. (Combination drug with *phenylpropanolamine*; decongestant, nonnarcotic antitussive, and expectorant drug).

Robitussin Cold & Cough (ENT) (generic *pseudoephedrine, dextromethorphan, guaifenesin*). Combination decongestant, nonnarcotic antitussive, and expectorant drug. Liqui-gels: 30 mg/10 mg/200 mg. [roh-bih-TUH-sihn].

Robitussin Cough Calmers, Robitussin Pediatric (ENT). Nonnarcotic antitussive drug. For dosage, see *dextromethorphan*. [roh-bih-TUH-sihn]. 210

Robitussin DAC (ENT) (generic *pseudoephedrine, codeine, guaifenesin*). Combination decongestant, narcotic antitussive, and expectorant drug. Syrup: 30 mg/10 mg/100 mg. [roh-bih-TUH-sihn].

Robitussin-DM (ENT) (generic *dextromethorphan, guaifenesin*). Combination nonnarcotic antitussive and expectorant drug. Liquid: 10 mg/100 mg. [roh-bih-TUH-sihn].

Robitussin Maximum Strength Cough & Cold, Robitussin Pediatric Cough & Cold (ENT) (generic *pseudoephedrine, dextromethorphan*). Combination decon-

gestant and nonnarcotic antitussive drug. Liquid: 15 mg/7.5 mg, 30 mg/15 mg. [roh-bih-TUH-sihn].

Robitussin Night Relief (ENT) (generic *pseudoephedrine, pyrilamine, dextromethorphan, acetaminophen*). Combination decongestant, antihistamine, nonnarcotic antitussive, and analgesic drug. Liquid: 10 mg/8.3 mg/5 mg/108.3 mg. [roh-bih-TUH-sihn].

Robitussin PE (ENT) (generic *pseudoephedrine, guaifenesin*). Combination decongestant and expectorant drug. Syrup: 30 mg/100 mg. [roh-bih-TUH-sihn].

Rocaltrol (Uro). Used to treat patients on dialysis who have hypocalcemia. For dosage, see *calcitriol*. [roh-KEHL-trawl]. 111

Rocephin (Antibio). Cephalosporin antibiotic used to treat various types of bacterial infections, including *Streptococcus, Staphylococcus, H. influenzae, E. coli*, and gonorrhea and Lyme disease. For dosage, see *ceftriaxone*. [roh-SEH-fihn]. 316

rocuronium (Zemuron) (Anes, Resp). Muscle relaxant drug used during surgery; used to treat patients who are intubated and on the ventilator. Intravenous: 10 mg/mL. [roh-kyour-OH-nee-uhm]. 199, 370

rofecoxib (Vioxx) (Analges, OB/GYN, Ortho). Nonsteroidal anti-inflammatory drug and cyclooxygenase-2 inhibitor used to treat pain; used to treat dysmenorrhea; used to treat rheumatoid arthritis and osteoarthritis. Liquid: 12.5 mg/5 mL, 25 mg/5 mL. Tablet: 12.5 mg, 25 mg, 50 mg. [roh-feh-KAWK-sihb]. 140, 255, 305

Roferon-A (Antivir, Chemo). Antiviral drug used to treat hepatitis C, cytomegalovirus, and herpes eye infections; chemotherapy drug used to treat leukemia, bladder cancer, non-Hodgkin's lymphoma, cutaneous T-cell lymphoma, and Kaposi's sarcoma. For dosage, see *interferon alfa-2a*. 133, 330

Roferon-A (Derm, OB/GYN). Antiviral drug used to treat condyloma acuminatum/genital warts. For dosage, see *interferon alfa-2a*.

Rogaine, Rogaine Extra Strength (Derm) (generic *minoxidil*). Topical vasodilator used to treat male and female pattern baldness. Liquid: 2%, 5%. [ROH-gayn]. 99

Rohypnol (Psych). Illegal drug not approved for use in the United States. So-called "date-rape drug." [roh-HIP-nawl]. 293

Rolaids (GI) (generic *calcium, magnesium*). Combination antacid. Tablet: 220 mg/45 mg. 117

Roman numerals in drug dosages. 71

Romazicon (Emerg, Psych). Benzodiazepine antagonist used to reverse an overdose of a benzodiazepine antianxiety drug. For dosage, see *flumazenil*. [roh-MEH-zeh-kawn]. 182, 293

Rondec Chewable Tablets (ENT) (generic *pseudoephedrine, brompheniramine*). Combination decongestant and antihistamine drug. Chewable tablets: 60 mg/4 mg. [RAWN-dehk].

Rondec-DM (ENT) (generic *pseudoephedrine, carbinoxamine, dextromethorphan*). Combination decongestant, antihistamine, and nonnarcotic antitussive drug. Drops: 25 mg/2 mg/4 mg. Syrup: 60 mg/4 mg/15 mg. [RAWN-dehk]. 213

Rondec Oral Drops, Rondec Tablets (ENT) (generic *pseudoephedrine, carbinoxamine*). Combination decongestant and antihistamine. Drops: 25 mg/2 mg. Tablet: 60 mg/4 mg. [RAWN-dehk].

(Rondomycin) (Antibio). No longer on the market. (Generic name *methacycline*; tetracyline-type antibiotic).

ropinirole (Requip) (Neuro). Used to treat Parkinson's disease. Tablet: 0.25 mg, 0.5 mg, 1 mg, 2 mg, 5 mg. [roh-PIH-neh-rohl]. 269

ropivacaine (Naropin) (Anes). Local, regional nerve block, and epidural anesthetic. Injection: 2 mg/mL, 5 mg/mL, 7.5 mg/mL, 10 mg/mL. [roh-PIH-vah-kayn]. 368

roquinimex (Linomide) (Chemo). Used to treat leukemia patients who have undergone bone marrow transplantation. Orphan drug. 362

rose bengal (Rosets) (Oph). Used to show corneal abrasions. Dye strips.

Rosets (Oph). Used to show corneal abrasions. Dye strips.

rosiglitazone (Avandia) (Endo, OB/GYN). Oral antidiabetic drug; also used to treat the elevated insulin levels caused by polycystic ovary syndrome. Tablet: 2 mg, 4 mg, 8 mg. [roh-sig-LIH-tah-zohn]. 240

(RotaShield) (GI). No longer on the market. (Generic name *rotavirus vaccine*; used to prevent rotavirus diarrhea in infants).

route of administration.
endotracheal. 42, 179
gastrostomy. 40
inhalation. 40
intra-arterial. 42
intra-articular. 42
intracardiac. 42, 179
intradermal. 43
intramuscular. 41
intrathecal. 43
intravenous. 179, 374
jejunostomy. 40
nasogastric (NG) tube. 39
oral. 38
parenteral. 40
rectal. 40
subcutaneous. 41
sublingual. 39
topical. 40
transdermal. 40
umbilical artery/vein. 43
vaginal. 40

Rovamycine (Antivir). Used to treat *Cryptosporidium parvum* in AIDS patients. For dosage, see *spiramycin*. Orphan drug. 332

Rowasa (GI). Anti-inflammatory-type drug used to treat ulcerative colitis. For dosage, see *mesalamine*. [roh-WAH-sah]. 126

Roxanol, Roxanol 100, Roxanol Rescudose, Roxanol T (Analges, Anes, Cardio, OB/GYN). Narcotic analgesic drug used to treat moderate-to-severe pain; used as a preoperative drug to sedate and supplement anesthesia; used to treat dyspnea in patients with congestive heart failure; used to treat the pain of childbirth. (Schedule II drug). For dosage, see *morphine*. [RAWK-seh-nawl]. 173, 297

roxatidine (Roxin (GI). Used to treat peptic ulcers. Investigational drug. 134

Roxiam (Psych). Used to treat psychosis. Generic: *remoxipride*. Investigational drug. 284

Roxicet, Roxicet 5/500 (Analges) (generic *acetaminophen, oxycodone*). Combination narcotic and nonnarcotic analgesic drug. (Schedule II drug). Tablet: 5 mg/325 mg, 5 mg/500 mg. Liquid: 5 mg/325 mg. [RAWK-sih-seht]. 303

Roxicodone, Roxicodone Intensol (Analges, Neuro). Narcotic analgesic used to treat moderate-to-severe pain; used to treat neuralgia from herpes zoster infection (shingles). (Schedule II drug). For dosage, see *oxycodone*. [rawk-see-KOH-dohn]. 276, 297

Roxilox (Analges) (generic *oxycodone, acetaminophen*). Combination narcotic and nonnarcotic analgesic drug. (Schedule II drug). Capsule: 5 mg/500 mg. [RAWK-sih-lawks]. 303

Roxin (GI) (generic *roxatidine*). Used to treat peptic ulcers. Investigational drug. 134

Roxiprin (Analges) (generic *aspirin, oxycodone*). Combination narcotic and nonnarcotic analgesic drug. (Schedule II drug). Tablet: 4.5 mg/325 mg. [RAWK-sih-prihn]. 302

RU-486 (OB/GYN). See *mifepristone*.

Rubex (Chemo). Chemotherapy antibiotic used to treat lung cancer, gastric cancer, thyroid cancer, breast cancer, ovarian cancer, bone cancer, bladder cancer, leukemia, Hodgkin's disease, non-Hodgkin's lymphoma, and Wilm's tumor. For dosage, see *doxorubicin*. [ROO-behks]. 342

Rx, definition of. 6

Rythmol (Cardio). Used to treat ventricular arrhythmias. For dosage, see *propafenone*. [RIHTH-mawl]. 159

s̄ (symbol for *without*).

SA (abbreviation for *sustained action*). Part of the trade name of drug.

Sabril (Neuro) (generic *vigabatrin*). Investigational drug used to treat epilepsy; orphan drug used to treat infantile spasms. 265

safety, margin of. See *margin of safety*.

Saizen (Derm, Endo). Used to maintain nitrogen balance in patients with severe burns; growth hormone replacement for adults and children with growth failure; also used to treat growth failure in infants who are small for gestational age. For dosage, see *somatropin*. 230

Salagen (ENT). Used to treat dry mouth from salivary gland dysfunction after radiation for head and neck cancer. For dosage, see *pilocarpine*. [SEH-lah-jehn].

salicylates (Analges, Ortho). Class of anti-inflammatory drugs like aspirin; used to treat pain; used to treat osteoarthritis and rheumatoid arthritis. 138, 299

salicylic acid (Clearasil Medicated Deep Cleanser, Pernox Lathering Abradant Scrub, PROPApH Foaming Face Wash, PROPApH Peel-off Acne Mask) (Derm). Topical keratolytic drug used to treat acne vulgaris. Liquid: 0.5%, 2%. Lotion. Mask: 2%. 83

salicylic acid (Compound W, Dr Scholl's Clear Away Plantar, Dr Scholl's Wart Remover, DuoFilm, DuoPlant, Wart-Off) (Derm). Topical keratolytic drug used to treat warts. Disk: 40%. Gel: 17%. Liquid: 17%. Patch: 40%. 91

salmeterol (Serevent, Serevent Diskus) (Resp). Bronchodilator. Aerosol inhaler: 25 mcg/puff. Diskus (inhaled powder): 50 mcg. [sehl-MEE-teh-rawl]. 193

salsalate (Disalcid) (Analges, Ortho). Salicylate nonaspirin drug used to treat pain; used to treat the pain and inflammation of osteoarthritis and rheumatoid arthritis. Tablet: 500 mg, 750 mg. [SEHL-seh-layt]. 138, 300

(Saluron) (Uro). No longer on the market. (Generic name *hydroflumethiazide*; thiazide diuretic).

Salutensin, Salutensin-Demi (Cardio) (generic *reserpine, hydroflumethiazide*). Combination antihypertensive and diuretic drug. Tablet: 0.125 mg/25 mg, 0.125 mg/50 mg. [sehl-yoo-TEHN-sihn]. 167

Sandimmune (Cardio, GI, Uro). Immunosuppressant drug given after organ transplant to prevent rejection of the donor heart, liver, or kidney. For dosage, see *cyclosporine*. [SEHND-ih-myoon].

Sandostatin, Sandostatin LAR Depot (Endo). Used to inhibit the overproduction of growth hormone in adults with acromegaly. For dosage, see *octreotide*. [sehn-doh-STEH-tihn]. 230

Sandostatin, Sandostatin LAR Depot (GI). Slows intestinal transit time; used to treat severe diarrhea caused by irritable bowel syndrome, AIDS, carcinoid tumors, VIPomas, short bowel syndrome, dumping syndrome, or chemotherapy. For dosage, see *octreotide*. [sehn-doh-STEH-tihn]. 134, 328

SangCya (Cardio, GI, Uro). Immunosuppressant drug given after organ transplantation to prevent rejection of the donor heart, liver, or kidney. For dosage, see *cyclosporine*. [sehng-SY-ah].

Sanorex (Ortho). Used to treat Duchenne's muscular dystrophy. Orphan drug.

Sansert (Analges). Used to treat migraine headaches. For dosage, see *methysergide*. [SEHN-sehrt]. 307

Santyl (Derm) (generic *collagenase*). Topical enzyme drug used to debride burns and wounds. Ointment. [SEHN-tuhl]. 96

saquinavir (Fortovase, Invirase) (Antivir). Protease inhibitor drug used to treat AIDS. Capsule: 200 mg. [sah-KWIH-nah-veer]. 325

Sarafem (OB/GYN). Selective serotonin reuptake inhibitor antidepressant used to treat premenstrual dysphoric disorder. For dosage, see *fluoxetine*. [SEH-rah-fehm]. 254

sargramostim (Leukine) (Antivir, Chemo). Granulocyte macrophage colony-stimulating factor used to increase white blood cell count in AIDS patients receiving zidovudine; used to stimulate white blood cell count after chemotherapy or with bone marrow transplant. Intravenous (powder to be reconstituted): 250 mcg/mL, 600 mcg/mL. [sawr-GREH-moh-stihm]. 332, 362

saw palmetto (Uro). Dietary supplement used to treat benign prostatic hypertrophy. 109

scabies (mites), drugs used to treat. 95

Scalpicin (Derm) (generic *hydrocortisone*). Topical corticosteroid anti-inflammatory drug. Liquid: 1%. [SKEHL-pih-sihn]. 92

schedule drugs. 16, 18, 60

schedule, drug dosage. 71

Scleromate (Cardio, GI). Sclerosing drug used to treat varicose veins; used to stop bleeding from esophageal varices. For dosage, see *morrhuate*. [SKLEH-roh-mayt].

Sclerosol Intrapleural Aerosol (Chemo, Resp). Powdered sclerosing drug administered via chest tube into the lung to treat malignant pleural effusion and pneumothorax. For dosage, see *talc*. [SKLEH-roh-sawl].

Scopace (GI). Antiemetic drug used to treat motion sickness; used to decrease peristalsis in patients with irritable bowel syndrome. For dosage, see *scopolamine*. 135

Scopace (Neuro). Anticholinergic drug used to treat muscle spasticity in Parkinson's disease. For dosage, see *scopolamine*.

scopolamine (Isopto Hyoscine) (Oph). Topical mydriatic drug. Ophthalmic solution: 0.25%. [skoh-PAWL-ah-meen]. 223

scopolamine (Scopace) (Neuro). Anticholinergic drug used to treat muscle spasticity in Parkinson's disease. Tablet: 0.4 mg. [skoh-PAWL-ah-meen].

scopolamine (Scopace, Transderm-Scop) (GI). Antiemetic drug used to treat motion sickness; used to decrease peristalsis in patients with irritable bowel syndrome. Tablet: 0.4 mg. Transdermal patch: 1.5 mg. [skoh-PAWL-ah-meen]. 128, 135

Scoville units. 91

Scriptene (Antivir) (generic *didanosine, zidovudine*). Combination nucleoside reverse transcriptase inhibitor drug used to treat AIDS. Investigational drug. 325

seal limbs. 15

Sebizon (Derm) (generic *sulfacetamide*). Topical anti-infective drug used to treat seborrheic dermatitis. Lotion: 10%. [SEH-beh-zohn]. 100

secobarbital (Seconal Sodium Pulvules) (Anes, Neuro). Barbiturate used to provide preoperative sedation; used for short-term treatment of insomnia. (Schedule II drug). Capsule: 100 mg. [seh-koh-BAR-beh-tawl]. 272, 371

Seconal Sodium Pulvules (Anes, Neuro). Barbiturate used to provide preoperative sedation; used for short-term treatment of insomnia. (Schedule II

drug). For dosage, see *secobarbital*. [SEH-koh-nawl]. 272, 371

secretin (Psych). Used to treat pediatric autism. Orphan drug.

Sectral (Cardio). Cardioselective beta-blocker used to treat hypertension and ventricular arrhythmias. For dosage, see *acebutolol*. [SEHK-trawl]. 160, 162

seizures. See *epilepsy*.

(Seldane) (ENT). No longer on the market. (Generic name *terfenadine*; antihistamine). Historical Notes feature.

Selecor (Cardio) (generic *celiprolol*). Selective beta$_2$-blocker for hypertension and angina pectoris. Investigational drug.

selective beta-blockers. Subclass of beta-blocker drugs. See *beta-blockers*.

selective estrogen receptor modulator (SERM) (OB/GYN, Ortho). Class of drugs used to prevent and treat osteoporosis in menopause. 144

selective norepinephrine reuptake inhibitors (SNRI) (Psych). Class of antidepressant drugs. Investigational drugs. 287

selective serotonin reuptake inhibitors (SSRI) (Psych). Class of antidepressant drugs. 286

selegiline (Carbex, Eldepryl) (Neuro, Psych). Used to treat Parkinson's disease. Pending use to treat depression. Capsule: 5 mg. Tablet: 5 mg. Transdermal patch (Pending). [seh-LEH-gih-leen]. 269

sennosides (ex-lax, ex-lax chocolated, Fletcher's Castoria, Maximum Strength ex-lax, Senokot, SenokotXTRA) (GI). Irritant/stimulant laxative. Granules: 15 mg/5 mL, 20 mg/5 mL. Tablet: 8.6 mg, 15 mg, 17 mg, 25 mg. Syrup: 8.8 mg/5 mL. Chocolated tablet: 15 mg. 124

Senokot, SenokotXTRA (GI). Irritant/stimulant laxative. For dosage, see *sennosides*. [SEH-noh-kawt]. 124

Senokot-S (GI) (generic *docusate, senna*). Combination stool softener and irritant/stimulant laxative. Tablet: 50 mg/8.6 mg. [SEH-noh-kawt]. 125

(Senolax) (GI). No longer on the market. (Irritant/stimulant laxative).

Sensorcaine, Sensorcaine MPF, Sensorcaine MPF Spinal (Anes). Local, regional nerve block, epidural, and spinal anesthetic. For dosage, see *bupivacaine*. 368

Sensorcaine (Dental, Oph, Ortho). Local anesthetic used before dental procedures; used in eye surgery; used to treat osteoarthritis or rheumatoid arthritis. For dosage, see *bupivacaine*.

Septocaine (Anes) (generic *articaine, epinephrine*). Used for infiltration and nerve block anesthesia in dentistry. Injection. 371

Septopal (Ortho). Antibiotic used to treat osteomyelitis. For dosage, see *gentamicin*. [SEPH-toh-pawl]. 148

Septra, Septra DS, Septra IV (Antibio) (generic *sulfamethoxazole, trimethoprim*). Combination antibiotic and sulfonamide anti-infective drug used to treat a variety of bacterial infections, including traveler's diarrhea; used to treat *Pneumocystis carinii* pneumonia in AIDS patients. Liquid: 200 mg/40 mg per 5 mL. Tablet: 400 mg/80 mg, 800 mg/160 mg. Intravenous: 80 mg/16 mg per 5 mL; 400 mg/80 mg per 5 mL. [SEHP-trah]. 106, 329, 330

septuplets, McCaughey. 245

Sequels. Part of the trade name of drug, indicating a slow-release capsule.

Ser-Ap-Es (Cardio) (generic *hydralazine, reserpine, hydrochlorothiazide*). Combination antihypertensive and a diuretic drug. Tablet: 25 mg/0.1 mg/15 mg. 167

Serax (Psych). Benzodiazepine drug used to treat anxiety and neurosis; used to treat alcohol withdrawal. (Schedule IV drug). For dosage, see *oxazepam*. [SEER-acks]. 281

Serentil (Psych). Phenothiazine drug used to treat schizophrenia; used to treat behavioral problems in patients with mental retardation or chronic brain syndrome; used to treat anxiety and depression in alcoholism; used to treat anxiety. For dosage, see *mesoridazine*. [seh-REHN-tihl]. 283

Serevent, Serevent Diskus (Resp). Bronchodilator. For dosage, see *salmeterol*. [SEHR-eh-vehnt]. 193

Serlect (Psych). Used to treat psychosis. Generic: *sertindole*. Investigational drug. 284

SERM. See *selective estrogen receptor modulator*.

sermorelin (Geref) (Antivir, Endo, OB/GYN). Used to treat AIDS wasting syndrome; used to treat growth hormone deficiency; used to treat infertility due to failure to ovulate. Orphan drug. 230, 244, 327

Seromycin Pulvules (Resp). Used to treat tuberculosis. For dosage, see *cycloserine*. [seh-roh-MY-sihn]. 197

Serophene (OB/GYN). Ovulation-stimulating hormone used to treat infertility. For dosage, see *clomiphene*. [SEH-roh-feen]. 244

Seroquel (Psych). Drug used to treat psychosis and schizophrenia. For dosage, see *quetiapine*. [SEHR-oh-kwel]. 284

Serostim (Antivir, Endo). Growth hormone replacement for adults and children with growth failure; used to treat growth failure of infants who are small for gestational age; used to treat AIDS wasting syndrome. For dosage, see *somatropin*. [SEHR-oh-stihm]. 328

serotonin (neurotransmitter). 306

sertindole (Serlect) (Psych). Used to treat psychosis. Investigational drug. 284

sertraline (Zoloft) (OB/GYN). Selective serotonin reuptake inhibitor used to treat premenstrual dysphoric disorder. Tablet: 25 mg, 50 mg, 100 mg. Liquid: 20 mg/mL. [SEHR-trah-leen]. 255

sertraline (Zoloft) (Psych). Selective serotonin reuptake inhibitor antidepressant used to treat depression; used to treat panic disorder; used to treat obsessive-compulsive disorder; used to treat post-traumatic stress disorder; used to treat social anxiety disorder. Tablet: 25 mg, 50 mg, 100 mg. Liquid: 20 mg/mL. [SEHR-trah-leen]. 287, 289, 290

Serzone (Psych). Antidepressant. For dosage, see *nefazodone*. [SEHR-zohn]. 288

sevelamer (Renagel) (Uro). Used to decrease serum phosphorus levels in hemodialysis patients with end-stage renal disease. Capsule: 403 mg. [seh-VEH-lah-meer]. 112

sevoflurane (Ultane) (Anes). Used to induce and maintain general anesthesia. Inhaled gas. [see-voh-FLOHR-ayn]. 370

sexually transmitted disease (STDs), drugs used to treat.

sheep's wool. 7

shingles, drugs used to treat. 275, 276

SI (abbreviation for *International System of Units*).

SIADH, drugs used to treat. 231

Sibelium (Neuro). Used to treat alternating hemiplegia. For dosage, see *flunarizine*. 275

(Siblin) (GI). No longer on the market. (Irritant/stimulant laxative).

sibutramine (Meridia) (GI). Appetite suppressant used to treat obesity. (Schedule IV drug). Capsule: 5 mg, 10 mg, 15 mg. [sih-BYOO-trah-meen]. 129

side effect. 51

Sig. Abbreviation for Latin word *signetur* which means *write on the label*. 78

sildenafil (Viagra) (Uro). Used to treat impotence due to erectile dysfunction. Tablet: 25 mg, 50 mg, 100 mg. [sihl-DEH-nah-fihl]. 109

Silvadene (Derm) (generic *silver sulfadiazine*). Topical antibacterial drug used to treat severe burns. Cream. [SIHL-vah-deen]. 97

silver nitrate (chemical formula $AgNO_3$) (Derm, ENT, OB/GYN). Topical drug used to cauterize skin lesions (warts, granulation tissue); used to cauterize small blood vessels (to stop nosebleeds and oozing from the umbilical cord in newborns). Liquid: 10%, 25%, 50%. Ointment: 10%.

silver nitrate (Oph). Topical antibiotic used to prevent gonorrhea-caused blindness in newborns. Ophthalmic solution: 1%. 258

silver sulfadiazine (Silvadene) (Derm).   Topical antibacterial drug used to treat severe burns. Cream. 97

simethicone (Extra Strength Gas-X, Gas-X, Maalox Anti-Gas, Maximum Strength Mylanta Gas, Mylanta Gas, Mylicon, Phazyme, Phazyme 95, Phazyme 125) (GI).   Anti-gas drug. Capsule: 125 mg. Chewable tablet: 40 mg, 80 mg, 125 mg. Oral drops: 40 mg/0.6 mL. Tablet: 60, 95 mg. 118

Similac Low-Iron, Similac PM 60/40 Low-Iron, Similac with Iron (GI).   Infant formula. Liquid, powder (to be reconstituted).

Simpson, James. 366

Simulect (Uro).   Immunosuppressant monoclonal antibody given after kidney transplantation to prevent rejection of the donor kidney.   For dosage, see *basiliximab*. [SIH-muh-lehkt]. 110

simvastatin (Zocor) (Cardio).   HMG-CoA reductase inhibitor drug used to treat hypercholesterolemia. Tablet: 5 mg, 10 mg, 20 mg, 40 mg, 80 mg. [sihm-vah-STEH-tihn].170

Sinarest Extra Strength, Sinarest Sinus (ENT) (generic *pseudoephedrine, chlorpheniramine, acetaminophen*). Combination decongestant, antihistamine, and analgesic drug. Tablet: 30 mg/2 mg/325 mg, 30 mg/2 mg/500 mg.

Sinarest 12 Hour (ENT).   Decongestant.   For dosage, see *oxymetazoline*. 206

Sine-Aid IB (ENT) (generic *pseudoephedrine, ibuprofen*). Combination decongestant and analgesic drug. Caplet: 30 mg/200 mg.

Sinemet-10/100,   Sinemet-25/100,   Sinemet-25/250, Sinemet CR (Neuro) (generic *carbidopa, levodopa*). Combination drug used to treat Parkinson's disease. Tablet: 10 mg/100 mg, 25 mg/100 mg, 25 mg/250 mg, 50 mg/200 mg. [SIH-neh-meht]. 270

Sine-Off Maximum Strength No Drowsiness Formula (ENT) (generic *pseudoephedrine, acetaminophen*). Combination decongestant and analgesic drug. Caplet: 30 mg/500 mg.

Sine-Off Sinus Medicine (ENT) (generic *pseudoephedrine, chlorpheniramine, acetaminophen*).   Combination decongestant, antihistamine, and analgesic drug. Caplet: 30 mg/2 mg/500 mg.

Sinequan, Sinequan Concentrate (Analges, Derm, Diab, Neuro, Ortho).   Tricyclic antidepressant used to treat migraines; used to treat urticaria; used to treat diabetic neuropathy; used to treat postherpetic neuralgia; used to treat phantom limb pain. For dosage, see *doxepin*. [SIH-neh-kwan]. 98, 147, 241, 275, 282, 307

Sinequan, Sinequan Concentrate (Psych).   Tricyclic antidepressant; used to treat depression; also used to

treat anxiety and neurosis.   For dosage, see *doxepin*. [SIHN-eh-kwan]. 285

Sinex (ENT).   Decongestant.   For dosage, see *phenylephrine*. 206

Singulair (Resp).   Leukotriene receptor blocker used to prevent and treat asthma.   For dosage, see *montelukast*. [SIHN-gyoo-lehr]. 196

Sinus Excedrin Extra Strength (ENT) (generic *pseudoephedrine, acetaminophen*).   Combination decongestant and analgesic drug. Caplet: 30 mg/500 mg. Tablet: 30 mg/500 mg.

Sinutab Maximum Strength Sinus Allergy (ENT) (generic *pseudoephedrine, chlorpheniramine, acetaminophen*).   Combination decongestant, antihistamine, and analgesic drug. Caplet: 30 mg/2 mg/500 mg. Tablet: 30 mg/2 mg/500 mg.

Sinutab Non-Drying (ENT) (generic *pseudoephedrine, guaifenesin*).   Combination decongestant and expectorant drug. Capsule: 30 mg/200 mg.

Sinutab Without Drowsiness (ENT) (generic *pseudoephedrine, acetaminophen*).   Combination decongestant and analgesic drug. Tablet: 30 mg/325 mg.

sirolimus (Rapamune) (Derm).   Immunsuppressant drug used to treat severe, disabling psoriasis. Liquid: 1 mg/mL. Tablet: 1 mg. 87

sirolimus (Rapamune) (Uro).   Immunosuppressant drug given after kidney transplant to prevent rejection of the donor kidney. Liquid: 1 mg/mL. 110

6-MP.   See *mercaptopurine*.

Skelaxin (Ortho).   Skeletal muscle relaxant used to treat minor muscle spasms associated with injuries. For dosage, see *metaxalone*. [skeh-LEHK-sihn]. 144

skeletal muscle relaxants (Ortho).   Class of drugs used to treat muscular spasm and spasticity. 144

Skelid (Ortho).   Inhibits the breakdown of bone; used to treat Paget's disease.   For dosage, see *tiludronate*. 148

skin, drugs used to treat the.   See *dermatology drugs*.

SL (abbreviation for *sublingual*).

Sleep-eze 3 (Neuro).   Antihistamine drug sleep aid. For dosage, see *diphenhydramine*.

Slo-bid Gyrocaps (Resp).   Bronchodilator.   For dosage, see *theophylline*. 193

Slo-Phyllin, Slo-Phyllin Gyrocaps (Resp).   Bronchodilator; used to prevent apnea in premature infants.   For dosage, see *theophylline*. 193

Slo-Phyllin GG (Resp) (generic *theophylline, guaifenesin*).   Combination bronchodilator and expectorant drug. Capsule: 150 mg/90 mg. Liquid: 150 mg/90 mg. [SLAW-fih-lihn *or* SLOH-fih-lihn]. 195

Slow-K (Uro).   Potassium supplement used to replace potassium loss caused by diuretics. Tablet: 8 mEq. 105

slow-release tablet. See *tablet.*

SMA Iron Fortified, SMA Lo-Iron Infant Formula (GI). Infant formula. Liquid, powder (to be reconstituted).

smoking, drugs used to help patients stop. 199

SMX (abbreviation for *sulfamethoxazole*). See *sulfamethoxazole.*

SNRI (abbreviation for *selective norepinephrine reuptake inhibitors*).

social anxiety disorder, drugs used to treat. 290

sodium bicarbonate (Emerg). Used to treat metabolic acidosis during cardiac arrest. Intravenous: 4.2% (0.5 mEq/mL), 5% (0.6 mEq/mL), 7.5% (0.9 mEq/mL), 8.4% (1 mEq/mL). 181

sodium bicarbonate (GI). Used to neutralize acid as an ingredient in some antacids. See *Alka-Seltzer, Bromo Seltzer.* 117

sodium hyaluronate (AMO Vitrax, Amvisc, Amvisc Plus, Healon, Healon GV) (Oph). Injected into the eye during eye surgery to keep the anterior chamber expanded and replace intraocular fluid. Intraocular injection: 10 mg/mL, 12 mg/mL, 14 mg/mL, 16 mg/mL, 30 mg/mL.

sodium hyaluronate (Supartz) (Ortho). Used to maintain the lubricating quality of the synovial fluid in patients with osteoarthritis. Intra-articular: 125 mg/2.5 mL. [soh-dee-uhm hy-ehl-yoo-RAW-nayt]. 141

(Sodium P. A. S.) (Resp). No longer on the market. (Generic name *para-aminosalicylic acid*; used to treat tuberculosis).

sodium tetradecyl (Sotradecol) (Cardio, GI). Sclerosing drug used to treat varicose veins; used to stop bleeding from esophageal varices. Intravenous (injection into the varicose vein or esophageal varix): 1%, 3%. [soh-dee-uhm teh-trah-DEH-kuhl]. 135, 174

sodium thiosalicylate (Rexolate) (Ortho). Salicylate nonaspirin drug used to treat gout. Intramuscular: 50 mg/mL. [SOH-dee-uhm thy-oh-sah-LIH-seh-layt]. 146

Solaraze (Derm) (generic *diclofenac*). Nonsteroidal anti-inflammatory drug used to treat actinic keratoses. Gel: 3%. 98

Solarcaine Aloe Extra Burn Relief (Derm) (generic *lidocaine*). Topical anesthetic. Cream: 0.5%. Gel: 0.5%. Spray: 0.5%. 94

Solarcaine, Solarcaine Medicated First Aid (Derm) (generic *benzocaine*). Topical anesthetic. Lotion. Spray: 20%. 94

Solfoton (Neuro). Barbiturate used to treat tonic-clonic and partial seizures; used to treat status epilepticus; used to treat the seizures of eclampsia during pregnancy; used to treat insomnia. (Schedule IV drug). For dosage, see *phenobarbital.* 264, 267, 272

Solganal (Ortho). Gold compound used to treat rheumatoid arthritis. For dosage, see *aurothioglucose.* [SOHL-geh-nawl]. 142

soluble T4 (Antivir). Used to treat AIDS. Orphan drug. 326

Solu-Cortef (Endo). Injected corticosteroid anti-inflammatory drug used to treat severe inflammation in various body systems. For dosage, see *hydrocortisone.* [sawl-yoo-KOHR-tehf]. 232

Solu-Medrol (Endo). Injected corticosteroid anti-inflammatory used to treat severe inflammation in various body systems. For dosage, see *methylprednisolone.* [sawl-yoo-MEH-drawl]. 232

(Solurex, Solurex LA) (Ortho). No longer on the market. (Generic name *dexamethasone*; corticosteroid anti-inflammatory drug injected in joint).

solution (drug form). 35

Soma (Ortho). Skeletal muscle relaxant used to treat minor muscle spasms associated with injuries. For dosage, see *carisoprodol.* [SOH-mah]. 144

Soma Compound (Ortho) (generic *aspirin, carisoprodol*). Combination analgesic and skeletal muscle relaxant drug. Tablet: 325 mg/200 mg. [SOH-mah]. 146

Soma Compound with Codeine (Ortho) (generic *aspirin, carisoprodol, codeine*). Combination analgesic, narcotic analgesic, and skeletal muscle relaxant. Tablet: 325 mg/16 mg/200 mg. {SOH-mah]. 146

Somagard (Endo). Used to treat precocious puberty. For dosage, see *deslorelin.*

Somatrel (Endo). Used to diagnose lack of growth hormone due to pituitary gland malfunction. Orphan drug.

somatrem (Protropin) (Endo). Growth hormone replacement. Subcutaneous or intravenous (powder to be reconstituted): 5 mg, 10 mg. 230

somatropin (BioTropin, Serostim) (Antivir). Used to treat AIDS wasting syndrome. Orphan drug. 328

somatropin (Genotropin, Genotropin MiniQuick, Humatrope, Norditropin, Nutropin, Nutropin AQ, Nutropin Depot, Saizen, Serostim) (Antivir, Endo, OB/GYN). Growth hormone replacement for adults and children with growth failure; used to treat growth failure of infants who are small for gestational age; used to treat AIDS wasting syndrome (Serostim only); orphan drug used to stimulate ovulation in infertility (Norditropin). Subcutaneous (powder to be reconstituted): 0.2 mg, 0.4 mg, 0.6 mg, 0.8 mg, 1 mg, 1.2 mg, 1.4 mg, 1.5 mg, 1.6 mg, 1.8 mg, 2 mg, 4 mg (12 IU), 5 mg (15 IU), 5.8 mg (17.4 IU), 6 mg (18 IU), 8 mg (24 IU), 10 mg (30 IU), 12 mg (36 IU), 13.5 mg, 13.8 mg (41.4 IU), 18 mg, 22.5 mg, 24 mg (72 IU). Subcutaneous: 5 mg/1.6 mL, 10 mg/1.5 mL, 15 mg/1.5 mL. Intramuscular (powder to be reconstituted): 5 mg (15IU). [soh-mah-TROH-pihn]. 230, 244

Sominex (Neuro). Antihistamine drug sleep aid. For dosage, see *diphenhydramine*. [SAW-mih-nehks]. 273

Sominex Pain Relief (Neuro) (generic *acetaminophen, diphenhydramine*). Combination analgesic and antihistamine drug sleep aid. Tablet: 500 mg/25 mg. [SAW-mih-nehks]. 273

Sonata (Neuro). Nonbarbiturate drug used to treat insomnia. (Schedule IV drug). For dosage, see *zaleplon*. [soh-NAH-tah]. 272

Sorbitrate (Cardio). Nitrate drug used to prevent and treat angina pectoris. For dosage, see *isosorbide dinitrate*. [SOHR-bih-trayt]. 156

Sorbsan (Derm). Topical absorbent calcium fibers used to absorb drainage from burns, skin ulcers, and wounds. Wound packing fibers. 96

Soriatane (Derm). Oral vitamin A-type drug used to treat psoriasis. For dosage, see *acitretin*. [SOH-ree-ah-tayn]. 87

sorivudine (Bravavir) (Antivir). Used to treat herpes zoster infection (shingles). Orphan drug. 330

sotalol (Betapace, Betapace AF) (Cardio). Nonselective beta-blocker used to treat ventricular arrhythmias. Tablet: 80 mg, 120 mg, 160 mg, 240 mg. [SOH-tah-lawl]. 160

Sotradecol (Cardio, GI). Sclerosing drug used to treat varicose veins; used to stop bleeding from esophageal varices. Intravenous. For dosage, see *sodium tetradecyl*. 135, 174

Soyalac (GI). Infant soy formula. Liquid, powder (to be reconstituted).

(Spanidin) (Uro). No longer on the market. (Generic name *gusperimus*; used to treat rejection of kidney transplant).

Spansule. Part of the trade name of drug, indicating a slow-release capsule. 65

sparfloxacin (Zagam) (Antibio). Fluoroquinolone antibiotic used to treat a variety of infections, including community-acquired pneumonia, *H. influenzae, S. pneumoniae,* and *Klebsiella*. Tablet: 200 mg. [spahr-FLAWK-sah-sihn]. 318

(Sparine) (Psych). No longer on the market. (Generic name *promazine*; phenothiazine antipsychotic drug).

Spartaject (Chemo). Alkylating chemotherapy orphan drug used to treat brain cancer. For dosage, see *busulfan*. 341

Spec-T (ENT) (generic *benzocaine*). Topical anesthetic used to treat sore throats. Lozenge: 10 mg.

Spectazole (Derm) (generic *econazole*). Topical antifungal and antiyeast drug. Cream: 1%. [SPEHK-tah-zohl]. 89

spectinomycin (Trobicin) (Antibio). Antibiotic used to treat gonorrhea. Intramuscular: 400 mg/mL. [spehk-tih-noh-MY-sihn]. 319

Spectracef (Antibio). Cephalosporin antibiotic used to treat bronchitis, pharyngitis, tonsillitis, and skin infections. For dosage, see *cefditoren*. [SPEHK-trah-sehf]. 315

(Spectrobid) (Antibio). No longer on the market. (Generic name *bacampicillin*; penicillin-type antibiotic).

spelling of drug names. 22

Spexil (Antibio). Antibiotic similar to spectinomycin. Investigational drug. 321

Spheramine (Neuro). Used to treat Parkinson's disease. Generic: *allogeneic human retinal pigment epithelial cells*. Orphan drug. 270

spiramycin (Rovamycine) (Antivir). Used to treat *Cryptosporidium parvum* in AIDS patients. Orphan drug. 332

spironolactone (Aldactone) (Uro). Potassium-sparing diuretic. Tablet: 25 mg, 50 mg, 100 mg. [spih-raw-noh-LEHK-tohn]. 104

Sporanox (Antifung). Used to treat severe topical and systemic fungal and yeast infections. For dosage, see *itraconazole*. [SPOHR-eh-nawks]. 90, 334, 335

Sporidin-G (Antivir). Cow immunoglobulin used to treat *Cryptosporidium parvum* gastrointestinal tract infection in patients with AIDS. For dosage, see *bovine immunoglobulin*. 331

Sportscreme Ice Gel (Ortho). Topical irritant drug used to mask the pain of arthritis and muscular aches. Gel. 148

Sprinkle. Part of the trade name of drug, indicating that a capsule can be opened and the contents sprinkled on food. 66

SQ (abbreviation meaning *subcutaneous*). 41

SR (abbreviation for *slow release*). Part of the trade name of drug. 66

SSKI (ENT). Expectorant. For dosage, see *potassium iodide*.

SSRI (abbreviation for *selective serotonin reuptake inhibitors*).

Stadol, Stadol NS (Analges, OB/GYN). Narcotic analgesic drug used to treat moderate-to-severe pain; used to treat pain during labor and delivery. (Schedule IV drug). For dosage, see *butorphanol*. [STAY-dawl]. 297

staging of cancer. 338

stanozolol (Winstrol) (Chemo, Endo). Anabolic steroid used to treat metastatic breast cancer; used to treat hereditary angioedema; also used illegally by athletes. Tablet: 2 mg. [steh-NAW-zoh-lawl]. 234

(Staphcillin) (Antibio).   No longer on the market. (Generic name *methicillin*; penicillin-type antibiotic).

Starlix (Diab).   Oral antidiabetic drug.   For dosage, see *nateglinide*. [STAHR-lihks]. 240

Starry Night, The (oil painting). 153

Staticin (Derm) (generic *erythromycin*).   Topical drug used to treat acne vulgaris. Liquid: 1.5%, 2%. [STEH-tih-sihn]. 84

statins (Cardio).   Brief term for the class of HMG-CoA reductase inhibitor drugs used to treat hyper-cholesterolemia. The generic names of all of the drugs in this class end with *-statin*. 170

stavudine (d4T) (Zerit) (Antivir).   Nucleoside reverse transcriptase inhibitor drug used to treat AIDS. Capsule: 15 mg, 20 mg, 30 mg, 40 mg. Liquid (powder to be reconstituted): 1 mg/mL. [STEH-vyoo-dine]. 324

STD (abbreviation *for sexually transmitted disease*).   See *sexually transmitted diseases*.

Stelazine (Psych).   Phenothiazine drug used to treat psychosis; used to treat anxiety.   For dosage, see *trifluoperazine*. [STEHL-ah-zeen]. 282

Stemgen (Chemo).   Used to increase the number of blood progenitor cells collected during pheresis prior to chemotherapy or bone marrow transplant. For dosage, see *ancestim*. 361

Stenorol (Misc).   Used to treat systemic sclerosis. For dosage, see *halofuginone*.

Step 2 (Derm).   Topical drug used to treat pediculosis (lice). Creme rinse. 96

Sterecyt (Chemo).   Chemotherapy drug used to treat non-Hodgkin's lymphoma.   For dosage, see *prednimustine*.

Steritalc (Chemo, Resp).   Powdered sclerosing drug administered via chest tube into the lung to treat malignant pleural effusion and pneumothorax. For dosage, see *talc*. [STEH-ree-tehlk].

steroid, anabolic.

steroid.   See *corticosteroid*.

(Stilphostrol) (Chemo).   No longer on the market. (Generic name *diethylstilbestrol;* hormonal chemotherapy drug).

Stimate (Endo, Hem, Uro).   Antidiuretic hormone replacement used to treat diabetes insipidus, bleeding in hemophiliacs, and enuresis.   For dosage, see *desmopressin*. 111, 188, 231

St. Joseph Adult Chewable Aspirin (Cardio, Hem, Neuro).   Salicylate drug used to treat current myocardial infarction and prevent repeat myocardial infarction; anticoagulant; used to prevent transient ischemic attacks and strokes.   For dosage, see *aspirin*. 158

(St. Joseph Cold Tablets for Children) (ENT).   No longer on the market. (Combination drug with *phenylpropanolamine;* decongestant and analgesic drug).

St. Joseph Cough Suppressant (ENT).   Nonnarcotic antitussive drug.   For dosage, see *dextromethorphan*.

stool softener.   See *laxative*.

Storz Sulf (Oph).   Topical sulfonamide anti-infective drug used to treat bacterial eye infections.   For dosage, see *sulfacetamide*. 218

Streptase (Cardio, Hem).   Thrombolytic enzyme used to dissolve blood clots from a myocardial infarction, pulmonary embolus, or deep venous thrombosis.   For dosage, see *streptokinase*. 174, 188

streptokinase (Streptase) (Cardio, Hem).   Thrombolytic enzyme used to dissolve blood clots from a myocardial infarction, pulmonary embolus, or deep venous thrombosis. Intravenous (powder to be reconstituted): 250,000 IU; 750,000 IU; 1,500,000 IU. [strehp-toh-KY-nays]. 174, 188

streptomycin (Antivir, Resp).   Aminoglycoside antibiotic used to treat *Mycobacterium avium-intracellulare* in AIDS patients; used to treat tuberculosis. Intramuscular: 400 mg/mL. [strehp-toh-ZOH-sihn]. 197, 329

streptozocin (Zanosar) (Chemo).   Alkylating chemotherapy drug used to treat pancreatic cancer. Intravenous (powder to be reconstituted): 1 g (100 mg/mL). [strehp-toh-ZOH-sihn] 341

Stresstabs + Iron (Misc).   Multivitamin with iron nutritional supplement. Tablet.

Stri-Dex Anti-Bacterial Foaming Wash (Derm) (generic *triclosan*).   Topical antiseptic used to treat acne vulgaris. Liquid: 1%. 83

subcu (abbreviation for *subcutaneous*). 41

subcutaneous route, administration of drugs by the. 41

Sublimaze (Anes).   Preoperative narcotic drug used to provide sedation; used to induce and maintain general anesthesia. (Schedule II drug).   For dosage, see *fentanyl*. [SUHB-leh-mays]. 369

sublingual route, administration of drugs by the. 39

Suboxone (Analges, Psych) (Generic names *buprenorphine, naloxone*).   Combination narcotic and narcotic antagonist drug used to treat narcotic addiction. Orphan drug. 294

subQ (abbreviation for *subcutaneous*). 41

substitution, generic drug for trade name drug. 30, 78

Subutex (Analges, Psych).   Used to treat narcotic addiction.   For dosage, see *buprenorphine*. [SUH-byoo-tehks]. 293, 308

Suby's Solution G (Uro).   Used to dissolve phosphate stones in the bladder. Irrigation solution (via catheter). 112

succimer (Chemet) (Emerg, Neuro, Uro).   Chelating drug used to treat arsenic, lead, and mercury poisoning and lead encephalopathy; used to treat cystine kidney stones. Capsule: 100 mg. 112, 277

succinimides (Neuro).   Class of drugs used to treat epilepsy. 264

succinylcholine (Anectine, Anectine Flo-Pack, Quelicin) (Anes, Resp).   Muscle relaxant drug used during surgery; used to treat patients who are intubated and on the ventilator. Intravenous: 20 mg/mL, 50 mg/mL. Intravenous (powder to be reconstituted): 500 mg, 1 g. [suhk-sih-nuhl-KOH-leen]. 199, 370

sucralfate (Carafate) (GI).   Used to treat peptic ulcers by binding directly to the ulcer site. Suspension: 1 g/10 mL. Tablet: 1 g. [SUHL-kreh-fayt]. 119

sucralfate (Carafate) (Chemo).   Used to treat oral mucositis in patients receiving radiation therapy for head and neck cancer. Suspension: 1 g/10 mL. Tablet: 1 g. [SUHL-kreh-fayt]. 350

Sucrets, Sucrets Children's Sore Throat, Sucrets Maximum Strength (ENT) (generic *dyclonine*).   Topical anesthetic used to treat sore throats. Lozenge: 1.2 mg, 3 mg. Throat spray: 0.1%.

Sucrets Cough Control, Sucrets 4-Hour Cough (ENT).   Nonnarcotic antitussive drug.   For dosage, see *dextromethorphan*. 210

Sudafed, Sudafed 12 Hour (ENT).   Decongestant. For dosage, see *pseudoephedrine*. 206

Sudafed Cold & Cough (ENT) (generic *pseudoephedrine, dextromethorphan, guaifenesin*).   Combination decongestant, nonnarcotic antitussive, and expectorant drug. Liquid Caps: 30 mg/10 mg/100 mg.

Sudafed Plus (ENT) (generic *pseudoephedrine, chlorpheniramine*).   Combination decongestant and antihistamine drug. Tablet: 60 mg/4 mg.

Sudafed Severe Cold (ENT) (generic *pseudoephedrine, dextromethorphan, acetaminophen*).   Combination decongestant, nonnarcotic antitussive, and analgesic drug. Caplet: 30 mg/15 mg/500 mg. Tablet: 30 mg/15 mg/500 mg.

Sufenta (Analges, Anes, OB/GYN, Resp).   Narcotic used to induce and maintain general anesthesia; used to treat pain during labor and delivery; used to sedate patients who are intubated and on the ventilator. (Schedule II drug).   For dosage, see *sufentanil*. [soo-FEHN-tah]. 199, 298, 369

sufentanil (Sufenta) (Analges, Anes, OB/GYN, Resp).   Narcotic used to induce and maintain general anesthesia; used to treat pain during labor and delivery; used to sedate patients who are intubated and on the ventilator. (Schedule II drug). Intravenous: 50 mcg/mL. [soo-FEHN-tah-nill]. 199, 298, 369

suicide attempt, drugs used to treat. 182

suicide attempts, Accutane and. 53, 85

(Sulamyd) (Oph).   No longer on the market. (Generic name *sulfacetamide*; topical sulfa anti-infective drug for the eye).

Sular (Cardio).   Calcium channel blocker used to treat hypertension.   For dosage, see *nisoldipine*. [SOO-lahr]. 163

sulconazole (Exelderm) (Derm).   Topical antifungal drug. Cream: 1%. Liquid: 1%. [suhl-KAW-neh-zohl]. 89

sulfacetamide (Bleph-10, Cetamide, Ocusulf-10, Storz Sulf, Sulster) (Oph).   Topical sulfonamide anti-infective drug used to treat bacterial eye infections. Ophthalmic solution: 1%, 10%, 30%. Ophthalmic ointment: 10%. [suhl-fah-SEE-tah-mide]. 218

sulfacetamide (Sebizon) (Derm).   Topical anti-infective drug used to treat seborrheic dermatitis. Lotion: 10%. [suhl-fah-SEE-tah-mide]. 100

(sulfacytine) (Uro).   No longer on the market. (Trade name *Renoquid*; sulfonamide drug used to treat urinary tract infections).

sulfadiazine (Antibio).   Sulfonamide drug used to treat a variety of bacterial infections, including urinary tract infections and otitis media; orphan drug used to treat *Toxoplasma gondii* encephalitis in AIDS patients. Tablet: 500 mg. [suhl-fah-DY-ah-zeen]. 106, 312, 332

sulfa drugs.   See *sulfonamides*.

(sulfamethizole) (Antibio, Uro).   No longer on the market. (Trade name *Thiosulfil Forte*; sulfonamide anti-infective drug).

sulfamethoxazole (SMX) (Gantanol) (Antibio).   Sulfonamide drug used to treat a variety of bacterial infections, including urinary tract infection and otitis media. Tablet: 500 mg. [suhl-fah-meh-THAWK-sah-zohl]. 106, 312

Sulfamylon (Derm) (generic *mafenide*).   Topical antibacterial drug used to treat severe burns. Cream, liquid. [suhl-fah-MY-lawn]. 97

(sulfanilamide) (OB/GYN).   No longer on the market. (Trade name *AVC*; topical sulfa drug for vaginal yeast infections).

sulfasalazine (Azulfidine, Azulfidine EN-tabs) (GI, Ortho).   Anti-inflammatory-type drug used to treat ulcerative colitis and Crohn's disease; used to treat rheumatoid arthritis. Tablet: 500 mg. [suhl-fah-SEH-lah-zeen]. 126, 142

sulfinpyrazone (Anturane) (Ortho).   Used to treat gout. Capsule: 200 mg. Tablet: 100 mg. [suhl-feh-PY-rah-zohn]. 146

sulfisoxazole (Gantrisin) (Oph).   Topical sulfonamide anti-infective used to treat bacterial eye infections. Ophthalmic solution: 4%. [suhl-feh-SAWK-seh-zohl]. 213

sulfisoxazole (Gantrisin Pediatric) (Antibio).   Sulfonamide used to treat a variety of bacterial infections, including urinary tract and otitis media. Liquid: 500 mg/5 mL. Tablet: 500 mg. [suhl-feh-SAWK-seh-zohl]. 106, 312

sulfonamide drugs (Antibio, Oph, Uro). Class of anti-infective drugs used to treat urinary tract infections, eye infections, and other types of infections. [suhl-FAW-neh-mide] 106, 312

sulfonamide drugs discovered. Historical Notes feature. 312

Sulfoxyl Regular, Sulfoxyl Strong (Derm) (generic *benzoyl peroxide, sulfur*). Topical combination antibiotic and keratolytic drug used to treat acne vulgaris. Lotion: 5%/2%, 10%/2%. [suhl-FAWK-sihl]. 84

sulindac (Clinoril) (Analges, Ortho). Nonsteroidal anti-inflammatory drug used to treat bursitis, gout, osteoarthritis, rheumatoid arthritis, and tendinitis. Tablet: 150 mg, 200 mg. [soo-LIHN-dack]. 139, 146, 304

Sulster Solution (Oph) (generic name *prednisolone, sulfacetamide*). Topical combination corticosteroid and sulfa anti-infective drug. Ophthalmic solution: 0.25%/10%. 218

(Sultrin) (OB/GYN). No longer on the market. (Generic name *triple sulfa*; topical sulfa drug used to treat vaginal infections).

sumatriptan (Imitrex) (Analges). Serotonin receptor agonist drug used to treat migraine headaches and cluster headaches. Tablet: 25 mg, 50 mg, 100 mg. Nasal spray: 5 mg, 20 mg. Subcutaneous: 12 mg/mL. [soo-mah-TRIP-tehn]. 306

Summer's Eve Medicated Douche (OB/GYN). Antibacterial povidone-iodine vaginal douche. Douche: 0.30%.

Sumycin, Sumycin 250, Sumycin 500 (Antibio). Antibiotic used to treat a variety of infections, including acne vulgaris, *H. pylori* of the gastrointestinal tract, *Chlamydia*, gonorrhea, and syphilis. For dosage, see *tetracycline*. [soo-MY-sihn]. 84, 120, 317

Supartz (Ortho). Used to maintain the lubricating quality of synovial fluid in patients with osteoarthritis. For dosage, see *sodium hyaluronate*.

"super aspirin." General term used by the media to refer to cyclooxygenase-2 inhibitors used to treat osteoarthritis and rheumatoid arthritis or, alternatively, to the platelet aggregation inhibitor abciximab (ReoPro).

Suplena (GI). Liquid nutritional supplement formulated for patients with renal disease. Liquid.

suppository. 37

Supprelin (Endo). Used to treat precocious puberty. For dosage, see *histrelin*. [soo-PRAY-lihn].

Suprane (Anes). Used to induce and maintain general anesthesia. Inhaled gas. [SOO-prayn]. 370

Suprax (Antibio). Cephalosporin antibiotic used to treat various types of bacterial infections, including *Streptococcus, E. coli, H. influenzae*, and gonorrhea. For dosage, see *cefixime*. [SOO-pracks]. 316

suprofen (Profenal) (Oph). Topical nonsteroidal anti-inflammatory drug used only during eye surgery to prevent miosis. Ophthalmic solution: 1%. [soo-PROH-fehn].

suramin (Metaret) (Chemo). Chemotherapy drug used to treat prostate cancer. Orphan drug. 348

Surfak Liquigels (GI). Stool softener laxative. For dosage, see *docusate*. 125

Surgicel (Hem). Topical hemostatic drug used to control bleeding during surgery. Strip. Surgical Nu-knit.

Surmontil (Psych). Tricyclic antidepressant. For dosage, see *trimipramine*. [sehr-MAWN-till]. 286

Survanta (Resp). Natural lung surfactant used to prevent and treat respiratory distress syndrome in premature newborns. For dosage, see *beractant*. [sehr-VEHN-tah]. 201

suspension (drug form). 37

Sustacal, Sustacal Basic, Sustacal Plus (GI). Liquid nutritional supplement. Liquid. Powder (to be reconstituted). Pudding.

Sustagen (GI). Liquid nutritional supplement. Powder (to be reconstituted).

Sustaire (Resp). Bronchodilator. For dosage, see *theophylline*. 193

Sustiva (Antivir). Nonnucleoside reverse transcriptase inhibitor drug used to treat AIDS. For dosage, see *efavirenz*. [suhs-TEE-vah]. 325

(sutilains) (Derm). No longer on the market. (Trade name *Travase*; topical drug used to debride burns and wounds).

swish and swallow. 211

Symlin (Diab). Given to patients with type I and type II diabetes mellitus to delay gastric emptying and improve blood sugar control. For dosage, see *pramlintide*.

Symmetrel (Antivir, Neuro, Resp). Used to treat influenza A virus respiratory tract infection; used to treat Parkinson's disease. For dosage, see *amantadine*. [SIH-meh-trell]. 268, 330

Synagis (Antivir). Monoclonal antibody used to treat respiratory syncytial virus. For dosage, see *palivizumab*. [SIH-nah-jihs].

Synalar, Synalar-HP (Derm) (generic *fluocinolone*). Topical corticosteroid anti-inflammatory drug. Cream: 0.01%, 0.025%, 0.2%. Liquid: 0.01%. Ointment: 0.025%. [SIH-neh-lawr]. 92

Synalgos-DC (Analges) (generic *dihydrocodeine, aspirin, caffeine*). Combination narcotic, nonnarcotic drug, and caffeine drug. (Schedule III drug). Capsule: 16 mg/356.4 mg/30 mg. [sih-NEHL-gohs]. 302

Synarel (Endo, OB/GYN). Hormonal drug used to treat precocious puberty in boys and girls; used to treat endometriosis. For dosage, see *nafarelin*. [SIHN-ah-rehl]. 248

Synercid (Antibio) (generic *dalfopristin, quinupristin*). Combination antibiotic drug used to treat life-threatening bacterial infections from *Staphylococcus* and vancomycin-resistant bacteria. Intravenous: 350 mg/500 mg per 10 mL. [SIH-nehr-sihd]. 320

synergism. 56

Synovir (Antivir). Used to treat AIDS wasting syndrom. For dosage, see *thalidomide*.

SYNSORB Cd (Antivir). Used to treat *Clostridium difficile* AIDS-related diarrhea. Investigational drug. 328

Synthroid (Endo). Thyroid hormone replacement. For dosage, see *levothyroxine*. [SIN-throyd]. 229

Syntocinon (OB/GYN). Used to stimulate uterine contractions; used to treat postpartum uterine bleeding; used to treat incomplete abortion. For dosage, see *oxytocin*. [sihn-TOH-seh-nawn]. 246, 248

Synvisc (Ortho). Used to maintain the lubricating quality of the synovial fluid in patients with osteoarthritis. For dosage, see *hyaluronic acid derivative*. [SIHN-vihsk].

syphilis, drugs used to treat. 258

syringe, insulin. 63, 239

syringe, tuberculin (TB). 66

syrup. 36

systemic effect. 50

tablet.
   enteric. 34
   long-acting (LA). 34
   scored. 33
   slow-release (SR). 34

Tabloid (Chemo). Pure antagonist chemotherapy drug used to treat leukemia. For dosage, see *thioguanine*. 339

Tabron (Misc). Multivitamin with iron nutritional supplement. Tablet.

(Tacaryl) (GI). No longer on the market. (Generic name *methdilazine*; antiemetic drug).

(Tace) (Chemo, OB/GYN). No longer on the market. (Generic name *chlorotrianisene*; hormonal chemotherapy drug, estrogen replacement for menopause).

Tac-40 (Endo, Ortho). Corticosteroid anti-inflammatory drug used to treat severe inflammation in various body systems; injected into a joint to treat osteoarthritis and rheumatoid arthritis. For dosage, see *triamcinolone*. 233

tacrine (Cognex) (Neuro). Cholinesterase inhibitor used to treat Alzheimer's disease. Capsule: 10 mg, 20 mg, 30 mg, 40 mg. [TEH-kreen]. 271

tacrolimus (Prograf) (Cardio, GI, Uro). Immunosuppressant drug given after organ transplant to prevent rejection of the donor heart, liver, or kidney. Capsule: 1 mg. Intravenous: 5 mg/mL. [tah-kroh-LY-muhs]. 110, 135, 174

tacrolimus (Protopic) (Derm). Topical nonsteroidal anti-inflammatory drug used to treat eczema. Ointment: 0.03%, 0.1%. [tah-kroh-LY-muhs]. 100

Tac-3 (Derm). Corticosteroid anti-inflammatory drug injected into skin lesions. For dosage, see *triamcinolone*. 92

Tagamet, Tagamet 200 HB (Derm, GI). H_2 blocker used in conjunction with standard antihistamines to treat chronic itching and hives; used to treat peptic ulcers and *H. pylori* infection. For dosage, see *cimetidine*. [TEH-gah-meht]. 94, 118

TA-HPV (Chemo). Recombinant DNA human papillomavirus drug used to treat cervical cancer. Orphan drug. 362

Talacen (Analges) (generic *acetaminophen, pentazocine*). Combination nonnarcotic and narcotic analgesic drug used to treat moderate-to-severe pain. (Schedule IV drug). Tablet: 650 mg/25 mg. [TEHL-ah-sehn]. 303

talc (Sclerosol Intrapleural Aerosol, Steritalc) (Chemo, Resp). Sclerosing drug administered via chest tube into the lung to treat malignant pleural effusion and pneumothorax. Powder.

Talwin (Analges, Anes). Narcotic analgesic drug used to treat moderate-to-severe pain; used as a preoperative drug to sedate. (Schedule IV drug). For dosage, see *pentazocine*. [TAWL-whin]. 298, 371

Talwin Compound (Analges) (generic *aspirin, pentazocine*). Combination nonnarcotic and narcotic analgesic drug used to treat moderate-to-severe pain. (Schedule IV drug). Tablet: 325 mg/12.5 mg. [TAWL-whin]. 302

Talwin NX (Analges) (generic *naloxone, pentazocine*). Combination narcotic antagonist and narcotic drug used to treat moderate-to-severe pain. (Schedule IV drug). Tablet: 0.5 mg/50 mg. [TAWL-whin]. 303

Tambocor (Cardio). Used to treat atrial and ventricular arrhythmias. For dosage, see *flecainide*. [TEHM-boh-kohr]. 159

Tamiflu (Antivir). Antiviral drug used to prevent and treat influenza A virus infections. For dosage, see *oseltamivir*. [TEH-meh-floo]. 330

tamoxifen (Nolvadex) (Chemo, Endo). Hormonal chemotherapy drug used to treat breast cancer; used to treat gynecomastia in men. Tablet: 10 mg, 20 mg. [tah-MAWK-sih-fehn]. 343

tamsulosin (Flomax) (Uro). Alpha$_1$-receptor blocker used to treat benign prostatic hypertrophy. Capsule: 0.4 mg. [tehm-soo-LOH-sihn]. 109

tannic acid (Zilactin Medicated) (ENT).   Topical drug used to form a protective covering over canker sores and cold sores in and around the mouth. Gel: 7%.

Tantum (Chemo).   Used to prevent oral mucositis in patients receiving radiation therapy for head and neck cancer.   For dosage, see *benzydamine*. 350

Tao (Antibio).   Macrolide antibiotic used to treat respiratory tract infections and pneumonia.   For dosage, see *troleandomycin*. [TAY-oh].

Tapazole (Endo).   Antithyroid drug used to treat hyperthyroidism.   For dosage, see *methimazole*. [TEH-peh-zawl]. 230

Tarabine PFS (Chemo).   Pyrimidine antagonist chemotherapy drug used to treat leukemia.   For dosage, see *cytarabine*. [TEH-rah-been]. 340

(Taractan) (Psych).   No longer on the market. (Generic name *chlorprothixene*; antipsychotic drug).

tardive dyskinesia.   In Depth feature.

Targocid (Antibio).   Vancomycin-type antibiotic. Investigational drug. 321

target organ.   51

Targretin (Chemo, Derm).   Oral and topical drug used to treat the cancerous skin lesions of cutaneous T-cell lymphoma.   For dosage, see *bexarotene*. [TAWR-greh-tihn]. 98, 347

Tasmar (Neuro).   COMT inhibitor used to treat Parkinson's disease.   For dosage, see *tolcapone*. [TEHZ-mahr]. 269

Tavist (Derm, ENT).   Antihistamine used to treat allergic rhinitis and allergic reactions with hives and itching.   For dosage, see *clemastine*. 207

(Tavist D) (ENT).   No longer on the market. (Combination drug with *phenylpropanolamine*; decongestant and antihistamine drug).

Taxol (Chemo, Uro).   Mitosis inhibitor chemotherapy drug used to treat breast cancer, ovarian cancer, lung cancer, head and neck cancer, gastrointestinal tract cancer, pancreatic cancer, prostatic cancer, non-Hodgkin's lymphoma, and Kaposi's sarcoma; used to treat polycystic kidney disease.   For dosage, see *paclitaxel*. [TACK-sawl]. 112, 344

Taxotere (Chemo).   Mitosis inhibitor chemotherapy drug used to treat breast cancer, lung cancer, head and neck cancer, gastric cancer, pancreatic cancer, ovarian cancer, prostatic cancer, bladder cancer, malignant melanoma, and non-Hodgkin's lymphoma. For dosage, see *docetaxel*. [TACK-soh-teer]. 344

tazarotene (Tazorac) (Derm).   Topical vitamin A-type drug used to treat acne vulgaris and psoriasis. Cream: 0.05%, 0.1%. Gel: 0.05%, 0.1%. [teh-ZEH-roh-teen]. 84, 86

Tazicef (Antibio).   Cephalosporin antibiotic used to treat a variety of bacterial infections, including *Strep-*

tococcus, *Staphylococcus*, *E. coli*, and *H. influenzae*. For dosage, see *ceftazidime*. [TEH-zih-sehf]. 316

Tazidime (Antibio).   Cephalosporin antibiotic used to treat a variety of bacterial infections, including *Streptococcus*, *Staphylococcus*, *E. coli*, and *H. influenzae*. For dosage, see *ceftazidime*. [TEH-zih-dime]. 316

Tazorac (Derm) (generic *tazarotene*).   Topical vitamin A-type drug used to treat acne vulgaris and psoriasis. Cream: 0.05%, 0.1%. Gel: 0.05%, 0.1%. [TEH-zoh-rack]. 84, 86

TB (abbreviation for *tuberculosis*).   See *tuberculosis*.

TB syringe.   See *tuberculin syringe*.

TCA (abbreviation for *tricyclic antidepressant*).   See *tricyclic antidepressants*.

Tears Naturale, Tears Naturale Free, Tears Naturale II, Tears Plus, Tears Renewed (Oph).   Artificial tears. Drops.

teceleukin (Chemo).   Interleukin-2 chemotherapy drug used to treat malignant melanoma and renal cancer. Orphan drug.   [teh-kee-LOO-kihn]. 361

Teczem (Cardio) (generic *diltiazem, enalapril*).   Combination antihypertensive drug. Tablet: 180 mg/5 mg. 166

(Tedral) (Resp).   No longer on the market. (Generic name *theophylline, ephedrine, phenobarbital*; combination bronchodilator and sedative).

tegaserod (Zelmac) (GI).   A 5-HT$_4$ (serotonin) blocker used to treat irritable bowel syndrome in women. Tablet: 6 mg. 135

(Tegison) (Derm).   No longer on the market. (Generic name *etretinate*; vitamin A-type drug used to treat psoriasis).

(Tegopen) (Antibio).   No longer on the market. (Generic name *cloxacillin*; penicillin-type antibiotic).

Tegretol, Tegretol-XR (Neuro, Psych).   Anticonvulsant drug used to treat tonic-clonic and partial seizures; used to treat trigeminal neuralgia; used to treat schizophrenia; used to treat manic-depressive disorder.   For dosage, see *carbamazepine*. [TEH-greh-tawl]. 265, 283, 289

Tegrin for Psoriasis, Tegrin Medicated, Tegrin Medicated for Psoriasis (Derm) (generic *coal tar*).   Topical drug used to treat psoriasis. Cream: 5%. Lotion: 5%. Shampoo: 7%. Soap: 5%. [TEH-grihn]. 86

Tegrin-LT (Derm).   Topical drug used to treat pediculosis (lice). Shampoo. 96

teicoplanin (Targocid) (Antibio).   Antibiotic similar to vancomycin. Investigational drug. 321

Teladar (Derm) (generic *betamethasone*).   Topical corticosteroid anti-inflammatory drug. Cream: 0.05%. 92

(Teldrin 12-Hour Allergy Relief) (ENT).   No longer on the market. (Combination drug with *phen-*

ylpropanolamine; decongestant and antihistamine drug).

telithromycin (Ketek) (Antibio, Resp).   Ketolide class of antibiotic used to treat community-acquired pneumonia. Tablet: 400 mg. [teh-lith-roh-MY-sihn].

telmisartan (Micardis) (Cardio).   Angiotensin II receptor blocker used to treat hypertension. Tablet: 40 mg, 80 mg. 164

(Temaril) (GI).   No longer on the market. (Generic name *trimeprazine;* antiemetic drug).

temazepam (Restoril) (Neuro).   Nonbarbiturate benzodiazepine drug used to treat insomnia. (Schedule IV drug). Capsule: 7.5 mg, 15 mg, 30 mg. [teh-MEH-zeh-pahm]. 272

Tembid.   Part of the trade name of a drug, indicating sustained-release tablet. 65

Temodal (Chemo).   Chemotherapy drug used to treat metastatic melanoma.   For dosage, see *temozolomide.* 348

Temodar (Chemo).   Chemotherapy drug used to treat brain cancer.   For dosage, see *temozolomide.* [TEH-moh-dahr]. 248

temoporfin (Foscan) (Chemo).   Chemotherapy drug used to treat head and neck cancer. Orphan drug. 248

Temovate (Derm) (generic *clobetasol*).   Topical corticosteroid anti-inflammatory drug. Cream: 0.05%. Gel: 0.05%. Liquid: 0.05%. Ointment: 0.05%. [TEH-moh-vayt]. 92

temozolomide (Temodal, Temodar) (Chemo).   Chemotherapy drug used to treat metastatic melanoma and brain cancer. Capsule: 5 mg, 20 mg, 100 mg, 250 mg. [teh-moh-ZOH-loh-mide]. 348

Tempra 1, Tempra 2, Tempra 3 (Analges).   Nonnarcotic nonaspirin analgesic drug used to treat fever and pain in children.   For dosage, see *acetaminophen.* 301

tenecteplase (TNKase) (Cardio, Hem).   Tissue plasminogen activator used to dissolve blood clots from myocardial infarction. Intravenous (powder to be reconstituted): 50 mg. [teh-NEHK-teh-plays]. 174, 188

Tenex (Cardio, Psych).   Alpha$_2$-receptor blocker used to treat hypertension; used to treat withdrawal from heroin; an orphan drug used to treat fragile X syndrome.   For dosage, see *guanfacine.* 165, 293

tenidap (Enable) (Ortho).   Anti-inflammatory cytokine inhibitor used to treat rheumatoid arthritis. Investigational drug. 148

teniposide (Vumon) (Chemo).   Mitosis inhibitor chemotherapy drug used to treat leukemia. Intravenous: 10 mg/mL. [teh-NIH-poh-side]. 344

Ten-K (Uro).   Potassium supplement used to replace potassium loss caused by diuretics. Tablet: 10 mEq. 105

tenofovir (Viread) (Antivir).   Nucleotide reverse transcriptase inhibitor drug used to treat AIDS. Tablet: 300 mg. [teh-NOH-foh-veer]. 324

Tenoretic 50, Tenoretic 100 (Cardio) (generic *atenolol, chlorthalidone*).   Combination beta-blocker antihypertensive and diuretic drug. Tablet: 50 mg/25 mg, 100 mg/25 mg. [teh-noh-REH-tihk]. 167

Tenormin (Analges, GI, Psych).   Cardioselective beta-blocker drug used to treat migraine headaches; used to prevent rebleeding from esophageal varices in patients with cirrhosis; used to treat alcohol withdrawal syndrome and performance anxiety.   For dosage, see *atenolol.* [teh-NOHR-mihn]. 132, 290, 306

Tenormin (Cardio).   Cardioselective beta-blocker drug used to treat angina pectoris, hypertension, and ventricular arrhythmias; used to prevent repeat myocardial infarction.   For dosage, see *atenolol.* [teh-NOHR-mihn]. 157, 158, 160, 162

Tenovil (Antivir) (generic *interleukin-10*).   Used to treat AIDS. Investigational drug. 326

Tensilon (Neuro).   Anticholinesterase drug used to diagnose (not treat) myasthenia gravis.   For dosage, see *edrophonium.* [TEHN-sih-lawn]. 275

Tenuate, Tenuate Dospan (GI).   Appetite suppressant used to treat obesity. (Schedule IV drug).   For dosage, see *diethylpropion.* [TEH-yoo-ate]. 129

Tequin (Antibio).   Fluoroquinolone antibiotic used to treat many types of infections; used to treat Legionnaire's disease.   For dosage, see *gatifloxacin.* [TEH-kwihn]. 105, 198, 318

Terazol 3, Terazol 7 (OB/GYN) (generic *terconazole*).   Topical drug used to treat vaginal yeast infections. Vaginal cream: 0.4%, 0.6%. Vaginal suppository: 80 mg. [TEH-reh-zohl]. 256

terazosin (Hytrin) (Cardio, Uro).   Alpha$_1$-receptor blocker used to treat hypertension; used to treat benign prostatic hypertrophy. Capsule: 1 mg, 2 mg, 5 mg, 10 mg. [teh-rah-ZOH-sihn]. 109, 165

terbinafine (Lamisil AT, Lamisil DermGel) (Derm).   Topical antifungal drug. Cream: 1%. Gel: 1%. Spray: 1%. [tehr-BIH-neh-fine]. 89

terbinafine (Lamisil) (Antifung).   Oral drug used to treat severe topical fungal infections. Tablet: 250 mg. [tehr-BIH-neh-fine]. 334

terbutaline (Brethaire, Bricanyl) (Resp).   Bronchodilator. Aerosol inhaler: 200 mcg/puff. Tablet: 2.5 mg, 5 mg. Subcutaneous: 1 mg/mL. [tehr-BYOO-tah-leen]. 193

(terbutaline) (OB/GYN).   No longer used to stop premature labor contractions. (Trade name *Bricanyl*).

terconazole (Terazol 3, Terazol 7) (OB/GYN).   Topical drug used to treat vaginal yeast infections. Vaginal cream: 0.4%, 0.6%. Vaginal suppository: 80 mg. [tehr-KAW-neh-zohl]. 256

(terfenadine) (ENT). No longer on the market. (Trade name *Seldane*; antihistamine).

terlipressin (Glypressin) (GI). Sclerosing drug used to to stop bleeding from esophageal varices. Intravenous (injected into the esophageal varix). [tehr-lih-PREH-sihn]. 135

terodiline (Micturin) (Uro). Used to treat urinary incontinence. Investigational drug. 112

terpin hydrate (ENT). Expectorant. Liquid: 85 mg/5 mL. 210

(Terra-Cortril) (Oph). No longer on the market. (Combination corticosteroid and antibiotic drug for the eye).

Terramycin IM (Antibio, OB/GYN). Tetracycline antibiotic used to treat a variety of infections, including gonorrhea, syphilis, and *Chlamydia*. For dosage, see *oxytetracycline*. [teh-rah-MY-sihn]. 317

Teslac (Chemo). Hormonal chemotherapy drug used to treat breast cancer. (Schedule III drug). For dosage, see *testolactone*. [TEHS-lack] 343

TESPA. See *thiotepa*.

Tessalon, Tessalon Perles (ENT). Nonnarcotic antitussive drug. For dosage, see *benzonatate*. [TEH-seh-lawn]. 210

testing.
  animal drug. 27
  control group in drug. 28
  human drug. 27
  in vitro drug. 27
  in vivo drug. 27
  new drug. 27
  volunteers for drug. 28

Testoderm, Testoderm TTS (Endo). Male sex hormone used to treat the lack of production of testosterone due to absence, injury, or malfunction of the testes or malfunction of the pituitary gland; used to treat delayed puberty in boys. For dosage, see *testosterone*. [TEHS-toh-dehrm].

testolactone (Teslac) (Chemo). Hormonal chemotherapy drug used to treat breast cancer. (Schedule III drug). Tablet: 50 mg. [tehs-toh-LACK-tohn]. 343

Testopel (Endo). Male sex hormone used to treat the lack of production of testosterone due to absence, injury, or malfunction of the testes or malfunction of the pituitary gland; used to treat delayed puberty in boys. For dosage, see *testosterone*. [TEHS-toh-pehl].

testosterone (AndroGel, Theraderm Testosterone Transdermal System) (Antivir). Used to treat AIDS wasting syndrome. Orphan drug. 327

testosterone (Androderm, Delatestryl, Depo-Testosterone, Testoderm, Testoderm TTS, Testopel) (Endo).

Male sex hormone used to treat the lack of production of testosterone due to absence, injury, or malfunction of the testes or malfunction of the pituitary gland; used to treat delayed puberty in boys. Intramuscular: 100 mg/mL, 200 mg/mL. Sublingual: (orphan drug). Transdermal patch: 2.5 mg/ 24 hr, 4 mg/24 hr, 5 mg/24 hr, 6 mg/24 hr. Pellets (implanted under the skin): 75 mg. [tehs-TAW-steh-rohn].

testosterone (AndroGel) (Endo). Topical male sex hormone used to treat lack of production of testosterone due to absence, injury, or malfunction of the testes or malfunction of the pituitary gland. Gel: 1%. [tehs-TAW-steh-rohn].

testosterone (Delatestryl) (Chemo). Male sex hormone used to treat breast cancer in women. Intramuscular: 200 mg/mL. [tehs-TAW-steh-rohn]. 343

Testred (Chemo, Endo). Male sex hormone used to treat breast cancer in women; used to treat the lack of production of testosterone due to absence, injury, or malfunction of the testes or malfunction of the pituitary gland; used to treat delayed puberty in boys. For dosage, see *methyltestosterone*. [TEHS-trehd]. 343

tetrabenazine (Neuro, Psych). Used to treat Huntington's chorea; used to treat tardive dyskinesia side effects of antipsychotic drugs. Orphan drug. 277, 284

tetracaine (Pontocaine) (Anes). Spinal/epidural anesthetic drug. Injection: 0.2%, 0.3%, 1%. [TEH-trah-kayn]. 368

tetracaine (Pontocaine) (ENT, GI, Resp). Topical anesthetic applied to the nose and throat prior to laryngoscopy, esophagoscopy, and bronchoscopy. Liquid: 2%. [TEH-trah-kayn].

tetracaine (Pontocaine, Viractin) (Derm). Topical anesthetic. Cream: 2%. Gel: 2%. Ointment: 1%. [TEH-trah-kayn]. 94

tetracaine (Oph). Topical anesthetic drug for the eyes. Ophthalmic solution: 0.5%. [TEH-trah-kayn].

tetracyclic antidepressants (Psych). Class of drugs used to treat depression. 286

tetracycline (Achromycin) (Derm). Topical antibiotic used to treat acne vulgaris. Ointment: 3%. [teh-trah-SY-kleen]. 84

tetracycline (Actisite) (ENT). Topical drug used to treat periodontitis in the mouth. Fiber packing. [teh-trah-SY-kleen].

tetracycline (Panmycin, Sumycin, Sumycin 250, Sumycin 500, Tetracyn, Tetracyn 500, Tetralan) (Antibio). Antibiotic used to treat a variety of infections, including acne vulgaris, *H. pylori* of the gastrointestinal tract, *Chlamydia*, gonorrhea, and syphilis. Capsule: 100 mg, 250 mg, 500 mg. Tablet: 250 mg, 500 mg. Liquid: 125 mg/5 mL. [teh-trah-SY-kleen]. 84, 120, 317

tetracyclines (Antibio). Class of antibiotics. 317

Tetracyn, Tetracyn 500 (Antibio). Antibiotic used to treat a variety of infections, including acne vulgaris, *H. pylori* of the gastrointestinal tract, *Chlamydia*, gonorrhea, and syphilis. For dosage, see *tetracycline*. [TEH-trah-sihn]. 84, 120, 317

tetrahydrozoline (ENT). Decongestant. Drops: 0.05%, 0.1%. Spray: 0.05%, 0.1%. [teh-trah-hy-DRAW-zoh-leen]. 206

tetrahydrozoline (Collyrium Fresh, Eyesine, Murine Plus, Optigene 3, Tetrasine, Tetrasine Extra, Visine Allergy Relief) (Oph). Topical decongestant/vasoconstrictor used to treat irritation and allergy symptoms in the eyes. Ophthalmic solution: 0.05%. [teh-trah-hy-DRAW-zoh-leen].

Tetralan (Antibio). Antibiotic used to treat a variety of infections, including acne vulgaris, *H. pylori* of the gastrointestinal tract, *Chlamydia*, gonorrhea, and syphilis. For dosage, see *tetracycline*. [TEH-trah-lehn]. 84, 317

Tetrasine (Oph). Topical decongestant/vasoconstrictor used to treat irritation and allergy symptoms in the eyes. For dosage, see *tetrahydrozoline*. [TEH-trah-seen].

Teveten (Cardio). Angiotensin II receptor blocker used to treat hypertension. For dosage, see *eprosartan*. 164

thalidomide, history of. Historical Notes feature. 15, 328

thalidomide (Thalomid) (Antivir, Chemo, GI). Used to treat AIDS wasting syndrome; used to treat aphthous stomatitis in AIDS patients; used to treat brain cancer, multiple myeloma, and Kaposi's sarcoma; used to prevent graft-versus-host disease after bone marrow transplantation; used to treat Crohn's disease. Orphan drug. (Synovir). Capsule: 50 mg. [theh-LIH-doh-mide]. 135, 328, 348, 362

Thalomid (Antivir, Chemo, GI). Used to treat AIDS wasting syndrome; used to treat aphthous stomatitis in AIDS patients; used to treat brain cancer, multiple myeloma, and Kaposi's sarcoma; used to prevent graft-versus-host disease after bone marrow transplantation; used to treat Crohn's disease. For dosage, see *thalidomide*. 135, 327, 348, 362

Tham (Emerg). Used to treat metabolic acidosis during cardiac arrest. For dosage, see *tromethamine*. 181

THC (abbreviation for *delta-9-tetrahydrocannabinol*). See *dronabinol*. 128

Theobid Duracaps (Resp). Bronchodilator. For dosage, see *theophylline*. 193

Theo-Dur (Resp). Bronchodilator. For dosage, see *theophylline*. 193

Theolair, Theolair-SR (Resp). Bronchodilator; used to prevent apnea in premature infants. For dosage, see *theophylline*. 193

theophylline (Accurbron, Bronkodyl, Elixophyllin, Quibron-T Dividose, Quibron-T/SR Dividose, Respbid, Slo-bid Gyrocaps, Slo-Phyllin, Slo-Phyllin Gyrocaps, Sustaire, Theobid Duracaps, Theo-Dur, Theolair, Theolair-SR, Theovent, T-Phyl, Uniphyl) (Resp). Bronchodilator; used to prevent apnea in premature infants. Capsule: 60 mg, 100 mg, 125 mg, 130 mg, 200 mg, 250 mg, 260 mg, 300 mg. Liquid: 80 mg/15 mL, 150 mg/15 mL Tablet: 100 mg, 125 mg, 200 mg, 250 mg, 300 mg, 400 mg, 450 mg, 500 mg, 600 mg. [thee-AW-feh-lihn]. 193

(Theo-24) (Resp). No longer on the market. (Generic name *theophylline*; bronchodilator).

Theovent (Resp). Bronchodilator. For dosage, see *theophylline*. [THEE-oh-vehnt]. 193

TheraCys (Chemo). Chemotherapy drug used to treat bladder cancer. For dosage, see *BCG*. [THEH-rah-sihs]. 347

Theraderm Testosterone Transdermal System (Antivir). Used to treat AIDS wasting syndrome. For dosage, see *testosterone*. 328

Therafectin (Ortho). Used to treat rheumatoid arthritis. Investigational drug. 147

TheraFlu Flu and Cold Medicine (ENT) (generic *pseudoephedrine, chlorpheniramine, acetaminophen*). Combination decongestant, antihistamine, and analgesic drug. Powder (to be dissolved in hot water): 60 mg/4 mg/650 mg.

TheraFlu Flu, Cold & Cough (ENT) (generic *pseudoephedrine, chlorpheniramine, dextromethorphan, acetaminophen*). Combination decongestant, antihistamine, nonnarcotic antitussive, and analgesic drug. Powder (to be mixed with water): 60 mg/4 mg/20 mg/650 mg.

TheraFlu Non-Drowsy Flu, Cold & Cough Maximum Strength (ENT) (generic *pseudoephedrine, dextromethorphan, acetaminophen*). Combination decongestant, nonnarcotic antitussive, and analgesic drug. Powder (to be mixed with water): 60 mg/30 mg/1000 mg.

TheraFlu Non-Drowsy Formula Maximum Strength (ENT) (generic *pseudoephedrine, dextromethorphan, acetaminophen*). Combination decongestant, nonnarcotic antitussive, and analgesic drug. Caplet: 30 mg/15 mg/500 mg.

Theragran Hematinic Tablet (Misc). Multivitamin with iron nutritional supplement. Tablet.

Theragran Stress Formula (Misc). Multivitamin with iron nutritional supplement. Tablet.

Theragyn (Chemo). Monoclonal antibody chemotherapy drug used to treat ovarian cancer. Orphan drug. 346

therapeutic effect. 51

therapeutic index (TI). 53, 66

Therapeutic Mineral Ice, Therapeutic Mineral Ice Exercise Formula (Ortho). Topical irritant drug used to mask the pain of arthritis and muscular aches. Gel.

Theratope-STn (Chemo). Cancer vaccine. Investigational drug. 349

thiazide diuretics (Uro). Class of drugs used to excrete sodium and water from the body.

thiethylperazine (Torecan) (GI). Antiemetic drug. Tablet: 10 mg. Intramuscular: 5 mg/mL. [thy-eh-thul-PEH-rah-zeen]. 127

thioguanine (Tabloid) (Chemo). Purine antagonist chemotherapy drug used to treat leukemia. Tablet: 40 mg. [thy-oh-GWAH-neen]. 339

Thiola (Uro). Used to prevent the formation of cystine kidney stones in patients with cystinuria. For dosage, see *tiopronin*. 112

thiopental (Pentothal) (Anes). Barbiturate used to induce and maintain general anesthesia. Intravenous: 20 mg/mL (2%), 25 mg/mL (2.5%). [thy-oh-PEHN-tawl]. 367, 369

Thioplex (Chemo). Alkylating chemotherapy drug used to treat breast cancer, ovarian cancer, and Hodgkin's disease. For dosage, see *thiotepa*. [THY-oh-plehks]. 341

thioridazine (Mellaril, Mellaril-S) (Psych). Phenothiazine drug used to treat psychosis, used to treat anxiety; used as short-term treatment for explosive, impulsive behavior and mood lability in children; used to treat attention-deficit/hyperactivity disorder. Tablet: 10 mg, 15 mg, 25 mg, 50 mg, 100 mg, 150 mg, 200 mg. Liquid: 30 mg/mL, 100 mg/mL. Suspension: 25 mg/5 mL, 100 mg/5 mL. [thy-oh-RIH-dah-zeen]. 283, 292

(Thiosulfil Forte) (Antibio, Uro). No longer on the market. (Generic name *sulfamethizole*; sulfonamide anti-infective drug).

thiotepa (Thioplex) (Chemo). Alkylating chemotherapy drug used to treat breast cancer, ovarian cancer, and Hodgkin's disease. Intravenous, intracavitary, or intravesical (powder to be reconstituted): 15 mg. [thy-oh-TEH-pah]. 341

thiothixene (Navane) (Psych). Used to treat psychosis. Capsule: 1 mg, 2 mg, 5 mg, 10 mg, 20 mg. Liquid: 5 mg/mL. 284

Thorazine. Historical Notes feature. 283

Thorazine, Thorazine Spansules (GI). Antiemetic drug; used to treat nausea and vomiting caused by chemotherapy; used to treat intractable hiccoughs. For dosage, see *chlorpromazine*. [THOR-ah-zeen]. 127

Thorazine, Thorazine Spansules (Psych). Phenothiazine drug used to treat psychosis; used to treat manic-depressive disorder; used as short-term treatment for explosive, impulsive behavior and mood lability in children; used to treat attention-

deficit/hyperactivity disorder. For dosage, see *chlorpromazine*. [THOR-ah-zeen]. 283, 289, 292

3HT. See *lamivudine*.

Threostat (Neuro). Used to treat the spasticity associated with amyotrophic lateral sclerosis. For dosage, see *L-threonin*. 276

Thrombate III (Hem). Used to treat patients with antithrombin III deficiency. For dosage, see *antithrombin III*.

thrombin (Thrombostat, Thrombogen) (Hem). Topical hemostatic drug used to control oozing bleeding. Powder.

Thrombogen (Hem). Topical hemostatic drug used to control oozing bleeding. Powder.

thrombolytic drugs. 187

Thrombostat (Hem). Topical hemostatic drug used to control oozing bleeding. Powder.

thrush. 210

thymalfasin (Zadaxin) (Chemo, GI). Chemotherapy drug used to treat liver cancer; used to treat hepatitis B. Orphan drug. 135, 348

Thymitaq (Chemo). Chemotherapy drug used to treat head and neck cancer, lung cancer, gastric cancer, pancreatic cancer, and colon cancer. For dosage, see *nolatrexed*.

Thymoglobulin (Chemo, Uro). Immunoglobulin used to treat rejection of donor kidney after organ transplantation; orphan drug used to treat myelodysplastic syndrome. Intravenous: 25 mg. [thy-moh-GLAW-byoo-lihn].

thymopentin (Timunox) (Antivir). Used to treat AIDS. Investigational drug. 326

(thyroglobulin) (Endo). No longer on the market. (Trade name *Proloid*; thyroid hormone replacement).

thyroid gland dysfunction, drugs used to treat. 229

Thyrolar (Endo). Thyroid hormone replacement used to treat hypothyroidism. For dosage, see *liotrix*. [THY-roh-lawr]. 229

TI (abbreviation for *therapeutic index*). See *index, therapeutic*.

tiagabine (Gabitril Filmtabs) (Neuro). Anticonvulsant drug used to treat simple and complex partial seizures. Tablet: 2 mg, 4 mg, 12 mg, 16 mg. [tee-ah-GEH-been]. 265

Tiamate (Cardio). Calcium channel blocker used to treat angina pectoris, hypertension, and atrial and ventricular arrhythmias; used to treat Raynaud's disease. For dosage, see *diltiazem*. 157, 160, 163

tiapride (Psych). Used to treat Tourette's syndrome. Orphan drug.

tiazofurin (Tiazole) (Chemo). Chemotherapy drug used to treat leukemia. Orphan drug. 348

Tiazole (Chemo). Chemotherapy drug used to treat leukemia. For dosage, see *tiazofurin*. 348

tibolone (Livial, Xyvion) (OB/GYN). Steroid that stimulates estrogen, progesterone, and androgen receptors; used to treat menopause in women who cannot or will not take estrogen hormone replacement therapy. Investigational drug. 253

Ticar (Antibio). Penicillin-type antibiotic used to treat a variety of infections, including *Pseudomonas aeruginosa* and *E. coli*. For dosage, see *ticarcillin*. [TY-kawr]. 313

ticarcillin (Ticar) (Antibio). Penicillin-type antibiotic used to treat a variety of infections, including *Pseudomonas aeruginosa* and *E. coli*. Intramuscular or intravenous (powder to be reconstituted): 1 g, 3 g, 6 g. [TY-kawr-sill-ehn]. 313

TICE BCG (Chemo). Chemotherapy drug used to treat bladder cancer. For dosage, see *BCG*. 347

TICE BCG (Resp). Immunization drug used to treat children who are around persons with untreated or poorly treated tuberculosis. Multi-tine device.

Ticlid (Hem, Neuro). Platelet aggregation inhibitor used to prevent blood clots and reduce the risk of stroke in patients with a previous history of stroke. For dosage, see *ticlopidine*. [TY-klihd]. 187, 277

ticlopidine (Ticlid) (Hem, Neuro). Platelet aggregation inhibitor used to prevent blood clots and reduce the risk of stroke in patients with a previous history of stroke. Tablet: 250 mg. [ty-KLOH-peh-deen]. 187, 277

ticonazole (Monistat 1, Vagistat-1) (OB/GYN). Topical antiyeast drug used to treat vaginal infections. Vaginal ointment: 6.5%. [ty-KAW-neh-zohl].

t.i.d. (abbreviation meaning *three times a day*).

Tigan (GI). Antiemetic drug. For dosage, see *trimethobenzamide*. [TY-gehn]. 127

Tikosyn (Cardio). Used to treat atrial arrhythmias. For dosage, see *dofetilide*. [TEE-koh-sihn].

Tilade (Resp). Mast cell stabilizer used to prevent acute asthma attacks. For dosage, see *nedocromil*. [TY-layd]. 197

tiludronate (Skelid) (Ortho). Inhibits the breakdown of bone; used to treat Paget's disease. Tablet: 240 mg. 148

Timentin (Antibio) (generic *ticarcillin, clavulanic acid*). Combination penicillin-type antibiotoic and beta-lactimase inhibitor drug. Intravenous (powder to be reconstituted): 3 g/0.1 mg. [ty-MEHN-tihn]. 320

Timolide 10-25 (Cardio) (generic *timolol, hydrochlorothiazide*). Combination beta-blocker antihypertensive and diuretic drug. Tablet: 10 mg/25 mg. [TIH-moh-lide]. 167

timolol (Blocadren) (Analges, Ortho, Psych). Nonselective beta-blocker used to treat migraine headaches; used to treat essential familial tremors; used to treat performance anxiety. Tablet: 5 mg, 10 mg, 20 mg. [TIH-moh-lawl]. 146, 306

timolol (Blocadren) (Cardio). Nonselective beta-blocker used to treat hypertension and ventricular arrhythmias; used to prevent a repeat myocardial infarction. Tablet: 5 mg, 10 mg, 20 mg. [TIH-moh-lawl]. 158, 160, 162

timolol (Betimol, Timoptic, Timoptic-XE) (Oph). Topical beta-receptor blocker used to treat glaucoma. Ophthalmic solution: 0.25%, 0.5%. Ocudose/Ocumeter. [TIH-moh-lawl]. 221

Timoptic, Timoptic-XE (Oph). Topical beta-receptor blocker used to treat glaucoma. For dosage, see *timolol*. [tih-MAWP-tihk]. 221

Timunox (Antivir). Used to treat AIDS. For dosage, see *thymopentin*. [TIH-myoo-nawks]. 326

Tinactin, Tinactin for Jock Itch (Derm) (generic *tolnaftate*). Topical antifungal drug. Cream: 1%. Liquid: 1%. Powder: 1%. Spray: 1%. [tih-NEHK-tihn]. 89

(Tindal) (Psych). No longer on the market. (Generic name *acetophenazine*; phenothiazine antipsychotic drug).

tine test (Aplitest, Tine Test PPD) (Resp). Screening test device with multiple tines coated with purified protein derivative (PPD) from *Mycobacterium tuberculosis* to test for tuberculosis. Tine test: 5 TU/unit.

Tine Test PPD (Resp). Screening test device with multiple tines coated with purified protein derivative (PPD) from *Mycobacterium tuberculosis* to test for tuberculosis. For dosage, see *tine test*.

tinea corporis. See *ringworm*.

tinea cruris. See *jock itch*.

tinea pedis. See *athlete's foot*.

Ting (Derm) (generic *miconazole*). Topical antifungal drug. Cream: 1%. 89

tinzaparin (Innohep) (Hem). Low molecular weight heparin anticoagulant. Subcutaneous: 20,000 IU/mL. [tihn-SEH-peh-rihn].

tioconazole (Monistat-1, Vagistat-1) (OB/GYN). Topical drug used to treat vaginal yeast infections. Vaginal ointment: 6.5%. [ty-oh-KAW-neh-zohl]. 256

tiopronin (Thiola) (Uro). Used to prevent the formation of cystine kidney stones in patients with cystinuria. Tablet: 100 mg.

tiratricol (Triacana) (Endo). Used to suppress the release of thyroid-stimulating hormone from the pituitary gland of patients with thyroid cancer. Orphan drug. 230

tirilazad (Neuro). Antioxidant that helps tissue survive after a central nervous system injury. Investigational drug.

tirofiban (Aggrastat) (Cardio, Hem). Platelet aggregation inhibitor used to prevent blood clots in patients with unstable angina or myocardial infarction, or who are undergoing angioplasty or atherectomy. Intravenous: 50 mcg/mL, 250 mcg/mL. 174, 187

Tisit, Tisit Blue (Derm). Topical drug used to treat pediculosis (lice). Gel, liquid, shampoo. 96

tissue plasminogen activators (tPA) (Hem). Class of drugs that dissolve blood clots. 188

Titradose. Part of the trade name of drug, indicating a scored, dividable tablet. 66

Titralac, Titralac Extra Strength (GI). Calcium-containing antacid. Chewable tablet: 420 mg, 750 mg. [TIH-treh-lack]. 116

Titralac Plus (GI) (generic *calcium, simethicone*). Combination antacid and anti-gas drug. Tablet: 420 mg/20 mg. Liquid: 500 mg/20 mg. [TIH-treh-lack]. 117

titrate. 66

tizanidine (Zanaflex) (Neuro, Ortho). Skeletal muscle relaxant used to treat severe muscle spasticity associated with multiple sclerosis, cerebral palsy, stroke, or spinal cord injury. Tablet: 4 mg. [ty-ZEH-nih-deen]. 145, 277

TMP (abbreviation for *trimethoprim*). See *trimethoprim*.

TNKase (Cardio, Hem). Tissue plasminogen activator used to dissolve blood clots from myocardial infarction. For dosage, see *tenecteplase*. 174, 188

TOBI (Antibio). Aminoglycoside antibiotic used to treat a variety of bacterial infections, including *Staphylococcus, E. coli, Pseudomonas,* and *Klebsiella;* used to treat cystic fibrosis patients with *Pseudomonas* infection. For dosage, see *tobramycin*. 317

TobraDex Ophthalmic Suspension (Oph) (generic *dexamethasone, tobramycin*). Topical combination corticosteroid and antibiotic drug. Ophthalmic suspension: 0.1%/0.3%. [TOH-brah-dehks].

tobramycin (Nebcin, Nebcin Pediatric, TOBI) (Antibio). Aminoglycoside antibiotic used to treat a variety of bacterial infections, including *Staphylococcus, E. coli, Pseudomonas,* and *Klebsiella;* used to treat cystic fibrosis patients with *Pseudomonas* infection. [toh-brah-MY-sihn]. 317

tobramycin (Defy, Tobrex) (Oph). Topical antibiotic used to treat bacterial eye infections. Ophthalmic solution: 0.3%. Ophthalmic ointment: 3 mg/g. [toh-brah-MY-sihn].

Tobrex (Oph). Topical antibiotic used to treat bacterial eye infections. For dosage, see *tobramycin*. [TOH-brehks]. 218

tocainide (Tonocard) (Cardio). Used to treat ventricular arrhythmias. Tablet: 400 mg, 600 mg. 159

tocolytic drugs (OB/GYN). Class of drugs used to stop premature/preterm labor. 246

Tofranil, Tofranil-PM (Analges, Diab, Neuro, Ortho). Tricyclic antidepressant used to treat migraines; used to treat diabetic neuropathy; used to treat postherpetic neuralgia; used to treat phantom limb pain. For dosage, see *imipramine*. [TOH-frah-nill]. 147, 241, 276, 307

Tofranil, Tofranil-PM (Psych, Uro). Tricyclic antidepressant used to treat depression; used to treat panic disorder; used to treat anorexia nervosa and bulimia nervosa; used to treat childhood bedwetting. For dosage, see *imipramine*. [TOH-frah-nill]. 111, 286, 289, 291

tolazamide (Tolinase) (Diab). Oral antidiabetic drug. Tablet: 100 mg, 200 mg, 500 mg. [toh-LEH-zah-mide]. 240

tolazoline (Priscoline) (Cardio). Used to treat persistent pulmonary hypertension in newborns with persistent fetal circulation. Intravenous: 25 mg/mL. [toh-LEH-zoh-leen]. 174

tolbutamide (Orinase) (Diab). Oral antidiabetic drug. Tablet: 500 mg. [tohl-BYOO-tah-mide]. 240

tolcapone (Tasmar) (Neuro). COMT inhibitor used to treat Parkinson's disease. Tablet: 100 mg, 200 mg. 269

Tolectin 200, Tolectin 600, Tolectin DS (Analges, Ortho). Nonsteroidal anti-inflammatory drug used to treat osteoarthritis and rheumatoid arthritis. For dosage, see *tolmetin*. [toh-LEHK-tihn]. 139, 304

Tolinase (Diab). Oral antidiabetic drug. For dosage, see *tolazamide*. [TOH-lih-nays]. 240

tolmetin (Tolectin 200, Tolectin 600, Tolectin DS) (Analges, Ortho). Nonsteroidal anti-inflammatory drug used to treat osteoarthritis and rheumatoid arthritis. Capsule: 400 mg. Tablet: 200 mg, 600 mg. 139, 304

tolnaftate (Absorbine Athlete's Foot Cream, Absorbine Footcare, Aftate for Athlete's Foot, Aftate for Jock Itch, Tinactin, Tinactin for Jock Itch) (Derm). Topical antifungal drug. Cream: 1%. Gel: 1%. Liquid: 1%. Powder: 1%. Spray: 1%. [tohl-NEHF-tayt]. 89

tolrestat (Alredase) (Diab). Used to treat diabetic neuropathy and retinopathy. Investigational drug. 241

tolterodine (Detrol, Detrol LA) (Uro). Used to treat overactive bladder. Tablet: 1 mg, 2 mg, 4 mg. [tohl-TEH-roh-dohn]. 112

Tonocard (Cardio). Used to treat ventricular arrhythmias. For dosage, see *tocainide*. [TOH-noh-kawrd]. 159

Topamax (Neuro). Anticonvulsant drug used to treat tonic-clonic and simple and complex partial seizures; used to treat Lennox–Gestaut syndrome. For dosage, see *topiramate*. [TOH-pah-macks]. 265

topical route, administration of drugs by the. 40

Topicort, Topicort LP (Derm) (generic *desoximetasone*). Topical corticosteroid anti-inflammatory drug. Cream: 0.05%, 0.25%. Gel: 0.05%. Ointment: 0.25%. [TAW-pih-kohrt]. 92

(Topicycline) (Derm). No longer on the market. (Generic name *tetracycline*; topical antibiotic used to treat acne vulgaris).

topiramate (Topamax) (Neuro). Anticonvulsant drug used to treat tonic-clonic and simple and complex partial seizures; used to treat Lennox–Gestaut syndrome. Sprinkle capsule: 15 mg, 25 mg. Tablet: 25 mg, 100 mg, 200 mg. [toh-PEER-ah-mayt]. 265

Toposar (Chemo). Mitosis inhibitor chemotherapy drug used to treat lung cancer, testicular cancer, liver cancer, ovarian cancer, uterine cancer, breast cancer, gastric cancer, leukemia, Hodgkin's disease, non-Hodgkin's lymphoma, rhabdomyosarcoma, and Kaposi's sarcoma. For dosage, see *etoposide*. [TOH-poh-sawr]. 344

topotecan (Hycamtin) (Chemo). Mitosis inhibitor chemotherapy drug used to treat lung cancer and ovarian cancer. Intravenous (powder to be reconstituted): 4 mg. [toh-poh-TEE-kehn]. 344

Toprol-XL (Analges, Ortho, Psych). Cardioselective beta-blocker used to treat migraine headaches; used to treat essential familial tremor; used to treat the side effects of muscle restlessness from antipsychotic drugs. For dosage, see *metoprolol*. [TOH-prawl]. 146, 294, 306

Toprol-XL (Cardio). Cardioselective beta-blocker used to treat angina pectoris, congestive heart failure, hypertension, and ventricular arrhythmias; used to prevent repeat myocardial infarction. For dosage, see *metoprolol*. [TOH-prawl]. 157, 158, 160

Toradol (Analges). Nonsteroidal anti-inflammatory drug used to treat pain; used to treat migraine headaches. For dosage, see *ketorolac*. [TOHR-ah-dawl]. 304, 307

Torecan (GI). Antiemetic drug. For dosage, see *thiethylperazine*. [TOHR-eh-kehn]. 127

toremifene (Fareston) (Chemo). Hormonal chemotherapy drug used to treat breast cancer. Tablet: 60 mg. [tohr-EH-mih-feen]. 343

Tornalate (Resp). Bronchodilator. For dosage, see *bitolterol*. [TOHR-neh-layt]. 193

torsemide (Demadex) (Uro). Loop diuretic. Tablet: 5 mg, 10 mg, 20 mg, 100 mg. Intravenous: 10 mg/mL. [TOHR-seh-mide]. 104

Totacillin (Antibio). Penicillin-type antibiotic used to treat various types of bacterial infections, including *E. coli* and gonorrhea; used to prevent subacute bacterial endocarditis. For dosage, see *ampicillin*. [toh-TEH-lah-sill-ehn]. 313

total parenteral nutrition (TPN) (I.V.).   Intravenous fluid of amino acids, electrolytes, vitamins, and minerals. 376

Tourette's syndrome, drugs used to treat. 293

toxic effect. 53

toxicology. 1

TPA (abbreviation for *tissue plasminogen activator*). See *tissue plasminogen activator*.

T-Phyl (Resp). Bronchodilator. For dosage, see *theophylline*. 193

TPN (abbreviation for *total parenteral nutrition*).   See *total parenteral nutrition*.

Trac Tabs 2X (Uro) (generic *L-hyoscyamine, methenamine, methylene blue*). Combination urinary tract antispasmodic and anti-infective drug. Tablet. 107

Tracleer (Resp). Endothelin receptor blocker used to dilate the pulmonary blood vessels in patients with pulmonary arterial hypertension. For dosage, see *bosentan*. 198

Tracrium (Anes, Resp). Muscle relaxant drug used during surgery; used to treat patients who are intubated and on the ventilator. For dosage, see *atracurium*. [TREH-kree-uhm]. 199, 370

Tracy, Margaret.

trade name of drug. 22

(Tral) (GI). No longer on the market. (Generic name *hexocyclium*; gastrointestinal antispasmodic drug).

tramadol (Ultram) (Analges). Nonnarcotic analgesic drug used to treat moderate-to-severe pain. Tablet: 50 mg. [TREH-mah-dawl]. 299

(Trancopal) (Psych). No longer on the market. (Generic name *chlormezanone*; antianxiety drug).

Trandate (Cardio). Alpha$_1$ and nonselective beta-receptor blocker used to treat hypertension and hypertensive crisis. For dosage, see *labetalol*. [TREHN- dayt]. 165

Trandate (Endo). Alpha$_1$ and nonselective beta-receptor blocker used to treat hypertension caused by pheochromocytoma of the adrenal medulla. For dosage, see *labetalol*. [TREHN-dayt]. 168

trandolapril (Mavik) (Cardio). Angiotensin-converting enzyme inhibitor used to treat hypertension. Tablet: 1 mg, 2 mg, 4 mg. [trehn-DOH-lah-prihl]. 164

tranexamic acid (Cyklokapron) (Hem). Hemostatic drug used to prevent or treat hemorrhage in hemophiliac patients; used during tooth extractions in hemophiliac patients. Tablet: 500 mg. Intravenous: 100 mg/mL. [treh-nehk-SEH-mihk EH-sehd].

tranquilizers.

major. See *antipsychotic drugs*.

minor. See *antianxiety drugs*.

transdermal patch. 38

transdermal route, administration of drugs by the. 40

Transderm-Nitro (Cardio).   Nitrate drug used to prevent and treat angina pectoris.   For dosage, see *nitroglycerin.* 156

Transderm-Scop (GI).   Antiemetic drug used to treat motion sickness; used to decrease peristalsis in irritable bowel syndrome.   For dosage, see *scopolamine.* 128

Tranxene, Tranxene-SD, Tranxene-SD Half Strength, Tranxene-T (Neuro, Psych).   Benzodiazepine drug used to treat anxiety and neurosis; used to treat alcohol withdrawal, used to treat partial seizures. (Schedule IV drug).   For dosage, see *clorazepate.* [TREHN-zeen]. 264, 281

tranylcypromine (Parnate) (Psych).   MAO inhibitor used to treat depression. Tablet: 10 mg. [trah-nihl-SIH-proh-meen]. 288

trastuzumab (Herceptin) (Chemo).   Human monoclonal antibody used to treat breast cancer and pancreatic cancer. Intravenous (powder to be reconstituted): 440 mg. 346

Trasylol (Hem).   Hemostatic drug that decreases perioperative blood loss in patients undergoing coronary artery bypass grafting.   For dosage, see *aprotinin.* 172

TraumaCal (GI).   Liquid nutrional supplement formulated for patients with severe stress from disease or trauma. Liquid.

(Travase) (Derm).   No longer on the market. (Generic name *sutilains;* topical drug used to debride burns and wounds).

Travasol 2.75%, Travasol 3.5%, Travasol 4.25%, Travasol 5.5%, Travasol 8.5%, Travasol 10% (I.V.).   Intravenous fluids for total parenteral nutrition. 378

Travasorb, Travasorb HN, Travasorb MCT, Travasorb STD (GI).   Liquid nutritional supplement. Powder (to be reconstituted).

Travasorb Hepatic Diet (GI).   Liquid nutritional supplement formulated for patients with liver failure. Powder (to be reconstituted).

Travatan (Oph).   Topical drug used to treat glaucoma.   For dosage, see *travoprost.* [TREH-vah-tehn]. 222

travoprost (Travatan) (Oph).   Topical drug used to treat glaucoma. Ophthalmic solution: 0.004%. [TREH-voh-prawst]. 222

trazodone (Desyrel, Desyrel Dividose) (Psych). Tetracyclic antidepressant used to treat depression; used to treat panic disorder. Tablet: 50 mg, 100 mg, 150 mg, 300 mg. [TREH-zoh-dohn]. 288, 289

Trecator-SC (Resp).   Used to treat tuberculosis. For dosage, see *ethionamide.* 197

Trelstar Depot (Chemo).   Hormonal chemotherapy drug used to treat prostate cancer.   For dosage, see *triptorelin.* [TREHL-stawr DEE-poh]. 344

tremors,   drugs used to treat. 146

Trental (Cardio).   Used to improve circulation in the legs of patients with peripheral vascular disease by decreasing blood viscosity.   For dosage, see *pentoxifylline.* [TREHN-tawl].

treosulfan (Ovastat) (Chemo).   Chemotherapy drug used to treat ovarian cancer. Orphan drug. 348

Treponema pallidum.

treprostinil (Remodulin) (Resp).   Vasodilator used to treat pulmonary arterial hypertension. Subcutaneous: Administered continously via a MiniMed microinfusion device. [treh-PRAW-steh-nihl]. 198

tretinoin (Avita, Renova, Retin-A, Retin-A Micro) (Derm).   Topical vitamin A-type drug used to treat acne vulgaris; used to treat facial wrinkles and areas of hyperpigmentation. Cream: 0.02%, 0.025%, 0.05%, 0.1%. Gel: 0.025%, 0.1%. Liquid: 0.05%. [tree-teh-NOH-ihn]. 84

tretinoin (Oph).   Used to treat squamous metaplasia of the cornea. Orphan drug. [tree-teh-NOH-ihn].

tretinoin (Atragen, Vesanoid) (Chemo).   Vitamin A-type chemotherapy drug used to treat leukemia; investigational drug used to treat Kaposi's sarcoma and non-Hodgkin's lymphoma. Capsule: 10 mg. [tree-teh-NOH-ihn]. 348

Trexan (Analges).   Narcotic antagonist used to block the effect of narcotics as ongoing treatment for former narcotic-dependent patients.   For dosage, see *naltrexone.* [TREHK-sehn]. 182, 308

Triacana (Endo).   Used to suppress the release of thyroid-stimulating hormone from the pituitary gland of patients with thyroid cancer.   For dosage, see *tiratricol.* 230

triacetin (Fungoid, Fungoid Creme, Fungoid Tincture) (Derm).   Topical antifungal drug. Cream, liquid. [try-ah-SEE-tihn]. 89

(Triam-A, Triam Forte) (Ortho).   No longer on the market. (Generic name *triamcinolone;* corticosteroid anti-inflammatory drug injected into a joint to treat osteoarthritis and rheumatoid arthritis).

triamcinolone (Aristocort, Aristocort A, Flutex, Kenalog, Kenalog-H) (Derm).   Topical corticosteroid anti-inflammatory drug. Cream: 0.025%, 0.1%, 0.5%. Lotion: 0.025%, 0.1%. Ointment: 0.025%, 0.1%, 0.5%. Spray. [try-ehm-SIH-nah-lohn]. 92

triamcinolone (Aristocort, Aristocort Forte, Aristospan Intra-articular, Kenacort, Kenalog-40, Tac-40, Trilog, Trilone) (Chemo, Endo, Ortho).   Corticosteroid anti-inflammatory drug used to treat severe inflammation in various body systems; used to treat Addison's disease; injected into a joint to treat osteoarthritis and rheumatoid arthritis; used to treat leukemia and lymphoma. Tablet: 4 mg, 8 mg. Syrup: 4 mg/5 mL. Intra-articular or intramuscular: 20 mg/mL, 40 mg/mL. [try-ehm-SIH-nah-lohn]. 93, 141, 232, 233, 351

triamcinolone (Aristocort Intralesional, Aristospan Intralesional, Kenalog-10, Tac-3) (Derm). Corticosteroid anti-inflammatory drug injected into skin lesions. Intradermal: 3 mg/mL, 5 mg/mL, 10 mg/mL, 25 mg/mL. [try-ehm-SIH-nah-lohn]. 92

triamcinolone (Azmacort) (Resp). Corticosteroid used to prevent acute asthma attacks. Aerosol inhaler: 100 mcg/puff. [try-ehm-SIH-nah-lohn]. 196

triamcinolone (Kenalog in Orabase) (ENT). Topical corticosteroid drug used to treat ulcers and inflammation in the mouth. Paste: 0.1%. [try-ehm-SIH-nah-lohn]. 208

triamcinolone (Nasacort, Nasacort AQ, Tri-Nasal) (ENT). Topical intranasal corticosteroid used to treat allergic rhinitis. Aerosol nasal inhaler: 55 mcg/spray. Spray: 50 mcg/spray, 55 mcg/spray. [try-ehm-SIH-nah-lohn]. 208

(Triaminic, Triaminic Allergy, Triaminic Cold & Allergy) (ENT). No longer on the market. (Combination drug with *phenylpropanolamine;* decongestant and antihistamine drug).

Triaminic AM Decongestant Formula, Triaminic Infant Oral Decongestant (ENT). Decongestant. For dosage, see *pseudoepherine.* [try-ah-MIH-nihk]. 206

Triaminic AM Cough & Decongestant (ENT) (generic *pseudoephedrine, dextromethorphan*). Combination decongestant and nonnarcotic antitussive drug. Liquid: 15 mg/7.5 mg. [try-ah-MIH-nihk].

(Triaminic-DM) (ENT). No longer on the market. (Combination drug with *phenylpropanolamine;* decongestant and nonnarcotic antitussive drug).

(Triaminic Expectorant) (ENT). No longer on the market. (Combination drug with *phenylpropanolamine;* decongestant and expectorant drug).

(Triaminic Expectorant with Codeine) (ENT). No longer on the market. (Combination drug with *phenylpropanolamine;* decongestant, narcotic antitussive, and expectorant drug).

Triaminic Nite Light, Triaminic Nite Time Maximum Strength (ENT) (generic *pseudoephedrine, chlorpheniramine, dextromethorphan*). Combination decongestant, antihistamine, and nonnarcotic antitussive drug. Liquid: 15 mg/1 mg/7.5 mg. [try-ah-MIH-nihk].

Triaminic Severe Cold & Fever (ENT) (generic *pseudoephedrine, chlorpheniramine, dextromethorphan, aceta-*

minophen). Combination decongestant, antihistamine, nonnarcotic antitussive, and analgesic drug. Liquid: 15 mg/1 mg/7.5 mg/180 mg. [try-ah-MIH-nihk].

Triaminic Sore Throat Formula (ENT) (generic *pseudoephedrine, dextromethorphan, acetaminophen*). Combination decongestant, nonnarcotic antitussive, and analgesic drug. Liquid: 15 mg/7.5 mg/160 mg. [try-ah-MIH-nihk].

(Triaminic-12) (ENT). No longer on the market. (Combination drug with *phenylpropanolamine;* decongestant and antihistamine drug).

(Triaminicol Multi-Symptom Relief, Triaminicol Multi-Symptom Relief Colds with Cough) (ENT). No longer on the market. (Combination drug with *phenylpropanolamine;* decongestant, antihistamine, and nonnarcotic antitussive drug).

triamterene (Dyrenium) (Uro). Potassium-sparing diuretic. Capsule: 50 mg, 100 mg. [try-EHM-teh-reen]. 104

Triavil 4-10, Triavil 4-25, Triavil 2-10, Triavil 2-25 (Psych) (generic *amitriptyline, perphenazine*). Combination antidepressant and antipsychotic drug. Tablet: 10 mg/2 mg, 25 mg/2 mg, 10 mg/4 mg, 25 mg/4 mg, 50 mg/4 mg. [TRY-ah-vill]. 293

Triaz (Derm) (generic *benzoyl peroxide*). Topical antibiotic used to treat acne vulgaris. Gel: 6%, 10%. Liquid: 10%. 83

triazolam (Halcion) (Neuro). Nonbarbiturate benzodiazepine drug used to treat insomnia. (Schedule IV drug). Tablet: 0.125 mg, 0.25 mg. [try-EH-zoh-lehm]. 272

Tri-Chlor (Derm) (generic *tricholoroacetic acid*). Topical drug used to treat warts. Liquid: 80%. 91

trichlormethiazide (Diurese, Metahydrin, Naqua) (Uro). Thiazide diuretic. Tablet: 4 mg. [try-klohr-meh-THY-ah-zide]. 103

trichloroacetic acid (Tri-Chlor) (Derm). Topical drug used to treat warts. Liquid: 80%. 91

Trichomonas vaginalis, drugs used to treat.

trichosanthin (Antivir). Antiviral drug used to treat AIDS. Investigational drug. 326

triclosan (Stri-Dex Anti-Bacterial Foaming Wash) (Derm). Topical antiseptic used to treat acne vulgaris. Liquid: 1%. [TRY-kloh-sehn]. 83

Tricodene Cough & Cold (ENT) (generic *pyrilamine, codeine*). Combination antihistamine and narcotic antitussive drug. Liquid: 12.5 mg/8.2 mg.

Tricor (Cardio). Used to treat hypercholesterolemia by decreasing low-density lipoproteins; used to treat hypertriglyceridemia by decreasing serum triglycerides and very low-density lipoprotein levels. For dosage, see *fenofibrate.* 171

tricyclic antidepressants. Historical Notes feature.

tricyclic antidepressants (Psych). Class of drugs used to treat depression. 285

Tridesilon (Derm) (generic *desonide*). Topical corticosteroid anti-inflammatory drug. Cream: 0.05%. Ointment: 0.05%. [try-DEH-sih-lawn]. 92

tridihexethyl (Pathilon) (GI). Antispasmodic drug used to treat spasm of smooth muscle of the bowel. Tablet: 25 mg. 122

Tridil (Cardio). Nitrate drug used to prevent and treat angina pectoris; used to treat hypertensive crisis. For dosage, see *nitroglycerin*. [TRY-dihl]. 156, 168

Tridione (Neuro). Anticonvulsant drug used to treat absence seizures. For dosage, see *trimethadione*. [try-DY-ohn]. 265

trifluoperazine (Stelazine) (Psych). Phenothiazine drug used to treat psychosis; used to treat anxiety. Tablet: 1 mg, 2 mg, 5 mg, 10 mg. Liquid: 10 mg/mL. Intramuscular: 2 mg/mL. [try-floo-oh-PEH-rah-zeen]. 282, 283

(triflupromazine) (GI, Psych). No longer on the market. (Trade name *Vesprin*; phenothiazine antipsychotic drug; also antiemetic drug).

trifluridine (Viroptic) (Oph). Topical antiviral drug used to treat herpes simplex infection of eyes. Ophthalmic solution: 1%. [try-FLOOR-eh-deen]. 219

TriHemic 600 (Cardio). Combination iron, intrinsic factor, vitamin B_{12}, vitamin C, and folic acid drug used to treat iron deficiency anemia and pernicious anemia. Tablet: 115 mg/75 mg/25 mcg/600 mg/1 mg. 174

trihexyphenidyl (Artane) (Neuro). Anticholinergic drug used to treat Parkinson's disease. Capsule: 5 mg. Tablet: 2 mg, 5 mg. Liquid: 2 mg/5 mL. [try-hehk-seh-FEH-nah-dill]. 269

Trilafon (GI). Phenothiazine drug used to treat nausea and vomiting; used to treat intractable hiccoughs. For dosage, see *perphenazine*. [TRIHL-ah-fawn]. 127

Trilafon (Psych). Phenothiazine drug used to treat psychosis. For dosage, see *perphenazine*. [TRIHL-ah-fawn]. 283

Trileptal (Neuro). Anticonvulsant used to treat partial seizures. For dosage, see *oxcarbazepine*. [try-LEHP-tawl]. 265

Tri-Levlen (OB/GYN) (generic *levonorgestrel, ethinyl estradiol*). Triphasic combination progestins and estrogen oral contraceptive. Tablet: 0.05 mg/30 mcg then 0.075 mg/40 mcg then 0.125 mg/30 mcg. [try-LEHV-lehn]. 251

Trilisate (Analges, Ortho) (generic *choline salicylate, magnesium salicylate*). Combination salicylate drug used to treat pain and inflammation; used to treat osteoarthritis and rheumatoid arthritis. Liquid: 500 mg/5 mL. Tablet: 500 mg, 750 mg, 1000 mg. [TRIH-lih-sayt]. 138, 302

Trilog (Endo, Ortho). Corticosteroid anti-inflammatory drug used to treat severe inflammation in various body systems; injected into a joint to treat osteoarthritis and rheumatoid arthritis. For dosage, see *triamcinolone*. [TRY-lawg]. 233

Trilone (Endo, Ortho). Corticosteroid anti-inflammatory drug used to treat severe inflammation in various body systems; injected into a joint to treat osteoarthritis and rheumatoid arthritis. For dosage, see *triamcinolone*. [TRY-lohn]. 233

(trimeprazine) (GI). No longer on the market. (Trade name *Temaril*; antiemetic drug).

trimethadione (Tridione) (Neuro). Anticonvulsant drug used to treat absence seizures. Capsule: 300 mg. Dulcets chewable tablet: 150 mg. [try-meh-thah-DY-ohn]. 265

trimethaphan (Arfonad) (Cardio). Peripheral vasodilator used to treat hypertensive crisis. Intravenous: 50 mg/mL. 168

trimethobenzamide (Tigan) (GI). Antiemetic drug. Capsule: 100 mg, 250 mg. Suppository: 100 mg, 200 mg. Intramuscular: 100 mg/mL. [try-meh-thoh-BEHN-zah-mide]. 127

trimethoprim (TMP) (Primsol, Proloprim) (Antibio, Uro). Antibiotic used to treat urinary tract and other types of infections. Tablet: 100 mg, 200 mg. Liquid: 50 mg/5 mL. [try-MEH-thoh-prihm]. 106

trimetrexate (NeuTrexin) (Antivir, Chemo). Used to treat *Pneumocystis carinii* pneumonia in AIDS patients; chemotherapy drug used to treat bone cancer, head and neck cancer, colon cancer, rectal cancer, pancreatic cancer, and lung cancer. Orphan drug. 328, 348

trimipramine (Surmontil) (Psych). Tricyclic antidepressant. Capsule: 25 mg, 50 mg, 100 mg. [treh-MIH-prah-meen]. 286

Trimox (Antibio). Penicillin-type antibiotic used to treat various types of bacterial infections, including *Streptococcus, H. influenzae, E. coli,* gonorrhea, and *Chlamydia*; used prophylactically to prevent subacute bacterial endocarditis in at-risk patients undergoing dental or surgical procedures; used to treat *H. pylori* infection of the gastrointestinal tract. For dosage, see *amoxicillin*. [TRY-mawks]. 313

(Trimpex) (Antibio). No longer on the market. (Generic name *trimethoprim*; antibiotic).

Trinalin Repetabs (ENT) (generic *pseudoephedrine, azatadine*). Combination decongestant and antihistamine drug. Tablet: 120 mg/1 mg. [TRIH-nah-lihn]. 213

Trinam (Cardio) (generic *vascular endothelial growth factor gene*). This drug is contained within a biodegradable device. It is used to prevent intimal hyperplasia within blood vessels that have been surgically anastomosed. Implanted biodegradable collar with reservoir. 174

Tri-Nasal (ENT). Topical intranasal corticosteroid used to treat allergic rhinitis. For dosage, see *triamcinolone*. 208

Tri-Norinyl (OB/GYN) (generic *norethindrone, ethinyl estradiol*). Triphasic combination progestins and estrogen oral contraceptive. Tablet: 0.5 mg/35 mcg then 1 mg/35 mcg then 0.5 mg/35 mcg. [try-NOHR-eh-nill]. 251

Trinsicon (Cardio). Combination iron, intrinsic factor, vitamin B$_{12}$, vitamin C, and folic acid drug used to treat iron deficiency anemia and pernicious anemia. Capsule: 110 mg/240 mg/15 mcg/75 mg/0.5 mg. [TRIHN-sih-kawn]. 174

Triostat (Endo). Thyroid hormone replacement. For dosage, see *liothyronine*. [TREE-oh-steht]. 229

trioxsalen (Trisoralen) (Derm). Oral drug used in conjunction with ultraviolet light to treat hypopigmented areas of skin in patients with vitiligo. Tablet: 5 mg. [try-AWK-sah-lehn]. 100

triphasic oral contraceptives (OB/GYN). Class of drugs for oral contraception using three different levels of progesterone per month. 250

Triphasil (OB/GYN) (generic *levonorgestrel, ethinyl estradiol*). Triphasic combination progestins and estrogen oral contraceptive. Tablet: 0.05 mg/30 mcg then 0.075 mg/40 mcg then 0.125 mg/30 mcg. [try-FAY-sill]. 251

(triple sulfa) (OB/GYN). No longer on the market. (Trade name *Sultrin*; topical sulfa drug used to treat vaginal infections).

Triple X (Derm). Topical drug used to treat pediculosis (lice).

triptorelin (Decapeptyl) (Chemo). Chemotherapy drug used to treat ovarian cancer. Orphan drug. 343

triptorelin (Trelstar Depot) (Chemo). Hormonal chemotherapy drug used to treat prostate cancer. Intramuscular: 3.75 mg microgranules. [trip-toh-RAY-lihn]. 344

Trisenox (Chemo). Chemotherapy drug used to treat leukemia; used as an orphan drug to treat multiple myeloma. For dosage, see *arsenic trioxide*. [TRY-seh-nawks]. 347

Trisoralen (Derm). Oral drug used in conjunction with ultraviolet light to treat hypopigmented areas of skin in patients with vitiligo. For dosage, see *trioxsalen*. [try-soh-RAY-lehn]. 100

Tritec (GI) (generic *bismuth, ranitidine*). Combination antibacterial and H$_2$ blocker drug used to treat peptic ulcers caused by *H. pylori* infection. Tablet: 400 mg. [TRY-tehk]. 120

Trivora-28 (OB/GYN) (generic *levonorgestrel, ethinyl estradiol*). Triphasic combination progestins and estrogen oral contraceptive. Tablet: 0.05 mg/30 mcg then 0.075 mg/40 mcg then 0.125 mg/30 mcg. [TRY-voh-rah]. 251

Trizivir (Antivir) (generic, *abacavir, lamivudine, zidovudine*). Combination nucleoside reverse transcriptase inhibitor drug used to treat AIDS. Tablet: 300 mg/150 mg/300 mg. [TRY-zih-veer]. 325

Trobicin (Antibio). Antibiotic used to treat gonorrhea. For dosage, see *spectinomycin*. [TROH-bih-sihn]. 319

troche. 35

(troglitazone) (Endo). No longer on the market. (Trade name *Rezulin*; oral antidiabetic drug).

troleandomycin (Tao) (Antibio). Macrolide antibiotic used to treat respiratory tract infections and pneumonia. Capsule: 250 mg. [troh-lee-ehn-doh-MY-sihn].

tromethamine (Tham) (Emerg). Used to treat metabolic acidosis during cardiac arrest. Intravenous: 150 mEq/500 mL. [troh-MEH-thah-meen]. 181

Tronolane (GI) (generic *pramoxine*). Topical anesthetic drug used to treat hemorrhoids. Cream: 1%. [TRAW-noh-layn]. 134

Tronolane (GI) (generic *zinc oxide*). Topical drug used to treat hemorrhoids. Suppository: 11%. [TRAW-noh-layn]. 135

Tronothane (Derm) (generic *pramoxine*). Topical anesthetic. Cream: 1%. [TRAW-noh-thayn]. 94

TrophAmine 6%, TrophAmine 10% (I.V.). Intravenous fluids for total parenteral nutrition. 378

tropicamide (Mydriacyl) (Oph). Topical mydriatic drug. Ophthalmic solution: 0.5%, 1%. 223

trospectomycin (Spexil) (Antibio). Antibiotic similar to spectinomycin. Investigational drug. 321

trough levels of drug. 66

trovafloxacin (Trovan) (Antibio). Fluoroquinolone antibiotic used to treat a variety of infections, including *S. aureus, E. coli, Pseudomonas, H. influenzae*, and community-acquired pneumonia; used to treat Legionnaire's disease. Tablet: 100 mg, 200 mg. Intravenous: 5 mg/mL. [troh-vah-FLAWK-sah-sihn]. 198, 318

Trovan (Antibio). Fluoroquinolone antibiotic used to treat a variety of infections, including *S. aureus, E. coli, Pseudomonas, H. influenzae*, and community-acquired pneumonia; used to treat Legionnaire's disease.   For dosage, see *trovafloxacin*. [TROH-vehn]. 198, 318

Trovert (Endo).   Used to treat acromegaly. Orphan drug. 230

Trufill n-BCA (Neuro).   Cyanoacrylate compound used to block a cerebral arteriovenous malformation prior to surgery.

Trugene test (Antivir).   A test rather than a drug. Used to tell which AIDS drugs are no longer effective for an individual patient because the virus has undergone mutation while in that patient's body. 332

Trusopt (Oph).   Topical carbonic anhydrase inhibitor drug used to treat glaucoma.   For dosage, see *dorzolamide*. [TROO-sawpt]. 221

trypsin (Dermuspray, Granulderm, Granulex, GranuMed) (Derm).   Topical enzyme drug used to debride burns and wounds. Spray. 96

T/Scalp (Derm) (generic *hydrocortisone*).   Topical corticosteroid anti-inflammatory drug. Liquid: 1%. 92

T-Stat (Derm) (generic *erythromycin*).   Topical antibiotic used to treat acne vulgaris. Liquid: 1.5%, 2%. 84

T-tube administration.

tuberculin syringe. 66

tuberculosis.

drugs used to treat. 197
Focus on Healthcare Issues feature. 198
Historical Notes feature. 197
tests for. 202

Tubersol (Resp).   Diagnostic test that uses purified protein derivative (PPD) from *Mycobacterium tuberculosis* injected under the skin to test for tuberculosis. For dosage, see *Mantoux test*.

tubocurarine (Anes).   Muscle relaxant drug used during surgery. Intramuscular and intravenous: 3 mg/mL (20 units). [too-boh-kyour-AH-reen]. 370

Tuinal Pulvules (Neuro) (generic *amobarbital, secobarbital*).   Combination barbiturate drug used for short-term treatment of insomnia. (Schedule II drug). Capsule: 50 mg/50 mg, 100 mg/100 mg. [TOO-eh-nawl]. 272

tumor necrosis factor (Antivir).   Used to treat AIDS. Investigational drug. 326

Tums, Tums Ultra, Extra Strength Tums E-X (GI).   Calcium-containing antacid. Chewable tablet: 500 mg, 750 mg, 1000 mg. 116

Tussi-Organidin NR, Tussi-Organidin-S NR (ENT) (generic *codeine, guaifenesin*).   Combination narcotic antitussive and expectorant drug. Liquid: 10 mg/100 mg. [TUH-see-ohr-GEH-nih-dihn]. 213

(Tuss-Ornade) (ENT).   No longer on the market. (Combination drug with *phenylpropanolamine*; decongestant and nonnarcotic antitussive drug).

Twinrix (GI) (generic *inactivated hepatitis A, recombinant hepatitis B*).   Combination hepatitis A and hepatitis B vaccine. Intramuscular: 720 EL.U./20 mcg per mL. 135

Tylenol cyanide murders.   Historical Notes feature. 301

Tylenol, Tylenol Arthritis, Tylenol Extended Relief, Tylenol Extra Strength, Tylenol Junior Strength, Tylenol Regular Strength, Children's Tylenol, Children's Tylenol Soft Chews, Infants' Drops Tylenol (Analges, Ortho).   Nonnarcotic nonaspirin analgesic drug used to treat fever and pain in children and adults; used to treat the pain of osteoarthritis in adults.   For dosage, see *acetaminophen*. [TY-leh-nawl]. 139, 301

Tylenol Cold No Drowsiness (ENT) (generic *pseudoephedrine, dextromethorphan, acetaminophen*).   Combination decongestant, nonnarcotic antitussive, and analgesic drug. Caplet: 30 mg/15 mg/325 mg. Gelcaps: 30 mg/15 mg/325 mg. [TY-leh-nawl].

Tylenol Flu Maximum Strength (ENT) (generic *pseudoephedrine, dextromethorphan, acetaminophen*).   Combination decongestant, nonnarcotic antitussive, and analgesic drug. Gelcap: 30 mg/15 mg/500 mg. [TY-leh-nawl].

Tylenol Flu Night Time Maximum Strength (ENT) (generic *pseudoephedrine, diphenhydramine, acetaminophen*).   Combination decongestant, antihistamine, and analgesic. Powder (to be dissolved in water): 60 mg/50 mg/1000 mg. [TY-leh-nawl].

Tylenol Severe Allergy (ENT) (generic *diphenhydramine, acetaminophen*).   Combination antihistamine and analgesic drug. Caplet: 12.5 mg/500 mg. [TY-leh-nawl].

Tylenol with Codeine (Analges) (generic *codeine, acetaminophen*).   Combination narcotic and nonnarcotic analgesic drug. (Schedule V drug). Liquid: 12 mg/120 mg per 15 mL. [TY-leh-nawl]. 303

Tylenol with Codeine No. 2 (Analges) (generic *codeine, acetaminophen*).   Combination narcotic and nonnarcotic analgesic drug. (Schedule III drug). Tablet: 15 mg/300 mg. [TY-leh-nawl]. 303

Tylenol with Codeine No. 3 (Analges) (generic *codeine, acetaminophen*).   Combination narcotic and nonnarcotic analgesic drug. (Schedule III drug). Tablet: 30 mg/300 mg. [TY-leh-nawl]. 303

Tylenol with Codeine No. 4 (Analges) (generic *codeine, acetaminophen*).   Combination narcotic and nonnarcotic analgesic drug. (Schedule III drug). Tablet: 60 mg/300 mg. [TY-leh-nawl]. 303

Tylox (Analges) (generic *oxycodone, acetaminophen*).   Combination narcotic and nonnarcotic analgesic drug. (Schedule II drug). Capsule: 5 mg/500 mg. [TY-lawks]. 303

tyloxapol (Enuclene) (Oph).   Solution to clean and wet an artificial eye. Ophthalmic solution: 0.25%. [ty-LAWK-sah-pohl].

Tympagesic (ENT) (generic *benzocaine*).   Topical anesthetic for the ear. Drops. [TIHM-peh-JEE-sihk].

U-100 (Diab).   Dosage indication on insulin; 100 units of insulin per milliliter. 239

U-500 (Diab).   Dosage indication on insulin; 500 units of insulin per milliliter. 239

Ucephan (Misc) (generic *benzoate, phenylacetate*). Combination drug used to prevent and treat increased levels of ammonia in the blood in patients with abnormalities of the enzymes that produce urea. Orphan drug.

Uendex (Resp).   Inhaled drug used to treat cystic fibrosis.   For dosage, see *dextran sulfate*. [yoo-EHN-dehks].

ulcerative colitis, drugs used to treat. 126

ulcers, drugs used to treat peptic. 116

ulcers, drugs used to treat skin. 96

Ultane (Anes).   Used to induce and maintain general anesthesia. Inhaled gas. 370

Ultiva (Anes).   Narcotic used to induce and maintain general anesthesia.   For dosage, see *remifentanil*. [uhl-TEE-vah]. 369

Ultracal (GI).   Liquid nutritional supplement. Liquid.

Ultracet (Analges) (generic *tramadol, acetaminophen*). Combination nonnarcotic analgesic drug. Tablet: 37.5 mg/325 mg. [UHL-trah-seht]. 302

(Ultralente Iletin) (Diab).   No longer on the market. (Long-acting insulin).

Ultram (Analges).   Nonnarcotic analgesic drug used to treat moderate-to-severe pain.   For dosage, see *tramadol*. [UHL-trahm]. 299

Ultrase MT12, Ultrase MT 18, Ultrase MT 20 (GI) (generic *amylase, lipase, protease*).   Combination drug replacement therapy for digestive enzymes. Capsule, tablet: 20,000 units/4500 units/25,000 units;   39,000   units/12,000   units/39,000   units; 58,500 units/18,000 units/58,500 units; 65,000 units/ 20,000 units/65,000 units. [UHL-trays]. 135

Ultra Tears (Oph).   Artificial tears. Drops.

Ultravate (Derm) (generic *halobetasol*).   Topical corticosteroid anti-inflammatory drug. Cream: 0.05%. Ointment: 0.05%. [UHL-trah-vayt]. 92

ultraviolet light. See *PUVA*. 88

umbilical artery/vein route, administration of drugs by the. 43

umbilical cord blood (I.V.).   Intravenous stem cells blood product derived from the placenta/umbilical

cord of newborns. Focus on Healthcare Issues feature. 380

Unasyn (Antibio) (generic *ampicillin, sulbactam*). Combination penicillin-type antibiotic and beta-lactamase inhibitor drug. Intramuscular or intravenous (powder to be reconstituted): 1 g/0.5 g, 2 g/1 g. [YOO-nah-sihn]. 320

Unguentine Plus (Derm) (generic *lidocaine*).   Topical anesthetic. Cream: 2%. [UHN-gwihn-teen]. 94

Unicard (Cardio) (generic *dilevalol*).   Beta-blocker used to treat hypertension. Investigational drug. 173

Unipen (Antibio).   Penicillin-type antibiotic used to treat a variety of bacterial infections, including staphylococci.   For dosage, see *nafcillin*. [YOO-nih-pehn]. 313

Uniphyl (Resp).   Bronchodilator.   For dosage, see *theophylline*. [YOO-nil-fihl]. 193

Unisom Nighttime Sleep-Aid (Neuro).   Sleep aid. For dosage, see *doxylamine*. [YOO-neh-sawm].

Unisom with Pain Relief (Neuro) (generic *acetaminophen, diphenhydramine*).   Combination analgesic and antihistamine sleep aid. Tablet: 650 mg/50 mg. [YOO-neh-sawm].

unit of blood.

Unit, International (IU). 69

United States Adopted Names Council. 22

United States Clean Air Act. 194

United States Pharmacopeia (USP). 14

Unithroid (Endo).   Thyroid hormone replacement. For dosage, see *levothyroxine*. 229

units, drug. 70

Univasc (Cardio).   Angiotensin-converting enzyme inhibitor used to treat hypertension.   For dosage, see *moexipril*. [YOO-nih-vehsk]. 163

unoprostone (Rescula) (Oph).   Topical drug used to treat glaucoma. Ophthalmic solution: 0.15%. [yoo-noh-PRAW-stohn]. 222

urea (Ureaphil) (Endo, Neuro, OB/GYN, Oph).   Diuretic used to treat syndrome of inappropriate antidiuretic hormone; used to treat increased intracranial pressure; used to induce abortion; used to treat increased intraocular pressure. Intravenous: 40 g/150 mL. [yoo-REE-ah]. 231, 255, 277

Ureaphil (Endo, Neuro, OB/GYN, Ophth).   Diuretic used to treat syndrome of inappropriate antidiuretic hormone; used to treat increased intracranial pressure; used to induce abortion; used to treat increased intraocular pressure.   For dosage, see *urea*. [yoo-REE-ah-fill]. 231, 255, 277

(Urecholine) (Uro).   No longer on the market. (Generic name *bethanechol*; urinary antispasmodic drug).

Urex (Antibio, Uro). Anti-infective drug only used to treat urinary tract infections. For dosage, see *methenamine*. [YOUR-ehks]. 106, 319

urinary retention, drugs used to treat. 107

urinary tract drugs. 102

urinary tract infections, drugs used to treat. 105

urine, pregnant mares'. 252

Urised (Uro) (generic *L-hyoscyamine, methenamine, methylene blue*). Combination urinary tract antispasmodic and anti-infective drug. Tablet. [YOUR-ih-sehd]. 107

Urispas (Uro). Antispasmodic drug used to treat urinary frequency and urgency. For dosage, see *flavoxate*. [YOUR-ih-spehs]. 107

(Urobiotic) (Uro). No longer on the market. (Combination antibiotic, sulfonamide anti-infective, and analgesic drug).

Urocit-K (Ortho, Uro). Used to prevent the formation of uric acid kidney stones in patients with gout. For dosage, see *potassium citrate*. 112, 146

urofollitropin (Fertinex, Metrodin) (Endo, OB/GYN). Ovulation-stimulating hormone drug used to treat infertility; orphan drug used to treat low sperm count and infertility in men with pituitary gland malfunction. Subcutaneous (powder to be reconstituted): 75 IU, 150 IU. [your-oh-foh-lih-TROH-pihn]. 244

urogastrone (Oph). Used to promote healing after corneal transplant. Orphan drug.

Urogesic (Uro). Urinary tract analgesic. For dosage, see *phenazopyridine*. [your-oh-JEE-sihk]. 107

Urogesic Blue (Uro) (generic *L-hyoscyamine, methenamine, methylene blue*). Combination urinary tract antispasmodic and anti-infective drug. Tablet. [your-oh-JEE-sihk]. 107

(urokinase) (Cardio, Hem, Resp). No longer on the market. (Generic name *Abbokinase*; thrombolytic enzyme).

Urolene Blue (Uro). Used to treat oxalate kidney stones. For dosage, see *methylene blue*. [YOOR-oh-leen bloo]. 112

UroXatral (Uro). Alpha$_1$-receptor blocker used to treat benign prostatic hypertrophy. For dosage, see *alfuzosin*. 109

ursodiol (Actigall) (GI). Used to dissolve gallstones. Capsule: 300 mg. [EHR-soh-dy-awl]. 129

USP (abbreviation for *United States Pharmacopeia*). See *United States Pharmacopoeia*.

UTI (abbreviation for *urinary tract infection*). See *urinary tract infection*.

(Uticort) (Derm). No longer on the market. (Generic name *betamethasone*; topical corticosteroid).

Uvadex (Derm) (generic *methoxsalen*). Topical drug used in conjunction with ultraviolet light to darken hypopigmented areas of skin in vitiligo. Liquid: 20 mcg/mL. Lotion: 1%. [YOO-vah-dehks].

vaccination (misc). 3

vaccine, anthrax (Antibio). Class of drugs used to prevent anthrax infection. 321

vaccine, HIV/AIDS (Antivir). Class of drugs used to prevent HIV infection. 327

Vagifem (OB/GYN). Hormone replacement therapy used to treat atrophic vaginitis of menopause. For dosage, see *estradiol hemihydrate*. [VEH-juh-fehm]. 252

vaginal infections, drugs used to treat. 256

vaginal route, administration of drugs by the. 40

Vagisil (OB/GYN) (generic *benzocaine, lanolin*). Topical combination anesthetic and lanolin for the perineal area. Cream. [VEH-gih-sihl].

Vagistat-1 (OB/GYN) (generic *tioconazole*). Topical drug used to treat vaginal yeast infections. Vaginal ointment: 6.5%. [VEH-jeh-steht]. 256

valacyclovir (Valtrex) (Antivir, Derm, OB/GYN). Drug used to treat herpes zoster virus infections; used to treat genital herpes (condyloma acuminatum). Tablet: 500 mg, 1 g. [veh-lah-SY-kloh-veer]. 330

Valcyte (Antivir). Antiviral drug used to treat cytomegalovirus retinitis. For dosage, see *valganciclovir*. [VEHL-site]. 330

valdecoxib (Bextra) (Analges, OB/GYN, Ortho). Nonsteroidal anti-inflammatory and cyclooxygenase-2 inhibitor drug used to treat dysmenorrhea; used to treat osteoarthritis and rheumatoid arthritis. Tablet: 10 mg. [vehl-deh-CAWK-sihb]. 140, 255, 305

Valergen 20, Valergen 40 (Chemo, OB/GYN). Hormonal chemotherapy drug used to treat prostate carcinoma; hormone replacement therapy used to treat the symptoms of menopause. For dosage, see *estradiol valerate*. [VAH-lehr-gehn]. 252

valganciclovir (Cymeval, Valcyte) (Antivir). Antiviral drug used to treat cytomegalovirus retinitis. Tablet: 450 mg. [vahl-gehn-SIHK-kloh-veer]. 330

(Valisone, Valisone Reduced Strength) (Derm). No longer on the market. (Generic name *betamethasone*; topical corticosteroid anti-inflammatory drug).

Valium (Anes). Benzodiazepine drug used preoperatively to decrease anxiety and provide sedation. (Schedule IV drug). For dosage, see *diazepam*. [VEH-lee-uhm]. 371

Valium (Emerg, Neuro, Psych). Benzodiazepine drug used to treat status epilepticus and acute alcohol withdrawal. (Schedule IV drug). For dosage, see *diazepam*. [VEH-lee-uhm].

Valium (Neuro, Ortho). Benzodiazepine drug used as a skeletal muscle relaxant to treat minor muscle spasms associated with injuries; used to treat severe muscle spasticity associated with multiple sclerosis, cerebral palsy, stroke, or spinal cord injury; used to treat epilepsy. (Schedule IV drug).   For dosage, see *diazepam*. [VEH-lee-uhm]. 144, 264

Valium (Psych).   Benzodiazepine drug used to treat anxiety and neurosis; used to treat panic disorder; used to treat alcohol withdrawal. (Schedule IV drug).   For dosage, see *diazepam*. [VEH-lee-uhm]. 281

(Valmid) (Neuro).   No longer on the market. (Generic name *ethinamate*; nonbarbiturate used to treat insomnia).

(Valpin) (GI).   No longer on the market. (Generic name *anisotropine*; GI antispasmodic drug).

valproic acid (Depacon, Depakene, Depakote, Depakote ER) (Analges, Neuro, Psych).   Used to treat migraine headaches, used to treat absence and complex partial seizures; used to treat the mania of manic-depressive disorder. Capsule: 125 mg. Tablet: 125 mg, 250 mg, 500 mg. Liquid: 250 mg/5 mL. Intravenous: 100 mg/mL. [vehl-PROH-ick EH-sihd]. 265, 288, 307

valrubicin (Valstar) (Chemo).   Chemotherapy antibiotic used to treat bladder cancer. Intravesical injection: 40 mg/mL. [vehl-ROO-beh-sihn]. 342

valsartan (Diovan) (Cardio).   Angiotensin II receptor blocker used to treat congestive heart failure and hypertension. Capsule: 80 mg, 160 mg. [vehl-SAWR-tehn]. 155, 164

Valstar (Chemo).   Chemotherapy antibiotic used to treat bladder cancer.   For dosage, see *valrubicin*. [VEHL-stawr]. 342

Valtrex (Antivir, Derm, OB/GYN).   Antiviral drug used to treat herpes zoster virus infections and genital herpes (condyloma acuminatum).   For dosage, see *valacyclovir*. [VEHL-trehks]. 330

Vancenase AQ 84, Vancenase Pockethaler (ENT). Topical intranasal corticosteroid used to treat allergic rhinitis.   For dosage, see *beclomethasone*. [VEHN-seh-nays]. 208

Vanceril, Vanceril Double Strength (Resp).   Inhaled corticosteroid used to prevent acute asthma attacks. For dosage, see *beclomethasone*. [VEHN-seh-rihl].

Vancocin (Antibio).   Antibiotic used to treat a variety of bacterial infections, including *Staphylococcus*, methicillin-resistant staphylococcus (MRSA), *C. difficile*, and antibiotic-associated pseudomembranous colitis.   For dosage, see *vancomycin*. [VEHN-koh-sihn]. 319

Vancoled (Antibio).   Antibiotic used to treat a variety of bacterial infections, including *Staphylococcus*, methicillin-resistant staphylococcus (MRSA), *C. difficile*,

and antibiotic-associated pseudomembranous colitis. For dosage, see *vancomycin*. [VEHN-koh-lehd]. 319

vancomycin (Vancocin, Vancoled) (Antibio).   Antibiotic used to treat a variety of bacterial infections, including *Staphylococcus*, methicillin-resistant staphylococcus (MRSA), *C. difficile*, and antibiotic-associated pseudomembranous colitis. Pulvule: 125 mg, 250 mg. Liquid (powder to be reconstituted): 1 g. Intravenous (powder to be reconstituted): 1 g. [vehn-koh-MY-sihn]. 319

van Gogh, Vincent. 153

Vaniqa (Derm) (generic *eflornithine*).   Topical drug that slows the growth of unwanted facial hair in women. Cream: 13.9%. [VEH-nih-kwah].

Vanlev (Cardio).   Drug that acts as an angiotensin-converting enzyme inhibitor but also inhibits neutral endopeptidase, another enzyme that regulates the blood pressure.   For dosage, see *omapatrilat*. 165

Vanquish (Analges) (generic *acetaminophen, aspirin, caffeine*).   Combination nonnarcotic analgesic and caffeine drug. Caplet: 227 mg/194 mg/33 mg. [VEHN-kwish]. 302

Vantin (Antibio).   Cephalosporin antibiotic used to treat various types of bacterial infections, including *H. influenzae*, staphylococci, *E. coli*, and gonorrhea. For dosage, see *cefpodoxime*. [VEHN-tihn]. 316

Vaqta (GI).   Hepatitis A vaccine.   For dosage, see *hepatitis A vaccine*.

varicose veins, drugs used to treat.

Vascor (Cardio).   Calcium channel blocker used to treat angina pectoris.   For dosage, see *bepridil*. [VEHS-kohr]. 157

Vaseretic 5-12.5, Vaseretic 10-25 (Cardio) (generic *enalapril, hydrochlorothiazide*).   Combination angiotensin-converting enzyme inhibitor antihypertensive and diuretic drug. Tablet: 5 mg/12.5 mg, 10 mg/25 mg. [vay-seh-REH-tihk]. 167

(Vasocidin) (Oph).   No longer on the market. (Combination corticosteroid and anti-infective sulfa drug).

Vasocine (Oph) (generic name *prednisolone, sulfacetamide*).   Topical combination corticosteroid and sulfa anti-infective drug. Ophthalmic ointment: 0.5%/10%. [VAY-soh-seen].

Vasoclear, Vasoclear A Solution (Oph).   Topical decongestant/vasoconstrictor used to treat irritation and allergy symptoms in the eyes.   For dosage, see *naphazoline*. [VAY-soh-kleer].

Vasocon Regular (Oph).   Topical decongestant/vasoconstrictor used to treat irritation and allergy symptoms in the eyes.   For dosage, see *naphazoline*. [VAY-soh-kawn].

Vasodilan (Cardio).   Peripheral vasodilator used to treat peripheral vascular disease and Raynaud's disease. For dosage, see *isoxsuprine*. [vay-soh-DY-lehn]. 168, 173

vasodilators (Cardio). Class of drugs used to dilate blood vessels. 66, 168

(Vasomax) (Uro). No longer on the market. (Used to treat male impotence).

vasopeptidase inhibitors (VPIs) (Cardio). Class of drugs used to treat hypertension and congestive heart failure. 165

vasopressin (Pitressin) (Endo). Antidiuretic hormone replacement used to treat diabetes insipidus. Intramuscular or subcutaneous: 20 pressor units/mL. [vay-soh-PREH-sihn]. 231

vasopressors (Emerg). Class of drugs used to constrict blood vessels and raise the blood pressure during emergency resuscitation. 181

Vasosulf (Oph) (generic name *phenylephrine, sulfacetamide*). Topical combination decongestant and sulfa anti-infective drug. Ophthalmic solution: 0.125%/15%. [VAY-soh-suhlf].

Vasotec, Vasotec I.V. (Cardio, Uro). Angiotensin-converting enzyme inhibitor drug used to treat hypertension and congestive heart failure; used to treat hypertensive crisis; used to treat diabetic nephropathy. For dosage, see *enalapril*. [VAY-soh-tehk]. 111, 154, 163, 167

Vasoxyl (Anes). Vasopressor used to treat hypotension that occurs with spinal anesthesia. For dosage, see *methoxamine*. [vay-SAWK-sihl]. 371

VaxSyn HIV-1 (Antivir). Used to treat AIDS. Orphan drug. 326

(V-Cillin K) (Antibio). No longer on the market. (Generic name *penicillin V*; penicillin-type antibiotic).

VCR. See *vincristine*.

Vectrin (Antibio). Tetracycline-type antibiotic used to treat a variety of infections, including acne vulgaris, gonorrhea, syphilis, and *Chlamydia*; used to treat malignant pleural effusion. For dosage, see *minocycline*. [VEHK-trihn]. 84, 317

vecuronium (Norcuron) (Anes, Resp). Muscle relaxant drug used during surgery; used to treat patients who are intubated and on the ventilator. Intravenous (powder to be reconstituted): 10 mg, 20 mg. [veh-kyour-OH-nee-uhm]. 199, 370

Veetids (Antibio). Penicillin antibiotic used to treat various types of bacterial infections, including *Streptococcus*, *Staphylococcus*, *Pneumococcus*, and Lyme disease. For dosage, see *penicillin V*. [VEE-tihds]. 313

Velban (Chemo). Mitosis inhibitor chemotherapy drug used to treat Hodgkin's disease, cutaneous T-cell lymphoma, testicular cancer, and Kaposi's sarcoma. For dosage, see *vinblastine*. [VEHL-behn]. 344

velnacrine (Mentane) (Neuro). Cholinesterase inhibitor used to treat Alzheimer's disease. Investigational drug. 271

Velosef (Antibio). Cephalosporin antibiotic used to treat a variety of bacterial infections, including *Streptococcus, Staphylococcus, E. coli*, and *H. influenzae*. For dosage, see *cephradine*. [VEHL-oh-sehf]. 315

Velosulin BR (Diab). Fast-acting regular insulin. Subcutaneous: 100 units/mL. [veh-LAW-soo-lihn]. 238

venlafaxine (Effexor, Effexor XR) (Psych). Antidepressant used to treat depression; used to treat anxiety. Capsule: 3.75 mg, 75 mg, 150 mg. Tablet: 25 mg, 37.5 mg, 50 mg, 75 mg, 100 mg. [vehn-lah-FEHK-seen]. 282, 288

Venofer (Hem, Uro). Used to treat iron deficiency anemia in hemodialysis patients. For dosage, see *iron sucrose*. [VEH-noh-fehr]. 111, 189

ventilator patients, drugs used to treat. 199

Ventolin HFA, Ventolin Nebules, Ventolin Rotacaps (Resp). Bronchodilator. For dosage, see *albuterol*. [VEHN-toh-lihn]. 193

VePesid (Chemo). Mitosis inhibitor chemotherapy drug used to treat lung cancer, testicular cancer, liver cancer, ovarian cancer, uterine cancer, breast cancer, gastric cancer, leukemia, Hodgkin's disease, non-Hodgkin's lymphoma, rhabdomyosarcoma, and Kaposi's sarcoma. For dosage, see *etoposide*. [veh-PEH-sihd]. 344

verapamil (Calan, Verelan) (Analges). Calcium channel blocker used to treat migraine headaches. Capsule: 100 mg, 120 mg, 180 mg, 200 mg, 240 mg, 300 mg, 360 mg. Tablet: 40 mg, 80 mg, 120 mg, 180 mg, 240 mg. Intravenous: 5 mg/2 mL. [veh-REH-pah-mill]. 306

verapamil (Calan, Calan SR, Covera-HS, Isoptin SR, Verelan, Verelan PM) (Cardio). Calcium channel blocker used to treat angina pectoris, congestive heart failure, hypertension, and atrial and ventricular arrhythmias. Capsule: 100 mg, 120 mg, 180 mg, 200 mg, 240 mg, 300 mg, 360 mg. Tablet: 40 mg, 80 mg, 120 mg, 180 mg, 240 mg. Intravenous: 5 mg/2 mL. [veh-REH-pah-mill]. 154, 157, 160, 163

verbal order. See *order*.

Verelan (Analges). Calcium channel blocker used to treat migraine headaches. For dosage, see *verapamil*. [VEER-eh-lehn]. 306

Verelan, Verelan PM (Cardio). Calcium channel blocker used to treat angina pectoris, congestive heart failure, hypertension, and atrial and ventricular arrhythmias. For dosage, see *verapamil*. [VEER-eh-lehn]. 154, 157, 160, 163

Vermox (Misc). Used to treat pinworms, round-worms, and hookworms. For dosage, see *meben-dazole*. [VEHR-mawks].

verrucae (common warts), drugs used to treat. 92

Versed (Anes, Resp). Preoperative drug used to pro-duce sedation; used to induce and maintain general anesthesia; used to sedate patients who are intu-bated and on a ventilator. For dosage, see *midazo-lam*. [vehr-SEHD]. 199, 369

verteporfin (Visudyne) (Oph). Used to treat macular degeneration. The drug is administered intra-venously and then the eyes are exposed to a red laser light to activate the drug. It is also used to treat ocular histoplasmosis.

vertigo, drugs used to treat. 128

Vesanoid (Chemo). Vitamin A-type chemotherapy drug used to treat leukemia. For dosage, see *tretinoin*. [VEH-seh-noyd]. 348

vesnarinone (Arkin-Z) (Cardio). Used to treat con-gestive heart failure. Investigational drug. 174

(Vesprin) (GI, Psych). No longer on the market. (Generic name *triflupromazine*; antipsychotic drug; also used as antiemetic).

Vestra (Psych). First drug of a new class of selective norepinephrine reuptake inhibitor (SNRI) antide-pressants used to treat depression. Generic: *reboxe-tine*. Investigational drug.

Vexol (Oph). Topical corticosteroid used to treat in-flammation of the eyes. For dosage, see *rim-exolone*. [VEHK-sawl]. 219

Viadur (Chemo). Hormonal chemotherapy drug used to treat prostatic cancer. For dosage, see *leu-prolide*. [VY-ah-dehr]. 343

Viagra (Uro). Used to treat impotence due to erectile dysfunction. For dosage, see *sildenafil*. [vy-EH-grah]. 109

vial. 66, 67

Vibramycin, Vibramycin IV (Antibio). Tetracycline-type antibiotic used to treat a variety of infections, including traveler's diarrhea, gonorrhea, syphilis, and *Chlamydia*; used to treat cutaneous or inhaled anthrax from bioterrorism. For dosage, see *doxy-cycline*. [vy-brah-MY-sihn]. 98, 123, 317

Vibra-Tabs (Antibio). Tetracycline-type antibiotic used to treat a variety of infections, including trav-eler's diarrhea, gonorrhea, syphilis, and *Chlamydia*; used to treat cutaneous or inhaled anthrax from bioterrorism. For dosage, see *doxycycline*. [VY-brah-tehbs]. 98, 123, 317

Vicks Children's Chloraseptic, Vicks Chloraseptic Sore Throat (ENT) (generic *benzocaine*). Topical anesthetic used to treat sore throats. Lozenge: 5 mg, 6 mg.

Vicks Children's NyQuil Nighttime Cold/Cough, Vicks Pediatric Formula 44D Multi-Symptom Cough & Cold (ENT) (generic *pseudoephedrine, chlor-pheniramine, dextromethorphan*). Combination de-congestant, antihistamine, and nonnarcotic anti-tussive drug. Liquid: 10 mg/0.67 mg/5 mg.

Vicks DayQuil (ENT) (generic *pseudoephedrine, dex-tromethorphan, guaifenesin*). Combination decon-gestant, nonnarcotic antitussive, and expectorant drug. LiquiCap: 30 mg/10 mg/100 mg. Liquid: 10 mg/3.3 mg/33.3 mg.

(Vicks DayQuil Allergy Relief 4-Hour Liquid Gel-caps) (ENT). No longer on the market. (Combina-tion drug with *phenylpropanolamine*; decongestant and antihistamine drug).

(Vicks DayQuil Allergy Relief 12 Hour) (ENT). No longer on the market. (Combination drug with *phenyl-propanolamine*; decongestant and antihistamine drug).

(Vicks DayQuil Sinus Pressure & Congestion Relief) (ENT). No longer on the market. (Combination drug with *phenylpropanolamine*; decongestant and ex-pectorant drug).

Vicks DayQuil Sinus Pressure & Pain Relief (ENT) (generic *pseudoephedrine, acetaminophen*). Combi-nation decongestant and analgesic drug. Caplet: 30 mg/500 mg.

(Vicks Dry Hacking Cough) (ENT). Nonnarcotic an-titussive drug. No longer on the market. (Combina-tion drug with *phenylpropanolamine*; antitussive and decongestant).

Vicks Formula 44 Cough Control Discs (ENT) (generic *benzocaine, dextromethorphan*). Combination topi-cal anesthetic and nonnarcotic antitussive drug. Lozenge: 1.25 mg/5 mg, 2 mg/5 mg, 10 mg/10 mg, 15 mg/7.5 mg.

Vicks 44E (ENT) (generic *dextromethorphan, guaifenesin*). Combination nonnarcotic antitussive and expecto-rant drug. Liquid: 6.7 mg/66.7 mg.

Vicks 44M Cold, Flu & Cough (ENT) (generic *pseu-doephedrine, chlorpheniramine, dextromethorphan, aceta-minophen*). Combination decongestant, antihista-mine, nonnarcotic antitussive, and analgesic drug. LiquiCaps: 30 mg/2 mg/10 mg/250 mg.

Vicks 44 Non-Drowsy Cold & Cough, Vicks Formula 44D Cough & Decongestant, Vicks 44D Cough & Head Congestion, Vicks Pediatric Formula 44D Cough & Decongestant (ENT) (generic *pseu-doephedrine, dextromethorphan*). Combination de-congestant and nonnarcotic antitussive drug. LiquiCaps: 60 mg/30 mg. Liquid: 10 mg/5 mg, 20 mg/10 mg.

Vicks Inhaler (ENT). Nasal inhaler decongestant. For dosage, see *desoxyephedrine*. 206

Vicks NyQuil, Vicks NyQuil Multi-Symptom (ENT) (generic *pseudoephedrine, doxylamine, dextromethorphan, acetaminophen*). Combination decongestant, antihistamine, nonnarcotic antitussive, and analgesic drug. LiquiCaps: 30 mg/6.25 mg/10 mg/250 mg. Liquid: 10 mg/2.1 mg/5 mg/167 mg.

Vicks Sinex 12-Hour (ENT). Decongestant. For dosage, see *oxymetazoline.* 206

Vicks VapoRub (ENT). Topical irritant and aromatic drug used to treat the muscle aches and stuffy nose of the common cold. Cream.

Vicodin, Vicodin ES, Vicodin HP (Analges) (generic *hydrocodone, acetaminophen*). Combination narcotic and nonnarcotic analgesic drug. Tablet: 5 mg/500 mg, 7.5 mg/750 mg, 10 mg/660 mg. [VY-koh-dihn]. 303

Vicodin Tuss (ENT) (generic *hydrocodone, guaifenesin*). Combination narcotic antitussive and expectorant drug. Syrup: 5 mg/100 mg. [VY-koh-dihn TUHS]. 213

Vicoprofen (Analges) (generic *hydrocodone, ibuprofen*). Combination narcotic and nonsteroidal anti-inflammatory drug analgesic. (Schedule III drug). Tablet: 7.5 mg/200 mg. [vy-koh-PROH-fehn]. 303

vidarabine (Ara-A, Vira-A) (Antivir, OB/GYN, Oph). Topical antiviral drug used to treat herpes simplex and herpes zoster infection of the vagina and eyes. Ophthalmic ointment: 3%. [vih-DEH-rah-been]. 219

Videx, Videx EC (Antivir). Nucleoside reverse transcriptase inhibitor drug used to treat AIDS. For dosage, see *didanosine.* [VY-dehks]. 324

vigabatrin (Sabril) (Neuro). Investigational drug used to treat epilepsy; Orphan drug used to treat infantile spasms. 265

viloxazine (Catatrol) (Neuro, Psych). Bicyclic antidepressant. Orphan drug for treating narcolepsy. Investigational drug for treating depression. 274

vinblastine (Velban) (Chemo). Mitosis inhibitor chemotherapy drug used to treat Hodgkin's disease, cutaneous T-cell lymphoma, testicular cancer, and Kaposi's sarcoma. Intravenous: 1 mg/mL, (powder to be reconstituted) 10 mg. [vihn-BLEH-steen]. 344

Vinca (plant) (periwinkle).

Vincasar PFS (Chemo). Mitosis inhibitor chemotherapy drug used to treat breast cancer, bladder cancer, Hodgkin's disease, non-Hodgkin's lymphoma, rhabdomyosarcoma, Wilms' tumor, and Kaposi's sarcoma. For dosage, see *vincristine.* [VIHN-kah-sawr]. 112, 344

vincristine (Vincasar PFS) (Chemo). Mitosis inhibitor chemotherapy drug used to treat breast cancer, bladder cancer, Hodgkin's disease, non-Hodgkin's lymphoma, rhabdomyosarcoma, Wilms' tumor, and Kaposi's sarcoma. Intravenous: 1 mg/mL. [vihn-KRIHS-teen]. 112, 344

vindesine (Eldisine) (Chemo). Chemotherapy drug. Investigational drug. 344

vinorelbine (Navelbine) (Chemo). Mitosis inhibitor chemotherapy drug used to treat lung cancer, breast cancer, uterine cancer, and Kaposi's sarcoma. Intravenous: 10 mg/mL. 344

(Vioform) (Derm). No longer on the market. (Generic name *clioquinol*; topical antifungal drug).

Viokase (GI) (generic *amylase, lipase, protease*). Combination drug replacement therapy for digestive enzymes. Tablet: 30,000 units/8000 units/30,000 units. Powder (to be reconstituted). [VY-oh-kays].

Vioxx (Analges, OB/GYN, Ortho). Nonsteroidal anti-inflammatory drug and cyclooxygenase-2 inhibitor used to treat pain; used to treat dysmenorrhea; used to treat osteoarthritis and rheumatoid arthritis. For dosage, see *rofecoxib.* [VY-awks]. 140, 255, 305

Vira-A (Antivir, OB/GYN, Oph). Topical antiviral drug used to treat herpes simplex and herpes zoster infection of eye or vagina. For dosage, see *vidarabine.* 219

Viracept (Antivir). Protease inhibitor drug used to treat AIDS. For dosage, see *nelfinavir.* [VEER-ah-sehpt]. 325

Viractin (Derm) (generic *tetracaine*). Topical anesthetic. Cream: 2%. Gel: 2%. [veer-AHK-tihn]. 94

viral infections, drugs used to treat.
topical. 90
systemic. 323

Viramune (Antivir). Nonnucleoside reverse transcriptase inhibitor drug used to treat AIDS. For dosage, see *nevirapine.* [VEER-ah-myoon]. 325

Virazole (Antivir). Antiviral drug used to treat respiratory syncytial virus. For dosage, see *ribavirin.* [VEER-ah-zohl]. 331

Viread (Antivir). Nucleotide reverse transcriptase inhibitor drug used to treat AIDS. For dosage, see *tenofovir.* [VEH-reed]. 324

Virilon, Virilon IM (Chemo, Endo). Male sex hormone used to treat breast cancer in women; used to treat the lack of production of testosterone due to absence, injury, or malfunction of the testes or malfunction of the pituitary gland; used to treat delayed puberty in boys. For dosage, see *methyltestosterone.* [VEER-eh-lawn]. 343

Viroptic (Oph). Topical antiviral drug used to treat herpes simplex infection of eyes. For dosage, see *trifluridine.* [veer-AWP-tihk]. 219

virulizin (Chemo). Used to treat Kaposi's sarcoma. Investigational drug.

Viscoat (Oph) (generic *chondroitin, sodium hyaluronate*). Aqueous humor replacement injected during surgery. Intraocular injection: 40 mg/30 mg per mL.

Visine Allergy Relief (Oph). Topical decongestant/vasoconstrictor used to treat irritation and allergy symptoms in the eyes. For dosage, see *tetrahydrozoline*. [VY-zeen].

Visine L.R. (Oph). Topical decongestant/vasoconstrictor used to treat irritation and allergy symptoms in the eyes. For dosage, see *oxymetazoline*. [VY-zeen].

Visken (Cardio). Nonselective beta-blocker used to treat hypertension and ventricular arrhythmias. For dosage, see *pindolol*. [VIHS-kihn]. 160, 162

Vistaril (Anes). Drug used preoperatively to produce sedation and relieve anxiety. For dosage, see *hydroxyzine*. [VIH-stah-rill]. 371

Vistaril (Derm). Drug used to treat severe itching. For dosage, see *hydroxyzine*. [VIHS-tah-rihl].

Vistaril (GI). Drug used to treat severe nausea and vomiting. For dosage, see *hydroxyzine*. [VIHS-tah-rihl]. 127

Vistaril (Psych). Drug used to treat anxiety and neurosis; used to treat hysteria; used to treat alcohol withdrawal. For dosage, see *hydroxyzine*. [VIHS-tah-rihl]. 282

Vistide (Antivir, Oph). Antiviral drug used to treat cytomegalovirus retinitis in AIDS patients. For dosage, see *cidofovir*. [VIHS-tide]. 329

Visudyne (Oph). Used to treat macular degeneration. The drug is administered intravenously and then the eyes are exposed to a red laser light to activate the drug. It is also used to treat ocular histoplasmosis. For dosage, see *verteporfin*. [VIHS-yoo-dine].

vitamin A-type drugs (Derm). Class of drugs used to treat acne vulgaris and psoriasis. 84, 86, 87

vitamin B₁₂. See *cyanocobalamin*.

vitamin C. See *ascorbic acid*.

vitamin D-type drugs (Derm). Class of drugs used to treat psoriasis. 86

vitamin K (AquaMEPHYTON, Mephyton) (Hem). Used to treat patients with clotting factor deficiency; used to restore normal blood clotting times in patients who have had an overdose of anticoagulants other than heparin; given prophylactically to newborns to prevent hemorrhagic disease of the newborn. Tablet: 5 mg. Subcutaneous, intramuscular, or intravenous: 2 mg/mL, 10 mg/mL. 189

vitamins, fat-soluble (A, D, E, K).

Vitrasert (Antivir, Oph). Antiviral drug used to treat cytomegalovirus retinitis in AIDS patients. For dosage, see *ganciclovir*. 329

Vitravene (Antivir, Oph). Antiviral drug used to treat cytomegalovirus retinitis in AIDS patients. For dosage, see *fomivirsen*. [VIH-trah-veen]. 329

Vivactil (Analges, Diab, Neuro, Ortho). Tricyclic antidepressant used to treat migraines; used to treat diabetic neuropathy; used to treat postherpetic neuralgia; used to treat obstructive sleep apnea; used to treat phantom limb pain. For dosage, see *protriptyline*. [vy-VACK-tehl]. 147, 241, 277, 307

Vivactil (Psych). Tricyclic antidepressant used to treat depression. For dosage, see *protriptyline*. [vy-VACK-tehl]. 286

Vivelle, Vivelle-Dot (OB/GYN, Ortho). Hormone replacement therapy used to treat the symptoms of menopause; used to prevent and treat osteoporosis. For dosage, see *estradiol*. [vy-VEHL]. 252

Vivonex T.E.N. (GI). Liquid nutritional supplement. Powder (to be reconstituted).

VLB. See *vinblastine*.

VM-26. See *teniposide*.

V.O. or **VO.** Abbreviation for *verbal order*.

Voltaren, Voltaren-XR (Analges, OB/GYN, Ortho). Nonsteroidal anti-inflammatory drug used to treat pain; used to treat dysmenorrhea; used to treat osteoarthritis and rheumatoid arthritis. For dosage, see *diclofenac*. [vohl-TEH-rehn]. 139, 255, 304

Voltaren (Oph). Topical nonsteroidal anti-inflammatory drug used to treat inflammation in the eyes. For dosage, see *diclofenac*. [vohl-TEH-rehn]. 219

volunteers for drug testing. 28

vomiting, drugs used to treat. 127

vomiting center. 127

(Vontrol) (GI). No longer on the market. (Generic name *diphenidol*; antiemetic drug used to treat motion sickness).

VP-16, VP-16-213. See *etoposide*.

Vumon (Chemo). Mitosis inhibitor chemotherapy drug used to treat leukemia. For dosage, see *teniposide*. 344

Waksman, Selman. 197

warfarin (Coumadin) (Hem). Anticoagulant. Tablet: 1 mg, 2 mg, 2.5 mg, 3 mg, 4 mg, 5 mg, 6 mg, 7.5 mg, 10 mg. [WAR-feh-rihn]. 186

Wart-Off (Derm) (generic *salicylic acid*). Topical keratolytic drug used to treat warts. Liquid: 17%. 91

warts, drugs used to treat. 91

wasting syndrome. See *AIDS wasting syndrome*.

Welchol (Cardio). Bile acid sequestrant used to treat hypercholesterolemia. For dosage, see *colesevelam*. [WEHL-kawl]. 169

Wellbutrin, Wellbutrin SR (GI, Psych). Antidepressant used to treat depression; used to treat obesity.

For dosage, see *bupropion*. [wehl-BYOO-trihn]. 129, 288

Wellcovorin (Chemo).   Cytoprotective drug used to prevent toxicity in patients receiving high-dose methotrexate.   For dosage, see *leucovorin*. [WEHL-koh-voh-rihn]. 350

Westcort (Derm) (generic *hydrocortisone*).   Topical corticosteroid anti-inflammatory drug. Cream: 0.2%. Ointment: 0.2%. 92

Wigraine (Analges) (generic *ergotamine, caffeine*). Combination vasoconstrictor drug used to treat migraine headaches. Tablet: 1 mg/100 mg. [Y-grayn]. 307

WinRho SDF (OB/GYN).   Immunoglobulin used after abortion, amniocentesis, or chorionic villus sampling to treat Rh-negative mother with an Rh-positive baby to prevent hemorrhagic disease of the newborn in a subsequent pregnancy. Intramuscular or intravenous (powder to be reconstituted): 600 IU, 1500 IU, 5000 IU, 120 mcg, 300 mcg, 1000 mcg.

Winstrol (Chemo, Endo).   Anabolic steroid used to treat metastatic breast cancer; used to treat hereditary angioedema; also used illegally by athletes. For dosage, see *stanozolol*. [WIHN-strohl]. 234

wolfsbane (herb for repelling vampires). 6

Women's Tylenol Multi-Symptom Menstrual Relief (OB/GYN) (generic *acetaminophen, pamabrom*). Combination analgesic and diuretic used to treat premenstrual dysphoric disorder and dysmenorrhea. Caplet: 500 mg/25 mg.

Wyamine (Anes).   Vasopressor used to treat hypotension that occurs with spinal anesthesia.   For dosage, see *mephentermine*. [Y-ah-meen]. 371

(Wyamycin S) (Antibio).   No longer on the market. (Generic name *erythromycin*; antibiotic).

Wyanoids Relief Factor (GI) (generic *cocoa butter, shark liver oil*).   Topical drug used to treat hemorrhoids. Suppository. [Y-ah-noyds]. 135

Wycillin (Antibio).   Penicillin antibiotic used to treat various types of bacterial infections, including *Streptococcus, Pneumococcus, Staphylococcus*, gonorrhea, and syphilis; used to treat cutaneous and inhaled anthrax from bioterrorism.   For dosage, see *penicillin G procaine*. [y-SIHL-ihn]. 313

Wygesic (Analges) (generic *propoxyphene, acetaminophen*).   Combination narcotic and nonnarcotic analgesic drug. (Schedule IV drug). Tablet: 65 mg/650 mg. [y-JEE-sihk]. 303

Wymox (Antibio).   Penicillin-type antibiotic used to treat various types of bacterial infections, including *Streptococcus, H. influenzae, E. coli*, gonorrhea, and *Chlamydia*; used prophylactically to prevent subacute bacterial endocarditis in at-risk patients under-

going dental or surgical procedures; used to treat *H. pylori* infection of the gastrointestinal tract.   For dosage, see *amoxicillin*. [Y-mawks]. 120, 313

Wytensin (Cardio).   Alpha$_2$-receptor blocker used to treat hypertension.   For dosage, see *guanabenz*. [y-TEHN-sihn]. 165

Xalatan (Oph).   Topical drug used to treat glaucoma. For dosage, see *lantanoprost*. [ZAH-lah-tehn]. 222

Xanax (OB/GYN, Psych).   Benzodiazepine drug used to treat anxiety and neurosis; used to treat panic disorder; used to treat premenstrual dysphoric disorder. (Schedule IV drug).   For dosage, see *alprazolam*. [ZEH-nacks]. 254, 281, 289

Xanelim (Derm).   Monoclonal antibody used to treat severe psoriasis.   For dosage, see *efalizumab*. 87

Xeloda (Chemo).   Pyrimidine antagonist chemotherapy drug used to treat breast cancer and colon cancer. For dosage, see *capecitabine*. [zeh-LOH-da]. 339

Xenical (GI).   Lipase inhibitor used to treat obesity. For dosage, see *orlistat*. [ZEH-nih-kehl]. 129

Xerecept (Neuro).   Used to treat edema around a brain tumor.   For dosage, see *corticotropin-releasing factor*. [ZEER-eh-sehpt]. 275

Xigris (Antibio).   Used to treat severe sepsis.   For dosage, see *drotrecogin*. [ZY-grihs]. 321

Xomazyme-H65 (Chemo).   Immunosuppressant used to prevent rejection after bone marrow transplant. Orphan drug. 362

Xomazyme-791 (Chemo).   Chemotherapy drug used to treat colon and rectal cancer. Orphan drug. 348

Xopenex (Resp).   Bronchodilator.   For dosage, see *levalbuterol*. [ZOH-peh-nehks]. 193

X-Prep Bowel Evacuant Kit-1 (GI) (generic *senna, senna/docusate, bisacodyl*).   Bowel evacuant/enema. Oral liquid, oral tablets, suppository. 126

X-Prep Bowel Evacuant Kit-2 (GI) (generic *senna, magnesium citrate, bisacodyl*).   Bowel evacuant/enema. Oral liquid, granules, and suppository. 126

X-Prep Liquid (GI) (generic *senna*).   Bowel evacuant. Oral liquid. 126

XR (abbreviation for *extended release*). 67

Xylocaine (Derm) (generic *lidocaine*).   Topical anesthetic. Liquid. Ointment: 2.5%. Spray. [ZY-loh-kayn]. 94

Xylocaine (Oph).   Anesthetic injected into the eye to produce corneal anesthesia and akinesis during eye surgery.   For dosage, see *lidocaine*. [ZY-loh-kayn].

Xylocaine (Uro).   Topical anesthetic applied to the urethra prior to cystoscopic procedures. Jelly: 2%. [ZY-loh-kayn]. 111

Xylocaine, Xylocaine MPF (Anes).   Local, regional nerve block, epidural, and spinal anesthetic.   For dosage, see *lidocaine*. [ZY-loh-kayn]. 367, 368

Xylocaine, Xylocaine 10% Oral, Xylocaine Viscous 2% (ENT) (generic *lidocaine*). Topical oral anesthetic. Oral liquid: 2%, 4%. Spray: 10%. [ZY-loh-kayn].

Xylocaine HCl IV for Cardiac Arrhythmias (Cardio). Used to treat ventricular arrhythmias. For dosage, see *lidocaine*. [ZY-loh-kayn]. 159, 180

xylometazoline (Otrivin, Otrivin Pediatric Nasal Drops) (ENT). Decongestant. Drops: 0.05%, 0.1%. Spray: 0.05%, 0.1%. [zy-loh-meh-tah-ZOH-leen]. 206

Xyrem (Neuro). Used to treat narcolepsy. For dosage, see *oxybate*. [ZY-rehm]. 274

Xyvion (OB/GYN). Steroid that stimulates estrogen, progesterone, and androgen receptors; used to treat menopause in women who cannot or will not take estrogen hormone replacement therapy. Investigational drug. 253

Yasmin (OB/GYN) (generic *drospirenone, ethinyl estradiol*). Monophasic combination progestins and estrogen used to treat premenstrual dysphoric disorder. Tablet: 3 mg/30 mcg. [YEHZ-mihn].

yeast infections, drugs used to treat.
topical. 90
systemic. 335

Yodoxin (GI). Used to treat intestinal amebiasis. For dosage, see *iodoquinol*. [yoh-DAWK-sihn]. 133, 319

Yutopar (OB/GYN). Used to stop preterm labor contractions. For dosage, see *ritodrine*. [YOO-toh-pawr]. 246

Zadaxin (Chemo, GI). Chemotherapy drug used to treat liver cancer; used to treat hepatitis B. For dosage, see *thymalfasin*. [zah-DEHK-sihn]. 135, 348

Zaditor (Oph). Topical mast cell stabilizer used to treat allergy symptoms in the eyes. For dosage, see *ketotifen*. [ZEH-dih-tohr]. 220

zafirlukast (Accolate) (Resp). Leukotriene receptor blocker used to prevent and treat asthma. Tablet: 10 mg, 20 mg. 196

Zagam (Antibio). Fluoroquinolone antibiotic used to treat a variety of infections, including community-acquired pneumonia, *H. influenzae, S. pneumoniae,* and *Klebsiella*. For dosage, see *sparfloxacin*. 318

zalcitabine (ddC) (Hivid) (Antivir). Nucleoside reverse transcriptase inhibitor drug used to treat AIDS. Tablet: 0.375 mg, 0.75 mg. [zehl-SIH-tah-been]. 324

zaleplon (Sonata) (Neuro). Nonbarbiturate drug used to treat insomnia. (Schedule IV drug). Capsule: 5 mg, 10 mg. [ZEHL-eh-plawn]. 272

Zanaflex (Neuro, Ortho). Skeletal muscle relaxant used to treat severe muscle spasticity associated with multiple sclerosis, cerebral palsy, stroke, or spinal cord injury. For dosage, see *tizanidine*. [ZEH-neh-flehks]. 145, 277

zanamivir (Relenza) (Antivir). Antiviral drug used to treat influenza A virus infection. Powder for inhalation: 5 mg. [ZAH-neh-mih-veer]. 330

Zanosar (Chemo). Alkylating chemotherapy drug used to treat pancreatic cancer. For dosage, see *streptozocin*. [ZEH-noh-sawr]. 341

Zantac, Zantac 75, Zantac EFFERdose, Zantac GELdose (GI). H_2 blocker used to treat peptic ulcers and *H. pylori* infection. For dosage, see *ranitidine*. [ZEHN-tack]. 118

Zarontin (Neuro). Anticonvulsant drug used to treat absence seizures. For dosage, see *ethosuximide*. [zah-RAWN-tihn]. 264

Zaroxolyn (Uro). Thiazide-like diuretic. For dosage, see *metolazone*. [zah-RAWK-seh-lihn]. 103

Zebeta (Cardio). Cardioselective beta-blocker used to treat angina pectoris, hypertension, and ventricular arrhythmias. For dosage, see *bisoprolol*. 157, 160, 162

Zefazone (Antibio). Cephalosporin antibiotic used to treat a variety of bacterial infections, including staphylococci, *E. coli,* and *H. influenzae*. For dosage, see *cefmetazole*. [ZEH-fah-zohn]. 316

Zelmac (GI). A 5-HT$_4$ (serotonin) blocker used to treat irritable bowel syndrome in women. For dosage, see *tegaserod*. 135

Zemuron (Anes, Resp). Muscle relaxant drug used during surgery; used to treat patients who are intubated and on the ventilator. For dosage, see *rocuronium*. [ZEH-myour-awn]. 199, 370

Zenapax (Chemo, Uro). Immunosuppressant monoclonal antibody given after bone marrow transplant to prevent rejection; given after kidney transplantation to prevent rejection of the donor kidney. For dosage, see *daclizumab*. [ZEE-nah-pehks]. 110, 362

Zerit (Antivir). Nucleoside reverse transcriptase inhibitor drug used to treat AIDS. For dosage, see *stavudine*. [ZEH-riht]. 324

Zestoretic (Cardio) (generic *lisinopril, hydrochlorothiazide*). Combination angiotensin-converting enzyme inhibitor antihypertensive and diuretic drug. Tablet: 10 mg/12.5 mg, 20 mg/12.5 mg. [zehs-toh-REH-tihk]. 167

Zestril (Cardio). Angiotensin-converting enzyme inhibitor drug used to treat congestive heart failure and hypertension; used to improve survival rate after myocardial infarction. For dosage, see *lisinopril*. [ZEH-strihl]. 154, 158, 163

Zetar (Derm) (generic *coal tar*). Topical drug used to treat psoriasis. Shampoo: 1%. [ZEE-tawr]. 86

Ziac (Cardio) (generic *bisoprolol, hydrochlorothiazide*). Combination beta-blocker antihypertensive and diuretic drug. Tablet: 2.5 mg/6.25 mg, 5 mg/6.25 mg, 10 mg/6.25 mg. [ZY-ack]. 167

Ziagen (Antivir). Nucleoside reverse transcriptase inhibitor drug used to treat AIDS. For dosage, see *abacavir*. [ZY-ah-jehn]. 324

ziconotide (Analges). Used to treat intractable pain. Investigational drug. 309

zidovudine (AZT) (Aztec, Retrovir) (Antivir). Nucleoside reverse transcriptase inhibitor drug used to treat AIDS; investigational drug used to treat AIDS. Capsule: 100 mg. Tablet: 300 mg. Syrup: 50 mg/5 mL. Intravenous: 10 mg/mL. [zee-doh-VYOO-deen]. 324

Zilactin-B Medicated (ENT) (generic *benzocaine*). Topical anesthetic for the mouth. Gel: 10%. [ZIH-lack-tihn]. 213

Zilactin-L (Derm) (generic *lidocaine*). Topical anesthetic. Liquid: 2.5%. [ZIH-lack-tihn]. 94

Zilactin Medicated (ENT) (generic *tannic acid*). Topical drug used to form a protective covering over canker sores and cold sores in and around the mouth. Gel: 7%. [ZIH-lack-tihn].

zileuton (Zyflo) (Resp). Leukotriene receptor blocker used to prevent and treat asthma. Tablet: 600 mg. [zih-loo-tohn]. 196

Zinacef (Antibio). Cephalosporin antibiotic used to treat various types of infections, including *Streptococcus, Staphylococcus, H. influenzae, E. coli*, and gonorrhea. For dosage, see *cefuroxime*. [ZIH-neh-sehf]. 316

zinc acetate (Galzin). Used to treat Wilson's disease. Orphan drug.

Zincfrin (Oph). Topical decongestant/vasoconstrictor used to treat irritation and allergy symptoms in the eyes. For dosage, see *phenylephrine*. [ZINK-frihn].

zinc oxide (Derm). Topical astringent used to dry oozing skin, irritation, and diaper rash. Common ingredient in many topical combination drugs. Ointment. 95

zinc oxide (Nupercainal, Tronolane) (GI). Topical drug used to treat hemorrhoids. Suppository. 135

Zinecard (Cardio). Cytoprotective drug used to prevent renal toxicity in patients receiving doxorubicin chemotherapy. For dosage, see *dexrazoxane*. [ZIH-neh-kawrd]. 173, 350

Zintevir (Antivir). Antiviral drug used to treat AIDS. Investigational drug. 326

ziprasidone (Geodon) (Psych). Drug used to treat psychosis and schizophrenia. Capsule: 20 mg, 40 mg, 60 mg, 80 mg. Intramuscular: (Pending). [zih-PREH-sih-dohn].

Ziradryl (Derm) (generic *diphenhydramine, zinc oxide*). Topical combination antihistamine/antipruritic and astringent drug. Lotion: 1%/2%. [ZEER-ah-drihl]. 94

Zithromax (Antibio). Macrolide antibiotic used to treat a variety of infections, including community-acquired pneumonia, *H. influenzae*, gonorrhea, *Chlamydia*, and Legionnaire's disease. For dosage, see *azithromycin*. [ZIH-throh-macks]. 198, 319

Zocor (Cardio). HMG-CoA reductase inhibitor drug used to treat hypercholesterolemia. For dosage, see *simvastatin*. [ZOH-kohr]. 170

Zofran (GI). Antiemetic drug; used to treat nausea and vomiting caused by chemotherapy. For dosage, see *ondansetron*. [ZOH-frehn].

Zoladex (Chemo, OB/GYN). Hormonal chemotherapy drug used to treat breast cancer; used to treat prostate cancer; used to treat endometriosis. For dosage, see *goserelin*. [ZOHL-ah-dehks]. 248, 343

zoledronic acid (Zometa) (Chemo, Ortho). Bone resorption inhibitor used to treat hypercalcemia caused by malignancy; investigational drug used to treat Paget's disease and metastatic bone lesions. Intravenous (powder to be reconstituted): 4 mg. [zohl-eh-DRAW-nick EH-sihd]. 148, 363

Zolicef (Antibio). Cephalosporin antibiotic used to treat a variety of bacterial infections, including *Streptococcus, Staphylococcus, E. coli*, and *H. influenzae*. For dosage, see *cefazolin*. [ZOH-lih-sehf]. 315

zolmitriptan (Zomig, Zomig ZMT) (Analges). Serotonin receptor agonist drug used to treat migraine headaches. Tablet/orally disintegrating tablet: 2.5 mg, 5 mg. [zohl-meh-TRIP-tehn]. 306

Zoloft (OB/GYN). Selective serotonin reuptake inhibitor antidepressant used to treat premenstrual dysphoric disorder. For dosage, see *sertraline*. [ZOH-lawft]. 255

Zoloft (Psych). Selective serotonin reuptake inhibitor antidepressant used to treat depression; used to treat panic disorder; used to treat obsessive-compulsive disorder; used to treat posttraumatic stress disorder; used to treat social anxiety disorder. For dosage, see *sertraline*. [ZOH-lawft]. 287, 289, 290

zolpidem (Ambien) (Neuro). Nonbarbiturate drug used to treat insomnia. (Schedule IV drug). Tablet: 5 mg, 10 mg. [zohl-pih-dehm]. 272

Zometa (Chemo, Ortho) (generic *zoledronic acid*). Bone resorption inhibitor used to treat hypercalcemia caused by malignancy; investigational drug used to treat Paget's disease and metastatic bone lesions. For dosage, see *zoledronic acid*. 148, 363

Zomig, Zomig ZMT (Analges). Serotonin receptor agonist drug used to treat migraine headaches. For dosage, see *zolmitriptan*. [ZOH-mihg]. 306

Zonalon (Derm) (generic *doxepin*).   Topical antihistamine/antipruritic drug. Cream: 5%. [ZOH-nah-lawn]. 93

Zonegran (Neuro).   Anticonvulsant drug used to treat partial seizures.   For dosage, see *zonisamide*. [ZOH-neh-grehn]. 265

zonisamide (Zonegran) (Neuro).   Anticonvulsant drug used to treat partial seizures. Capsule 100 mg. [zoh-NIH-sah-mide].265

ZORprin (Analges, Ortho).   Salicylate drug used to relieve fever and pain in children and adults; used to treat the pain and inflammation of osteoarthritis and rheumatoid arthritis in adults.   For dosage, see *aspirin*. [ZOHR-prihn]. 300

Zostrix, Zostrix-HP (Derm, Ortho) (generic *capsaicin*). Topical irritant drug used to mask the pain of herpes zoster virus lesions (shingles); used to mask the pain of arthritis. Cream: 0.025%, 0.075%. [ZOH-stricks]. 91, 147

Zosyn (Antibio) (generic *piperacillin, tazobactam*). Combination penicillin-type antibiotic and beta-lactamase inhibitor drug. Intravenous (powder to be reconstituted): 2 g/0.25 g, 3 g/375 g, 4 g/0.5 g. [ZOH-sihn]. 320

Zovia 1/35E, Zovia 1/50E (OB/GYN) (generic *ethynodiol, ethinyl estradiol*).   Monophasic combination progestins and estrogen oral contraceptive. Tablet: 35 mcg/1 mg, 50 mcg/1 mg. [ZOH-vee-ah]. 250

Zovirax (Antivir, Derm, OB/GYN).   Used to treat herpes simplex virus and herpes zoster virus infections; used to treat AIDS.   For dosage, see *acyclovir*. [zoh-VY-racks]. 91, 330

Zovirax (OB/GYN) (generic *acyclovir*).   Topical antiviral drug used to treat herpes simplex type 2 virus lesions. Ointment: 5%. [zoh-VY-racks]. 259

Zurase (Chemo).   Used to prevent hyperuricemia and tumor lysis syndrome in patients receiving chemotherapy. Orphan drug. 363

Zyban (Psych, Resp).   Antidepressant; Non-nicotine aid used to help patients stop smoking.   For dosage, see *bupropion*. [ZY-behn]. 200

Zydone (Analges) (generic *hydrocodone, acetaminophen*). Combination narcotic and nonnarcotic analgesic drug. (Schedule III drug).   Tablet: 7.5 mg/400 mg, 10 mg/400 mg. [ZY-dohn]. 303

Zyflo (Resp).   Leukotriene receptor blocker used to prevent and treat asthma.   For dosage, see *zileuton*. 196

Zyloprim (Chemo, Ortho).   Used to treat cancer patients with elevated uric acid; used to treat gout. For dosage, see *allopurinol*. [ZY-loh-prihm]. 146, 361

Zymase (GI) (generic *amylase, lipase, protease*).   Combination drug replacement therapy for digestive enzymes. Capsule: 24,000 units/12,000 units/24,000 units. 135

Zyprexa, Zyprexa Zydis (Neuro, Psych).   Drug used to treat the dementia of Alzheimer's disease; used to treat psychosis and schizophrenia; used to treat the mania of manic-depressive disorder.   For dosage, see *olanzapine*. [zy-PREHK-sah]. 271, 284, 288

Zyrkamine (Chemo).   Chemotherapy drug used to treat non-Hodgkin's lymphoma.   For dosage, see *mitoguazone*. 348

Zyrtec (Derm, ENT).   Antihistamine used to treat allergic rhinitis and allergic reactions with hives and itching.   For dosage, see *cetirizine*. [ZUHR-tehk]. 207

Zyrtec-D 12 Hour (ENT) (generic *cetirizine, pseudoephedrine*).   Combination antihistamine and decongestant drug. Tablet: 5 mg/120 mg. [ZUHR-tehk]. 213

Zyvox (Antibio).   Antibiotic used to treat a variety of bacterial infections, including *Staphylococcus*, *Streptococcus*, community-acquired pneumonia; used to treat methicillin-resistant *Staphylococcus aureus* (MRSA); used to treat vancomycin-resistant *Enterococcus*.   For dosage, see *linezolid*. [ZY-vawks]. 319